Everything
You Need to
Know about
Diseases

Springhouse Corporation
Springhouse, PA

STAFF

Senior Publisher
Matthew Cahill

Clinical Manager
Cindy Tryniszewski, RN, MSN

Art Director
John Hubbard

Senior Editor
Michael Shaw

Editors
Marcia Andrews, Kathy Goldberg, Peter H. Johnson

Copy Editors
Cynthia C. Breuninger (manager), Priscilla DeWitt, Mary T. Durkin, Lynette High, Christina P. Ponczek, Doris Weinstock

Designers
Stephanie Peters (senior associate art director), Lesley Weissman-Cook (book designer), Donald G. Knauss, Elaine Ezrow, Linda Franklin, Lorraine Lostracco-Carbo, Mary Ludwicki, Kaaren Mitchel

Manufacturing
Deborah Meiris (director), Pat Dorshaw, T.A. Landis

Production Coordinator
Margaret A. Rastiello

Editorial Assistants
Mary Madden, Beverly Lane

© 1996 by Springhouse Corporation. All rights reserved. No part of this publication may be used or reproduced in any manner whatsoever without written permission except for brief quotations embodied in critical articles and reviews. For information, write Springhouse Corporation, 1111 Bethlehem Pike, P.O. Box 908, Springhouse, PA 19477-0908. Authorization to photocopy items for internal or personal use, or for the internal or personal use of specific clients, is granted by Springhouse Corporation for users registered with the Copyright Clearance Center (CCC) Transactional Reporting Service, provided that the fee of $.75 per page is paid directly to CCC, 27 Congress St., Salem MA 01970. For those organizations that have been granted a photocopy license by CCC, a separate system of payment has been arranged. The fee code for users of the Transactional Reporting Service is 0874348226/96 $00.00 + .75.
Printed in the United States of America.

EYNKD-010595

℞ A member of the Reed Elsevier plc group

Library of Congress Cataloging-in-Publication Data
Everything you need to know about diseases.
    p. cm.
    Includes index.
1.Medicine, Popular.   I. Springhouse Corporation.
RC81.E915   1996
616 — dc20   95-6697
ISBN0-87434-822-6   CIP

CONTENTS

ADVISORY BOARD

CONTRIBUTORS & CONSULTANTS

Virginia P. Arcangelo, RN, PhD, MSN, CRNP, Nurse Practitioner, Thomas Jefferson University Hospital, Philadelphia

John P. Atkinson, MD, Chairman of Internal Medicine, Professor of Microbiology and Immunology, Washington University School of Medicine, St. Louis

Charold L. Baer, RN, PhD, Professor, Department of Adult Health and Illness, Oregon Health Sciences University School of Nursing, Portland

Katherine G. Baker, RN, MN, Clinical Specialist, UCLA Center for Health Sciences

Ardelina Albano Baldonado, RN, PhD, Associate Professor, Assistant Dean and Director, Undergraduate Program, Marcella Niehoff School of Nursing, Loyola University of Chicago

Edmund Martin Barbour, MD, Associate Clinical Professor of Medicine, Wayne State University, Detroit

Jo Anne Bennett, RN, MA, CNA, Adjunct Instructor, Lienhard School of Nursing, Pace University, Pleasantville, NY

Margaret Hamilton Birney, RN, MSN, Lecturer, College of Nursing, Wayne State University, Detroit

Nora Lynn Bollinger, RN, MSN, Oncology Clinical Nurse Specialist, Walter Reed Army Medical Center, Washington, DC

Ann L. Boutcher, RN,C, MSN, Nurse Genetic Counselor, Genecare Medical Genetics Center, Chapel Hill, NC

Barbara Gross Braverman, RN, MSN, CS, Psychiatric Clinical Nurse Specialist, Medical College of Pennsylvania, Philadelphia; Geropsychiatric Clinical Nurse Specialist, Abington (PA) Memorial Hospital

Christine S. Breu, RN, MN, Research Associate, University of California, Los Angeles

Lawrence W. Brown, MD, FAAN, FAAP, Associate Professor of Pediatrics and Neurology, Medical College of Pennsylvania, Philadelphia

Lillian S. Brunner, MSN, ScD, LittD, FAAN, Nurse-Author, Brunner Associates, Berwyn, PA

Brian P. Burlew, MD, FCCP, Pulmonologist, St. Luke's Hospital, Bethlehem, PA

Linda Byers, RN,C, BSN, MS, Director of Clinical Services, Community Action, Family Planning Program, San Marcos, TX

G. Carpenter, MD, Associate Professor of Pediatrics, Thomas Jefferson University, Philadelphia

Gerald Charnogursky, MD, Medical Director, Joslin Center for Diabetes at MacNeal Hospital, Berwyn, IL; Clinical Assistant Professor of Medicine, Loyola University, Chicago

JoAnn Coleman, RN, MS, CS, OCN, Clinical Nurse Specialist, Gastrointestinal Surgery, Johns Hopkins Hospital, Baltimore

Rae Conley, RN, MSN, Clinical Nurse Specialist, Thomas Jefferson University Hospital, Philadelphia

Robert B. Cooper, MD, Assistant Attending Physician and Clinical Assistant Professor of Medicine, The New York Hospital, Cornell Medical Center

Jerome M. Cotler, MD, Professor, Orthopaedic Surgery, Jefferson Medical College of Thomas Jefferson University, Philadelphia

Robert L. Cox, MD, Clinical Consultant, Infectious Diseases, Porter Memorial Hospital, Rocky Mountain Hospital, Denver; Swedish Medical Center, Craig Hospital, Englewood, CO

Stella Doherty, RN, MSN, former Nursing Services Consultant for Tuberculosis, Commonwealth of Pennsylvania, Pennsylvania Department of Health, Division of Acute Infectious Disease Control, Harrisburg

Richard M. Donner, MD, Pediatric Cardiologist and Chief of Department, St. Christopher's Hospital for Children; Department of Pediatrics, Temple University School of Medicine, Philadelphia

Brian B. Doyle, MD, Director, Anxiety Disorders Program, Georgetown University School of Medicine, Washington, DC

Phyllis Dubendorf, RN, MSN, CCRN, CNRN, Clinical Nurse Specialist, Thomas Jefferson University Hospital, Philadelphia

Stephen C. Duck, MD, Associate Professor, Pediatrics, Northwestern University Medical School, Evanston, IL

Stanley J. Dudrick, MD, FACS, Program Director and Associate Chairman, St. Mary's Hospital, Department of Surgery, Waterbury, CT

Roland D. Eavey, MD, FAAP, FACS, Director, ENT Pediatric Services, Massachusetts Eye and Ear Infirmary, Boston

Michael D. Ellis, MD, FACOG, Attending Physician, Abington (PA) Memorial Hospital; President, Ellis, Michaelson, McDonald, Frangipane & Associates, Abington, PA

Lori S. Farmer, RN, MS, ARNP, Director of Genetic and Perinatal Counseling, Fayetteville (NC) Diagnostic Center

Mary Ellen Florence, RN, PhD, Assistant Professor of Nursing, Stockton State College, Pomona, NJ

Bernadette M. Forget, RN, MSN, BS, Head Nurse, Dermatology, Yale-New Haven Hospital, New Haven, CT

Anna Gawlinski, RN, MSN, CCRN, Cardiovascular Clinical Nurse Specialist, UCLA Medical Center

Donald P. Goldsmith, MD, Associate Professor of Pediatrics, Temple University School of Medicine, Philadelphia; Director, Rheumatic Diseases Center, St. Christopher's Hospital for Children, Philadelphia

Christine Grady, RN, MSN, CNS, Clinical Specialist, Immunology, Allergy, and Infectious Disease, National Institutes of Health Clinical Center, Bethesda, MD

Donna H. Groh, RN, MSN, Assistant Director of Nursing, Children's Hospital of Los Angeles

Arnold W. Gurevitch, MD, Chief, Division of Dermatology, Harbor-UCLA Medical Center; Professor of Clinical Medicine, Harbor-UCLA School of Medicine, Torrance, CA

Sundaram Hariharan, MD, Assistant Professor of Internal Medicine (Nephrology), University of Cincinnati

Mary L. Harris, MD, Assistant Professor of Medicine, Johns Hopkins Medical Institutions, Baltimore

Susan J. Hart, RN,C, MSN, CCRN, Adjunct Professor, Seton Hall University College of Nursing, South Orange, NJ; Staff Nurse, Morristown (NJ) Memorial Hospital

Rebecca G. Hathaway, RN, MSN, Assistant Director of Nursing, Assistant Clinical Professor, UCLA Medical Center, UCLA School of Nursing

Laura Lucia Hayman, RN, PhD, Chair and Program Director, Nursing of Children, University of Pennsylvania School of Nursing, Philadelphia

Eddie R. Hedrick, BS, MT(ASCP), Manager, Infection Control Department, University of Missouri-Columbia Hospital and Clinics

Patricia Turk Horvath, RN, MSN, Corporate Health Programs Coordinator, The Standard Oil Company (Ohio), Cleveland

Mitchell M. Jacobson, MD, Clinical Professor, University of Wisconsin Medical School, Madison; Associate Clinical Professor of Medicine, Medical College of Wisconsin, Milwaukee

Karen Jantzi, RN, MSN, Psychiatric Coordinator, Indian Creek Foundation, Harleysville, PA

William M. Keane, MD, Surgeon, Pennsylvania Hospital, Philadelphia; Assistant Clinical Professor, University of Pennsylvania School of Medicine, Philadelphia

Paul M. Kirschenfeld, MD, FACP, FCCP, Medical Director, Intensive Care Unit; Program Director, Internal Medicine Residency Program, Atlantic City (NJ) Medical Center

Ruth S. Kitson, RN, BAA(N), MBA, Director of Nursing, Critical Care, Toronto Western Hospital

Nancy L. Konstantinides, RN,C, MS, Metabolic Nurse Specialist, University of Minnesota Hospital and Clinics, Minneapolis

Mary Ann Lafferty-Della Valle, PhD, Research Associate, Department of Human Genetics, School of Medicine, and Lecturer, School of Nursing, University of Pennsylvania, Philadelphia

Peter G. Lavine, MD, Director, Coronary Care Unit, Crozer-Chester Medical Center, Chester, PA

Dennis E. Leavelle, MD, Associate Professor and Consultant, Mayo Medical Laboratories, Mayo Clinic, Rochester, Minn.

Harold I. Lief, MD, Professor Emeritus of Psychiatry, University of Pennsylvania School of Medicine, Philadelphia; Psychiatrist, Pennsylvania Hospital, Philadelphia

Herbert A. Luscombe, MD, Professor and Chairman Emeritus, Department of Dermatology, Jefferson Medical College of Thomas Jefferson University, Philadelphia

Neil MacIntyre, MD, Assistant Professor of Medicine, Duke University Medical Center, Durham, NC

Linda L. Martin, RN, MSN, Pulmonary Clinical Nurse Specialist, University of Virginia Medical Center, Charlottesville

Celestine B. Mason, RN, BSN, MA, Associate Professor, Pacific Lutheran University, Tacoma, WA

Edwina A. McConnell, RN, MS, Independent Nurse Consultant; Staff Nurse, Madison (WI) General Hospital

Karen E. Michael, RN, MSN, Case Manager, Greater Atlantic Health Service, Philadelphia

Attila Nakeeb, MD, Senior Resident, Department of Surgery, Johns Hopkins Hospital, Baltimore

Judith L. Nerad, MD, Assistant Professor of Medicine, Loyola University Medical Center, Maywood, IL

Brenda M. Nevidjon, RN, MSN, Cancer Program Manager, Providence Medical Center, Seattle

Thaddeus S. Nowinski, MD, Clinical Associate Professor, Thomas Jefferson University, Philadelphia; Associate Surgeon, Wills Eye Hospital, Philadelphia

John J. O'Shea, MD, Chief, Lymphocyte Cell Biology Section, Arthritis and Rheumatism Branch, National Institute of Arthritis and Musculoskeletal and Skin Diseases, National Institutes of Health, Bethesda, MD

Mary Pasdur, RN, MSN, OCN, Clinical Nurse Specialist, M.D. Anderson Cancer Center, Houston

Adele W. Pike, RN, MSN, Clinical Nurse, National Institutes of Health, Clinical Center, Bethesda, MD

Katherine S. Puls, RN, MS, CNM, Nurse Midwife in Private Practice, Women's Alternative Health Care of Barrington, IL

Iris M. Reyes, MD, Assistant Professor, Department of Emergency Medicine, Hospital of the University of Pennsylvania, Philadelphia

Marilyn A. Roderick, MD, RN, BSN, Physician, General Practice, Redwood City, CA

Allan Ronald, MD, FRCPS, Professor of Internal Medicine, University of Manitoba, Winnipeg, Canada

Barbara C. Rynerson, RN,C, MS, Associate Professor, University of North Carolina at Chapel Hill

Linda Patti Sarna, RN, MN, Assistant Clinical Professor, UCLA School of Nursing

Kristine A. Scordo, RN, PhD, Clinical Director, Clinical Nurse Specialist, The Cardiology Center of Cincinnati

Marilyn R. Shahan, RN, MS, Nurse Epidemiologist, Denver Department of Health and Hospitals, Disease Control Service

Susan Budassi Sheehy, RN, MSN, CEN, Assistant Director, Trauma Service, St. Joseph Hospital, Tacoma, WA; Associate Clinical Professor, University of Washington School of Nursing, Seattle

Brenda K. Shelton, RN, MS, CCRN, OCN, Critical Care Clinical Nurse Specialist, Johns Hopkins Hospital Oncology Center, Baltimore

Bryan P. Simmons, MD, Medical Director, Infection Control, Methodist Hospitals of Memphis

Marilyn Sawyer Sommers, RN, PhD, CCRN, Assistant Professor, College of Nursing and Health, University of Cincinnati

Brenda M. Splitz, RN, MSN, ANP, Adult Clinical Coordinator, Nurse Practitioner Program; and Adjunct Faculty for Health Care Sciences, George Washington University Hospital, Washington, DC

Charlene Wandel Stanich, RN, MN, Associate Vice President, Medical Nursing, Presbyterian-University Hospital, Pittsburgh

Johanna K. Stiesmeyer, RN, MS, CCRN, Critical Care Clinical Educator, El Camino Hospital, Mountain View, CA

Warren Summer, MD, Section Chief, Pulmonary-Critical Care Medicine, Louisiana State University Medical Center, New Orleans

Basia Belza Tack, RN, MSN, ANP, Professor, School of Nursing, University of Washington, Seattle

Maureen R. Tierney, MD, MSc, Fellowship Director and Attending Physician, Infectious Disease Unit, Massachusetts General Hospital, Boston

Richard W. Tureck, MD, Professor of Obstetrics and Gynecology; Director, In Vitro Fertilization/Embryo Transfer Program, University of Pennsylvania School of Medicine, Philadelphia

Sharon McBride Valente, RN, MS, CS, FAAN, Adjunct Assistant Professor, University of Southern California, Department of Nursing, Los Angeles; Clinical Specialist in Mental Health in Private Practice, Los Angeles

Susan VanDeVelde-Coke, EN, MA, MNS, Director of Nursing, Health Sciences Center, Winnipeg, Manitoba, Canada

Mary Mishler Voga, RN, MSN, CHN, Course Coordinator and Instructor, Helene Fuld School of Nursing, Camden, NJ

Jennifer Vonnahme, RN, MA, OCN, Instructor of Clinical Nursing, College of Nursing and Health, University of Cincinnati

Peggy L. Wagner, RN, MSN, CCRN, Cardiovascular Clinical Nurse Specialist, St. Michael Hospital, Milwaukee

Joni Walton, RN, MSN, CRTT, RRT, Critical Care Clinical Nurse Specialist, St. Luke's Hospital, Kansas City, MO

Juanita Watson, RN, MSN, Director, Department of Continuing Education, Saint Agnes Medical Center, Philadelphia

Patricia D. Weiskittel, RN, MSN, CNN, Clinical Nurse Specialist, University Hospital, Cincinnati

Joanne F. White, RN, MNEd, Associate Dean, School of Nursing, Duquesne University, Pittsburgh

John K. Wiley, MD, FACS, Associate Clinical Professor of Neurosurgery, Wright State University School of Medicine, Dayton, OH; Neurosurgery, Inc., Dayton, OH

Mary R. Zimmerman, RN, BSN, MS, Director of Nursing, Madison (WI) General Hospital

FOREWORD

Never before has there been a greater need for accurate and trustworthy medical information for the general public. Although medical and scientific literature brims with the latest theories, insights, and findings, many medical references for the layperson lack authority and are not genuinely helpful. More than ever, it's crucial for people to understand and participate fully in their medical care for it to succeed. Consider, for instance, the many challenges that lie ahead not only for doctors but also for every health-conscious person.

The AIDS epidemic continues

Right now, the best efforts of the world's medical researchers have only slowed the progress of this killer. Until scientists achieve a cure, continued public education and prevention remain our best strategy for curbing this deadly syndrome.

Infections on the rise

In the mid-20th century, the development of antibiotics enabled us to control and cure many deadly bacterial infections. Today we must deal with the problem of increasing bacterial resistance to antibiotics. In addition, new microbes have recently been discovered, bringing new health threats — such as Lyme disease and Legionnaires' disease — in their wake and contributing to other longstanding disorders, such as peptic ulcers.

Heart disease: Still the leading killer

Today we possess unprecedented knowledge about risk factors for heart disease and how to eliminate them. We know that public education is critical in our efforts to screen for and eliminate such risk factors as smoking, high blood pressure, high cholesterol levels, and a lack of physical exercise. We also know that nutritional factors play a key role. Despite this knowledge and the best efforts of our doctors, heart disease remains the leading cause of death in the United States and Canada.

Cancer

The long sought-after cancer "cure" still eludes us. As cancer researchers explore the human genome in earnest, the true complexity of the problem becomes apparent. As our understanding grows, we realize more clearly than ever before that prevention and early detection continue to be our best defense against most cancers.

The changing health care climate

In the United States, the delivery of health care is evolving. In effect, medical care is increasingly moving out of the hospital and into the doctor's office, outpatient settings, and patients' homes. Along with these changes comes the need for all of us to be more knowledgeable about our care and, if we or a family member become ill, to learn as much as we can about the condition.

How this book can help you

Everything You Need to Know about Diseases will help you become more knowledgeable about your health — and about virtually any illness that you or a loved one may have. Prepared with the help of more than 100 doctors and medical authorities, this comprehensive reference covers over 500 illnesses and conditions — including heart disease, cancer, the common cold, AIDS, and Alzheimer's disease. It also covers hearing loss, nutritional disorders, ulcers, the flu, anemia, Lyme disease, injuries of all kinds, asthma, stroke, tuberculosis, diabetes, PMS, herpes, and hundreds more.

For each of these illnesses, you'll find clear answers, usually in a page or two, to these essential questions:

- What causes the condition?
- What are the symptoms?
- How is the condition diagnosed?
- How is it treated?
- What can a person with the condition do to get better, to aid in its treatment, and to relieve any discomfort?

Besides this core information, you'll find many special features, each of them marked by a small picture. For instance, you'll find:

- *Prevention Tips:* how you can avoid getting an illness or, if you have one, how to prevent a recurrence
- *Self-Help:* what you can do to feel better or adjust to your illness
- *Advice for Caregivers:* what you can do — step by step — if you're caring for someone who has an illness
- *Straight Talk:* easy-to-understand answers to commonly asked questions about medical ailments and conditions
- *Insight into Illness:* why an illness occurs and how it develops — all clearly explained and often illustrated
- *Traveler's Advisory:* how to avoid getting sick if you're traveling to parts of the world where certain illnesses are prevalent.

With all of these features, *Everything You Need to Know about Diseases* will prove indispensable time and time again. There's no book for the general public that rivals its thoroughness, helpfulness, and reliability. Don't let your home be without it.

Robert B. Cooper, MD
Assistant Attending Physician and
Clinical Assistant Professor of Medicine
The New York Hospital/Cornell Medical Center

1

HEART AND BLOOD VESSEL DISORDERS

AORTIC ANEURYSM OF THE ABDOMEN

What do doctors call this condition?

Abdominal aortic aneurysm

What is this condition?

An aortic aneurysm of the abdomen is an abnormal bulge in the wall of the aorta, the body's main artery. It generally occurs where this big artery branches to carry blood to the legs. Such aneurysms are four times more common in men than in women and most prevalent between ages 50 and 80.

Over half of all people with untreated abdominal aneurysms die, primarily from a rupture of the bulge, within 2 years of diagnosis. About 15% survive beyond 5 years.

What causes it?

About 95% of aortic aneurysms of the abdomen result from arteriosclerosis (hardening of the arteries). These aneurysms develop slowly. Blood pressure within the aorta progressively weakens the vessel walls and enlarges the aneurysm.

What are its symptoms?

Although aortic aneurysms of the abdomen usually don't cause symptoms, most are evident (unless the person is obese) as a pulsating mass near the naval. Sometimes it's tender.

Lower back pain that radiates to the side and groin from pressure on lumbar nerves may signify that the aneurysm has grown and is about to rupture.

Rupture of an aneurysm may cause severe, persistent abdominal and back pain. Twenty percent of people whose aneurysms rupture die immediately. In some cases, signs of hemorrhage — such as weakness, sweating, a fast pulse, and low blood pressure — may be subtle. People with a rupture may remain in stable condition for hours before going into shock.

How is it diagnosed?

Because an aortic aneurysm of the abdomen rarely produces symptoms, it's often detected accidentally on an X-ray or during a routine physical exam. An ultrasound test can determine aneurysm size,

SELF-HELP

Living with an aneurysm

Whether you're awaiting surgery or not, here are some tips to help you function safely and comfortably at home.

Slow down
Don't give up all activity, but do cut back enough to keep your blood pressure at a safe and steady level. For instance, taking a stroll around your neighborhood or in the park may be better for you than jogging.

Monitor your blood pressure
Learn to take your blood pressure regularly — as your nurse or doctor showed you. (Or ask someone else to take it for you.) Write down the results. Follow your doctor's guidelines for acceptable levels. Be sure to notify the doctor if your blood pressure is higher or lower than those levels.

Eat sensibly
Keep your blood pressure on an even keel by eating sensibly. For example, follow a low-salt, low-fat diet. Losing weight may help too.

Check your circulation
Examine your legs every day for changes in color and temperature and for numbness or tingling sensations. Tell your doctor if you notice any changes.

Avoid infection
Protect yourself from complications caused by poor circulation in your legs. Keep your skin clean, dry, and free of scratches that bacteria could enter.

Wash your feet in warm, soapy water every day. Then dry them thoroughly by blotting them with a towel. Be sure to dry between the toes. Check your feet daily for cuts, cracks, blisters, or red, swollen areas. Call your doctor if you cut your foot, even slightly.

Avoid wearing tight shoes or clothing that may further restrict your circulation. And don't wear elastic garters, sit with your knees crossed, or walk barefoot.

Take your medicine
Make sure you understand exactly how and when to take your medicine. And if you have questions about any medicine, including possible side effects, call your doctor or pharmacist. Also consult them before you take any nonprescription medicine, such as cold remedies.

Recognize danger symptoms
Have someone call your doctor at once if you experience:
- a severe headache or chest or abdominal pain
- cool, clammy skin
- disorientation or unusual sleepiness
- extreme restlessness or anxiety.

---

shape, and location. Aortography (X-rays of the aorta after injection of a dye) shows the condition of vessels in the region of the aneurysm and the extent of the aneurysm.

How is it treated?
Usually, aortic aneurysm of the abdomen requires surgical removal of the aneurysm and replacement of the damaged aortic section with a Dacron graft. If the aneurysm is small and produces no symptoms, surgery may be delayed; however, small aneurysms may also rupture. Regular physical exams and ultrasound checks are necessary to detect

enlargement, which may forewarn of rupture. Large aneurysms or those that produce symptoms involve a significant risk of rupture and need immediate surgical repair. (See *Living with an aneurysm*.)

*A*ORTIC ANEURYSM OF THE CHEST

What do doctors call this condition?

Thoracic aortic aneurysm

What is it?

An aortic aneurysm of the chest is an abnormal widening of the aorta, the body's main artery. The heart pumps blood through the aorta to the rest of the body.

An aortic aneurysm may be *dissecting,* a hemorrhagic separation in the aortic wall; *saccular,* an outpouching of the arterial wall, with a narrow neck; or *fusiform,* a spindle-shaped enlargement involving the entire circumference of the aorta.

Some aneurysms progress to serious and, eventually, fatal complications, such as rupture of untreated thoracic dissecting aneurysm into the sac surrounding the heart (pericardium), with resulting tamponade (compression).

What causes it?

Commonly, an aortic aneurysm of the chest is caused by atherosclerosis (plaque buildup in the arteries), which weakens the aortic wall and gradually distends the lumen of the artery. The lining of the aorta may become torn. Other causes include infection of the aorta, congenital heart disorders, injury, syphilis, or high blood pressure. Aortic aneurysms of the chest are most common in men between ages 50 and 70.

What are its symptoms?

The most common symptom of aortic aneurysm of the chest is pain. In a dissecting aneurysm, such pain may have a sudden onset, with a tearing or ripping sensation in the thorax or the anterior chest. It may extend to the neck, shoulders, lower back, or abdomen.

Accompanying signs include fainting, pallor, sweating, shortness of breath, increased pulse rate, leg weakness or brief paralysis, and

Repairing an aortic aneurysm

A person with an aortic aneurysm — either of the abdomen or chest — may need emergency surgery called *aneurysmectomy*.

In this operation, the surgeon cuts into the sac of the aneurysm (below left). After removing the involved segment, the surgeon replaces it with biologically neutral graft material, such as Dacron (below center). Then the surgeon cleans the diseased tissue of plaque or clotted blood and sews this section around the graft (below right).

The section that once composed the aneurysm now covers the graft.

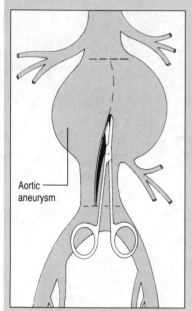

Aortic aneurysm

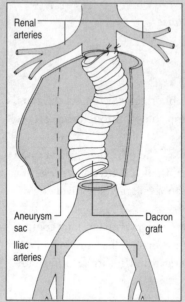

Renal arteries

Aneurysm sac

Iliac arteries

Dacron graft

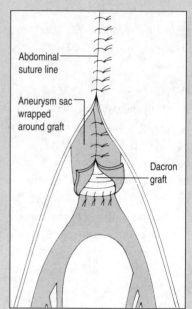

Abdominal suture line

Aneurysm sac wrapped around graft

Dacron graft

abrupt changes in pulses or blood pressure between arms and legs. The person appears to be in shock.

Effects of saccular or fusiform aortic aneurysms of the chest vary. They may include an ache in the shoulders, lower back, or abdomen; shortness of breath, coughing, or wheezing; hoarseness or loss of voice; and, possibly, numbness and tingling in the arms or legs and pain along the course of a nerve. Aneurysms may rupture.

How is it diagnosed?

Diagnosis relies on the person's history, signs and symptoms, and results of appropriate tests. In a person with no symptoms, diagnosis often occurs accidentally when chest X-rays show widening of the aorta. Other tests, such as aortography and an echocardiogram (an ultrasound test of the heart), help confirm the aneurysm.

How is it treated?

Dissecting aortic aneurysm is an emergency that requires prompt surgery and stabilizing measures: drugs to lower blood pressure and reduce the force of the heart's contractions, oxygen to help breathing, narcotics to relieve pain, intravenous fluids and, possibly, blood transfusions.

Surgery consists of removing the aneurysm, restoring normal blood flow through a Dacron or Teflon graft replacement and, with aortic valve insufficiency, replacing the aortic valve. (See *Repairing an aortic aneurysm.*)

ARTERIAL OCCLUSIVE DISEASE

What is this condition?

In arterial occlusive disease, the aorta and its major branches are blocked or become narrowed. This interrupts blood flow, usually to the legs and feet. The disorder may affect the carotid, vertebral, innominate, subclavian, mesenteric, and celiac arteries. (See *Sites of arterial occlusion*, page 8.)

Occlusions may be acute or chronic and often cause severe ischemia, skin ulcers, and gangrene.

Arterial occlusive disease is more common in males than females.

What causes it?

Arterial occlusive disease is a frequent complication of atherosclerosis (plaque buildup in the arteries). The blockage may develop from internal causes, such as blood clot formation or thrombosis, or external causes, such as injury or fracture. Predisposing factors include smoking; aging; conditions such as high blood pressure, high cholesterol or fat levels, and diabetes; and a family history of blood vessel disorders, heart attack, or stroke.

What are its symptoms?

Arterial occlusive disease may produce a wide variety of signs and symptoms, depending on which arteries are affected. For example, if occlusion occurs in arteries in the leg (such as the femoral artery), the person may may have pale, cool legs and pain in the feet. An impor-

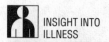

INSIGHT INTO
ILLNESS

Sites of arterial occlusion

This anatomic diagram can help you understand the arterial system. It shows the location of the aorta, its major branching arteries, and the body areas affected by the blood flow from these arteries. If you have arterial occlusive disease, your doctor can tell you exactly where the blockage has occurred.

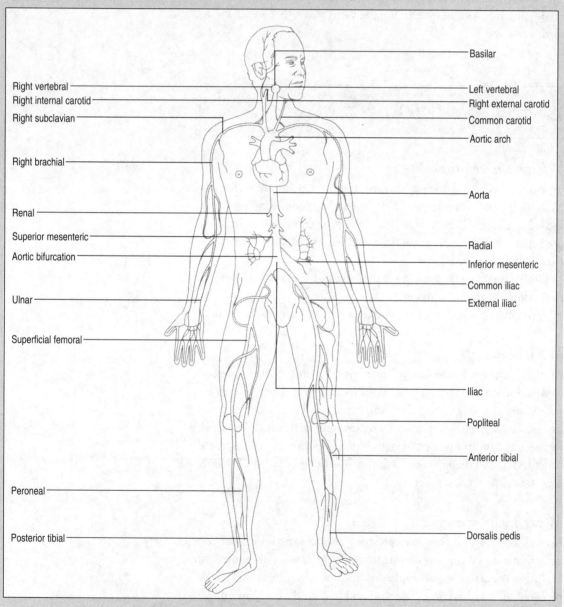

Understanding surgery for arterial occlusive disease

For a person with arterial occlusive disease, the doctor may recommend one of the operations described below.

Embolectomy
In this procedure, the surgeon uses a balloon-tipped catheter to remove plaque from the artery. Embolectomy is used mainly to treat a blockage of the mesenteric, femoral, or popliteal artery.

Thromboendarterectomy
In this operation, the surgeon opens the artery and removes the obstructing thrombus (atherosclerotic plaque) and the middle layer of the arterial wall. This procedure is usually done after angiography (X-rays of the artery) and is often used in conjunction with autogenous vein or Dacron bypass graft surgery.

Patch grafting
The doctor removes the thrombotic arterial segment and replaces it with an autogenous vein or a Dacron graft.

Bypass graft
In this operation, blood flow is diverted through an autogenous or woven Dacron graft to bypass the thrombotic arterial segment.

Lumbar sympathectomy
Depending on the condition of the sympathetic nervous system, this procedure may be done in someone who has had reconstructive surgery.

Amputation
This operation becomes necessary if arterial reconstructive surgery fails or if the person develops gangrene, uncontrollable infection, or intractable pain.

tant sign of arterial occlusive disease in the femoral artery is intermittent claudication, a pain in the calves upon exertion.

If the person develops an occlusion in the carotid artery, he or she may experience a transient ischemic attack — a sudden, brief episode of sensory and motor impairment, which may lead to a stroke.

How is it diagnosed?
Diagnosis of arterial occlusive disease is usually based on the person's history and physical exam. Supportive diagnostic tests include arteriography and an ultrasound scan.

How is it treated?
Generally, treatment of arterial occlusive disease depends on the cause, location, and size of the obstruction. For people with mild chronic disease, treatment usually consists of eliminating smoking, blood pressure control, and walking exercise. For people with carotid artery occlusion, drug therapy may begin with Persantine and aspirin. For those with intermittent claudication caused by chronic arte-

SELF-HELP

How to take care of your feet

If you have arterial occlusive disease, these guidelines on foot care and injury precautions can help you protect your feet from injury and subsequent infection.

Daily care

• Wash your feet daily with mild soap and warm water. (To prevent burns, never use hot water.) Dry your feet carefully, especially between the toes.
• If your skin is dry, apply lanolin ointment. If your feet tend to sweat, use a mild foot powder, making sure it doesn't cake.
• Inspect your feet daily — around the nails, between the toes, and on the soles. Look for corns, calluses, redness, swelling, bruises, or breaks in the skin.
• To treat corns or calluses, soak your feet, gently pat them dry with a towel, and apply lanolin ointment. Repeat these steps once or twice a day until you see improvement. If corns or calluses don't improve, visit a podiatrist.

Never use nonprescription corn remedies, and never cut corns or calluses with a razor or knife.

Special precautions

• Cut your toenails straight across and file them carefully to eliminate rough edges. Do this under good light after washing your feet. If your toenails are too thick to cut or if they tend to crack when cut, have a podiatrist cut them.

• Make sure new shoes fit comfortably and support, protect, and cover your feet completely. Break them in gradually.
• Never go barefoot.
• Don't use hot-water bottles, heating pads, or ice on your legs or feet. Decreased blood flow to the legs and feet reduces sensation in the feet; you could burn or chill them without feeling it.
• If a foot injury causes a break in the skin, wash the affected area with soap and water immediately and cover it with a dry sterile gauze bandage. Change the bandage daily and inspect the area for redness, swelling, and drainage.

When to notify the doctor

Call the doctor if any foot injury doesn't improve in 72 hours or if you notice any of these signs of poor circulation when examining your feet:
• new sores or ulcers that take unusually long to heal
• unusual, persistent warmth or coolness
• numbness or muscle weakness
• swelling that doesn't resolve after you raise your leg.

rial occlusive disease, Trental may improve blood flow through the capillaries.

Acute arterial occlusive disease usually requires surgery to restore circulation to the affected area. (See *Understanding surgery for arterial occlusive disease*, page 9.)

What can a person with arterial occlusive disease do?

• Avoid wearing tight clothing.
• Practice proper foot care to prevent infection. (See *How to take care of your feet*.)

BLOOD CLOT IN A VEIN

What do doctors call this condition?
Thrombophlebitis

What is this condition?
This acute condition is marked by inflammation and blood clot (thrombus) formation. The clot may occur in deep or surface veins.

A blood clot in a vein often begins with localized inflammation alone (phlebitis), but such inflammation rapidly provokes thrombus formation. This disorder is frequently progressive, leading to pulmonary embolism, a potentially deadly complication.

What causes it?
A thrombus occurs when a change in the inside lining of a blood vessel causes platelet aggregation and consequent fibrin entrapment of red and white blood cells and additional platelets. The rapidly expanding clot initiates a chemical inflammatory process in the inside lining of the vessel, which leads to fibrosis. The enlarging clot may block the vein partially or totally, or it may detach and move to lodge elsewhere in the circulation.

Although the cause of a deep-vein blood clot may be unknown, it usually results from damage to the vessel lining, accelerated blood clotting, and reduced blood flow. Predisposing factors are prolonged bed rest, trauma, surgery, childbirth, and use of oral contraceptives.

Causes of a superficial blood clot include trauma, infection, intravenous drug abuse, and chemical irritation due to extensive use of the intravenous route for medications and diagnostic tests.

What are its symptoms?
In both types of blood clot in a vein, the symptoms vary with the site and length of the affected vein. Although a deep-vein blood clot may cause no signs or symptoms, it may produce severe pain, fever, chills and, possibly, swelling and bluish discoloration of the affected arm or leg. A superficial blood clot produces visible and palpable signs, such as heat, pain, swelling, redness, tenderness, and hardening along the length of the affected vein. Extensive vein involvement may cause inflammation of the lymph glands.

SELF-HELP

Taking steps toward healthier legs

If you have a blood clot in a vein, improving the circulation in your legs can promote healing and prevent complications, such as pain and swelling. Here's how you can have healthier legs.

Raise your legs
Rest your legs with your feet propped up higher than your heart. This helps gravity to move excess fluid out of your legs.

When you sit — at your desk, for example — prop up your feet with a footstool.

Watch your diet
Eat plenty of fresh fruits, vegetables, and seafood. Avoid salty foods, which can increase swelling. Examples of salty foods include bacon, ham, corned beef, smoked fish, pickles, potato chips, and crackers.

When you shop, check package labels and choose products that are low in fat and salt.

Prevent infection
Wash your legs daily with soap and warm water to remove germs that could cause infection. Avoid using bath powders that could dry your skin.

Don't hesitate to call your doctor if you notice any signs of a leg infection, such as redness or swelling.

Exercise regularly
Get involved in swimming or other pool exercises, such as walking or jogging in water. Or ask your doctor to recommend other specific exercises for your legs.

Choose proper clothing
Avoid tight garments that could cut off circulation in your legs, such as garters, girdles, and knee-high hosiery. Wear elastic support stockings all day, every day.

Watch for warning signs
Make sure that you inspect your legs every morning. Call your doctor if you notice these warning signs and symptoms of poor circulation:
- discolored skin (for example, brownish skin or bluish red areas)
- sores
- scales
- increasing leg pain or swelling.

Follow your treatment plan
Take your blood thinner or other prescribed medication exactly as your doctor directs. And keep all appointments for follow-up visits with your doctor.

How is it diagnosed?
Some people may have signs of inflammation and, possibly, a positive Homans' sign (pain on dorsiflexion of the foot) during a physical exam; others have no symptoms. Consequently, essential lab tests include:
- *Doppler ultrasound* to identify reduced blood flow to a specific area and any obstruction to blood flow in the veins
- *plethysmography* to show decreased circulation in the affected area; more sensitive than ultrasound in detecting deep-vein blood clot
- *phlebography* to show filling defects and diverted blood flow (usually confirms the diagnosis).

SELF-HELP

Care and prevention of leg ulcers

A blood clot in a vein can lead to leg ulcers. If you get these ulcers, you can help them heal and prevent new ulcers from forming by learning about your condition and its required care.

What is a leg ulcer?

It's an area of dying skin. Leg ulcers can form wherever an artery becomes blocked or constricted. When this happens, not enough blood gets to the skin and the tissue beneath it to nourish the area. Instead, blood tends to pool in your leg veins — sometimes from a condition called venous insufficiency.

Pressure then builds up in these congested leg vessels, and blood supply to the tissues dwindles. As the condition worsens, the skin becomes fragile, and an infection may arise from injury, pressure, and irritation. As a result, leg ulcers may develop.

Improving your circulation

To improve circulation in your legs, wear elastic support stockings called *antiembolism stockings*. These hose will help to return blood to your heart. They'll also improve circulation to your existing ulcer and may help to keep new ones from forming.

Put your feet up. Rest and elevate your legs for as long and as often as your doctor directs. This will reduce your legs' needs for nutrients and oxygen and help to promote healing. Always raise your lower leg above heart level.

Promoting healing

Follow these measures to help your ulcer heal:
- Keep your ulcer clean to prevent infection. Always wash your hands before and after changing your dressing or touching the wound. This keeps the area germ-free.
- Follow your doctor's instructions exactly when changing your dressing and applying ointments or other medications.
- Be patient. Your ulcer may take 3 months to a year to heal.
- Check with your doctor if your ulcer grows larger, feels increasingly painful, or becomes foul-smelling.

Preventing ulcers

Follow these measures to prevent ulcers:
- Watch for signs of new ulcers — leg swelling, pain, and discolored skin that looks brownish or dark blue.
- Wear support stockings to help prevent ulcers and to help heal an existing ulcer.
- Be careful to avoid injury to your leg, which can lead to ulcer development. For example, avoid activities that involve rugged physical contact, such as roughhousing with children or dogs.
- Prevent falls in your bathtub by installing safety rails or a grab bar and placing a nonskid mat in the tub.
- Wear low, nonskid footwear whenever possible.

Diagnosis of a superficial blood clot in a vein is based on a physical exam (redness and warmth over the affected area, palpable vein, and pain during palpation or compression).

How is it treated?

The goals of treatment are to control blood clot development, prevent complications, relieve pain, and prevent recurrence of the disorder. Measures to relieve signs and symptoms include bed rest, with elevation of the affected arm or leg (see *Taking steps toward healthier legs*); warm, moist soaks to the affected area; and pain relievers as ordered. After a deep-vein blood clot begins to subside, the person may begin to move around wearing elastic support stockings that were applied before he or she got out of bed. Treatment may also include blood-thinning drugs (initially, heparin; later, warfarin) to prolong clotting time.

Therapy for a severe superficial blood clot in a vein may include an anti-inflammatory drug, such as Indocin, along with elastic support stockings, warm soaks, and leg elevation.

What can a person with a blood clot in a vein do?

▪ Be sure to have follow-up blood studies so that your doctor can monitor the effectiveness of drug therapy.
▪ If you're taking heparin, make sure you or a family member know how to give injections under the skin.
▪ Avoid prolonged sitting or standing to help prevent recurrence.
▪ To minimize impaired blood flow in the veins, apply and use elastic support stockings properly. (See *Care and prevention of leg ulcers,* page 13.) Report any complications such as cold, blue toes.

BUERGER'S DISEASE

What do doctors call this condition?
Thromboangiitis obliterans

What is this condition?
Buerger's disease — an inflammatory, occlusive condition — causes segmental lesions and subsequent blood clot (thrombus) formation in the small and medium arteries (and sometimes the veins), thereby reducing blood flow to the feet and legs. This disorder may produce ulceration and, eventually, gangrene.

What causes it?
Although the cause of Buerger's disease is unknown, it has been linked to smoking, suggesting a hypersensitivity reaction to nicotine. Incidence is highest among men of Jewish ancestry between the ages of 20 and 40 who smoke heavily.

What are its symptoms?

Buerger's disease typically causes intermittent claudication (cramplike pains) of the instep, which is aggravated by exercise and relieved by rest. During exposure to low temperature, the feet initially become cold, pale, and numb; later, they redden, become hot, and tingle.

Occasionally, Buerger's disease also affects the hands, possibly resulting in painful fingertip ulcers.

How is it diagnosed?

The person's history and physical exam strongly suggest Buerger's disease. Supportive diagnostic tests include arteriography (X-ray of the artery) and an ultrasound scan.

How is it treated?

The primary goals of treatment are to relieve symptoms and prevent complications. Such therapy may include an exercise program that uses gravity to fill and drain the blood vessels or, in severe disease, a surgical procedure called a *lumbar sympathectomy* (interruption of the sympathetic nervous system pathway) to increase blood supply to the skin. Amputation may be necessary for nonhealing ulcers, intractable pain, or gangrene. (See *Coping with Buerger's disease.*)

CARDIAC TAMPONADE

What is this condition?

In cardiac tamponade, blood enters the sac around the heart (called the pericardial sac) and puts pressure on the heart muscle, impairing heart function. A slow accumulation and rise in pressure may not produce immediate symptoms because the pericardial sac can gradually stretch to accommodate the increase in fluid. However, if fluid builds up rapidly, tamponade may be fatal.

What causes it?

Cardiac tamponade may be idiopathic or may result from:
- cancer, bacterial infections, tuberculosis and, rarely, acute rheumatic fever

 SELF-HELP

Coping with Buerger's disease

The following tips can prevent complications, help you avoid acute episodes, and make you more comfortable.

Quit smoking
Stop smoking permanently to make treatment more effective. Ask your doctor or nurse for the names of smoking cessation programs in your area.

Try not to set it off
Avoid triggering factors, such as emotional stress, exposure to extreme temperatures, and injuries.

Treat your feet
- Wear shoes that fit well and cotton or wool socks.
- Practice proper foot care. Inspect your feet daily for cuts, scratches, redness, and soreness. Seek medical care immediately after any injury.

Other treatments for cardiac tamponade

Depending on the cause, additional treatments for this condition include the following.

If tamponade is caused by injury

The doctor may order a blood transfusion. A surgeon may perform a thoracotomy (cutting into the chest wall) to drain reaccumulating fluid or to repair bleeding sites.

If tamponade is caused by drug therapy

For heparin-induced tamponade, the doctor may prescribe the heparin antagonist protamine sulfate. For warfarin-induced tamponade, he or she may prescribe vitamin K.

- hemorrhage from trauma (such as gunshot or stab wounds of the chest) or nontraumatic causes (such as rupture of the heart or great vessels)
- heart attack
- uremia (an excess of waste products in the blood produced by the metabolism of protein).

What are its symptoms?

Cardiac tamponade causes increased pressure in the veins (a person's neck veins become visibly distended), low blood pressure, muffled heart sounds, and pulsus paradoxus (a pulse that decreases during inspiration). The disorder may also cause pallor or bluish discoloration of the skin, anxiety, rapid heart rate, restlessness, and liver enlargement. The person typically sits upright and leans forward during the episode of tamponade.

How is it diagnosed?

A chest X-ray, an electrocardiogram, pulmonary artery catheterization, and an ultrasound test of the heart identify the effects of cardiac tamponade.

How is it treated?

The goal of treatment is to relieve pressure around the heart by removing accumulated blood or fluid. This may be achieved by a procedure called *pericardiocentesis* (needle aspiration of the pericardial cavity) or surgical creation of an opening in the pericardial sac (called a *pericardial window*).

The person's cardiac output (the amount of blood pumped out of the heart each minute) will be maintained with intravenous fluids, albumin, and an inotropic drug, such as Isuprel or Intropin. (See *Other treatments for cardiac tamponade*.)

CORONARY ARTERY DISEASE

What is this condition?

The dominant effect of this disease is the loss of oxygen and nutrients to the heart because of diminished blood flow through the heart's arteries. This disease is near epidemic in the Western world.

Coronary artery disease occurs more often in men than in women, in whites, and in middle-aged and elderly people. In the past, it rarely affected premenopausal women, but that's no longer the case — perhaps because many women now take oral contraceptives, smoke cigarettes, and are employed in stressful jobs that used to be held exclusively by men.

What causes it?

Atherosclerosis is the usual cause of coronary artery disease. In atherosclerosis, fatty and fibrous plaques narrow the interior channel of the heart's arteries. They reduce the volume of blood that can flow through the arteries, thereby damaging the heart. Plaque formation also predisposes a person to thrombosis (blood clot formation), which can provoke a heart attack.

Atherosclerosis usually develops in high-flow, high-pressure arteries, such as those in the heart, brain, and kidneys, and in the aorta. It has been linked to many risk factors: family history, high blood pressure, obesity, smoking, diabetes, stress, sedentary lifestyle, and high cholesterol and triglyceride levels.

Uncommon causes of reduced coronary artery blood flow include dissecting aneurysms, infectious vasculitis, syphilis, and congenital defects in the coronary vascular system. Coronary artery spasms may also impede blood flow.

What are its symptoms?

The classic symptom of coronary artery disease is angina, which results from inadequate flow of oxygen to the heart. Angina is described as a burning, squeezing, or tight feeling in the chest that may radiate to the left arm, neck, jaw, or shoulder blade. Typically, the person clenches his or her fist over the chest or rubs the left arm when describing the pain, which may be accompanied by nausea, vomiting, fainting, sweating, and cool arms and legs.

Anginal episodes most often follow physical exertion but may also follow emotional excitement, exposure to cold, or a large meal. (See *The three forms of angina.*) Severe and prolonged anginal pain generally suggests a heart attack.

How is it diagnosed?

The person's history — including the frequency and duration of angina and the presence of associated risk factors — is crucial in evalu-

INSIGHT INTO ILLNESS

The three forms of angina

Angina has three major forms:
- *stable angina:* chest pain that is predictable in frequency and duration and can be relieved with nitroglycerin and rest
- *unstable angina:* chest pain that increases in frequency and duration and is more easily induced
- *Prinzmetal's angina:* coronary artery spasm that occurs at unpredictable times.

SELF-HELP

Getting cholesterol under control

Changing your diet can help reduce your cholesterol level. You'll need to reduce the amount of saturated fats that you eat. This means cutting down drastically on eggs, dairy products, and fatty meats. Rely instead on poultry, fish, fruits, vegetables, and high-fiber breads. Use this list as a starting point for your new diet.

FOOD	ELIMINATE	SUBSTITUTE
Bread and cereals	Breads with whole eggs listed as a major ingredient	Oatmeal, multigrain, and bran cereals; whole-grain breads; rye bread
	Egg noodles	Pasta, rice
	Pies, cakes, doughnuts, biscuits, high-fat crackers and cookies	Angel food cake; low-fat cookies, crackers, and home-baked goods
Eggs and dairy products	Whole milk, 2% milk, imitation milk	Skim milk, 1% milk, buttermilk
	Cream, half-and-half, most nondairy creamers, whipped toppings	None
	Whole milk yogurt and cottage cheese	Nonfat or low-fat yogurt, low-fat (1% or 2%) cottage cheese
	Cheese, cream cheese, sour cream, light cream cheese, light sour cream	None
	Egg yolks	Egg whites
	Ice cream	Sherbet, frozen tofu
Fats and oils	Coconut, palm, and palm kernel oils	Unsaturated vegetable oils (corn, olive, canola, safflower, sesame, soybean, and sunflower)
	Butter, lard, bacon fat	Unsaturated margarine and shortening, diet margarine
	Dressings made with egg yolks	Low-fat mayonnaise, unsaturated or low-fat salad dressings
	Chocolate	Baking cocoa
Meat, fish, and poultry	Fatty cuts of beef, lamb, or pork	Lean cuts of beef, lamb, or pork
	Organ meats, spare ribs, cold cuts, sausage, hot dogs, bacon	Poultry
	Sardines, roe	Sole, salmon, mackerel

SELF-HELP

Tips for exercising safely

If you have coronary artery disease, the following tips will help you exercise safely. Remember that your goal is to pace yourself, not to overdo it.

What you should do
- If you've been inactive for a long time, return to exercise gradually.
- Take part in fitness activities, such as walking and swimming, rather than competitive sports such as tennis.
- Wait 2 to 3 hours after a heavy meal before exercising. A light snack warrants a 1- to 2-hour wait. Also avoid hot or cold showers immediately before or after exertion.
- Wear comfortable, lightweight clothes and shoes with adequate support. Dress in layers and remove articles of clothing as you warm up.

What you shouldn't do
- Don't exercise in extreme heat or cold, windy weather, high humidity, or heavy pollution, or at a high altitude.
- Don't exercise if you have a fever or don't feel well.

When to slow down
You may be exercising too hard if you have muscle cramps, side "stitch," and excessive shortness of breath or fatigue. Slow down.

When to stop exercising
Stop exercising and check with your doctor immediately if you experience chest pain, a cold sweat, dizziness, nausea or vomiting, heart palpitations, heart fluttering, or an abnormal heart rhythm.

ating coronary artery disease. Diagnostic test results include the following:
- *Electrocardiogram during angina* shows heart damage and, possibly, an irregular heart rhythm. It tends to be normal when the person is pain-free.
- *Treadmill or bicycle stress test* may provoke chest pain and signs of heart damage.
- *Coronary angiography* reveals coronary artery narrowing or blockage.
- *Myocardial perfusion imaging* (with thallium-201 or Cardiolite) during treadmill exercise detects damaged areas of the heart, seen as "cold spots."

How is it treated?
The goal of treatment is to either reduce the heart's oxygen demand or increase its oxygen supply. Drug therapy consists primarily of nitrates such as nitroglycerin (given beneath the tongue, orally, through the skin in patch form, or topically in ointment form), Isordil (given

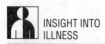

Pregnancy-related cardiomyopathy

Cardiomyopathy (an abnormally enlarged heart) may afflict women during the last trimester of pregnancy or within months after delivery.

Who and why
Doctors don't know why this happens, but they do know that it's most common in women over age 30 who've had two or more pregnancies — particularly those who are malnourished or those who have pregnancy-induced high blood pressure (preeclampsia).

A varied outcome
Treatment may reverse an enlarged heart and congestive heart failure in a pregnant woman, allowing the pregnancy to come to term. But if the heart remains enlarged despite treatment, the prognosis is poor.

beneath the tongue or orally), beta blockers (given orally), or calcium channel blockers (given orally).

Blocked coronary arteries may necessitate coronary artery bypass surgery and the use of vein grafts. In people with only partial blockage of the coronary arteries, the doctor may perform angioplasty, a procedure in which a catheter is used to compress fatty deposits and relieve blockages. Laser angioplasty, a newer procedure, corrects the blockage by melting fatty deposits.

Because coronary artery disease is so widespread, prevention is very important. Dietary restrictions aimed at reducing intake of calories (in obesity) and of salt, fats, and cholesterol serve to minimize the risk, especially when supplemented with regular exercise. (See *Getting cholesterol under control*, page 18.) Stopping smoking and reducing stress are also beneficial.

Other preventive actions include controlling high blood pressure, reducing triglyceride levels, and taking 2.5 grains of aspirin daily (to reduce the threat of blood clots).

What can a person with coronary artery disease do?
- Be sure to follow the prescribed drug therapy, exercise program, and diet. (See *Tips for exercising safely*, page 19.)
- Get regular, moderate exercise.
- Enroll in a self-help program to stop smoking.

DILATED CARDIOMYOPATHY

What is this condition?
Dilated cardiomyopathy is caused by extensively damaged heart muscle fibers. This disorder interferes with the heart's metabolism and greatly enlarges all four chambers of the heart, giving the heart a globular shape and causing it to contract poorly.

Dilated cardiomyopathy leads to intractable congestive heart failure, irregular heart rhythm, and emboli (blood clots or other material that is carried in the bloodstream). Because this disease usually isn't diagnosed until it's in the advanced stages, the prognosis is generally poor.

What causes it?

The cause of most cardiomyopathies is unknown. Dilated cardiomyopathy may occur as a primary heart disease or it may result from viruses, endocrine and electrolyte disorders, or nutritional deficiencies. Other causes include muscle disorders (myasthenia gravis, progressive muscular dystrophy, myotonic dystrophy), infiltrative disorders (hemochromatosis, amyloidosis, sarcoidosis), and sometimes pregnancy. (See *Pregnancy-related cardiomyopathy*.)

Cardiomyopathy may also be a complication of alcoholism. The condition may improve somewhat with abstinence but recurs when the person resumes drinking.

What are its symptoms?

In dilated cardiomyopathy, the heart ejects blood less efficiently than normal. Consequently, a large volume of blood remains in the left ventricle after its contraction, causing shortness of breath, fatigue, an irritating dry cough at night, swelling, liver engorgement, and swelling of the neck veins.

How is it diagnosed?

No single test confirms dilated cardiomyopathy. Diagnosis requires elimination of other possible causes of congestive heart failure and irregular heart rhythms. Tests include the following:
- *Electrocardiography* and *angiography* rule out ischemic heart disease; the electrocardiogram may also show an enlarged heart.
- *Chest X-ray* demonstrates an enlarged heart, lung congestion, or pleural effusion.

How is it treated?

Therapeutic goals include correcting the underlying causes and improving the heart's pumping ability with drugs, oxygen, and a sodium-restricted diet. (See *Living with dilated cardiomyopathy*.) Other options may include bed rest and steroids.

When these treatments fail, therapy may require a heart transplant for carefully selected people. Another option for selected individuals is cardiomyoplasty, a surgical procedure in which the latissimus dorsi muscle is wrapped around the ventricles. This helps the ventricle to effectively pump blood. A cardiomyostimulator delivers bursts of electrical impulses to contract the muscle.

 SELF-HELP

Living with dilated cardiomyopathy

Following these suggestions can make you more comfortable as you cope with this disease:
- Avoid alcohol to help alleviate symptoms.
- Cut down on salt in your diet.
- Watch for and report weight gain.
- Take Lanoxin as prescribed, and watch for side effects: appetite loss, nausea, vomiting, and yellow vision.
- Encourage family members to learn CPR.

HEART ATTACK

What do doctors call this condition?
Myocardial infarction

What is this condition?
In a heart attack, one of the heart's arteries fails to deliver enough blood to the part of the heart muscle it serves. The reduced blood flow causes destruction of localized areas of heart tissue.

If treatment is delayed, the person may die; almost half of sudden deaths from heart attack occur before the victims reach the hospital, within 1 hour after symptoms arise. (Typically, death stems from severe tissue damage or from complications.) The prognosis is better if vigorous treatment begins immediately.

What causes it?
Arteriosclerosis (hardening of the heart's arteries), which reduces the artery's blood flow, is usually the underlying cause of a heart attack. Risk factors include:
- a family history of heart disease
- high blood pressure
- smoking
- high cholesterol and triglyceride levels
- diabetes
- obesity or a diet high in saturated fats, carbohydrates, or salt
- a sedentary lifestyle
- aging
- drug use, especially cocaine
- stress or Type A personality.

Men are more susceptible to heart attacks than women, although the heart attack rate is rising in women — especially those who smoke or take oral contraceptives. (See *Resuming sex after a heart attack*, opposite, and *Walking the road to recovery*, page 24.)

What are its symptoms?
The chief symptom of a heart attack is persistent, crushing chest pain that may spread to the left arm, jaw, neck, or shoulder blades and may last 12 hours or longer. Typically, heart attack victims describe the pain as heavy, squeezing, or crushing. But some — particularly

SELF-HELP

Resuming sex after a heart attack

After you've been discharged from the hospital, you can expect to gradually resume most, if not all, of your usual activities, including sex. In fact, most people can resume having sex 3 to 4 weeks after a heart attack.

Sex is a moderate form of exercise, no more stressful than a brisk walk. However, sex that's accompanied by emotional distress can place a strain on your heart.

Read over the following guidelines. They can help you have a satisfying sex life. And be sure to discuss any related concerns with your doctor or nurse.

The right setting
Choose a quiet, familiar setting for sex. A strange environment may cause stress. Make sure the room temperature is comfortable. Excessive heat or cold makes your heart work harder.

When to have sex
Have sex when you're rested and relaxed. A good time is in the morning, after a good night's sleep.

When not to have sex
Don't have sex when you're tired or upset. Also avoid having sex after drinking a lot of alcohol. Alcohol expands your blood vessels, which makes your heart

work harder. And don't have sex after a big meal; wait a few hours.

Positioning for comfort
Choose positions that are relaxing and permit unrestricted breathing. Any position that's comfortable for you is okay.

Don't be afraid to experiment. At first, you may be more comfortable if your partner assumes a dominant role. You may also want to avoid positions that require you to use your arms to support yourself or your partner.

A few precautions
Ask your doctor if you should take nitroglycerin before having sex. This medication can prevent angina attacks during or after sex.

Remember, it's normal for your pulse and breathing rates to rise during sex. But they should return to normal within 15 minutes. Call your doctor at once if you have any of these symptoms after sex:
- sweating or palpitations for 15 minutes or longer
- breathlessness or a fast pulse rate for 15 minutes or longer
- chest pain that's not relieved by two or three nitroglycerin tablets (taken 5 minutes apart) or a rest period, or both
- sleeplessness after sex or extreme fatigue the next day.

elderly people and those with diabetes — don't experience pain. Others have mild pain that they, or their doctor, may mistake for indigestion. In people with hardening of the arteries, chest pain that grows more and more frequent, severe, or longer-lasting may signal an impending heart attack — especially if the pain isn't triggered by exertion, a heavy meal, or cold and wind.

Some heart attack victims also have a feeling of impending doom, fatigue, nausea, vomiting, shortness of breath, coolness in the arms

SELF-HELP

Walking the road to recovery

This simple daily walking program can help strengthen your heart and speed your recovery after a heart attack. Be sure to allow the full times for warm up and cool down.

To limber up your muscles, do stretching exercises, such as calf and shoulder stretches. For the calf stretch, place both hands on a wall, about shoulder height. Step with one foot toward the wall and lean against it, keeping your palms flat on the wall and your feet flat on the floor. Push against the wall until you feel a pull in your leg.

For the shoulder stretch, clasp your hands over your head and pull your shoulders backward.

WEEK	WARM UP	EXERCISE	COOL DOWN	TOTAL TIME
1	Stretch 2 minutes. Walk slowly 3 minutes.	Walk briskly 5 minutes.	Walk slowly 3 minutes. Stretch 2 minutes.	15 minutes
2	Stretch 2 minutes. Walk slowly 3 minutes.	Walk briskly 7 minutes.	Walk slowly 3 minutes. Stretch 2 minutes.	17 minutes
3	Stretch 2 minutes. Walk slowly 3 minutes.	Walk briskly 9 minutes.	Walk slowly 3 minutes. Stretch 2 minutes.	19 minutes
4	Stretch 2 minutes. Walk slowly 3 minutes.	Walk briskly 11 minutes.	Walk slowly 3 minutes. Stretch 2 minutes.	21 minutes
5	Stretch 2 minutes. Walk slowly 3 minutes.	Walk briskly 13 minutes.	Walk slowly 3 minutes. Stretch 2 minutes.	23 minutes
6	Stretch 2 minutes. Walk slowly 3 minutes.	Walk briskly 15 minutes.	Walk slowly 3 minutes. Stretch 2 minutes.	25 minutes
7	Stretch 2 minutes. Walk slowly 3 minutes.	Walk briskly 18 minutes.	Walk slowly 3 minutes. Stretch 2 minutes.	28 minutes
8	Stretch 2 minutes. Walk slowly 5 minutes.	Walk briskly 20 minutes.	Walk slowly 5 minutes. Stretch 2 minutes.	34 minutes
9	Stretch 2 minutes. Walk slowly 5 minutes.	Walk briskly 23 minutes.	Walk slowly 5 minutes. Stretch 2 minutes.	37 minutes
10	Stretch 2 minutes. Walk slowly 5 minutes.	Walk briskly 26 minutes.	Walk slowly 5 minutes. Stretch 2 minutes.	40 minutes
11	Stretch 2 minutes. Walk slowly 5 minutes.	Walk briskly 28 minutes.	Walk slowly 5 minutes. Stretch 2 minutes.	42 minutes
12	Stretch 2 minutes. Walk slowly 5 minutes.	Walk briskly 30 minutes.	Walk slowly 5 minutes. Stretch 2 minutes.	44 minutes

and legs, perspiration, anxiety, and restlessness. And some people have a "silent" heart attack, which causes no symptoms at all.

Complications

The most common complications of a heart attack are recurrent or persistent chest pain; irregular heart rhythms; failure of the heart's main chamber (left ventricle), causing heart failure or massive fluid buildup in the lungs; and failure of the heart to pump enough blood, causing shock.

Soon after a heart attack, a few people have potentially fatal complications — a blood clot in a vein, heart valve malfunction, rupture of the partition between the heart's chambers, and rupture of the heart muscle.

Up to several months after a heart attack, some people experience Dressler's syndrome — inflammation of the sac around the heart, accompanied by chest pain, fever, and possibly lung inflammation.

How is it diagnosed?

To confirm a heart attack, the doctor checks for persistent chest pain, characteristic electrocardiogram findings, and blood tests showing elevated levels of cardiac enzymes over a 72-hour period. A physical exam may reveal abnormal heart sounds.

When symptoms and physical exam results aren't clear-cut, the doctor assumes that the person has had a heart attack — to be on the safe side — until tests rule it out. To investigate further, these tests may be ordered:
- *12-lead electrocardiogram* — may reveal characteristic abnormalities during the first few hours after a heart attack
- *echocardiography* (a study of the heart's structure and motion) — may show abnormal motion of the ventricular wall in a heart attack that involves the entire wall of the heart.
- *technetium scans* — can identify badly damaged heart muscle by detecting emissions from the radioactive marker, an isotope of technetium, which looks like a "hot spot" on film. These scans help to pinpoint a recent heart attack.

How is it treated?

The goals of treatment are to relieve chest pain, stabilize the heart rhythm, ease the heart's workload, restore blood to the heart's arteries, and preserve heart muscle tissue. Irregular heart rhythms — the main problem during the first 48 hours after a heart attack — may require drugs and possibly a pacemaker. Rarely, a person requires car-

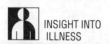

Understanding irregular heart rhythms

An irregular heart rhythm (also called a *cardiac arrhythmia*) is an abnormal change in the heart's rate, rhythm, or both. Various factors can disrupt normal conduction of the heart's electrical impulses.

The heart's conduction pathway is a system of specialized fibers that transmit rapid impulses through the heart's muscle cells, causing the heart to contract. When functioning properly, this pathway causes the two sides of the heart to beat synchronously and regularly. However, a disturbance in the conduction pathway can interrupt the heart's regular rate and rhythm.

Symptoms: From mild to life-threatening
Irregular heart rhythms alter the amount of blood pumped by the heart, which can lead to a wide range of symptoms and complications — from palpitations, dizziness, and fainting to a life-threatening blood clot in a vein or even cardiac arrest.

Treatment
An irregular heart rhythm may be treated with drugs that control the problem and procedures to manage it. Commonly used drugs include Lanoxin, Inderal, Isoptin, Cardioquin, and Pronestyl. However, be aware that these drugs can only control, not cure, the irregular heart rhythm.

Procedures used to manage an irregular heart rhythm include carotid sinus massage, Valsalva's maneuver, pacemaker insertion, electrocardioversion, and surgery.

Carotid sinus massage
In this procedure, the carotid sinus (where the common carotid artery forks), located on the side of the neck, is massaged for several seconds to try to restore a normal heart rhythm. Some people are taught to do this themselves when irregular rhythms occur.

Valsalva's maneuver
This procedure increases pressure in the chest, helping to restore a regular heart rhythm. To perform it, the person inhales deeply, holds his or her breath, and strains hard for at least 10 seconds before exhaling.

Pacemaker insertion
A pacemaker may be inserted into the heart. This device generates an electrical impulse that triggers the heart to contract and controls the heart rate. Usually, a temporary pacemaker is inserted first, remaining in place for up to several days until the irregular heart rhythm is controlled, a permanent pacemaker is inserted, or cardiac surgery is performed.

Electrocardioversion
In this procedure, the person first receives a sedative to induce sleep. Then an electrical current is delivered to the person's heart through paddles placed on his or her chest. This restores the person's normal heart rate and relieves symptoms.

Surgery
If the irregular heart rhythm can't be controlled by drugs or other conservative measures, the doctor may recommend surgery. Operations include open-heart surgery (to correct structural defects), permanent pacemaker implantation, or insertion of an implantable cardioverter-defibrillator. To insert this last device, the surgeon sews two small patches onto the heart's surface, and then tunnels thin wires attached to these patches under the skin to a pocket made in the abdomen — where the device is placed. The device automatically shocks the heart to restore a normal heart rhythm and rate when the heart has stopped beating or is beating irregularly.

dioversion, in which an electrical current is delivered to the heart in an attempt to restore a normal rhythm. (See *Understanding irregular heart rhythms.*)

To preserve heart muscle tissue, the doctor may administer thrombolytics (drugs that break up clots in the arteries) within 6 hours after heart attack symptoms arise. These drugs include streptokinase, alteplase, and urokinase.

Percutaneous transluminal coronary angioplasty may be another option. In this procedure, the doctor threads a thin, balloon-tipped catheter into the narrowed heart artery (if narrowing has caused the heart attack). After injecting contrast dye through the catheter to pinpoint the narrowed site, the doctor inflates the balloon catheter to expand and reopen the artery. If this procedure is done soon after symptoms begin, a thrombolytic drug may be injected directly into the artery.

Other treatments

After a heart attack, some people also receive:
- lidocaine, a drug used to control certain irregular heart rhythms
- other drugs, such as Pronestyl, Cardioquin, Bretylol, or Norpace
- the drug atropine or a temporary pacemaker if the heart rate is abnormally slow
- nitroglycerin, calcium channel blockers, or other drugs that relieve pain, redistribute blood to blood-starved areas of the heart, help the heart to pump more blood, and reduce the heart's workload
- heparin to prevent clotting
- morphine for pain relief and sedation
- drugs that improve heart contractions or raise blood pressure
- beta blockers, such as Inderal or Blocadren, after an acute heart attack to help prevent another heart attack
- aspirin to prevent clot formation (should be started within 24 hours after symptoms arise)
- bed rest with a bedside commode to rest the heart
- oxygen administration for 24 to 48 hours
- pulmonary artery catheterization to detect failure of the heart's left or right ventricle and to monitor the person's response to treatment. In this procedure, the doctor threads a thin, hollow tube through the heart and into the pulmonary artery to measure various pressures. (See *After a heart attack, what can you do?*)

 SELF-HELP

After a heart attack, what can you do?

To speed your recovery from a heart attack, follow these guidelines.

Comply with drug therapy
- Make sure you understand and follow the prescribed drug therapy plan and other treatment plans.
- Watch for and report signs of drug side effects. For example, if you're receiving Lanoxin, watch for appetite loss, nausea, vomiting, and yellow vision.
- Call the doctor if you have chest pain.

Eat a heart-friendly diet
Modify your diet, as directed by the doctor. Typical changes include cutting down on salt, fat, and cholesterol.

Other good moves
- If you smoke cigarettes, stop.
- Resume sexual activity gradually.
- Sign up for a cardiac rehabilitation program, as recommended by your doctor.

Complications of heart failure

Heart failure may lead to the following problems:
- fluid buildup in the lungs
- slow blood flow through the veins (for example, from prolonged bed rest), which increases the risk of a blood clot
- poor blood flow to the brain
- kidney problems, with severe imbalances of potassium, sodium, or other electrolytes.

HEART FAILURE

What is this condition?

In heart failure, the heart cannot pump enough blood to meet the body's needs. Usually, failure occurs in the left ventricle (the heart's main working chamber). But sometimes the right ventricle fails — either on its own or as a result of left-sided failure. Sometimes, both sides fail at the same time.

Although heart failure may be acute if it's caused by a heart attack, it's generally a chronic disorder associated with sodium and water retention by the kidneys.

New diagnostic tests and treatments have greatly improved the outlook for people with heart failure. But the prognosis still depends on the underlying cause and how it responds to treatment.

How heart failure progresses

When the left ventricle doesn't pump enough blood, compensatory mechanisms kick in to make sure that vital organs get enough blood. For example, the heartbeat grows stronger and faster, blood pressure rises, and venous return and blood volume increase.

But as left-sided failure worsens, these mechanisms fail. The left ventricle then enlarges and starts to malfunction, allowing blood to pool in the ventricle and another heart chamber, the atrium. Eventually, sodium and water enter the lungs, causing a buildup of fluid there known as *pulmonary edema*, a life-threatening emergency.

What causes it?

Causes of heart failure include:
- abnormality of the heart muscle, as occurs in a heart attack
- too little blood flow to the heart due to hardening of the arteries or disease of the heart muscle
- mechanical disturbances that impede filling of the ventricle (for instance, narrowing of a heart valve due to rheumatic heart disease or another heart disorder)
- disturbances in blood circulation that impair the heart's pumping ability (such as excessive workload from too much blood volume or pressure).

SELF-HELP

Planning low-salt meals

If you have heart failure, you'll need to reduce your salt (sodium) intake. Your doctor will tell you how many milligrams of salt you're allowed each day.

Things to do
- Read food labels for sodium content (200 milligrams of salt equals 80 milligrams of sodium chloride).
- Use herbs and spices to enhance the flavor of food. But realize that not all flavor enhancers are salt-free. Some, such as monosodium glutamate and horseradish, are notoriously high in sodium.
- Order baked, broiled, or roasted foods at restaurants and skip gravies, fruit juices, soups, and cheesy dressings.
- Include unsalted meat, broth, soups, and butter in your diet. Use special low-salt milk, canned vegetables, and baking powder.

Restrictions and warnings
- Avoid using salt in cooking and at the table.
- Stay away from salty foods, such as potato chips, pretzels, and snack crackers; canned soups and vegetables; prepared foods (for example, TV dinners and frozen entrees); lunch meats, cheeses, or pickles; and foods preserved in brine.
- Be aware that bottled soft drinks may be high in sodium. In low-calorie beverages, substituting sodium saccharin for sugar increases the sodium content even more.

Ask your doctor
Many over-the-counter medications contain sodium. Examples include Alka-Seltzer, Di-Gel, and Rolaids. Consult your doctor or pharmacist about the sodium content of over-the-counter medications before taking them.

Also seek your doctor's approval before using a salt substitute. Many products contain a salt other than sodium chloride. They may contain potassium or ammonium salts, which could be harmful if you have kidney or liver disease.

What are its symptoms?

Left-sided heart failure primarily causes respiratory symptoms; right-sided heart failure causes symptoms throughout the body. However, heart failure often affects both sides of the heart. (See *Complications of heart failure*.)

Symptoms of left-sided heart failure include shortness of breath, difficulty breathing except when upright, wheezing, coughing, oxygen shortage in the body, pale or bluish skin, palpitations, irregular heart rhythm, and increased blood pressure.

Symptoms of right-sided heart failure include swollen legs, liver and spleen enlargement, swollen neck veins, fluid buildup in the stomach, a swollen abdomen, slow weight gain, irregular heart rhythm, nausea, vomiting, appetite loss, weakness, fatigue, dizziness, and fainting episodes.

How is it diagnosed?

To diagnose heart failure, the doctor orders an electrocardiogram and a chest X-ray. The electrocardiogram usually reveals heart strain, an enlarged heart, or poor blood supply to the heart. It may also indicate an enlarged atrium, a fast heart rate, and premature heartbeats. A chest X-ray may show an enlarged heart, swelling of the space between tissues, and other characteristic findings.

To monitor the person's status, the doctor usually inserts a thin, hollow tube through the heart and into the pulmonary artery to monitor various pressures.

How is it treated?

The aim of treatment is to make the heart pump more effectively. To do this, the doctor tries to reverse the compensatory mechanisms that are causing the symptoms. To control heart failure quickly, the doctor may use the following treatments:

- diuretics (drugs that increase urine formation and excretion) to reduce total blood volume and relieve congestion in the circulation
- prolonged bed rest to rest the heart
- Lanoxin to strengthen the heart's contractions
- drugs that increase the heart's pumping capacity
- elastic support stockings to improve blood flow and prevent blood clots in leg veins.

What can a person with heart failure do?

- Avoid foods high in salt (sodium). (See *Planning low-salt meals,* page 29.)
- Take Lanoxin exactly as prescribed. Watch for and immediately report signs of toxicity, such as appetite loss, vomiting, and yellow vision.
- If you're taking a potassium-losing diuretic, be sure to take a prescribed potassium supplement and eat high-potassium foods, such as bananas, apricots, and orange juice.
- Notify the doctor promptly if your pulse is unusually irregular or drops below 60 beats per minute, or if you experience dizziness, shortness of breath (especially at night), blurred vision, a nagging dry cough, palpitations, increased fatigue, swollen ankles, decreased urine output, or a rapid weight gain (3 to 5 pounds [1.35 to 2.25 kilograms] in a week). (See *Living with heart failure.*)
- Get regular medical checkups.

SELF-HELP

Living with heart failure

Recognizing early symptoms of your condition is one way for you to monitor yourself and help prevent complications of heart failure. Keep your doctor posted on the symptoms you experience. Then follow the doctor's instructions. Of course, continue to follow your diet, activity, and medication plans as directed.

Common early symptoms of heart failure appear below. You'll also find tips for living with them.

If you have breathing difficulties
You may have trouble breathing when blood and fluids don't move fast enough through your lungs. You may feel short of breath with exertion, such as climbing the stairs or lifting a child. If this happens, stop what you're doing and steady yourself. Then rest until you feel better.

If you feel short of breath when you're resting or lying down, try raising your head with several pillows. Or, if you're short of breath when you get up after a nap or a night's sleep, sit up, dangle your legs over the bedside, and wiggle your feet and ankles. You can also stand up and walk around a bit to promote circulation.

If you notice swelling or weight gain
If your body doesn't get rid of extra salt and fluid, you may have swelling. If you press your finger to your skin and the impression remains briefly, you probably have some swelling.

You may also notice that your hands, ankles, or feet are puffy. Or you may see marks on your skin from the elastic in your socks or the rings on your fingers. To help reduce the swelling, raise your feet, ankles, or hands above the level of your heart.

Be sure to weigh yourself every day at about the same time, using the same scale and wearing the same amount of clothing. If you notice a sudden, unexplainable gain (of 2 pounds [1 kilogram] or more in a day), let your doctor know. He or she may prescribe medication or suggest other relief measures.

Other symptoms to watch for
Report these other symptoms to your doctor:
- a dry cough
- getting up frequently during the night to urinate
- increased weakness and fatigue
- upper abdominal pain or a bloated feeling.

A word of caution
Call your doctor right away if at any time you feel you can't breathe and your heart is pounding or if you cough up pink, frothy sputum.

HEART VALVE DISEASE

What is this condition?

In heart valve disease, three types of mechanical disruption can occur: stenosis (narrowing) of the valve opening, incomplete valve closure (insufficiency), or valve prolapse (the valve slips from its normal position). These disruptions can result from such disorders as endocarditis (infection of the inner lining of the heart muscle), congenital defects, and inflammation, and they can lead to heart failure.

Heart valve disease occurs in varying forms:

■ *Mitral insufficiency:* In this form, blood from the left ventricle flows back into the left atrium during the heart's contraction phase, causing the atrium to enlarge to accommodate the backflow. As a result, the left ventricle expands to accommodate the increased volume of blood from the atrium and to compensate for diminishing cardiac output. This eventually leads to ventricular failure.

■ *Mitral stenosis:* Narrowing of the valve by valvular abnormalities, fibrosis, or calcification blocks blood flow from the left atrium to the left ventricle. Consequently, left atrial volume and pressure rise and the chamber dilates. Greater resistance to blood flow causes pulmonary hypertension and right ventricular failure.

■ *Mitral valve prolapse:* One or both valve leaflets protrude into the left atrium. Mitral valve prolapse is the term used when anatomic prolapse is accompanied by symptoms unrelated to the valve abnormality.

■ *Aortic insufficiency:* Blood flows back into the left ventricle during the heart's relaxation phase, causing fluid overload in the ventricle, which enlarges. Excess fluids overload the left atrium and, finally, the pulmonary system. Left ventricular failure and pulmonary edema (fluid in the lungs) eventually result.

■ *Aortic stenosis:* Increased left ventricular pressure tries to overcome the resistance of the narrowed valve opening. The added workload increases the demand for oxygen, while diminished cardiac output reduces coronary artery perfusion and causes left ventricular failure.

■ *Pulmonic insufficiency:* Blood ejected during the heart's contraction phase flows back into the right ventricle during the heart's relaxation phase, causing fluid overload in the ventricle and, finally, right ventricular failure.

■ *Pulmonic stenosis:* Blocked right ventricular outflow causes the right ventricle to enlarge, eventually resulting in right ventricular failure.

■ *Tricuspid insufficiency:* Blood flows back into the right atrium during the heart's contraction phase, decreasing blood flow to the lungs and the left side of the heart. Fluid overload can eventually lead to right ventricular failure.

■ *Tricuspid stenosis:* Blocked blood flow from the right atrium to the right ventricle causes the right atrium to enlarge. Eventually, this leads to right ventricular failure.

What are its symptoms?

Signs and symptoms depend on which valve is affected. For example, a person with mitral stenosis may experience shortness of breath upon

STRAIGHT
TALK

Questions people ask after valve replacement

How will I know if my new heart valve is working?
You'll feel much better when your valve is working. If it malfunctions, you may have shortness of breath, chest pain, or dizziness. You may also notice that your hands and feet feel cold more frequently. If you experience these symptoms, contact your doctor.

When can I resume my normal activities?
In about 6 weeks. Soon after your surgery, you'll do simple exercises and motions in bed. Within 2 days, you'll be out of bed and sitting in a chair. Next, you'll take short walks and progress to two 10-minute walks a day. Then, you'll either do more walking or you'll get to pedal a stationary bike. When you leave the hospital, you should be able to do light chores.

For the first 3 to 4 weeks at home, try to climb only one flight of stairs a day.

For the first 5 weeks, don't drive a car. If you're a passenger, remember to wear a lap and shoulder belt. On long trips, stop hourly to walk and stretch your legs.

For the first 6 weeks (the time it takes your breast-bone wound to heal), don't lift, push, or pull anything heavier than 5 pounds (2.3 kilograms).

As for work, most patients recuperate at home until their 6-week follow-up exam. Then they return to their work schedule gradually, beginning with half days and working up to a full day.

Will using my microwave or having X-rays affect my new heart valve?
No. The manufacturer has designed your valve to operate safely around microwaves and X-rays.

---

exertion and while sleeping, weakness, fatigue, irregular heartbeats, and a chronic, nonproductive cough. A person with aortic insufficiency (also called *aortic regurgitation*) may experience shortness of breath upon exertion and when sleeping, night sweats, cough, fatigue, and anginal pain that may or may not be relieved by nitroglycerin.

If a heart valve disease leads to heart failure, the person will experience the signs and symptoms of heart failure. For more information, see pages 28 to 31.

How is it diagnosed?
To establish a diagnosis of heart valve disease, the doctor will explore the person's health history and perform a physical exam. If a valve problem is suspected, diagnostic tests, including catheterization of the heart, chest X-ray, echocardiography (ultrasound of the heart), and electrocardiography, may help the doctor pinpoint the disorder.

How is it treated?
Treatment depends on the nature and severity of the symptoms. For example, heart failure requires Lanoxin, diuretics, a salt-restricted

diet and, in severe cases, oxygen. Other measures may include blood-thinning drugs to prevent blood clot formation around diseased or replaced valves, antibiotics before and after surgery or dental care, and valvuloplasty.

If the person has severe signs and symptoms that can't be managed medically, open-heart surgery for valve replacement is indicated. (See *Questions people ask after valve replacement*, page 33.)

HIGH BLOOD PRESSURE

What do doctors call this condition?
Hypertension

What is this condition?
In high blood pressure, the blood exerts too much pressure against the walls of the arteries. When this condition persists, it eventually damages blood vessels and reduces blood flow to body tissues. This can damage the heart, kidneys, brain, and eyes.

If high blood pressure damages the heart and blood vessels, the risk of life-threatening complications — heart failure, a heart attack, or a stroke — increases. An episode of severely elevated blood pressure may lead to brain damage and even death.

High blood pressure affects 15% to 20% of adults in North America. It's a major cause of stroke, heart disease, and kidney failure. Fortunately, though, the outlook is good if the disorder is detected early and treatment starts before complications develop.

What causes it?
In most people, the cause of high blood pressure is unknown. However, researchers have identified certain risk factors — a family history of high blood pressure, race (most common in blacks), stress, obesity, a diet high in saturated fats or salt, tobacco use, a sedentary lifestyle, and aging.

Less commonly, high blood pressure is caused by an identifiable cause, such as:
- pregnancy
- neurologic disorders

- endocrine disorders — for example, Cushing's syndrome, primary hyperaldosteronism, or dysfunction of the thyroid, pituitary, or parathyroid glands
- disease of kidney vessels
- pheochromocytoma (a tumor of the adrenal gland)
- coarctation of the aorta (a congenital heart defect)
- use of oral contraceptives or other drugs, such as cocaine, epoetin alfa, and Sandimmune.

What are its symptoms?

High blood pressure rarely causes symptoms until blood vessels in the heart, brain, or kidneys change. Extremely high blood pressure damages the inner lining of small blood vessels, possibly leading to blood clots. When this happens, the effects of high blood pressure depend on the location of the damaged vessels:

- brain: stroke
- retina: blindness
- heart: heart attack
- kidneys: protein in the urine and, eventually, kidney failure.

High blood pressure makes the heart work harder, causing the left ventricle (the heart's main working chamber) to enlarge. Eventually, both the left and right ventricles may fail and fluid may build up in the lungs.

How is it diagnosed?

A blood pressure reading consists of two values. The first is *systolic pressure* — maximum pressure, or that exerted when the heart is beating. The second value is *diastolic pressure* — minimum pressure, or that exerted when the heart relaxes between beats. The doctor diagnoses high blood pressure after a series of blood pressure measurements above 140/90 in a person under age 50 or above 150/95 in a person over age 50.

The doctor also performs a physical exam, which may reveal abnormal sounds over certain arteries. An eye exam may reveal characteristic changes too.

The person's history and additional diagnostic studies may point to certain predisposing factors and help identify an underlying cause or complications. For example, intravenous pyelography (an X-ray study of the kidneys) can detect kidney shrinkage if high blood pressure has caused chronic kidney disease.

Questions people ask about high blood pressure

My father had high blood pressure, and now I have it. Could I have done anything to prevent getting it?
Probably not because the tendency to develop high blood pressure is inherited. However, people in high-risk families may be able to prevent it by decreasing salt in their diet and avoiding obesity from an early age, but this remains unproved.

If my blood pressure is normal, why can't I stop taking my medication?
Because even though your blood pressure falls within acceptable limits, it's not really normal — it's just controlled. If you stop taking your medication, your pressure may rise again. You may always need to take some medication. Of course, other measures, such as regular exercise, stress reduction, and a low-salt diet, may also help keep your blood pressure in check.

Can my blood pressure drop too low?
It might, if your treatment plan is changed — for example, if the doctor increases your drug dosage or gives you a different drug. So check your blood pressure regularly, and report any of these symptoms of low blood pressure to the doctor: dizziness, light-headedness, fatigue, and weakness.

I've heard that garlic helps lower high blood pressure. Can I use this instead of medication?
No. Although garlic is sold in various forms as a "treatment" for heart problems and high blood pressure, there is no documented evidence that it has succeeded in lowering blood pressure.

If the doctor suspects primary hyperaldosteronism as the cause of high blood pressure, the blood potassium level will be measured. To check for damage to the heart and blood vessels and other complications of high blood pressure, these tests may be ordered:

- *electrocardiogram*, which may show an enlarged left ventricle or decreased blood supply to this chamber
- *chest X-ray*, which may show an enlarged heart
- *echocardiography* (a study of heart motion and structure), which may show an enlarged left ventricle.

How is it treated?

To treat high blood pressure with no known cause, the doctor typically uses a stepped-care approach:

- *Step 1:* The person makes lifestyle changes, such as losing weight (if needed), limiting alcohol intake, exercising regularly, reducing salt intake, and stopping smoking.
- *Step 2:* If Step 1 measures fail to reduce blood pressure adequately, the person continues lifestyle modifications and starts drug therapy. Preferred drugs for lowering blood pressure include diuretics or beta

SELF-HELP

Cutting down on salt

You need to cut down on salt because too much salt causes your body to retain water. This can lead to high blood pressure or can worsen it. Even a moderate reduction in salt can lower blood pressure significantly.

Reducing your salt intake isn't hard to do. The following information and suggestions will help you get started.

Facts about salt
- Table salt is about 40% sodium.
- Americans consume about 20 times more salt than their bodies need.
- About three-fourths of the salt you consume is already in the foods and beverages you eat and drink.
- One teaspoon of salt contains 2 grams (2,000 milligrams) of sodium — the recommended daily amount for people with high blood pressure.
- You can reduce your intake to this level simply by not salting your food during cooking or before eating.
- Some people are so sensitive to salt that even a moderate amount causes their blood pressure to rise.
- The more salt you eat, the more medication you'll need to control your blood pressure if you're salt-sensitive.

Tips for reducing salt intake
Reducing your salt intake to a teaspoon or less a day is easy if you:
- read labels on medicines and food containers
- put away your salt shaker or, if you must use salt, use "light salt," which contains half the sodium of ordinary table salt

- buy fresh meats, fruits, and vegetables instead of canned, processed, and convenience foods
- substitute spices and lemon juice for salt
- watch out for sources of hidden sodium — for example, carbonated beverages, nondairy creamers, cookies, and cakes
- avoid salty foods, such as bacon, sausage, pretzels, potato chips, mustard, pickles, and some cheeses.

Know your sodium sources
Canned, prepared, and "fast" foods are loaded with sodium; so are condiments such as ketchup. Even some foods that don't taste salty contain high amounts of sodium. Consider the values below:

Food	Milligrams of sodium
1 can tomato soup	872
1 hot dog	639
1 cheeseburger	709
1 tablespoon ketchup	156
1 dill pickle	928
1 cup corn flakes	256

Other high-sodium sources include baking powder, baking soda, barbecue sauce, bouillon cubes, celery salt, chili sauce, cooking wine, garlic salt, onion salt, softened water, and soy sauce.

Surprisingly, many medicines and other nonfood items contain sodium, such as alkalizers for indigestion, laxatives, aspirin, cough medicine, mouthwash, and toothpaste.

blockers. If these drugs are ineffective or unacceptable, the doctor may prescribe angiotensin-converting enzyme inhibitors, calcium antagonists, alpha₁-receptor blockers, or alpha-beta blockers.

- *Step 3:* If the person still doesn't reach the desired blood pressure or make significant progress, the doctor increases the drug dosage, substitutes a drug in the same class, or adds a drug from a different class.

■ *Step 4:* If the person still fails to achieve the desired blood pressure or make significant progress, the doctor adds a second or third drug or a diuretic (if one isn't already prescribed).

If the cause of a person's high blood pressure is known, treatment aims at correcting the underlying cause and controlling the effects of high blood pressure.

What can a person with high blood pressure do?

■ Be sure to comply with prescribed therapy; uncontrolled high blood pressure may cause a stroke or a heart attack. (See *Questions people ask about high blood pressure,* page 36.)

■ Establish a daily routine for taking prescribed medication.

■ Notify the doctor if you experience side effects of medication.

■ Change your eating habits, as directed by the doctor. If you're obese, begin a weight-loss diet. Avoid high-sodium foods and table salt. (See *Cutting down on salt,* page 37.)

■ Avoid high-sodium antacids and over-the-counter cold and sinus medications, which contain substances that narrow the blood vessels.

■ As needed, make changes in your lifestyle — for example, by reducing stress and exercising regularly.

■ Have your doctor check your blood pressure at frequent, regular visits.

*H*YPERTROPHIC CARDIOMYOPATHY

What do doctors call this condition?
Idiopathic hypertrophic subaortic stenosis

What is this condition?
This primary disease of the heart is marked by disproportionate, asymmetrical thickening of the interventricular septum, the muscular wall that separates the heart's chambers. It may go undetected for years but may lead to potentially fatal heart failure.

What causes it?
This disorder results from defective cells in the heart muscle, a problem that may be genetic in origin. Signs and symptoms occur because

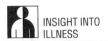

What happens in hypertrophic cardiomyopathy

In hypertrophic cardiomyopathy, the thickened heart muscle becomes inflexible, hindering normal expansion and contraction of the heart chambers. As a result, less blood can circulate with each heartbeat.

Valve function may deteriorate

Sometimes, the muscle between the ventricles thickens and bulges into the left ventricle, partially blocking the aortic valve and obstructing blood flow. This further reduces the amount of circulated blood. The anterior leaflet of the mitral valve (between the left atrium and the left ventricle) can also move into the outflow tract during ventricular contraction, reducing output even more.

Eventually — usually by adulthood — the heart can't supply enough oxygenated blood to meet the body's needs. As a result, the person may experi-

ence a variety of symptoms. Early symptoms include fainting, chest pain similar to angina, irregular heart rhythms, shortness of breath, and fatigue. These symptoms typically occur in adults after physical exertion or emotional stress.

Exercise can make things worse

Exercise and stress make the heart beat harder and faster and make the septal wall push harder, partially blocking the aortic valve. Fainting results from a sudden drop in the amount of blood leaving the heart, which deprives the brain of oxygen for a few seconds. A diminished blood supply in the coronary arteries and other heart structures leads to chest pain, irregular heart rhythms, fatigue, and shortness of breath.

As the disorder worsens and the heart no longer pumps effectively, congestive heart failure may result.

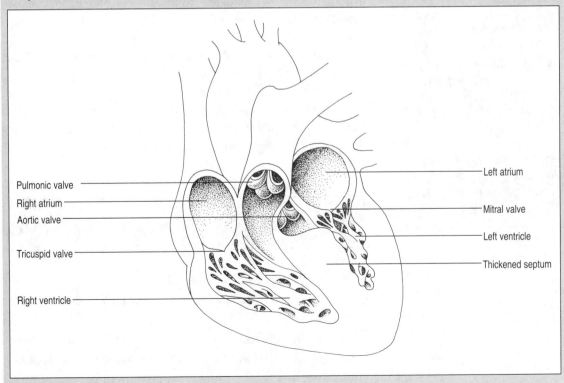

Living with hypertrophic cardiomyopathy

If you have this disease, your condition may remain stable for years. But to avoid serious problems, you must comply with your treatment plan and closely follow your doctor's advice. Here are some general guidelines.

Take it slow
• Avoid strenuous physical activities such as running. Fainting or cardiac arrest may follow what seemed to be a well-tolerated exercise.
• Encourage family members to learn CPR.

Avoid infections
Before dental work or surgery, be sure to take prescribed antibiotics to prevent infection of the heart lining.

Monitor your drug therapy
Don't stop taking Inderal suddenly; doing so could increase the demands on your heart.

the thickened heart muscle impedes the flow of blood in and out of the heart.

What are its symptoms?

Generally, symptoms don't appear until the disease is well advanced. The person may experience chest pains, irregular heart rhythms, shortness of breath, fainting, heart failure, and sudden death. (See *What happens in hypertrophic cardiomyopathy*, page 39.)

How is it diagnosed?

Diagnosis of hypertrophic cardiomyopathy depends on typical clinical findings and on test results:
• *Echocardiography* (most useful) shows increased thickness of the interventricular septum and abnormal motion of the heart valves.
• *Electrocardiography* usually reveals changes in the electrical impulses generated by the heart and altered heart rhythms.

How is it treated?

The goals of treatment are to relax the ventricle and to relieve obstructed blood flow in and out of the heart. The drug Inderal helps to slow the heart rate and relax the obstructing muscle, thereby promoting adequate filling of the heart's ventricle. This helps to reduce angina, fainting episodes, shortness of breath, and irregular heart rhythms. (See *Living with hypertrophic cardiomyopathy*.)

If drug therapy fails, surgery is indicated. Ventricular myotomy (removal of the enlarged septum) alone or combined with replacement of the mitral valve may ease obstructed blood flow and relieve symptoms. However, ventricular myotomy is a risky procedure.

INFLAMMATION OF THE HEART LINING

What do doctors call this condition?

Endocarditis, infective endocarditis, bacterial endocarditis

What is this condition?

Inflammation of the heart lining is an infection of the endocardium, heart valves, or a valve prosthesis, resulting from bacteria or fungi.

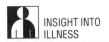
INSIGHT INTO
ILLNESS

How inflammation of the heart lining leads to embolism

Inflammation of the heart lining not only impairs heart valves, but also causes further complications. These arise when valve vegetations break away as emboli, travel through the bloodstream, and lodge in other organs, causing infarction. This flowchart shows the domino-like effect of this process, from infection to embolism.

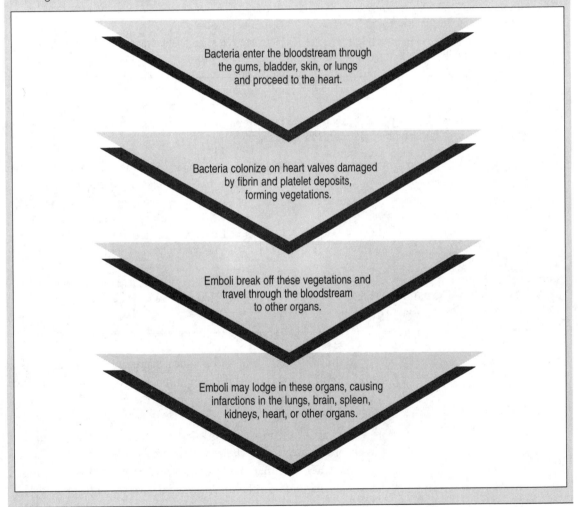

Bacteria enter the bloodstream through the gums, bladder, skin, or lungs and proceed to the heart.

Bacteria colonize on heart valves damaged by fibrin and platelet deposits, forming vegetations.

Emboli break off these vegetations and travel through the bloodstream to other organs.

Emboli may lodge in these organs, causing infarctions in the lungs, brain, spleen, kidneys, heart, or other organs.

The infection produces vegetative growths on the heart valves, the lining of a heart chamber, or the inside lining of a blood vessel that may embolize (break off and travel through the bloodstream) to the spleen, kidneys, central nervous system, and lungs. (See *How inflammation of the heart lining leads to embolism*.)

Warning signs in inflammatory heart disease

To prevent complications from inflammatory heart disease, you need to recognize the warning signs. They include chest pain, shortness of breath, unusual tiredness, sudden weight gain, and swollen hands or feet.

Don't be reluctant to tell your nurse or doctor about these warning signs, even though they may seem like nothing at first. The sooner you're treated, the better you'll feel.

Chest pain
If you have chest pain, tell your doctor right away. Describe where you feel the pain (for example, in the middle of your chest or on the left or right side) and how long the pain lasts. Then describe its intensity (for example, sharp or dull or pressing or burning).

Think of what, if anything, seems to bring on the pain, such as breathing or turning. Also think of what, if anything, seems to relieve it, such as lying down or sitting forward.

Shortness of breath
Here's a way to tell if you're more short of breath than usual. Try talking while you go about a daily activity, such as folding the laundry or weeding the garden. If you find you can't talk without getting out of breath, slow down and check with your doctor.

Unusual fatigue
Rate your usual activities on a scale of 1 to 10. Give a score of 10 to the ones that take the most effort. Now rate walking to the car, climbing the stairs, preparing dinner, and other activities.

If an activity is much harder to do than it used to be, or if yesterday's 5 becomes today's 10, check with your doctor.

Swelling and weight gain
Check your hands and feet for swelling. If they swell easily, tell your doctor.

Also check your weight each day at about the same time. Be sure to use the same scale and wear about the same amount of clothing. If you gain a lot of weight in a short time—say, 5 pounds (2.3 kilograms) in 1 week or 1 pound (0.5 kilogram) overnight—you could be retaining fluid. If this occurs, tell your doctor.

In this disorder, fibrin and platelets aggregate on the valve tissue and engulf circulating bacteria or fungi that flourish and produce vegetations. Such vegetations may cover the valve surfaces, causing ulcers and necrosis (tissue death).

Untreated, inflammation of the heart lining is usually fatal, but with proper treatment, the recovery rate is 70%. The prognosis is poorest when the inflammation causes severe valve damage, leading to insufficiency and heart failure, or when it involves a prosthetic valve.

What causes it?
Most cases of inflammation of the heart lining occur in intravenous drug abusers, people with prosthetic heart valves, and those with mitral valve prolapse. Other predisposing conditions include rheumatic heart disease, coarctation of the aorta, tetralogy of Fallot, subaortic

and aortic stenosis, ventricular septal defects, pulmonic stenosis, Marfan syndrome, and degenerative heart disease, especially calcific aortic stenosis. However, some people with an inflamed heart lining have no underlying heart disease.

What are its symptoms?

Early symptoms include malaise, weakness, fatigue, weight loss, loss of appetite, joint pain, sweating during the night, chills, valvular insufficiency and, in 90% of cases, an intermittent fever that may recur for weeks. When examining the person with a stethoscope, the doctor may hear a loud heart murmur.

In about 30% of people with the disorder, embolization (release of material into the bloodstream) from vegetating lesions or diseased valve tissue may produce:

- pain in the left upper area of the stomach, radiating to the left shoulder
- blood or pus in the urine, flank pain, and decreased urine output
- partial paralysis, inability to speak, or other nervous system deficits
- chest pain, shortness of breath, and a cough that may produce blood
- numbness and tingling in an arm, leg, finger, or toe.

Other signs may include an enlarged spleen, skin rash, and splinter hemorrhages under the nails. (See *Warning signs in inflammatory heart disease.*)

How is it diagnosed?

Three or more blood cultures in a 24- to 48-hour period identify the causative organism in up to 90% of people. The remaining 10% may have negative blood cultures, possibly suggesting fungal infection or infections that are hard to diagnose, such as *Haemophilus parainfluenzae.*

Echocardiography (an ultrasound test of the heart) may identify valvular damage; an electrocardiogram may show atrial fibrillation and other irregular heart rhythms that accompany valvular disease.

How is it treated?

Treatment tries to kill the infecting organism. Antibiotics should start promptly and continue for 4 to 6 weeks.

Supportive treatment includes bed rest, aspirin for fever and aches, and sufficient fluids. Severe valve damage may require corrective surgery if heart failure develops or in cases requiring that an in-

SELF-HELP

Living with inflammation of the heart lining

To help ensure a steady recovery from this condition, follow this advice.

During treatment

- Learn how to recognize symptoms of inflammation of the heart lining, and notify the doctor immediately if they occur.
- Watch for and report symptoms of embolization — blood in the urine, chest pain, pain in the left upper part of the stomach, or slight paralysis — which are common during the first 3 months of treatment for this disease.

After treatment

- Watch closely for fever, appetite loss, and other symptoms of relapse about 2 weeks after treatment stops.
- Avoid strenuous activities to prevent excessive physical exertion.
- Be sure to take prescribed antibiotics before, during, and after dental work, childbirth, and genitourinary, gastrointestinal, or gynecologic procedures.

fected prosthetic valve be replaced. (See *Living with inflammation of the heart lining*, page 43.)

INFLAMMATION OF THE HEART MUSCLE

What do doctors call this condition?
Myocarditis

What is this condition?
This disorder involves focal or diffuse inflammation of the cardiac muscle (myocardium). It may be acute or chronic and can occur at any age. Frequently, this disease fails to cause specific cardiovascular symptoms or electrocardiogram abnormalities, and recovery is usually spontaneous, without residual defects. Occasionally, it's complicated by heart failure. (See *How inflammation of the heart muscle develops.*)

What causes it?
Inflammation of the heart muscle is caused by:
- *viral infections,* such as coxsackievirus A and B strains and, possibly, polio, influenza, measles, German measles, adenoviruses, and echoviruses (most common causes in the United States)
- *bacterial infections,* such as diphtheria, tuberculosis, typhoid fever, tetanus, and staphylococcal, pneumococcal, and gonococcal infections
- *hypersensitive immune reactions,* such as acute rheumatic fever and postcardiotomy syndrome
- *radiation therapy* from large doses of radiation to the chest in treating lung or breast cancer
- *chemical poisons,* as in chronic alcoholism
- *parasitic infections,* especially South American trypanosomiasis (Chagas' disease) in infants and immunosuppressed adults, and toxoplasmosis
- *infections caused by parasitic worms,* such as trichinosis.

What are its symptoms?
Inflammation of the heart muscle usually causes nonspecific symptoms (such as fatigue, shortness of breath, palpitations, and fever)

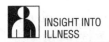

How inflammation of the heart muscle develops

Inflammation of the heart muscle can develop into severe complications. This flowchart shows the progression of this disorder to disabling heart disease, which can occur if treatment is delayed or is inadequate.

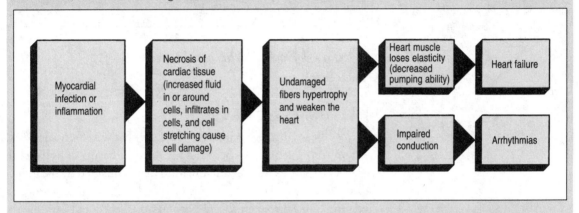

that reflect the accompanying infection. Occasionally, it may cause mild, continuous pressure or soreness in the chest.

How is it diagnosed?

The person's history commonly reveals recent febrile upper respiratory tract infection, viral pharyngitis, or tonsillitis. A physical exam detects irregular heart rhythms, abnormal heart sounds, and possibly a murmur.

An electrocardiogram typically shows abnormalities in heart rhythm. Stool and throat cultures may identify bacteria.

How is it treated?

Treatment includes antibiotics for bacterial infection, modified bed rest to decrease the heart's workload, and careful management of complications. (See *Understanding activity limitations*, page 46.)

Heart failure requires restricted physical activity to minimize myocardial oxygen consumption, supplemental oxygen therapy, restricted salt intake, diuretics to decrease fluid retention, and Lanoxin to increase myocardial contractility. However, Lanoxin must be used cautiously because some people with inflammation of the heart muscle may be sensitive to even small doses.

Understanding activity limitations

If you have uncomplicated inflammation of the heart muscle, be aware that activity limitations are temporary. In the meantime, you can engage in any hobbies or interests that are physically undemanding. As you recover, the doctor will instruct you to resume normal activities slowly and avoid competitive sports.

Irregular heart rhythms require prompt but cautious administration of antiarrhythmic drugs, such as Cardioquin or Pronestyl.

INFLAMMATION OF THE SAC AROUND THE HEART

What do doctors call this condition?
Pericarditis

What is this condition?
In this disease, the pericardium — the sac that envelops, supports, and protects the heart — becomes inflamed. It occurs in both acute and chronic forms. Acute inflammation may be marked by the build-up of fluid that may contain pus or blood. In chronic constrictive inflammation, the pericardium becomes thickened and fibrous, restricting heart motion. The prognosis depends on the underlying cause but is generally good in acute inflammation.

What causes it?
Common causes of this disease include:
- bacterial, fungal, or viral infection
- cancers (primary or spread from the lungs, breasts, or other organs)
- high-dose radiation to the chest
- uremia (an excess of waste products in the blood produced by the metabolism of protein)
- hypersensitivity or autoimmune disease, such as acute rheumatic fever (most common cause of inflammation of the sac around the heart in children), lupus, and rheumatoid arthritis
- injury to the pericardial sac, which may result from a heart attack (which later causes an autoimmune reaction in the pericardium), trauma, or surgery that leaves the pericardium intact but causes blood to leak into the pericardial cavity
- such drugs as Apresoline and Pronestyl.

What are its symptoms?
Acute inflammation of the sac around the heart typically produces a sharp and often sudden pain that usually starts over the sternum and

radiates to the neck, shoulders, back, and arms. However, unlike the pain of a heart attack, pericardial pain often increases with deep inspiration and decreases when the person sits up and leans forward.

A major complication of this disorder is pericardial effusion. (See *Symptoms of pericardial effusion*.)

How is it diagnosed?

Because inflammation of the sac around the heart often exists with other conditions, its diagnosis depends on typical signs and symptoms and elimination of other possible causes. When listening with a stethoscope, the doctor may hear a grating sound as the heart moves, called a *pericardial friction rub*. In addition, if acute inflammation has caused accumulation of fluid in the pericardial sac, the doctor may note changes in sounds produced by the heart — increased cardiac dullness, diminished or absent apical impulse, and distant heart sounds.

Diagnostic test results, such as white blood cell count and measurement of cardiac enzymes, may help to confirm inflammation and identify its cause. Open surgical drainage or cardiocentesis may be performed to obtain a culture of pericardial fluid. Culturing may help to identify a causative organism in bacterial or fungal inflammation. An electrocardiogram may show changes in heart rate and rhythm brought on by acute inflammation.

How is it treated?

The goal of treatment is to relieve symptoms and manage underlying systemic disease. When this condition is caused by a heart attack or follows heart surgery, treatment consists of bed rest as long as fever and pain persist and nonsteroidal anti-inflammatory drugs, such as aspirin and Indocin, to relieve pain and reduce inflammation. If these drugs fail to relieve symptoms, corticosteroids may be used.

Antibiotics, surgical drainage, or both may be needed to treat infectious inflammation of the sac around the heart. If cardiac tamponade (increased pressure on the heart muscle from fluid buildup) develops, the doctor may perform emergency pericardiocentesis. (See *What happens during pericardiocentesis*, page 48.)

Recurrent inflammation of the sac around the heart may require partial pericardiectomy, which creates a "window" that allows fluid to drain. In constrictive inflammation, total pericardiectomy (removal of the sac around the heart) may be necessary to permit adequate filling and contraction of the heart.

Symptoms of pericardial effusion

Pericardial effusion — fluid buildup in the membranes surrounding the heart — is the major complication of acute inflammation of the sac around the heart. This disorder may cause shortness of breath, difficulty breathing except when upright, a rapid heart rate, generalized chest pain, and a feeling of fullness in the chest.

Sudden effects

If the fluid accumulates rapidly, cardiac tamponade may develop. This condition causes pallor, clammy skin, low blood pressure, a decrease in blood pressure during slow inhalation, swollen neck veins and, eventually, cardiovascular collapse and death.

What happens during pericardiocentesis

Pericardiocentesis is done to relieve the pressure and discomfort caused by fluid that collects in the sac around the heart and restricts heart function. To accomplish this, the doctor removes fluid through a needle inserted in the pericardial cavity.

How it's done
Your chest will be cleansed with an antiseptic solution, draped to prevent infection, and then numbed with a local anesthetic. (If the procedure will be performed in the operating room, you may receive a general anesthetic.) Although you may feel some pressure as the needle is inserted, you won't feel pain. Electrocardiograph leads will be placed at various points on your skin to monitor your heart's activity; a member of the health care team will be available to monitor other indications of your progress.

After the doctor removes the needle, he or she may leave a flexible pericardial catheter temporarily in place so that excess pericardial fluid can be drained again, if necessary.

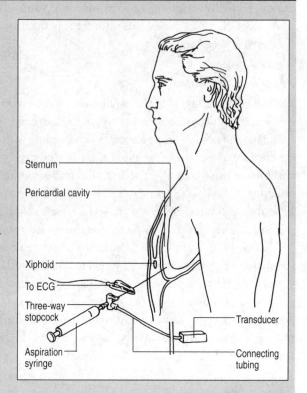

Sternum
Pericardial cavity
Xiphoid
To ECG
Three-way stopcock
Aspiration syringe
Transducer
Connecting tubing

PUMP FAILURE

What do doctors call this condition?
Cardiogenic shock

What is this condition?
Pump failure is a condition of diminished cardiac output that severely impairs the delivery of oxygen and vital nutrients to the body's organs and tissues. It reflects severe failure of the left ventricle, the heart's main chamber, and occurs as a serious complication in nearly 15% of all people hospitalized with a heart attack.

Pump failure typically strikes people in whom a heart attack has damaged more than 40% of the heart. The death rate may exceed 85%. Most people with pump failure die within 24 hours of onset. The prognosis for those who survive is poor.

What causes it?

Pump failure can result from any condition that causes significant left ventricular dysfunction with reduced cardiac output, such as a heart attack (most common), myocardial ischemia, papillary muscle dysfunction, or end-stage cardiomyopathy.

Dysfunction of the heart's left ventricle sets into motion a series of compensatory mechanisms that attempt to increase cardiac output and, in turn, maintain vital organ function. These compensatory responses initially stabilize the person but later cause deterioration with the rising oxygen demands of the already compromised heart.

What are its symptoms?

Signs of pump failure are caused by poor perfusion of blood throughout tissues: cold, pale, clammy skin; a drop in blood pressure; rapid heart rate; rapid, shallow breathing; low urine output; restlessness and mental confusion; narrowing pulse pressure; and bluish skin discoloration.

The left ventricle tries to compensate for heart damage. Eventually, compensatory mechanisms are overwhelmed by the heart's rising demand for oxygen.

How is it diagnosed?

The doctor listens to the heart for abnormal rhythms, faint heart sounds, and possibly, if the shock is caused by rupture of the ventricular septum or papillary muscles, a murmur. Other abnormal test findings include the following:

- *Pulmonary artery pressure monitoring* shows changes in pressures within the vessels of the heart and lungs.
- *Invasive arterial pressure monitoring* shows low blood pressure due to impaired ventricular ejection.
- *Arterial blood gas analysis* may show metabolic acidosis and hypoxia.
- *Electrocardiography* may reveal evidence of an acute heart attack, ischemia, or ventricular aneurysm.
- *Enzyme studies* may provide evidence of a heart attack or ischemia and suggest heart failure or shock.

How is it treated?

The aim of treatment is to enhance the heart's ability to function by increasing its output, improving heart muscle perfusion, and reducing the heart's workload with combinations of various drugs and mechanical-assist techniques. Drug therapy may include Intropin, Inocor or Dobutrex, Adrenalin, and Nitropress.

In some instances, the heart may be helped by an intra-aortic balloon pump. This surgically implanted device consists of a balloon attached to a large-diameter catheter and a pump that approximates the action of the heart in response to a signal from the electrocardiograph machine. It inflates during ventricular diastole to increase coronary artery perfusion, and deflates before systole, to reduce aortic pressure and resistance to ventricular flow. The end result is decreased ventricular workload.

RAYNAUD'S DISEASE

What is this condition?
Raynaud's disease is a circulatory disorder that affects the fingers and, sometimes, the toes. Small arteries that supply blood to the fingers and toes become increasingly sensitive to cold and other factors. When exposed to cold or stress, these arteries go into sudden, episodic spasms.

Raynaud's disease is most common in females, particularly between puberty and age 40. It's a harmless condition, requiring no specific treatment and causing no serious complications. However, Raynaud's phenomenon, a condition often associated with scleroderma and lupus, has a progressive course, leading to skin damage, gangrene, and amputation. Telling the two conditions apart is difficult, because some people who experience mild symptoms of Raynaud's disease for several years may later develop scleroderma or another serious condition.

What causes it?
Although the cause is unknown, several theories account for the reduced blood flow: extreme sensitivity of blood vessels to cold, increased blood vessel tone, and an abnormal immune response. (See *Questions people ask about Raynaud's disease*.)

STRAIGHT
TALK

Questions people ask about Raynaud's disease

I had my first attack shortly after I changed jobs. Could there be a connection?
Yes. The incidence of Raynaud's disease is unusually high in some occupations. Men and women who use vibrating tools — for example, dentists or road workers who operate pneumatic drills — are prone to the disorder. The incidence also rises among workers exposed to alternating hot and cold temperatures, such as meat packers and food processors.

How did I get Raynaud's disease?
The disorder has many causes. About 70% of people with this disease have some other medical problem that predisposes them to attacks. For example,

people with scleroderma — an autoimmune disease that affects the skin and other connective tissues — are especially prone to Raynaud's disease. In fact, Raynaud's disease may be the first sign that another disease process is at work.

Will I have Raynaud's attacks for the rest of my life?
Not necessarily. Some people recover — especially those who don't have related medical problems, such as arteriosclerosis. Of people who don't have related disorders, about 40% improve or recover completely, about 40% have the same symptoms year after year, and the remaining 20% get worse.

What are its symptoms?

After exposure to cold or stress, the skin on the fingers typically blanches, then becomes pale before changing to red and before changing from cold to normal temperature. Numbness and tingling may also occur. These symptoms are relieved by warmth.

How is it diagnosed?

Signs and symptoms that establish Raynaud's disease include skin color changes on both hands or feet induced by cold or stress, normal arterial pulses, and a history of symptoms lasting longer than 2 years.

How is it treated?

Initially, treatment consists of avoiding cold, mechanical, or chemical injury and stopping smoking. (See *Living with Raynaud's disease,* page 52.) Because drug side effects may be more bothersome than the disease itself, drug therapy is reserved for unusually severe symptoms. Sympathectomy (surgery to interrupt part of the sympathetic nerve pathways) may be helpful when conservative treatments fail to prevent skin ulcers.

SELF-HELP

Living with Raynaud's disease

Here are some tips for preventing or minimizing attacks of Raynaud's disease.

Identify what triggers your attacks

The most common triggers of Raynaud's disease are cold temperatures and emotional stress. If you aren't sure what causes your attacks, try keeping a diary. After each attack, jot down when it happened, your mood, your activity, the room temperature, and other possible clues. After 1 or 2 weeks, read your notes to see if you spot any patterns.

A sample diary entry might read: *"Tuesday, 8 p.m.:* Angry all day about increase in car insurance. Mild attack after taking ice cream from freezer."

Stay warm outside

When you go outdoors in cold weather, dress warmly in layers of clothing. Bundle up with a scarf, hat, and mittens — mittens keep your fingers warmer than gloves — even if you're just going to get the mail or take out the trash. To keep your body heat in, choose a coat that fits snugly at your neck and wrists, and put reflective inner soles in your shoes.

If you drive, let your car warm up before you start driving. This warms the seat and steering wheel.

Stay warm inside

Set thermostats for comfort. In the kitchen, wear oven mitts to remove food from the freezer, and try tongs to handle ice cubes. Wash vegetables and dishes in warm water. And hold cold drink glasses in insulated covers.

In the bedroom, use an electric mattress pad or blanket. Wear socks to bed, and keep a robe and slippers handy.

Practice healthful habits

Don't smoke — it can worsen attacks. Learn how to relax to relieve emotional stress. Don't let tensions build up. If necessary, see a counselor or join a support group. Get plenty of rest.

Other tips

- When your hands and fingers feel cold, try this exercise: Stretch your fingers wide apart. Like a softball pitcher, move your arms rapidly in a circular motion downward behind your body, then upward in front of you and back to the starting point. Do up to 80 revolutions a minute to warm your hands. Give yourself plenty of room.
- With severe symptoms, avoid activities that put pressure on sensitive fingers, such as typing, weeding, piano playing, snow skiing, and water sports (such as water skiing and swimming).
- Inspect your skin frequently and seek immediate care for signs of skin breakdown or infection.
- During an attack, protect yourself from injury. Don't touch anything hot or frozen, and avoid sharp objects that could cut you.

*R*HEUMATIC FEVER AND RHEUMATIC HEART DISEASE

What are these conditions?

Acute rheumatic fever is an inflammatory disease of childhood, often recurrent, that follows a strep infection. Rheumatic heart disease refers to the cardiac effects of rheumatic fever and includes pancarditis (inflammation of the heart muscle, heart lining, and sac around the heart) during the early acute phase and chronic heart valve disease later.

Long-term antibiotic therapy can minimize recurrence of rheumatic fever, reducing the risk of permanent heart damage and eventual valvular deformity. However, severe pancarditis occasionally causes fatal heart failure during the acute phase. (See *How rheumatic fever affects heart valves*, page 54.)

Rheumatic fever strikes most often during cool, damp weather in the winter and early spring. In the United States, it's most common in the northern states.

What causes them?

Rheumatic fever appears to be a reaction to a strep infection, in which antibodies manufactured to combat streptococci react and produce lesions at specific tissue sites, especially in the heart and joints. Fewer than 1% of people with strep infections ever contract rheumatic fever. Although rheumatic fever tends to run in families, this may merely reflect contributing environmental factors. For example, in lower socioeconomic groups, incidence is highest in children between ages 5 and 15, probably because of malnutrition and crowded living conditions.

What are the symptoms?

In 95% of cases, rheumatic fever characteristically occurs within a few days to 6 weeks of an initial strep infection. A temperature of at least 100.4° F (38° C) occurs, and most people complain of pain, swelling, and redness in the knees, ankles, elbows, or hips (polyarthritis).

In 5% of cases, rheumatic fever causes a nonirritating rash that gives rise to red lesions with blanched centers. It may also produce firm, movable, nontender nodules about 3 millimeters to 2 centimeters in diameter located just below the skin, usually near the elbows, knuckles, wrists, and knees. These nodules last for a few days to several weeks.

Later, rheumatic fever may cause transient chorea (involuntary body movements), which develops up to 6 months after the original strep infection. Mild chorea may produce hyperirritability, deteriorated handwriting, or inability to concentrate. Severe chorea causes

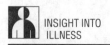

How rheumatic fever affects heart valves

Rheumatic fever causes changes in the mitral and aortic valves, two of the heart's four sets of valves. The valves swell, their leaflets become eroded along the closure line, and abnormal tissue growths called *vegetations* form along the inflamed leaflet edges. In many people, vegetations also form on adjacent leaflets that scar and partially fuse as they heal.

These illustrations show how rheumatic inflammation can affect a mitral valve, causing narrowing and backward blood flow through the valve.

Vegetations form on leaflets
In this view, the mitral valve leaflets are inflamed, with a thin line of vegetations along the delicate leaflet edges. These vegetations form when fibrin (the main component of a blood clot) and platelets (blood cells essential to blood clotting) build up on the damaged valve surface.

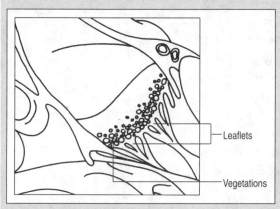

Narrowing reduces movement
Mitral stenosis (narrowing of the mitral valve) is the most common valvular defect in people with recurrent rheumatic fever. In this disorder, inflammation causes shrinkage of the chordae tendineae (cords that connect each valve leaflet to muscles in the heart chambers) as the leaflets fuse. This shrinkage reduces valve movement. The left atrium, one of the heart's four chambers, tries to force blood through the narrow valve opening into the left ventricle, the heart's main working chamber. Eventually, this causes the left atrium to enlarge, the lungs to become congested, and the right ventricle to enlarge and

eventually fail. Unfortunately, symptoms of mitral stenosis rarely appear until the valve opening narrows by about 50%.

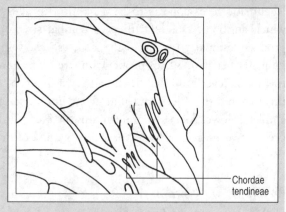

Blood flows backward
Some blood may flow backward into the atrium when the mitral valve narrows because the dysfunctional valve can't close tightly.

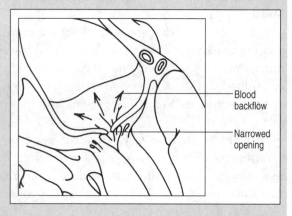

involuntary muscle spasms, poor muscle coordination, and weakness.

The most destructive effect of rheumatic fever is carditis, which develops in up to 50% of affected people and may affect the heart lining, heart muscle, sac around the heart, or heart valves. Inflammation of the sac around the heart may cause pain. Inflammation of the heart muscle leads to formation of a progressively fibrotic nodule and interstitial scars. Inflammation of the heart lining causes valve leaflets to swell and erode along their edges, and formation of beadlike vegetations composed of platelet and fibrin deposits. Severe rheumatic carditis may cause heart failure.

How are they diagnosed?

Diagnosis depends on recognition of one or more of the classic symptoms (carditis, polyarthritis, chorea, rash, or nodules beneath the skin) and a detailed history. Lab tests, such as white blood cell count and measurement of cardiac enzymes, support the diagnosis. Echocardiography (an ultrasound test of the heart) helps evaluate valvular damage, chamber size, and ventricular function.

How are they treated?

Effective management eliminates the strep infection, relieves symptoms, and prevents recurrence, reducing the chance of permanent heart damage. During the acute phase, treatment includes penicillin or erythromycin. Aspirin relieves fever and minimizes joint swelling and pain; if carditis is present or salicylates fail to relieve pain and inflammation, corticosteroids may be used. Supportive treatment requires strict bed rest for about 5 weeks during the acute phase with active carditis, followed by a progressive increase in physical activity. (See *Helping your child cope with rheumatic fever*, page 56.)

After the acute phase subsides, a monthly injection of penicillin or daily doses of oral Microsulfon or penicillin may be used to prevent recurrence. Such preventive treatment usually continues for 5 to 10 years. Severe mitral or aortic valve dysfunction causing persistent heart failure requires surgery to fix the heart valves, including commissurotomy (separation of the adherent, thickened leaflets of the mitral valve), valvuloplasty (inflation of a balloon within a valve), or valve replacement (with a prosthetic valve). Surgery is rarely necessary before late adolescence.

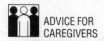

ADVICE FOR
CAREGIVERS

Helping your child cope with rheumatic fever

By monitoring your child closely and taking precautions, you can help to relieve symptoms, prevent disease recurrence, and lower the risk of permanent heart damage. Here are some guidelines to follow.

Watch for symptoms
- Watch for and report early signs of heart failure: shortness of breath and a hacking, nonproductive cough.
- Immediately report signs of recurrent strep infection: sudden sore throat, throat redness, swollen and tender glands in the neck, pain on swallowing, a temperature of 101° to 104° F (38.3° to 40° C), headache, and nausea.

Provide supportive care
- Make sure your child gets plenty of bed rest during the acute disease phase. Provide physically undemanding diversions. After this phase ends, spend as much time as possible with him or her to minimize boredom.

- Keep your child away from people with respiratory infections.
- Make sure your child brushes and flosses his or her teeth regularly to prevent gum infection.
- Arrange for your child to receive additional antibiotics before dental surgery.
- Make sure your child complies with prolonged antibiotic therapy and follow-up care.
- If possible, arrange for a tutor to help your child keep up with schoolwork during the long convalescence.

Take care of yourself
Remember, you're only human. Give yourself the time and opportunity to vent your frustrations during the long, tedious recovery period.

SHOCK FROM LOW BLOOD VOLUME

What do doctors call this condition?
Hypovolemic shock, hypovolemic shock syndrome

What is this condition?
In this type of shock, low blood volume causes circulatory problems and inadequate delivery of life-sustaining oxygen and nutrients to the body's vital organs and tissues. Without sufficient blood or fluid replacement, this condition may lead to irreversible brain and kidney damage, cardiac arrest and, ultimately, death.

What causes it?
This type of shock usually is caused by significant loss of blood — about one-fifth of the body's total. Such massive blood loss may re-

sult from gastrointestinal bleeding, hemorrhage, or any condition that reduces blood volume or other body fluids, such as severe burns.

What are its symptoms?

This condition causes low blood pressure, a rapid heart rate, rapid and shallow breathing, reduced urine output, and cold, pale, clammy skin.

How is it diagnosed?

No single symptom or diagnostic test establishes the diagnosis or severity of shock. Characteristic lab test findings include elevated amounts of certain elements in the blood, including potassium and lactate; changes in the physical characteristics of urine; decreased blood pH; decreased oxygen in blood in the arteries; and increased carbon dioxide in blood in the arteries.

In addition, gastroscopy (aspiration of gastric contents through a nasogastric tube) and X-rays identify internal bleeding sites; coagulation studies may detect bleeding from disseminated intravascular coagulation.

How is it treated?

Emergency treatment must include prompt and adequate blood and fluid replacement to restore blood volume and raise blood pressure.

Treatment may also include oxygen administration, control of bleeding by direct measures (such as applying pressure and elevating an extremity), and possibly surgery.

Without sufficient blood or fluid replacement, shock from low blood volume may lead to irreversible brain and kidney damage, cardiac arrest, and death.

Ventricular Aneurysm

What is this condition?

A ventricular aneurysm is an outpouching of the left ventricle that causes ventricular wall dysfunction. It occurs in people who've had a heart attack, developing within weeks after the attack or years later.

An untreated ventricular aneurysm can lead to irregular heart rhythms, systemic embolization (release of blood clots into the circulation), or congestive heart failure and is potentially fatal. Surgery

Caring for yourself after a ventricular aneurysm

Self-monitoring and compliance with therapy are crucial if you're recovering from a ventricular aneurysm. Be sure to:
- learn how to check your pulse for irregular rhythms and changes in the pulse rate
- follow your prescribed medication schedule — even during the night — and watch for drug side effects.
- involve your family — encourage them to learn CPR.

improves the prognosis in people with heart failure and in those who don't respond to other treatments.

What causes it?

When a heart attack destroys a large section of the left ventricle, the ventricular wall becomes a thin sheath of tissue. Under pressure, this thin layer stretches and forms a separate sac, an aneurysm.

What are its symptoms?

Ventricular aneurysm may cause irregular heart rhythms, palpitations, weakness on exertion, fatigue, and chest pain. This condition may also lead to heart failure. Ventricular aneurysms enlarge but rarely rupture.

How is it diagnosed?

The doctor will suspect ventricular aneurysm if a person has persistent heart rhythm disturbances affecting the ventricle, heart failure, or systemic embolization as well as a history of heart attack. Important diagnostic tests include the following:
- *Left ventriculography* reveals left ventricular enlargement, with an area of impaired movement and diminished cardiac function.
- *Chest X-ray* may demonstrate an abnormal bulge distorting the heart's contour if the aneurysm is large; the X-ray may be normal if the aneurysm is small.
- *Echocardiography* (an ultrasound test of the heart) shows abnormal motion in the left ventricular wall.

How is it treated?

Depending on the size of the aneurysm and the complications, treatment may involve only a routine medical exam to follow the person's condition or more aggressive measures. Emergency treatment of irregular heart rhythms includes drugs or cardioversion. Preventive treatment continues with drugs.

The most effective operation is aneurysmectomy (removal of the aneurysm), which restores adequate blood supply to the heart. (See *Caring for yourself after a ventricular aneurysm.*)

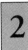

LUNG AND BREATHING DISORDERS

ADULT RESPIRATORY DISTRESS SYNDROME

What is this condition?

In this syndrome, fluid builds up in the lungs and causes them to stiffen. This impairs breathing, thereby reducing the amount of oxygen in the capillaries that supply the lungs. When severe, the syndrome can cause an unmanageable and ultimately fatal lack of oxygen. However, people who recover may have little or no permanent lung damage.

What causes it?

Adult respiratory distress syndrome is caused by:
- aspiration of stomach contents into the lungs
- infection, injury (such as a lung contusion, head injury, bone fracture with fat emboli), or too much oxygen
- viral, bacterial, or fungal pneumonia or microemboli (fat or air emboli or disseminated intravascular coagulation)
- drug overdose (barbiturates or narcotics) or blood transfusion
- smoke or chemical inhalation (nitrous oxide, chlorine, ammonia)
- hydrocarbon and paraquat (a toxic herbicide) ingestion
- pancreatitis or uremia
- near-drowning.

If the body can't remove the accumulated fluid, swelling within the lungs and narrowing of their airways develops. Oxygen deficiency is caused by fluid accumulation.

What are its symptoms?

Adult respiratory distress syndrome initially produces rapid, shallow breathing and shortness of breath within hours to days of the initial injury. Oxygen deficiency develops, causing an increased drive for breathing. Because of the effort required to expand the stiff lung, the person's chest retracts during breathing. As the person gets less oxygen, he or she becomes restless, apprehensive, and mentally sluggish.

Severe adult respiratory distress syndrome causes an overwhelming deficiency of oxygen which, if uncorrected, results in very low blood pressure, decreasing urine output and, eventually, heart attack.

Adult respiratory distress syndrome occurs when fluid builds up in the tissue and air sacs of the lungs and in the small airways, causing the lungs to stiffen.

How is it diagnosed?

Arterial blood gas analysis helps detect the syndrome. Other tests include pulmonary artery catheterization and chest X-rays.

Tests must rule out other lung disorders. To establish the cause of the illness, lab work includes cultures of sputum and blood specimens to detect infections; a toxicology screen for drug ingestion; and, if pancreatitis is a possibility, a serum amylase determination.

How is it treated?

When possible, treatment tries to correct the underlying cause of adult respiratory distress syndrome and to prevent progression and potentially fatal complications. Supportive medical care consists of administering humidified oxygen by a tight-fitting mask. Oxygen deficiency that doesn't respond adequately to these measures requires the use of a mechanical ventilator. Other supportive measures include fluid restriction, diuretics, and correction of electrolyte and acid-base abnormalities.

When adult respiratory distress syndrome requires a mechanical ventilator, drugs such as sedatives, narcotics, or the neuromuscular blockers Tubarine or Pavalon may be given to minimize restlessness and ease breathing.

When adult respiratory distress syndrome is caused by fat emboli or chemical injuries to the lungs, a short course of high-dose steroids may help if given early. Intravenous fluids and drugs may be given to maintain blood pressure. Infections require antibiotics.

ASBESTOSIS

What is this condition?

This lung condition is characterized by widespread filling and inflammation of the lung spaces with asbestos fibers. It can develop as long as 15 to 20 years after regular exposure to asbestos has ended. A potent cocarcinogen, asbestos aggravates the risk of lung cancer in cigarette smokers.

What causes it?

Asbestosis is caused by the inhalation of small asbestos fibers. These fibers move in the direction of airflow and penetrate the breathing passages. Sources include the mining and milling of asbestos, the construction industry (where asbestos is used in a prefabricated form), and the fireproofing and textile industries. Asbestos also has been used in the production of paints, plastics, and automobile brake and clutch linings.

Asbestos-related diseases develop in families of asbestos workers as a result of exposure to the fibrous dust shaken off workers' clothing at home. Asbestosis also strikes people who are exposed to fibrous dust or waste piles from nearby asbestos plants.

Inhaled fibers become encased in a brown, proteinlike sheath rich in iron — called *ferruginous bodies* or *asbestos bodies* — found in sputum and lung tissue.

Asbestos-related diseases occur in families of asbestos workers from exposure to fibrous dust shaken off workers' clothing at home. In the general public, such diseases result from exposure to fibrous dust or waste piles from nearby asbestos plants.

What are its symptoms?

The first symptom is usually shortness of breath on exertion, typically after 10 years' exposure. As lung damage becomes more extensive, this increases, until eventually the person is short of breath, even at rest. Advanced disease also causes a cough, chest pain, recurrent respiratory infections, and rapid breathing.

Asbestosis may cause complications, such as an enlarged heart and pulmonary hypertension. Club-shaped fingers commonly occur.

How is it diagnosed?

The person's history reveals occupational, family, or neighborhood exposure to asbestos fibers. A physical exam reveals characteristic, dry crackles at the bases of the lungs. An arterial blood gas test reveals a decreased oxygen level and a low carbon dioxide level. Finally, a chest X-ray and pulmonary function studies help diagnose this disease.

How is it treated?

This disease can't be cured. The goal of treatment is to relieve respiratory symptoms and, in advanced disease, to control the complications.

Respiratory symptoms may be relieved by chest physical therapy techniques such as controlled coughing. Aerosol therapy, inhaled mucolytics, and increased fluids (at least 3 quarts [3 liters] daily) may also help relieve respiratory symptoms. Diuretics, digitalis glycoside preparations, and salt restriction may be indicated for people with cor pulmonale. Oxygen deficiency requires oxygen administration by mask or by a mechanical ventilator. Respiratory infections require prompt administration of antibiotics.

What can a person with asbestosis do?

■ To prevent infections, avoid crowds and persons with infections and receive influenza and pneumococcal vaccines.

■ To improve your breathing, undergo physical reconditioning, conserve your energy in daily activities, and use relaxation techniques.

ATELECTASIS

What is this condition?

Atelectasis is the incomplete expansion of a lung, which may result in its partial or complete collapse. It causes oxygen deprivation.

Atelectasis may be chronic or acute and occurs to some degree in many people undergoing upper abdominal or chest surgery. The prognosis depends on prompt removal of any airway obstruction, relief of hypoxia (reduced oxygen supply to the tissues), and reexpansion of the collapsed lung.

What causes it?

Atelectasis often is caused by a breathing passageway blocked by mucus plugs. It's a common problem in people with chronic obstructive pulmonary disease, bronchiectasis, or cystic fibrosis and in those who smoke heavily. Atelectasis also may be caused by blockage with foreign bodies, lung cancer, and lung inflammation.

Other causes include respiratory distress syndrome of the newborn (hyaline membrane disease), too much oxygen, and fluid buildup in the lungs.

External compression, which inhibits full lung expansion, or any condition that makes deep breathing painful may also cause atelectasis. Such compression or pain may be caused by upper abdominal surgical incisions, rib fractures, chest pain, tight dressings around the chest, or obesity.

Atelectasis also may be caused by prolonged bed rest or mechanical ventilation. A drug overdose can also contribute to progressive atelectasis.

Atelectasis may be chronic or acute and occurs to some degree in many people recuperating from upper abdominal or chest surgery. It's often a problem in heavy smokers and in people with emphysema, chronic bronchitis, or cystic fibrosis.

What are its symptoms?

Symptoms vary with the cause of the collapsed lung, the degree of oxygen deprivation, and any underlying disease but generally include some shortness of breath. Atelectasis of a small area of the lung may produce only minor symptoms that subside without treatment. However, massive collapse can produce severe shortness of breath, anxiety, loss of skin color, sweating, peripheral circulatory collapse, rapid heartbeat, and chest retraction.

How is it diagnosed?

Diagnosis requires an accurate history, a physical exam, and a chest X-ray. The doctor listens to the chest for diminished or bronchial breath sounds. By tapping on the chest, while listening with a stethoscope, the doctor can tell if the lung is collapsed.

In widespread atelectasis, the chest X-ray shows characteristic changes in the lungs. If the cause is unknown, diagnostic procedures may include bronchoscopy to rule out an obstruction.

How is it treated?

Treatment includes incentive spirometry, mucus-destroying drugs, chest percussion, postural drainage, and frequent coughing and deep-breathing exercises. If these measures fail, bronchoscopy may be helpful in removing secretions. Humidity and drugs that expand the breathing passages can help.

Atelectasis from a lung tumor may require surgery or radiation therapy. People recovering from chest or abdominal surgery require pain relievers to allow deep breathing, which lowers the risk of atelectasis. (See *Advice for the person at risk for atelectasis.*)

 SELF-HELP

Advice for the person at risk for atelectasis

To prevent atelectasis after surgery, you can follow these practices:

- Cough and breathe deeply every 1 to 2 hours, as instructed by your doctor. To minimize pain during coughing exercises, hold a pillow tightly over the incision.
- Walk as soon as possible, as permitted by your doctor.
- Learn about and use postural drainage technique to remove secretions.
- Drink plenty of fluids to help remove secretions.
- Stop smoking and lose weight as needed.

BLACK LUNG

What do doctors call this condition?

Coal worker's pneumoconiosis, coal miner's disease, miner's asthma, anthracosis, anthracosilicosis

What is this condition?

A progressive lung disease, black lung occurs in two forms. Simple black lung is characterized by small opaque areas in the lung. In complicated black lung, also known as *progressive massive fibrosis,* masses of fibrous tissue occasionally develop in the lungs.

The risk of developing black lung depends on the duration of exposure to coal dust (usually 15 years or longer), the intensity of exposure (dust count, particle size), the location of the mine, the silica content of the coal (anthracite coal has the highest silica content), and the worker's susceptibility. Incidence of black lung is highest among anthracite coal miners in the eastern United States.

The prognosis varies. Simple asymptomatic disease is self-limiting, although progression to complicated black lung is more likely if black lung begins after a relatively short period of exposure. Complicated black lung may be disabling, resulting in severe respiratory and heart failure.

What causes it?

Black lung is caused by the inhalation and prolonged retention of coal dust particles. Simple black lung may cause focal emphysema (permanent dilation of small airways). Simple disease may progress to complicated black lung, involving one or both lungs. In this form of the disease, fibrous tissue masses enlarge and coalesce, causing gross destruction of structures in the lungs.

What are its symptoms?

Simple black lung causes no symptoms, especially in nonsmokers. Symptoms appear if complicated black lung develops and include shortness of breath on exertion and a cough that occasionally produces inky-black sputum. Other features of black lung include increasing shortness of breath and a cough that produces milky, gray, clear, or coal-flecked sputum. Recurrent lung infections produce yellow, green, or thick sputum.

Complications include pulmonary hypertension, an enlarged heart, and tuberculosis. In cigarette smokers, chronic bronchitis and emphysema may also complicate the disease.

How is it diagnosed?

The person's history reveals exposure to coal dust. A physical exam shows a barrel chest, hyperresonant lungs with diminished breath sounds, wheezes, and other abnormal lung sounds. In simple black lung, chest X-rays show small opacities, which may be present in all lung zones but are more prominent in the upper lung zones; in complicated black lung, one or more large opaque areas are seen.

Pulmonary function studies help to evaluate the person's breathing capacity. In addition, arterial blood gas studies provide information about the amount of oxygen and carbon dioxide in the blood.

How is it treated?

The goal of treatment is to relieve respiratory symptoms, to manage oxygen deficiency, and to avoid respiratory tract irritants and infections. (See *Coping with black lung.*) Treatment also includes careful observation for tuberculosis symptoms.

Respiratory symptoms may be relieved through therapy with drugs that widen the breathing passages (such as Theo-Dur or Aminophyllin), steroids (oral Orasone or an aerosol form), or Nasalcrom aerosol. Chest physical therapy techniques, such as controlled coughing, combined with chest percussion and vibration, help remove secretions.

Other measures include increased fluid intake (at least 3 quarts [liters] every day) and respiratory therapy techniques. In severe cases, it may be necessary to administer oxygen by mask if the person has chronic oxygen deprivation, or by mechanical ventilation. Respiratory infections require antibiotics.

 SELF-HELP

Coping with black lung

Take these steps to reduce the risk of further lung problems:
- To prevent infections, avoid crowds and people with respiratory infections.
- Be sure to get annual flu shots and Pneumovax (pneumococcal vaccine).
- Stay active to prevent your physical condition from deteriorating, but pace your activities.
- Practice relaxation techniques.

Bronchiectasis

What is this condition?

A condition marked by chronic abnormal dilation of bronchi and destruction of bronchial walls, bronchiectasis can occur throughout the tracheobronchial tree or can be confined to one segment or lobe of the lung. However, it usually affects both lungs in their lower lobes. Bronchiectasis is irreversible once established.

This disease has three forms: *cylindrical (fusiform)*, *varicose*, and *saccular (cystic)*. It affects people of both sexes and all ages. Because of the availability of antibiotics to treat acute respiratory tract infections, the incidence of bronchiectasis has dramatically decreased in the past 20 years. Its incidence is highest among Eskimos and the Maoris of New Zealand.

What causes it?

This disease is caused by conditions associated with repeated damage to bronchial walls and abnormal mucociliary clearance, which cause a breakdown of supporting tissue adjacent to airways. Such conditions include:

- cystic fibrosis
- immune disorders
- recurrent, inadequately treated bacterial respiratory tract infections, such as tuberculosis, and complications of measles, pneumonia, whooping cough, or flu
- a blocked breathing passage (by a foreign body, tumor, or narrowing) in association with recurrent infection
- inhalation of corrosive gas or repeated aspiration of gastric juices into the lungs
- congenital abnormalities (uncommon)

What are its symptoms?

Initially, bronchiectasis may cause no symptoms. When symptoms do arise, they're often attributed to other illnesses. The person usually complains of frequent bouts of pneumonia or coughing up blood. The classic symptom, however, is a chronic cough that produces copious, foul-smelling secretions, possibly totaling several cupfuls daily. Other symptoms include occasional wheezes, shortness of breath, sinus infections, weight loss, anemia, recurrent fever, chills, and other signs of infection.

How is it diagnosed?

A history of recurrent bronchial infections, pneumonia, and a bloody cough in a person whose chest X-rays show peribronchial thickening, collapsed areas of the lungs, and scattered cystic changes suggests bronchiectasis. A computed tomography scan (commonly called a CAT scan) helps diagnose the condition. A bronchoscopy can also be instrumental in pinpointing the site of any bleeding.

Other helpful lab tests include:

- *sputum culture* and *Gram stain* to identify predominant organisms
- *complete blood count* to detect anemia and leukocytosis
- *pulmonary function studies* to determine how well lungs are functioning and to detect hypoxemia (insufficient oxygen in the blood).

Bronchiectasis causes frequent bouts of pneumonia or coughing up blood. But the classic symptom is a chronic cough that produces large amounts of foul-smelling secretions that contain mucus and pus. The secretions may total several cupfuls daily.

How is it treated?

Treatment includes antibiotics, given orally or intravenously, for 7 to 10 days or until sputum production decreases. (See *Coping with bronchiectasis.*) Drugs that widen the breathing passages, combined with postural drainage and chest percussion, help remove secretions if the person has bronchospasm and thick, tenacious sputum. Bronchoscopy may be used to help mobilize secretions. Hypoxia requires oxygen therapy.

CHRONIC BRONCHITIS AND EMPHYSEMA

What are these conditions?

Chronic bronchitis and emphysema are characterized by chronically blocked breathing passages. Collectively, asthma, emphysema, and chronic bronchitis or any combination are called *chronic obstructive pulmonary disease.* Usually, more than one of these underlying conditions coexist; most often, bronchitis and emphysema occur together. (For information about asthma, see pages 693 to 698.)

The most common chronic lung diseases, chronic obstructive pulmonary diseases affect an estimated 17 million Americans, and their incidence is rising. They're more common in men than women, probably because, until recently, men were more likely to smoke heavily. Chronic bronchitis and emphysema don't always produce symptoms and cause only slight disability in many people. However, these diseases tend to worsen over time.

What causes them?

Predisposing factors include cigarette smoking, recurrent or chronic respiratory infections, air pollution, and allergies. Smoking is by far the most important of these factors. Smoking increases mucus production but impairs its removal from the airways, impedes the function of airway cells that digest disease-causing organisms, causes airway inflammation, destroys air sacs in the lungs, and leads to abnormal fibrous tissue growth in the bronchial tree. Early inflammatory changes may reverse themselves if the person stops smoking before lung destruction is extensive. Family and hereditary factors may also predispose a person to chronic bronchitis or emphysema.

 SELF-HELP

Coping with bronchiectasis

Perform coughing and deep-breathing exercises, as instructed, to promote good ventilation. Also note the following advice.

Loosen secretions
- Drink plenty of fluids to help you spit out secretions.
- Dispose of all secretions properly.

Protect airways
- If you smoke, stop. Smoking stimulates secretions and irritates the airways.
- Avoid air pollutants and people with upper respiratory tract infections.

Promote healing
- Get as much rest as possible.
- Eat balanced, high-protein meals to promote good health and tissue healing.
- Take medications (especially antibiotics) exactly as prescribed.

How to do controlled coughing exercises

Learning how to do coughing exercises will help you save energy and remove mucus from your airways. Here's what to do.

Preparing to cough

• Sit on the edge of your chair or bed. Put your feet flat on the floor, or use a stool if your feet don't touch the floor. Lean slightly forward.

• To help stimulate your cough reflex, slowly take a deep breath. Place your hands on your stomach. Breathe in through your nose, letting your stomach expand as far as it can.

• Next, purse your lips and slowly breathe out through your mouth. Concentrate on pulling your stomach inward. Try to exhale twice as long as you inhaled.

Ensuring productive cough

• Cough twice, keeping your mouth slightly open (once isn't enough). The first cough loosens mucus; the second cough helps remove it.

• Pause for a moment. Then breathe in through your nose by sniffing gently. Don't breathe deeply. If you do, the mucus you brought up may slide back into your lungs.

What are the symptoms?

The typical person with chronic bronchitis or emphysema is a long-term cigarette smoker who has no symptoms until middle age, when his or her ability to exercise or do strenuous work starts to decline and a productive cough begins. Subtle at first, these problems worsen with age and as the disease progresses. Eventually, they cause difficulty breathing on minimal exertion, frequent respiratory infections, oxygen deficiency in the blood, and abnormalities in pulmonary function. When advanced, chronic bronchitis and emphysema may cause chest deformities, overwhelming disability, heart enlargement, severe respiratory failure, and death.

How are they diagnosed?

A history of cigarette smoking plus the results of blood and pulmonary function studies help confirm these diseases.

How are they treated?

Treatment aims to relieve symptoms and prevent complications. Because most people with chronic bronchitis or emphysema receive outpatient treatment, they get comprehensive teaching to help them comply with therapy and understand the nature of these progressive diseases. If programs in pulmonary rehabilitation are available, they should consider enrolling.

What can a person with chronic bronchitis or emphysema do?

• Stop smoking and avoid other respiratory irritants.

• Install an air conditioner with an air filter in your home.

• If you're taking antibiotics to treat a respiratory infection, be sure to complete the entire prescribed course of therapy.

• Practice good oral hygiene to help prevent infection, and learn how to recognize early symptoms of infection. Avoid people with respiratory infections. Get Pneumovax (pneumococcal vaccine) and annual flu shots.

• To help remove secretions, learn how to cough effectively. (See *How to do controlled coughing exercises.*) If you have abundant, tenacious secretions, have a family member perform postural drainage (repositioning to drain fluids) and chest physical therapy. (Ask your doctor for instructions on these techniques.) If your secretions are thick, drink at least 6 eight-ounce glasses of fluid a day. A humidifier may aid secretion removal, especially in the winter.

SELF-HELP

How to overcome shortness of breath

When you're having trouble breathing, performing special exercises can help you feel better. Practice these exercises twice a day for 5 to 10 minutes until you get used to doing them.

Abdominal breathing

Lie comfortably on your back and place a pillow beneath your head. Bend your knees to relax your stomach.

Press one hand on your stomach lightly but with enough force to create slight pressure. Rest the other hand on your chest.

Now breathe slowly through your nose, using your stomach muscles. The hand on your stomach should rise when you inhale and fall when you exhale. The hand on your chest should remain almost still.

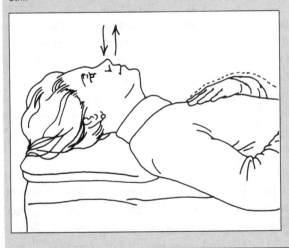

Pursed-lip breathing

Breathe in slowly through your nose to avoid gulping air. Hold your breath as you count to yourself, "one, 1,000; two, 1,000; three, 1,000."

Purse your lips as if you're going to whistle.

Now, breathe out slowly through pursed lips as you count to yourself, "one, 1,000; two, 1,000; three, 1,000; four, 1,000; five, 1,000; six, 1,000."

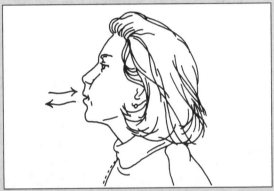

You should make a soft, whistling sound while you breathe out. Exhaling through pursed lips slows down your breathing and helps get rid of the stale air trapped in your lungs.

When performing pursed-lip breathing during activity, inhale before exerting yourself; exhale while performing the activity.

If the recommended counting rhythm feels awkward, find one that feels more comfortable. Keep in mind that you must breathe out longer than you breathe in.

• To strengthen your breathing muscles, take slow, deep breaths and exhale through pursed lips. (See *How to overcome shortness of breath*.)

• If you're receiving home oxygen therapy, make sure you or a family member knows how to use the equipment correctly. Don't increase the oxygen flow or concentration above what the doctor prescribes because too much oxygen may eliminate your respiratory drive and cause confusion and drowsiness. You probably won't need more than 2 to 3 liters per minute.

- Eat a balanced diet. Because you may tire easily when eating, eat frequent, small meals and consider using oxygen, delivered by a nasal cannula, during meals.
- Schedule rest periods throughout the day and exercise daily as directed by your doctor.

COLLAPSED LUNG

What do doctors call this condition?
Pneumothorax

What is this condition?
Collapsed lung is an accumulation of air or gas between the membranes that enclose the lungs. The amount of air or gas that's trapped determines the degree of lung collapse. In a *tension pneumothorax,* the air in the membranes is under higher pressure than air in the adjacent lung and blood vessels. Without prompt treatment, a tension or a large pneumothorax results in fatal lung and circulatory impairment.

Pneumothorax can also be classified as open or closed. In *open pneumothorax* (usually the result of injury), air flows between the lung membrane and the outside of the body. In *closed pneumothorax,* air reaches the membrane space directly from the lung.

What causes it?
Spontaneous pneumothorax usually occurs in otherwise healthy adults ages 20 to 40. It may be caused by air leakage from ruptured blebs (blisterlike accumulations of fluid) that are present at birth. It also may be caused by an emphysematous bleb that ruptures during exercise or coughing or from tuberculosis or cancer. The lung may also collapse spontaneously in interstitial lung disease.

Traumatic pneumothorax may be caused by chest surgery; a penetrating chest injury, such as a gunshot or knife wound; or the removal and analysis of lung tissue.

In tension pneumothorax, positive pressure in the lung membrane develops as a result of any of the causes of traumatic pneumothorax. When air enters the membrane through a tear in lung tissue and is unable to leave the same way, each inward breath traps air in the membrane, resulting in positive pressure. This in turn causes collapse of the lung and impaired return of blood through the veins. Decreased filling of the great veins of the chest diminishes cardiac output and lowers blood pressure.

What are its symptoms?

The cardinal features of a collapsed lung are sudden, sharp chest pain (exacerbated by movement of the chest, breathing, and coughing); asymmetrical chest wall movement; shortness of breath; and bluish skin discoloration. In moderate to severe pneumothorax, profound respiratory distress may develop, with signs of tension pneumothorax: weak and rapid pulse, pallor, neck vein distention, anxiety. Tension pneumothorax produces the most severe respiratory symptoms; a spontaneous pneumothorax that releases only a small amount of air into the lung membrane may cause no symptoms.

How is it diagnosed?

Sudden, sharp chest pain and shortness of breath suggest pneumothorax. A chest X-ray showing air in lung membrane confirms this diagnosis.

How is it treated?

Treatment is conservative for spontaneous pneumothorax in which no signs of increased membrane pressure (indicating tension pneumothorax) appear, lung collapse is less than 30%, and the person has no shortness of breath or other signs of distress. The treatment consists of bed rest; careful monitoring of blood pressure, pulse rate, and respirations; oxygen administration; and possibly, removal of air with a needle. If more than 30% of the lung has collapsed, a chest tube may be inserted to restore pressure.

Recurring spontaneous pneumothorax requires surgery. Traumatic and tension pneumothorax require chest tube drainage; traumatic pneumothorax may also require surgery.

Conservative treatment for a collapsed lung can consist of bed rest with careful monitoring of blood pressure, pulse rate, and respirations, plus oxygen administration and, possibly, removal of air with a needle.

COR PULMONALE

What is this condition?

A chronic heart condition, cor pulmonale is an enlargement of the right ventricle that results from various lung diseases, except those that primarily affect the left side of the heart, or congenital heart disease. Invariably, cor pulmonale follows some disorder of the lungs, pulmonary vessels, chest wall, or respiratory control center. For instance, chronic obstructive pulmonary disease produces pulmonary hypertension, which leads to right ventricular enlargement and failure. Because cor pulmonale generally occurs late during the course of chronic obstructive pulmonary disease and other irreversible diseases, the prognosis is generally poor.

Cor pulmonale accounts for about 25% of all types of heart failure.

What causes it?

Approximately 85% of people with cor pulmonale have chronic obstructive pulmonary disease. And 25% of people with chronic obstructive pulmonary disease eventually develop cor pulmonale.

Other respiratory disorders that produce cor pulmonale include:
- obstructive lung diseases, such as bronchiectasis and cystic fibrosis
- restrictive lung diseases, such as black lung and scleroderma
- loss of lung tissue after extensive lung surgery
- diseases of the lungs' blood vessels
- respiratory insufficiency without lung disease, as seen in muscular dystrophy and amyotrophic lateral sclerosis
- obesity hypoventilation syndrome (pickwickian syndrome) and upper airway obstruction
- living at high altitudes (chronic mountain sickness).

To compensate for the extra work needed to force blood through the lungs, the right ventricle dilates and enlarges. Eventually, this leads to right ventricular failure. Cor pulmonale accounts for about 25% of all types of heart failure.

Cor pulmonale is most common in areas of the world where the incidence of cigarette smoking and chronic obstructive pulmonary disease is high; it affects middle-aged to elderly men more often than women, but incidence in women is increasing. In children, cor pulmonale may be a complication of cystic fibrosis, upper airway obstruction, scleroderma, extensive bronchiectasis, or other disorders.

What are its symptoms?

At first, symptoms reflect the underlying disorder and occur mostly in the respiratory system. They include chronic cough, shortness of breath on exertion, wheezing respirations, fatigue, and weakness. As the disease progresses, symptoms include shortness of breath (even at rest) that worsens on exertion, rapid breathing, swelling, weakness, and discomfort in the right upper abdomen. A chest exam reveals findings characteristic of the underlying lung disease.

Drowsiness and alterations in consciousness may occur.

How is it diagnosed?

Pulmonary artery pressure measurements show increased right ventricular and pulmonary artery pressures as a result of increased pulmonary vascular resistance. Other useful diagnostic tests include echocardiography (ultrasound of the heart) or angiography, a chest X-ray, arterial blood gas analysis, electrocardiography, pulmonary function tests, and hematocrit.

How is it treated?

Treatment of cor pulmonale is designed to reduce oxygen deficiency, increase the person's exercise tolerance, and, when possible, correct the underlying condition. (See *Coping with cor pulmonale.*) In addition to bed rest, treatment may include administration of:

- digitalis glycosides (such as Lanoxin)
- antibiotics when respiratory infection is present
- potent pulmonary artery vasodilators (such as Hyperstat, Nipride, Aresoline, angiotensin-converting enzyme inhibitors, calcium channel blockers, or prostaglandins) in primary pulmonary hypertension
- oxygen by mask or, in acute cases, by a mechanical ventilator
- low-salt diet, restricted fluid intake, and diuretics, such as Lasix, to reduce swelling
- phlebotomy to reduce the red blood cell count
- anticoagulation with small doses of Calciparine to reduce the risk of thromboembolism.

 SELF-HELP

Coping with cor pulmonale

You can play an active role in your treatment by following these steps.

Follow the medication plan

- As instructed, check your radial pulse before taking Lanoxin or any digitalis glycoside. Report any change in pulse rate.
- Don't take nonprescribed medications, such as sedatives, that may depress your breathing.

Maintain a daily routine

- Eat a low-salt diet, weigh yourself daily, and watch for and immediately report swelling. To detect swelling, press the skin over your shin with a finger, hold it briefly, and then see if dimpling remains.
- Rest often and do breathing exercises regularly as instructed by your doctor.

Watch for infections

- Watch for and immediately report early signs of lung infection, such as increased sputum production, change in sputum color, increased coughing or wheezing, chest pain, fever, and tightness in the chest.
- Avoid crowds and people with respiratory infections, especially during the flu season.

CROUP

What is this condition?

Croup is a severe inflammation and obstruction of the upper airway, occurring as acute laryngotracheobronchitis (most common), laryngitis, and acute spasmodic laryngitis. Croup is a childhood disease affecting boys more often than girls, typically between ages 3 months and 3 years. It usually strikes during the winter. Up to 15% of children with croup have a strong family history of this condition. Recovery is usually complete.

What causes it?

Croup usually is caused by a viral infection. Parainfluenza viruses cause two-thirds of such infections; adenoviruses, respiratory syncytial virus, flu and measles viruses, and bacteria (pertussis and diphtheria) account for the rest.

What are its symptoms?

The onset of croup usually follows an upper respiratory tract infection. Symptoms include a harsh, high-pitched respiratory sound, hoarse or muffled vocal sounds, varying degrees of laryngeal obstruction and respiratory distress, and a characteristic sharp, barklike cough. These symptoms may last only a few hours or persist for a day or two. As it progresses, croup causes inflammatory swelling and, possibly, spasms that can block the upper airway and severely limit breathing.

Each form of croup has additional characteristics:

In *laryngotracheobronchitis,* the symptoms seem to worsen at night. Inflammation and swelling cause increasingly difficult exhalation, which frightens the child. Other characteristic features include fever, rattling sounds while exhaling, and scattered crackles.

Laryngitis, which is caused by vocal cord swelling, is usually mild and produces no respiratory distress except in infants. Early signs include a sore throat and cough.

Acute spasmodic laryngitis affects children between ages 1 and 3, particularly those with allergies and a family history of croup. It typically begins with mild to moderate hoarseness and a runny nose, followed by the characteristic cough and noisy inhalation (which often awaken the child at night), labored breathing with retractions, a rap-

STRAIGHT
TALK

Questions parents ask about croup

My child's barking cough at night sends me into a panic. What can I do right away to help my child breathe better?

One of the best ways to relieve a croup attack is to turn your bathroom into a temporary steamroom. Take your child into the bathroom, close the door, and turn on the hot water in the shower. Then sit outside the shower with him or her while steam fills the room. Let your child breathe in the steam for a few minutes. Don't let your child lie on his or her back, because this may obstruct the airway.

You can also take your child out into the cool night air (weather permitting and with proper clothing). The cool air may relieve his or her distress. If the barking cough occurs during the day, however, call the doctor.

My child seemed to be completely recovered but now seems sick again. What should I do?

Complications of croup, such as ear infections and pneumonia, can occur about 5 days after recovery. If your child develops an earache, productive cough, high fever, or increased shortness of breath, notify your doctor right away.

Can I do anything to prevent my child from getting croup again?

Unfortunately, you can't. Once a child has croup, he or she is likely to get it again with subsequent upper respiratory infections. But you can take steps to control croup attacks. At the first sign of a cold, use a humidifier or vaporizer to minimize airway irritation and break up congestion. Then closely watch your child for breathing difficulty and report any problems to the doctor right away.

Will my child outgrow these attacks?

Yes. Usually by age 3, or slightly older, a child is no longer susceptible to the most common form of croup, called *acute laryngotracheobronchitis*. This form tends to recur in children ages 3 months to 3 years, usually in the late fall or winter.

id pulse, and clammy skin. The child's understandable anxiety may lead to increasing shortness of breath. These severe symptoms diminish after several hours but reappear in a milder form on the next one or two nights. (See *Questions parents ask about croup*.)

How is it diagnosed?

When bacterial infection is the cause, throat cultures may identify organisms and also rule out diphtheria. A neck X-ray may show areas of upper airway narrowing and swelling. In evaluating the child, the doctor will look for foreign body obstruction (a common cause of croupy cough in young children) as well as masses and cysts.

How is it treated?

For most children with croup, home care with rest, cool humidification during sleep, and fever-reducing medicines such as Tylenol (or

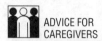

ADVICE FOR
CAREGIVERS

Tips for using a humidifier or vaporizer safely

A humidifier or vaporizer may help your child breathe easier. These devices add moisture to dry air, helping to soothe an irritated airway and break up congestion.

To ensure safety, most health professionals recommend using a cool mist humidifier. If you use a vaporizer instead, you must take precautions to prevent accidental steam burns. To use either unit, follow these guidelines:

- Read the manufacturer's directions carefully. Check the unit, especially the power cord, for signs of damage.
- Fill the unit's water tank to the right level with cool, clean tap water or distilled water. Assemble the unit as directed in the instruction booklet.
- If you use a humidifier, place the unit on a flat surface, several feet away from the child.

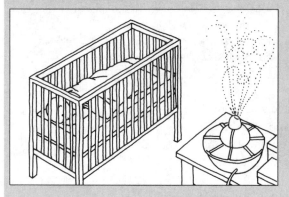

- If you use a vaporizer, you should place the unit on the floor or a secure table (not on a chair, where it might be knocked over and spill hot water). Don't point the steam vent directly at the child.

Prevent electrical hazards
Before plugging in either unit, make sure the power cord lies safely away from such objects as radiators or heaters. And make sure no one can step on or trip over it.

With either unit, periodically check to make sure it's working properly. Refill the water tank as necessary. Also, at least every hour, make sure your child's bed linen isn't damp with excess moisture. If it is, change the sheets, and move the unit slightly farther away from your child.

Unplug the power cord when you're not using the humidifier or vaporizer. And never move or tilt a unit without first turning it off and unplugging it.

Keep the unit clean
Empty and clean the humidifier or vaporizer daily. In a humidifier, germs can breed and thrive in any remaining water. In a vaporizer, mineral deposits from hard water may build up and block steam flow. Follow the manufacturer's directions for cleaning your unit. Then wipe it dry after each use.

another drug containing acetaminophen) relieve symptoms. (See *Tips for using a humidifier or vaporizer safely*.) However, severe breathing problems require hospitalization. The child usually recuperates in a mist tent, which provides constant humidification to help breathing. If bacterial infection is the cause, antibiotics are necessary. Oxygen therapy may also be required.

EPIGLOTTITIS

What is this condition?

This acute inflammation and swelling of the epiglottis, the lidlike flap that covers the larynx during swallowing of food and fluids, blocks the breathing passageways. It typically strikes children between ages 2 and 8. A critical emergency, epiglottitis can prove fatal in 8% to 12% of people unless it's recognized and treated promptly.

What causes it?

Epiglottitis usually is caused by infection with the bacterium *Haemophilus influenzae* type B and, occasionally, other bacteria.

What are its symptoms?

Sometimes preceded by an upper respiratory infection, epiglottitis may rapidly progress to completely block the upper breathing passages in 2 to 5 hours. Laryngeal obstruction results from inflammation and swelling of the epiglottis. Accompanying symptoms include high fever, high-pitched breathing, sore throat, difficulty swallowing, irritability, restlessness, and drooling. To relieve severe respiratory distress, the child with epiglottitis may hyperextend his or her neck, sit up, and lean forward with mouth open, tongue protruding, and nostrils flaring as he or she tries to breathe.

How is it diagnosed?

In acute epiglottitis, throat examination reveals a large, swollen, bright red epiglottis. Such an exam should follow lateral neck X-rays and, generally, should *not* be performed if suspected obstruction is great. Trained personnel (such as an anesthesiologist) should be on hand during the throat exam to insert an artificial airway if necessary.

How is it treated?

A child with acute epiglottitis and airway obstruction requires emergency hospitalization; he or she may need emergency endotracheal intubation or a tracheotomy and should be monitored in an intensive care unit. Respiratory distress that interferes with swallowing requires intravenous fluids to prevent dehydration. A child with acute epiglottitis should always receive a 10-day course of antibiotics.

An acute inflammation that tends to cause airway blockage, epiglottitis typically strikes children between ages 2 and 8. It can prove fatal in 8% to 12% of people unless recognized and treated promptly.

HEMOTHORAX

What is this condition?

In hemothorax, blood from damaged vessels enters the lungs. Depending on the amount of bleeding and the underlying cause, hemothorax may be associated with varying degrees of lung collapse.

What causes it?

Hemothorax usually is caused by blunt or penetrating chest injury, such as a gunshot wound. In fact, about 25% of people with such an injury have hemothorax. Less often, it is caused by chest surgery, pulmonary infarction, a tumor or dissecting aneurysm in the chest, or blood-thinning drugs.

What are its symptoms?

The person with hemothorax may experience chest pain, rapid breathing, and mild to severe shortness of breath, depending on the amount of blood in the lungs and associated disease. If respiratory failure results, the person may appear anxious, restless, possibly unresponsive, and blue in skin color; marked blood loss produces low blood pressure and shock. The affected side of the chest expands and stiffens, while the unaffected side rises and falls with the person's gasping respirations.

How is it diagnosed?

Characteristic symptoms with a history of trauma strongly suggest hemothorax. A doctor will examine the chest using a stethoscope. Other tests include thoracentesis, chest X-ray, and arterial blood gas studies.

How is it treated?

Treatment is designed to stabilize the person's condition, stop the bleeding, remove blood from the space around the lung, and reexpand the lung. Mild hemothorax usually clears in 10 to 14 days, requiring only observation for further bleeding. In severe hemothorax, fluid must be removed with a needle from the pleural cavity.

After the diagnosis is confirmed, a chest tube is inserted. If the chest tube doesn't improve the person's condition, a surgical proce-

Usually the result of blunt or penetrating chest injury, hemothorax may cause chest pain, rapid breathing, and difficulty breathing. If respiratory failure results, the person may seem anxious, restless, or unresponsive.

dure called a *thoracostomy* may be needed to remove blood and clots and to control bleeding.

*I*NFANT RESPIRATORY DISTRESS *S*YNDROME

What do doctors call this condition?

Respiratory distress syndrome, hyaline membrane disease

What is this condition?

Infant respiratory distress syndrome is the most common cause of death in newborns. In the United States alone, it kills 40,000 newborns every year. The syndrome occurs in premature infants and, if untreated, is fatal within 72 hours of birth in up to 14% of infants weighing less than 5½ pounds (2,500 grams). Aggressive management using mechanical ventilation can improve the prognosis, but a few infants who survive have lung problems. Mild infant respiratory distress syndrome slowly subsides after 3 days.

What causes it?

Infant respiratory distress syndrome occurs almost exclusively in infants born before the 37th week of development (60% of those born before the 28th week). It occurs more often in infants of diabetic mothers, those delivered by cesarean section, and those delivered suddenly after antepartum hemorrhage.

Although the breathing passages and alveoli (air sacs in the lungs) of an infant's respiratory system are present by the 27th week of gestation, the chest muscles are weak and the alveoli and capillary blood supply are immature. In respiratory distress syndrome, the premature infant develops widespread alveolar collapse due to lack of a substance called *surfactant*. This deficiency prevents the lungs from expanding and causes oxygen deficiency.

What are its symptoms?

While an infant with respiratory distress syndrome may breathe normally at first, he or she usually develops rapid, shallow respirations within minutes or hours of birth, with chest retractions, flaring nostrils, and audible grunting upon exhaling. The infant may also display low blood pressure, fluid retention, and decreased urine output. In severe disease, symptoms include absence of breathing, slow heart rate, and bluish skin discoloration.

How is it diagnosed?

While signs of respiratory distress in a premature infant during the first few hours of life strongly suggest respiratory distress syndrome, a chest X-ray and arterial blood gas analysis are necessary to confirm the diagnosis.

When a cesarean section is necessary before the 36th week of development, amniocentesis helps to assess prenatal lung development and, thus, the risk of infant respiratory distress syndrome.

How is it treated?

Treating a newborn with infant respiratory distress syndrome requires vigorous respiratory support. Warm, humidified, oxygen-enriched gases are given by oxygen hood or, if such treatment fails, by mechanical ventilation. Treatment also includes:

- a radiant infant warmer or isolette for regulation of body temperature
- intravenous fluids
- tube feedings or total parenteral nutrition if the infant is too weak to eat
- administration of surfactant by an endotracheal tube.

What can the parents of an infant with respiratory distress syndrome do?

- Learn about your infant's condition and, if possible, participate in care to promote normal parent-infant bonding.
- Be aware that full recovery may take up to 12 months.

Unless treated, infant respiratory distress syndrome is fatal within 72 hours of birth in nearly 15% of infants weighing less than 5½ pounds. Aggressive treatment can improve the prognosis.

LEGIONNAIRES' DISEASE

What is this condition?

Legionnaires' disease is an acute form of pneumonia produced by bacteria. It derives its name and notoriety from the peculiar, highly publicized disease that killed 29 of 182 victims at an American Legion convention in Philadelphia in July 1976.

This disease may occur epidemically or sporadically, usually in late summer or early fall. Its severity ranges from a mild illness, with or without pneumonitis, to severe pneumonia, with a mortality rate as high as 15%. A milder form called *Pontiac syndrome* subsides within a few days, but leaves the person fatigued for several weeks. It mimics Legionnaires' disease but produces few or no respiratory symptoms, no pneumonia, and no deaths.

What causes it?

The cause of Legionnaires' disease is the bacterium *Legionella pneumophila*, which probably is transmitted through the air. In past epidemics, it has spread through cooling towers or evaporation condensers in air-conditioning systems. However, *Legionella* also flourishes in soil and excavation sites. The disease doesn't spread from person to person.

Legionnaires' disease occurs more often in men than in women and is most likely to affect:

- middle-aged and elderly people
- immunocompromised people (particularly those receiving corticosteroids, for example, after transplantation), or those with lymphoma or other disorders associated with delayed hypersensitivity
- people with a chronic underlying disease, such as diabetes, chronic kidney failure, or chronic obstructive pulmonary disease
- alcoholics
- cigarette smokers (three to four times more likely to develop Legionnaires' disease than nonsmokers).

What are its symptoms?

Legionnaires' disease follows a predictable sequence, although it develops gradually or suddenly. After a 2- to 10-day incubation period, nonspecific symptoms appear, including diarrhea, loss of appetite, widespread muscle pain and generalized weakness, headache, recurrent chills, and an unremitting fever that develops within 12 to 48 hours and may reach 105° F (40.5° C). A cough then develops that eventually may produce grayish and, occasionally, blood-streaked sputum.

Other characteristic features include nausea, vomiting, disorientation, mental sluggishness, confusion, mild temporary amnesia, chest pain, rapid breathing, shortness of breath and, in 50% of people, a

Legionnaires' disease is probably transmitted by an airborne route. In past epidemics, it has spread through cooling towers or evaporation condensers in air-conditioning systems. But the agent that causes the disease also flourishes in soil and excavation sites.

slow heart rate. People who develop pneumonia may also experience reduced oxygen supply to body tissues.

How is it diagnosed?

The doctor focuses on possible sources of infection and predisposing conditions. In addition, a physical exam, chest X-ray, and blood studies can reveal evidence of Legionnaires' disease. Bronchial washings and blood, pleural fluid, and sputum tests rule out other infections.

Definitive test results, including the bacterial culture, aren't available until convalescence.

How is it treated?

Antibiotic treatment begins as soon as Legionnaires' disease is suspected and diagnostic material is collected. E-Mycin is the drug of choice, but if it's not effective alone, Rifadin can be added. If E-Mycin can't be given, Rifadin or Rifadin with Achromycin may be used.

Supportive therapy includes drugs to fight fever and improve blood circulation; oxygen administration by mask, cannula, or mechanical ventilation; and fluid replacement.

What can a person with Legionnaires' disease do?

As instructed by the doctor, continue to cough and do deep-breathing exercises until you recover completely.

LUNG ABSCESS

What is this condition?

Lung abscess is a lung infection accompanied by pus accumulation and tissue destruction. The abscess may be caused by bacteria and often has a well-defined border. The availability of effective antibiotics has made lung abscess much less common than it was in the past.

What causes it?

Lung abscess is a sign of a tissue-destroying pneumonia, often the result of aspiration of oropharyngeal contents. Poor oral hygiene with dental or gum disease is strongly associated with lung abscess.

What are its symptoms?

Symptoms of a lung abscess include a cough that may produce bloody or foul-smelling sputum, chest pain, shortness of breath, excessive sweating, chills, fever, headache, malaise, and weight loss. Complications include rupture of the abscess into the pleural space, which results in pus accumulating in the chest and, rarely, massive hemorrhage. Failure of an abscess to improve with antibiotic treatment suggests a possible underlying tumor or other causes of obstruction.

Treatment of a lung abscess consists of antibiotic therapy, often lasting for months, until X-rays show improvement or definite stability. Symptoms usually disappear in a few weeks.

How is it diagnosed?

The following techniques help diagnose a lung abscess:
- physical exam and chest X-ray
- biopsy of the suspected abscess
- bronchoscopy
- blood cultures, Gram stain, and culture of sputum.

How is it treated?

Treatment consists of antibiotic therapy, often lasting for months, until X-rays show improvement or definite stability. Symptoms usually disappear in a few weeks. Postural drainage may help a person to expel sputum accumulations; oxygen therapy may relieve a low level of oxygen in the blood. Poor response to therapy requires surgery to remove the abscess or the diseased section of the lung. All people with lung abscess need rigorous follow-up and serial chest X-rays.

PLEURAL EFFUSION AND EMPYEMA

What is this condition?

An excess of fluid in the pleural space is called *pleural effusion*. The pleural space refers to the thin space between the lung tissue and the membranous sac (called the *pleura*) that protects it.

Normally, this space contains a small amount of fluid that lubricates the pleural surfaces. Increased production or inadequate removal of this fluid causes a pleural effusion. The accumulation of pus and dead tissue in the pleural space is called *empyema*. Blood in the pleural space is called *hemothorax*, and chyle in this space is called *chylothorax*.

What causes it?

When an imbalance of pressures in the pleural capillaries occurs, excessive amounts of fluid can pass across intact capillaries. The result is known as *transudative pleural effusion*. Such effusions frequently are caused by heart failure, liver disease with ascites, peritoneal dialysis, and disorders resulting in too much blood in the vessels.

Exudative pleural effusions result when capillaries exhibit increased permeability, allowing fluid to leak into the pleural space. Exudative pleural effusions occur with tuberculosis, subdiaphragmatic abscess, pancreatitis, bacterial or fungal pneumonitis or empyema, malignant disease, pulmonary embolism with or without infarction, collagen diseases (lupus and rheumatoid arthritis), myxedema, and chest trauma.

Empyema is usually associated with infection in the pleural space.

What are its symptoms?

People with pleural effusion usually show symptoms from the underlying illness. Most people with large effusions, particularly those with underlying lung disease, complain of shortness of breath. Those with effusions associated with pleurisy complain of chest pain. People with empyema also develop fever and malaise.

How is it diagnosed?

Diagnosis depends on results from physical exam and chest X-ray. However, diagnosis also requires other tests to distinguish transudative from exudative effusions and to help pinpoint the underlying disorder. The most useful test is thoracentesis, in which a sample of pleural fluid is removed by needle and analyzed.

How is it treated?

Depending on the amount of fluid present, symptomatic effusion may require thoracentesis to remove fluid, or careful monitoring of the person's own reabsorption of the fluid. (For details, see *Learning about thoracentesis*.) Hemothorax requires drainage. Treatment of

Learning about thoracentesis

In thoracentesis, the doctor uses a needle to remove extra fluid from the area around your lung called the *pleural space*. A sample of this fluid will be sent to the lab, where it will be studied to find out what's causing your disorder.

The procedure is usually done in your hospital room, and it takes about 10 or 15 minutes.

Getting ready

The nurse will ask you to put on a hospital gown that opens down the back so the doctor can easily reach the right location for the procedure.

Then the nurse will take your vital signs (temperature, pulse rate, breathing rate, and blood pressure).

Next, the doctor will examine your back and chest and choose an area for inserting the needle. Then that area will be shaved and cleaned.

Just before the procedure, the nurse will help you to assume a special position. If the doctor decides to insert the needle into your back, you may sit on the edge of the bed and lean forward on the over-bed table. The nurse will help you rest your arms on a pillow and your feet on a stool (as shown below).

Or you may be asked to straddle a chair (as shown here).

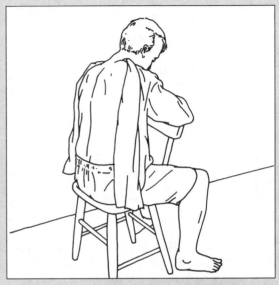

If the doctor decides to perform thoracentesis by obtaining a fluid sample from your chest, the nurse will help you sit up in bed with the head of your bed raised. This is called the *semi-Fowler's position*.

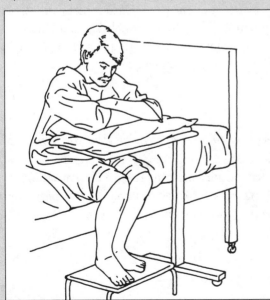

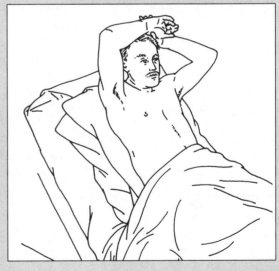

(continued)

Learning about thoracentesis *(continued)*

During the procedure

Immediately before thoracentesis, the doctor will clean your chest or back with a cold antiseptic solution. To numb the area, a local anesthetic will be injected. This may cause a slight stinging or burning sensation.

Then the doctor will perform thoracentesis by inserting a special needle between your ribs and into your chest cavity where the fluid lies.

You shouldn't feel much discomfort, but you may feel some pressure when the needle is inserted.

Don't move, and don't breathe deeply or cough when the needle's in place because this could damage your lung.

Be sure to let the doctor or nurse know if you feel short of breath, dizzy, weak, or sweaty or if your heart is racing.

Now the doctor will use the needle and a syringe to withdraw excess pleural fluid. If you have lots of fluid, a suction device may also be used. Usually, 1 to 2 quarts (liters) of fluid will be removed. If your lung holds more, you may need thoracentesis again later.

After the procedure

When the doctor removes the needle, you may feel the urge to cough. (Go ahead. It's safe to do so.) Then the doctor will apply pressure and a snug bandage to the site.

Immediately after thoracentesis, you'll have an X-ray to monitor your progress and check for complications. The nurse will check your vital signs frequently for the next few hours.

If the doctor withdrew a lot of fluid, you may notice that you're breathing more easily.

What to watch for

If you feel faint, tell the doctor. You may be given some oxygen. And be sure to report any other discomfort, such as difficult breathing, chest pain, or uncontrollable coughing. These can signal complications.

empyema requires insertion of one or more chest tubes after thoracentesis, to allow drainage of pus, and possibly surgical removal of the thick coating over the lung or rib resection to allow open drainage and lung expansion. Empyema also requires antibiotics. Associated hypoxia (low level of oxygen in the tissues) requires oxygen administration.

What can a person with pleural effusion and empyema do?

▪ As instructed, do deep-breathing exercises to promote lung expansion and use an incentive spirometer to promote deep breathing.

▪ If you developed pleural effusion as a complication of pneumonia or the flu, get prompt medical attention for chest colds.

PLEURISY

What do doctors call this condition?
Pleuritis

What is this condition?
Pleurisy is inflammation of the pleura, the serous membrane that lines the inside of the rib cage and envelops the lungs.

What causes it?
Pleurisy develops as a complication of pneumonia, tuberculosis, viruses, lupus, rheumatoid arthritis, uremia, Dressler's syndrome, cancer, pulmonary infarction, and chest injury.

What are its symptoms?
This disorder usually begins suddenly. Sharp, stabbing pain that increases with respiration may be so severe that it limits movement on the affected side during breathing. Shortness of breath also occurs. Other symptoms vary according to the underlying disease.

How is it diagnosed?
During the physical exam, the doctor will listen for a coarse, creaky sound during breathing called a *pleural friction rub*. Palpation over the affected area may reveal coarse vibration.

How is it treated?
Treatment generally focuses on relieving symptoms and includes anti-inflammatory agents, pain relievers, and bed rest. To control severe pain, the person may require local anesthesia (an intercostal nerve block of two or three intercostal nerves). If pleurisy occurs with pleural effusion, thoracentesis is required.

PNEUMONIA

What is this condition?

Pneumonia is an acute lung inflammation in which the lungs fill with a fibrous material, impairing gas exchange. With poor gas exchange, the blood has too much carbon dioxide and too little oxygen.

People with normal lungs and adequate immune defenses usually recover fully. However, pneumonia is the sixth leading cause of death in the United States.

Classifying pneumonia

Pneumonia can be classified by location or type, as well as cause.
- Location: *Bronchopneumonia* involves the lungs and small airways of the respiratory tract. *Lobular pneumonia* involves part of a lobe of the lung. *Lobar pneumonia* involves an entire lobe.
- Type: *Primary pneumonia* occurs when a person inhales or aspirates a disease-producing microorganism; it includes pneumococcal and viral pneumonia. *Secondary pneumonia* may occur in someone who's suffered lung damage from a noxious chemical or other insult, or it may be caused by the blood-borne spread of bacteria from a distant site.

What causes it?

Pneumonia can be caused by a virus, bacterium, fungus, protozoa, mycobacterium, mycoplasma, or rickettsia.

Certain factors can predispose a person to bacterial and viral pneumonia—chronic illness and debilitation, cancer (especially lung cancer), abdominal or chest surgery, atelectasis (the collapse of air sacs in the lung), the flu, common colds or other viral respiratory infections, chronic respiratory disease (such as emphysema, chronic bronchitis, asthma, bronchiectasis, or cystic fibrosis), smoking, malnutrition, alcoholism, sickle cell disease, tracheostomy, exposure to harmful gases, aspiration, and drugs that suppress the immune system.

Factors that predispose a person to aspiration pneumonia include old age, debilitation, nasogastric tube feedings, an impaired gag reflex, poor oral hygiene, and a decreased level of consciousness.

What are its symptoms?

In the early stage, a person with bacterial pneumonia may have these classic symptoms — coughing, sputum production, chest pain, shaking, chills, and fever.

On examination, the doctor may hear an abnormal breath sound called *crackles* and discover signs of *pleural effusion,* abnormal fluid buildup in the lungs. Effusion is responsible for fever, chest pain, shortness of breath, and a nonproductive cough.

Complications of pneumonia include respiratory failure, pus accumulation in the lungs, and lung abscess. Some people develop a bacterial infection in the blood; if the infection spreads to other parts of the body, it can lead to inflammation of the brain and spinal cord membranes, inflammation of the heart's interior lining, and inflammation of the sac surrounding the heart.

How is it diagnosed?

The doctor suspects pneumonia if the person has typical symptoms and physical exam results, along with a chest X-ray showing pulmonary infiltrates (abnormal substances in the lungs), and sputum containing acute inflammatory cells. If the person has pleural effusions, the doctor withdraws some fluid from the chest to analyze for signs of infection. Occasionally, the doctor obtains a sample of respiratory airway secretions or inserts an instrument called a *bronchoscope* into the airway to obtain materials for smear and culture. The person's response to antibiotics also provides important clues to the presence of pneumonia.

To speed recovery from pneumonia, supportive measures include a high-calorie diet, adequate fluid intake, bed rest, and pain relievers to reduce chest pain.

How is it treated?

Pneumonia is treated with antimicrobial drugs, which vary with the cause of the disease. Humidified oxygen therapy is given if the person has too little oxygen in the blood, and mechanical ventilation is used to treat respiratory failure. Other supportive measures include a high-calorie diet, adequate fluid intake, bed rest, and pain relievers to relieve chest pain. These supportive measures can increase the person's comfort, avoid complications, and speed recovery. To help remove secretions, the person may be taught to cough and perform deep-breathing exercises. (See *Questions people ask about pneumonia,* page 92.)

What can a person with pneumonia do?

- To avoid giving others your infection, dispose of secretions properly. Sneeze and cough into a disposable tissue.
- To prevent a recurrence of pneumonia, don't use antimicrobial drugs during minor viral infections, because this may lead to antibiotic-resistant bacteria in the upper airway. If you then develop pneu-

STRAIGHT
TALK

Questions people ask about pneumonia

I can't seem to stop coughing. Should I be taking cough medicine?
No, right now you need to cough. Coughing rids your lungs of excess mucus produced by your infection. Without coughing, these secretions will stay in your lungs, causing your infection to multiply and spread. If your cough keeps you awake at night or exhausts you, though, consult your doctor before your next appointment.

The doctor says I have "walking pneumonia." Does this mean I'm not very sick?
No. The term simply describes a pneumonia that causes mild symptoms. Even though your sickness hasn't forced you to bed, your infection is serious

and can spread further in you, as well as to others. That's why you should follow your treatment plan and take every precaution to avoid passing your infection to anyone else.

How long does pneumonia last? I've felt sick for what seems forever.
Complete recovery from pneumonia may take several weeks (especially if you're elderly, have another illness, or if the infection has spread). Your body uses a lot of energy fighting pneumonia. And like a runner after a marathon, your body needs time and rest to get back to normal. Don't sabotage your recovery by asking your body to do more than it can. Follow your doctor's instructions to rest regularly.

monia, you may need to take more toxic drugs to get rid of the organisms.

■ Get yearly flu shots and Pneumovax (pneumococcal vaccine) if you have asthma, chronic bronchitis, emphysema, chronic heart disease, or sickle cell disease.

PULMONARY EDEMA

What is this condition?
In pulmonary edema, fluid builds up in the spaces outside the lung's blood vessels (called *extravascular spaces*). In one form of this disorder, *cardiogenic pulmonary edema,* this accumulation is caused by rising pressure in the respiratory veins and tiny blood vessels called *capillaries.* A common complication of heart disorders, pulmonary edema can become a chronic condition, or it can develop quickly and rapidly become fatal.

What causes it?

Pulmonary edema usually is caused by failure of the left ventricle, the heart's main chamber, due to various types of heart disease. In these diseases, the damaged left ventricle requires increased filling pressures to pump enough blood to all the parts of the body. The increased pressures are transmitted to the heart's other chambers and to veins and capillaries in the lungs. Eventually, fluid in the blood vessels enters the spaces between the tissues of the lungs. This makes it harder for the lungs to expand and impedes the exchange of air and gases between the lungs and blood moving through lung capillaries.

Besides heart disease, other conditions that can predispose a person to pulmonary edema include:

- excessive amounts of intravenous fluids
- certain kidney diseases, extensive burns, liver disease, and nutritional deficiencies
- impaired lymphatic drainage of the lungs, as occurs in Hodgkin's disease
- impaired emptying of the heart's left upper chamber, as occurs in narrowing of the heart's mitral valve
- conditions that cause blockage of the respiratory veins.

What are its symptoms?

Early symptoms of pulmonary edema reflect poor lung expansion and extravascular fluid buildup. They include:

- shortness of breath on exertion
- sudden attacks of respiratory distress after several hours of sleep
- difficulty breathing except when in an upright position
- coughing.

On examination, the doctor may discover a rapid pulse, rapid breathing, an abnormal breath sound called *crackles*, an enlarged neck vein, and abnormal heart sounds.

With severe pulmonary edema, early symptoms may worsen as air sacs in the lungs and small respiratory airways fill with fluid. Breathing becomes labored and rapid, and coughing produces frothy, bloody sputum. The pulse quickens and the heart rhythm may become disturbed. The skin is cold, clammy, sweaty, and bluish. As the heart pumps less and less blood, the blood pressure drops and the pulse becomes thready.

How is it diagnosed?

The doctor makes a working diagnosis based on the person's symptoms and physical exam results and orders measurements of arterial blood gases, which usually show decreased oxygen with a variable carbon dioxide level. These measurements may also reveal a metabolic disturbance, such as respiratory alkalosis, respiratory acidosis, or metabolic acidosis. Chest X-rays typically reveal diffuse haziness in the lungs and, often, an enlarged heart and abnormal fluid buildup in the lungs.

The person may undergo a diagnostic procedure called *pulmonary artery catheterization* to help confirm failure of the left ventricle and rule out adult respiratory distress syndrome, which causes similar symptoms.

How is it treated?

Treatment of pulmonary edema aims to reduce the amount of extravascular lung fluid, to improve gas exchange and heart function and, if possible, to correct underlying disease.

Usually, the person receives high concentrations of oxygen. If an acceptable arterial blood oxygen level still can't be maintained, the person receives mechanical ventilation to improve oxygen delivery to the tissues and to treat acid-base disturbances.

The individual also may receive diuretics (for example, Lasix) to promote fluid elimination through urination, which in turn helps to reduce extravascular fluid.

To treat heart dysfunction, the person may receive a digitalis glycoside or other drugs that improve heart contraction. Some people also receive drugs that dilate the arteries such as Nipride. Morphine may be given to reduce anxiety, ease breathing, and improve blood flow from the pulmonary circulation to the arms and legs.

PULMONARY EMBOLISM AND INFARCTION

What is this condition?

Pulmonary embolism is the blockage of a pulmonary artery by foreign matter or a dislodged thrombus (a clotlike substance). The most common respiratory complication in hospital patients, pulmonary embolism strikes an estimated 6 million adults each year in the United States, causing 100,000 deaths.

Rarely, pulmonary embolism leads to localized destruction of lung tissue called pulmonary infarction by blocking the arterial blood supply. Infarction is more likely to happen in people with chronic heart or lung disease. Although pulmonary infarction may be so mild as to cause no symptoms, massive embolism (more than 50% blockage of the pulmonary arterial circulation) and infarction can be rapidly fatal.

What causes it?

Generally, pulmonary embolism is caused by dislodged thrombi that originate in a leg vein. More than half such thrombi arise in the deep veins of the legs and are usually multiple. Less commonly, thrombi originate in the veins of the pelvis, kidney, liver, heart, and arms. Thrombi form because of damage to the blood vessel wall, poor blood flow from the veins, or increased blood clotting. (See *How a clot travels from the leg to the lung.*)

Occasionally, the emboli contain air, fat, amniotic fluid, tumor cells, or talc (from drugs intended for oral use that are injected intravenously by addicts). Thrombi may turn into emboli spontaneously when clots dissolve, or they may be dislodged during injury, sudden muscle action, or a change in blood flow to the arms and legs. (See *Risk factors for pulmonary embolism,* page 96.)

What are its symptoms?

Total blockage of the main pulmonary artery is rapidly fatal. Smaller or fragmented emboli cause symptoms that vary with the size, number, and location of the emboli.

Usually, the first symptom of pulmonary embolism is labored breathing, which may be accompanied by chest pain. Other symptoms include a rapid pulse, a productive cough (sputum may be blood-tinged), slight fever, and fluid buildup in the lungs.

Less common symptoms include massive coughing up of blood, a rigid chest to avoid pain caused by movement, and leg swelling. A large embolus may cause bluish skin, fainting, and swollen neck veins.

Pulmonary embolism may also cause signs of circulatory collapse, such as a weak, rapid pulse and low blood pressure, along with signs of too little oxygen in the blood such as restlessness.

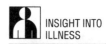 INSIGHT INTO ILLNESS

How a clot travels from the leg to the lung

A blood clot may form in a leg vein if a blood vessel is torn, if blood accumulates in the legs, or if the blood clots more easily than normal.

Then, if the clot breaks free, it will travel from the legs through progressively larger veins to the heart. The clot flows freely until it reaches the lungs, where the blood vessels again become small. Here it can cause a blockage, impeding blood flow to the lungs.

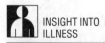

Risk factors for pulmonary embolism

Factors that predispose a person to pulmonary embolism include:

■ long-term immobility (such as from being bedridden)
■ chronic pulmonary disease (such as emphysema or chronic bronchitis)
■ congestive heart failure
■ atrial fibrillation (a type of irregular heartbeat)
■ thrombophlebitis (vein inflammation)
■ an increased number of red blood cells and bone marrow elements
■ an abnormally high platelet count
■ sickle cell disease
■ varicose veins
■ recent surgery
■ advanced age
■ pregnancy
■ leg or foot fractures or surgery
■ burns
■ obesity
■ blood vessel injury
■ cancer
■ use of oral contraceptives.

How is it diagnosed?

The doctor evaluates the person's history for factors that predispose to pulmonary embolism. The doctor also conducts a physical exam, listens for certain heart and chest sounds, and orders some or all of the following diagnostic tests:

■ *Chest X-ray* helps rule out other respiratory diseases and shows fluid buildup, areas of collapsed air sacs in the lungs, and signs that suggest pulmonary infarction.

■ *Lung scan* shows poor blood movement in areas beyond blocked vessels.

■ *Pulmonary angiography* (an X-ray study of lung circulation) is the most definitive test but poses some risk. It may be used if the doctor isn't sure of the diagnosis or to avoid unnecessary blood-thinning drugs in high-risk people.

■ *Electrocardiography* (a recording of the heart's electrical activity) helps distinguish pulmonary embolism from heart attack.

■ *Arterial blood gas measurements* sometimes show characteristic levels of arterial oxygen and carbon dioxide.

How is it treated?

Treatment aims to maintain cardiovascular and respiratory functions while the blockage resolves and to prevent more embolic episodes. Because most emboli resolve within 10 to 14 days, treatment consists of oxygen therapy, as needed, and the anticoagulant drug Calcilean to inhibit new thrombus formation. People with massive pulmonary embolism and shock may need clot-dissolving drugs, such as Abbokinase, Kabikinase, or Activase. Those with low blood pressure caused by emboli receive drugs called *vasopressors*, which stimulate muscle contraction in blood vessels. To treat infected emboli, the doctor looks for the source of the infection and prescribes antibiotics, not anticoagulants.

Surgery is required for people who can't take anticoagulants and in certain other situations. During surgery, the doctor may insert a device to filter blood returning to the heart and lungs.

What can a person with pulmonary embolism do?

■ If the doctor orders antiembolism stockings, be sure to apply them correctly. (See *How to apply antiembolism stockings.*)

■ If the doctor has prescribed the anticoagulant drug Coumadin, be aware that you may have to take it for 4 to 6 months. While taking

SELF-HELP

How to apply antiembolism stockings

To improve circulation in your lower legs, the doctor may want you to apply antiembolism stockings in the morning before getting out of bed and remove them at night after you're in bed. Follow these steps to apply the stockings.

Lightly dust your ankle with powder to ease stocking application.

Insert your hand into the stocking from the top, and grab the heel pocket from the inside. Turn the stocking inside out so the foot section is inside the stocking leg.

Hook the index and middle fingers of both your hands into the foot section. Ease the stocking over your toes, stretching it side to side as you move it up your foot. Point your toes to help ease on the stocking.

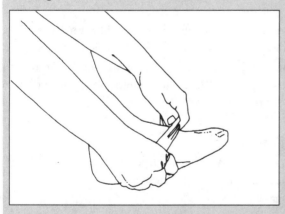

Center your heel in the stocking's heel pocket. Then, gather the loose material at your ankle, and slide the rest of the stocking up over your heel with short pulls, alternating front and back.

Insert your index and middle fingers into the gathered stocking at your ankle, and ease the stocking up your leg to the knee.

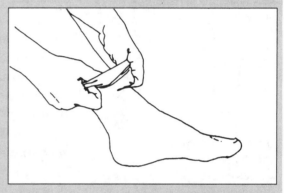

Stretch the stocking toward the knee, front and back, to distribute the material evenly. The stocking should fit snugly, with no wrinkles.

Make sure the top of the stocking is below the crease at the back of your knee. If the top of the stocking sits in the crease, it can put pressure on the vein and decrease circulation to your legs. Never let the stockings roll part way down your leg or bunch up in any way. This can create too much pressure on your leg veins.

this drug, watch for signs of bloody stools, blood in the urine, and large bruises. Take the drug exactly as ordered, and avoid taking any other drug (even for headaches or colds) or changing drug doses without consulting the doctor.

▪ Be sure to report for follow-up lab tests to monitor the effects of anticoagulant therapy.

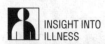

INSIGHT INTO
ILLNESS

Disorders that may cause pulmonary hypertension

High pulmonary artery pressure can be linked to the disorders below.

Disorders that damage lung tissue
- Chronic bronchitis and emphysema
- Sarcoidosis
- Pneumonia
- Lung cancer
- Scleroderma

Disorders that impair ventilation
- Obesity
- Kyphoscoliosis
- Obstructive sleep apnea

Disorders that obstruct blood vessels
- Pulmonary embolism
- Blood vessel inflammation

Disorders that affect the heart
- Congenital defects, such as patent ductus arteriosus, or atrial or ventricular septal defect
- Rheumatic valvular disease
- Mitral stenosis

PULMONARY HYPERTENSION

What is this condition?

Pulmonary hypertension occurs when pulmonary artery pressure rises above normal, but is not caused by aging or altitude. *Primary (idiopathic) pulmonary hypertension* is rare, occurring most often in women between ages 20 and 40; pregnant women have the highest mortality. *Secondary pulmonary hypertension* is caused by existing cardiac or pulmonary disease. The prognosis depends on the severity of the underlying disorder.

What causes it?

Primary pulmonary hypertension is thought to be caused by altered immune mechanisms. Secondary pulmonary hypertension is caused by oxygen deprivation from an underlying disease. (See *Disorders that may cause pulmonary hypertension.*)

What are its symptoms?

Most people complain of increasing shortness of breath on exertion, weakness, dizziness, and fatigue. Many also show signs of right-sided heart failure, including peripheral edema, ascites, neck vein distention, and liver enlargement. Other clinical effects vary according to the underlying disorder.

How is it diagnosed?

Diagnostic tests for pulmonary hypertension include the following:
- listening to the lungs through a stethoscope
- arterial blood gas analysis
- electrocardiography
- cardiac catheterization
- pulmonary angiography
- pulmonary function tests.

How is it treated?

Treatment usually includes oxygen therapy. For people with right ventricular failure, treatment also includes fluid restriction, digitalis glycosides to increase cardiac output, and diuretics to decrease intravascular volume and extravascular fluid accumulation. Of course, an important goal of treatment is correction of the underlying cause.

What can a person with pulmonary hypertension do?
- Avoid overexertion, and always rest between activities.
- Be sure to follow the prescribed diet and medication schedule.

RESPIRATORY ACIDOSIS

What is this condition?
An acid-base disturbance characterized by reduced alveolar ventilation, respiratory acidosis can be *acute* (caused by a sudden failure in ventilation) or *chronic* (as in long-term lung disease). The prognosis depends on the severity of the underlying disturbance as well as the person's general health.

What causes it?
Decreased ventilation reduces the body's excretion of carbon dioxide produced through metabolism. The retained carbon dioxide then combines with water to form an excess of carbonic acid, decreasing the blood pH. As a result, the concentration of hydrogen ions in body fluids (which directly reflects acidity) increases.

Some predisposing factors in respiratory acidosis are:
- *Drugs:* Narcotics, anesthetics, hypnotics, and sedatives decrease the sensitivity of the respiratory center.
- *Central nervous system trauma:* Spinal cord injury may impair ventilatory drive.
- *Chronic metabolic alkalosis:* The body attempts to normalize pH by decreasing alveolar ventilation.
- *Neuromuscular disease* (such as myasthenia gravis, Guillain-Barré syndrome, and poliomyelitis): Weakened muscles make breathing more difficult, reducing alveolar ventilation.

In addition, respiratory acidosis can be caused by airway obstruction or parenchymal lung disease, which interferes with alveolar ventilation; chronic obstructive pulmonary disease; asthma; severe adult respiratory distress syndrome; chronic bronchitis; large pneumothorax; extensive pneumonia; and pulmonary edema.

What are its symptoms?

Acute respiratory acidosis produces central nervous system disturbances that reflect changes in the pH of cerebrospinal fluid rather than increased carbon dioxide levels in cerebral circulation. Symptoms range from restlessness, confusion, and anxiety to sleepiness, with a fine or flapping tremor, or coma. The person may complain of headaches and exhibit shortness of breath and rapid breathing with papilledema and depressed reflexes. Unless the person is receiving oxygen, hypoxemia (low level of oxygen in the tissues) accompanies respiratory acidosis. This disorder may also cause cardiovascular abnormalities, such as a rapid heartbeat, high blood pressure, irregular atrial and ventricular beats and, in severe acidosis, low blood pressure with vasodilation (bounding pulses and warm periphery).

How is it diagnosed?

This condition is diagnosed by arterial blood gas analysis, which measures the levels of oxygen, carbon dioxide, and other gases in the blood.

How is it treated?

Effective treatment of respiratory acidosis is designed to correct the underlying source of alveolar hypoventilation.

Significantly reduced alveolar ventilation may require mechanical ventilation until the underlying condition can be treated. In chronic obstructive pulmonary disease, this includes bronchodilators, oxygen, corticosteroids and, frequently, antibiotics; drug therapy for conditions such as myasthenia gravis; removal of foreign bodies from the airway; antibiotics for pneumonia; dialysis or charcoal to remove toxic drugs; and correction of metabolic alkalosis.

Dangerously low blood pH levels (less than 7.15) can produce profound central nervous system and cardiovascular deterioration and may require administration of intravenous sodium bicarbonate. In chronic lung disease, an elevated carbon dioxide level may persist despite optimal treatment.

Acute respiratory acidosis causes central nervous system disturbances ranging from restlessness, confusion, and apprehension to sleepiness or even coma. Other symptoms may include headaches, labored breathing, depressed reflexes, a rapid pulse, high blood pressure, and heart arrhythmias.

RESPIRATORY ALKALOSIS

What is this condition?

Respiratory alkalosis is a condition marked by a decrease in the partial pressure of carbon dioxide of less than 35 millimeters of mercury, which is due to alveolar hyperventilation. Uncomplicated respiratory alkalosis leads to a decrease in hydrogen ion concentration, which causes elevated blood pH. Hypocapnia (decreased carbon dioxide in the blood) occurs when the elimination of carbon dioxide by the lungs exceeds the production of carbon dioxide in the cells.

What causes it?

Causes of respiratory alkalosis fall into two categories:
- *pulmonary:* pneumonia, interstitial lung disease, pulmonary blood vessel disease, and acute asthma
- *nonpulmonary:* anxiety, fever, aspirin toxicity, metabolic acidosis, central nervous system disease (inflammation or tumor), sepsis, liver failure, and pregnancy.

What are its symptoms?

The cardinal sign of respiratory alkalosis is deep, rapid breathing, possibly more than 40 breaths per minute. This hyperventilation usually leads to light-headedness or dizziness, agitation, numbness and tingling around the mouth, wrist and foot spasms, twitching, and weakness. Severe respiratory alkalosis may cause irregular heartbeats, seizures, or both.

How is it diagnosed?

This condition is diagnosed by arterial blood gas analysis, which measures the level of oxygen, carbon dioxide, and other gases in the blood.

How is it treated?

Treatment is designed to eradicate the underlying condition, for example, removal of ingested toxins, treatment of fever, and treatment of central nervous system disease. In severe respiratory alkalosis, the person may be instructed to breathe into a paper bag, which helps relieve acute anxiety and increases carbon dioxide levels.

SARCOIDOSIS

What is this condition?

Sarcoidosis is a multisystem, granulomatous disorder that produces swelling of the lymph nodes, lung problems, and skeletal, liver, eye, or skin lesions. It occurs most often in young adults (ages 20 to 40). In the United States, sarcoidosis occurs predominantly among blacks, affecting twice as many women as men.

Acute sarcoidosis usually resolves within 2 years. Chronic, progressive sarcoidosis, which is uncommon, is associated with pulmonary fibrosis and progressive pulmonary disability.

What causes it?

The cause of sarcoidosis is unknown, but the following possible causes have been considered:

- *hypersensitivity response* (possibly from T-cell imbalance) to such agents as atypical mycobacteria, fungi, and pine pollen
- *genetic predisposition* (suggested by a slightly higher incidence of sarcoidosis within the same family)
- *chemicals* (such as zirconium or beryllium) can lead to illnesses resembling sarcoidosis, suggesting an external cause for this disease.

What are its symptoms?

Initial symptoms include painful joints (wrists, ankles, and elbows), fatigue, malaise, and weight loss. Other symptoms vary according to the extent and location of the fibrosis:

- *respiratory:* breathlessness, cough (usually nonproductive), substernal pain; complications in advanced pulmonary disease include pulmonary hypertension and cor pulmonale
- *skin:* nodules with eruptions, extensive lesions on nasal mucous membranes
- *eye:* inflammation of the iris (common); glaucoma, blindness (rare)
- *lymphatic:* bilateral hilar and right paratracheal disease of the lymph nodes, and spleen enlargement
- *musculoskeletal:* weakness, joint and muscle pain, sunken lesions on fingers and toes

- *liver:* hepatitis, usually without symptoms
- *cardiovascular:* irregular heartbeats
- *central nervous system:* cranial or peripheral nerve palsies, meningitis, seizures, and diabetes insipidus.

How is it diagnosed?

Typical clinical features with appropriate lab data and X-ray findings suggest sarcoidosis. A positive Kveim-Siltzbach skin test supports the diagnosis. In this test, the person receives an injection of an antigen prepared from spleen or lymph node tissue from people with sarcoidosis. If the person has active sarcoidosis, granuloma develops at the injection site in 2 to 6 weeks. This reaction is considered positive when removal and analysis of skin tissue at the injection site shows discrete epithelioid cell granuloma.

Other relevant diagnostic tests include:
- chest X-ray
- removal and analysis of lymph node, skin, or lung tissue
- pulmonary function tests
- blood tests and arterial blood gas studies.

A negative tuberculin skin test, fungal serologies, and sputum cultures for mycobacteria and fungi, as well as negative biopsy cultures, help rule out infection.

How is it treated?

Sarcoidosis that produces no symptoms requires no treatment. However, sarcoidosis that causes eye, breathing, central nervous system, heart, or generalized symptoms (such as fever and weight loss) requires treatment with systemic or topical corticosteroids, as does sarcoidosis that produces a high level of calcium in the blood or destructive skin lesions. Such therapy is usually continued for 1 to 2 years, but some people may need lifelong treatment. (See *Coping with sarcoidosis.*) Other treatment includes a low-calcium diet and avoidance of direct exposure to sunlight in people with a high level of calcium in the blood.

 SELF-HELP

Coping with sarcoidosis

When sarcoidosis lingers, ask for support from family and friends so you can continue to take good care of yourself. Here's some additional advice:
- If you have too much calcium in your blood, eat a low-calcium diet.
- Be sure to comply with prescribed corticosteroid therapy.
- Get regular follow-up exams and treatment.
- If your vision is failing, ask your doctor for the names of community support and resource groups, and call the American Foundation for the Blind.

SILICOSIS

What is this condition?

Silicosis is a progressive disease characterized by nodular lesions, which frequently progress to fibrosis. It's the most common form of fibrotic lung disease.

Silicosis can be classified according to the severity of pulmonary disease and the speed of its onset and progression; it usually occurs as a simple illness that has no symptoms. *Acute silicosis* develops after 1 to 3 years in people who are exposed to high concentrations of silica (such as sand blasters and tunnel workers). *Accelerated silicosis* appears after an average of 10 years of exposure to lower concentrations of free silica. *Chronic silicosis* develops after 20 or more years of exposure to lower concentrations of free silica.

The prognosis is good, unless the disease progresses into the complicated fibrotic form, which causes respiratory insufficiency and cor pulmonale and is associated with pulmonary tuberculosis.

What causes it?

Silicosis is caused by the inhalation and pulmonary deposition of crystalline silica dust, mostly from quartz. The danger to the worker depends on the concentration of dust in the atmosphere, the percentage of free silica particles in the dust, and the duration of exposure.

Industrial sources of silica in its pure form include the manufacture of ceramics (flint) and building materials (sandstone). It occurs in mixed form in the production of construction materials (cement); it's found in powder form (silica flour) in paints, porcelain, scouring soaps, and wood fillers, and in the mining of gold, coal, lead, zinc, and iron. Foundry workers, boiler scalers, and stonecutters are all exposed to silica dust and, therefore, are at high risk for developing silicosis.

What are its symptoms?

Silicosis initially may cause no symptoms or it may produce shortness of breath on exertion, often attributed to being "out of shape" or "slowing down." If the disease progresses to the chronic and complicated stage, shortness of breath on exertion worsens, and other symptoms usually include rapid breathing and an insidious dry cough, which is most pronounced in the morning, appear.

Progression to the advanced stage causes shortness of breath on minimal exertion, worsening cough, and pulmonary hypertension. People with silicosis have a high incidence of tuberculosis.

Central nervous system changes, such as confusion, lack of energy, and a decrease in the rate and depth of breathing as the partial pressure of carbon dioxide increases, also occur in advanced silicosis. Other clinical features include malaise, disturbed sleep, and hoarseness.

How is it diagnosed?

The person's history reveals occupational exposure to silica dust. A physical exam is normal in simple silicosis; in chronic silicosis with conglomerate lesions, it may reveal signs of lung damage. Diagnostic tests include pulmonary function studies, chest X-rays, and arterial blood gas studies.

How is it treated?

The goal of treatment is to relieve respiratory symptoms, to manage oxygen deficiency and cor pulmonale, and to prevent respiratory tract irritation and infections. (See *Coping with silicosis.*) Treatment also includes careful observation for the development of tuberculosis. Respiratory symptoms may be relieved through daily use of bronchodilating sprays and increased fluid intake (at least 3 quarts [liters] daily). Steam inhalation and chest physical therapy techniques, such as controlled coughing and segmental bronchial drainage, with chest percussion and vibration, help clear secretions. In severe cases, it may be necessary to administer oxygen by cannula or mask (1 to 2 quarts [liters] per minute) for the person with chronic hypoxia (low level of oxygen in the tissues), or by mechanical ventilator. Respiratory infections require antibiotics.

 SELF-HELP

Coping with silicosis

You can improve your quality of life by consistently following this advice:
- To prevent infections, avoid crowds and people with respiratory infections, and receive annual flu shots and Pneumovax (pneumococcal vaccine).
- To increase your exercise tolerance, get regular activity.
- Plan daily activities to decrease the work of breathing. Pace yourself, rest often, and move slowly through your daily routine.

SUDDEN INFANT DEATH SYNDROME

What is this condition?

Also called *crib death*, sudden infant death syndrome is a medical mystery of early infancy. It kills apparently healthy infants, usually between ages 4 weeks and 7 months, for reasons that remain unexplained, even after an autopsy. Typically, parents put the infant to bed and later find him or her dead, often with no indications of a struggle or distress of any kind. Some infants may have had signs of a cold, but such symptoms are usually absent. Sudden infant death syndrome has occurred throughout history, all over the world, and in all climates.

Sudden infant death syndrome kills apparently healthy infants for reasons that remain unexplained. Research suggests that many of these infants may have had undetected abnormalities, such as an immature respiratory system and respiratory dysfunction.

What causes it?

Sudden infant death syndrome accounts for 7,500 to 8,000 deaths annually in the United States, making it one of the leading causes of infant death. Most of these deaths occur during the winter, in poor families, and among underweight babies and those born to mothers under age 20.

Although infants who die from this disorder often appear healthy, research suggests that many may have had undetected abnormalities, such as an immature respiratory system and respiratory dysfunction. In fact, the current thinking is that it may be caused by an abnormality in the control of breathing, which causes apnea (prolonged nonbreathing periods) with profound hypoxemia (decreased oxygen in the blood) and irregular heartbeats. Bottle feeding, instead of breastfeeding, and advanced parental age *don't* cause sudden infant death syndrome.

Although parents find some victims wedged in crib corners or with blankets wrapped around their heads, autopsies rule out suffocation as the cause of death. Even when blood-tinged sputum is found around the infant's mouth or on the crib sheets, autopsy shows an open airway, so choking on vomit is not the cause of death. Typically, these infants don't cry out and show no signs of having been disturbed in their sleep, although their positions or tangled blankets may suggest movement just before death, perhaps due to terminal spasm.

What are its symptoms?

Depending on how long the infant has been dead, the infant may have a mottled complexion with extreme bluish discoloration of the lips and fingertips, or pooling of blood in the legs and feet that looks like bruises. Pulse and respirations are absent, and the infant's diaper is wet and full of stools.

How is it diagnosed?

Diagnosis of sudden infant death syndrome requires an autopsy to rule out other causes of death. Characteristic histologic findings on autopsy include small or normal adrenal glands and petechiae over the visceral surfaces of the pleura, within the thymus (which is enlarged), and in the epicardium. Autopsy also reveals extremely well-preserved lymph structures and certain disease characteristics that suggest chronic hypoxemia, such as increased pulmonary artery smooth muscle. Examination also shows swollen, congestive lungs fully expanded in the pleural cavities, liquid (not clotted) blood in the heart, and curd from the stomach inside the windpipe.

How is it treated?

If the parents bring the infant to the emergency room, the doctor will decide whether to try to resuscitate him or her. In "aborted sudden infant death syndrome," an infant who is not breathing is successfully resuscitated. Such an infant, or any infant who had a sibling stricken by this disorder, should be tested for infantile apnea. If tests are positive, a home apnea monitor may be recommended.

Because most infants cannot be resuscitated, however, treatment focuses on emotional support for the family.

TUBERCULOSIS

What is this condition?

Tuberculosis is an acute or chronic infection caused by the bacterium *Mycobacterium tuberculosis*. In this disease, abnormal substances called *pulmonary infiltrates* accumulate, cavities develop, and masses of granulated tissue form within the lungs. These masses contain dead tissue with a crumbly-cheese appearance, along with excess fibrous connective tissue.

For people with tuberculosis strains that are sensitive to the usual antituberculosis drugs, correct treatment yields an excellent prognosis. However, in people with strains that resist two or more of the major drugs, the death rate is 50%.

Who's at risk for tuberculosis?

Researchers argue over the reasons for the increasing incidence of tuberculosis, but they agree that it's on the rise. And they can identify the people at highest risk.

Generally at risk are people living in crowded, poorly ventilated, unsanitary conditions, such as those in some prisons, tenement housing, or shelters for the homeless. Others at high risk include men (tuberculosis affects twice as many men as women); nonwhites (it's four times as common in nonwhites as in whites), the typical person with newly diagnosed tuberculosis being a single, homeless, nonwhite man; people in close contact with someone recently diagnosed with tuberculosis; those who've previously had the disease; and those with weak immune systems.

Specifically at risk are:
- black and Hispanic men between ages 25 and 44
- people with multiple sexual partners
- recent immigrants from Africa, Asia, Mexico, and South America
- people who've had all or part of their stomach surgically removed
- people with silicosis, diabetes, malnutrition, cancer, or diseases affecting the immune system
- drug and alcohol abusers
- patients in facilities for the chronically or mentally ill
- nursing home residents (who are 10 times more likely to contract tuberculosis than anyone in the general populace).

What causes it?

After exposure to *M. tuberculosis,* roughly 5% of infected people develop active tuberculosis within 1 year; the remainder have a dormant infection. The person's immune system usually controls the tubercle bacillus, a rounded nodule produced by *M. tuberculosis* infection, by killing it or walling it up in a tiny nodule. However, the bacterium may lie dormant within the tubercle for years, later reactivating and spreading. Although the main infection site is the lungs, mycobacteria commonly exist in other parts of the body.

Tuberculosis spreads through the air by droplets produced when an infected person coughs or sneezes. After inhalation, infection occurs if a tubercle bacillus settles in an alveolus (air sac in the lung). People living in crowded, poorly ventilated conditions are most likely to become infected with tuberculosis. (See *Who's at risk for tuberculosis?*)

What are its symptoms?

During the initial infection, tuberculosis rarely causes symptoms. However, some people have nonspecific symptoms, such as fatigue, weakness, appetite loss, weight loss, night sweats, and slight fever. During tuberculosis reactivation, the person may cough up sputum

Understanding tuberculin skin tests

A tuberculin skin test is a simple, painless way to screen for previous exposure to active tuberculosis.

The test procedure

You'll have the test while you're seated with your arm extended and supported. First, the doctor or nurse will clean the inside skin of your forearm with alcohol and allow it to dry completely.

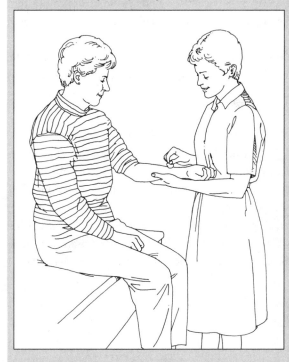

Then, if you're having the *Mantoux test,* the doctor or nurse will use a special syringe to inject a small amount of purified protein derivative of the tuberculosis bacilli under the skin of your forearm.

If you're having the *tine test,* the doctor or nurse will press a multipronged puncture device lightly onto your forearm skin to inject the test solution.

In 48 to 72 hours, either you or the doctor will evaluate the test findings. If the doctor wants you to note the test results, you'll be given a heavy paper card that has facsimile reactions embossed on it. You'll be asked to compare your skin reaction with the reactions shown on the card.

What do the findings mean?

A negative reaction (a normal finding) is no reaction or a reaction that's less than $1/5$ of an inch (5 millimeters) in diameter. A negative reaction means you haven't been exposed to tuberculosis. (Exceptions occur when very recent exposure precludes active immunity.)

A positive reaction is swelling of an area greater than $2/5$ of an inch (10 millimeters), with or without redness. This visible antigen-antibody reaction at the injection site shows that you've been exposed to tuberculosis.

Keep in mind that a positive reaction doesn't necessarily indicate active tuberculosis. Also, a person recently vaccinated with attenuated organisms (for example, bacillus Calmette-Guérin) will test positive even though he or she doesn't have tuberculosis.

filled with mucus and pus. Some people also cough up blood and have chest pain.

How is it diagnosed?

The doctor orders chest X-rays, a tuberculin skin test, and sputum smears and cultures to identify *M. tuberculosis.* The diagnosis must be precise, because several other diseases (such as lung cancer and lung abscess) may mimic tuberculosis.

Certain physical exam techniques and other diagnostic procedures aid the diagnosis. For instance, the doctor listens with a stetho-

SELF-HELP

Coping with tuberculosis

Besides your drug therapy, you should follow these guidelines:
- Get plenty of rest. To speed recovery, be sure to eat balanced meals. If you have a poor appetite, try eating small meals throughout the day rather than three large ones.
- Ask your doctor or pharmacist which medication side effects to watch for. Report these immediately.
- Be sure to get regular follow-up examinations.
- Learn about and watch for the symptoms of a recurrence of tuberculosis.
- Follow the prescribed long-term treatment schedule faithfully.
- Advise family members and others who have been exposed to you to ask their doctor whether they should have tuberculin tests.

scope for certain lung sounds and taps on the chest to detect dullness over the affected area.

In tuberculosis, a *chest X-ray* shows nodules, patchy infiltrates (mainly in the upper lobes of the lung), cavity formation, scar tissue, and calcium deposits. However, it may not be able to distinguish active from inactive tuberculosis.

A *tuberculin skin test* detects tuberculosis infection. Purified protein derivative or 5 tuberculin units are injected into the skin of the forearm. Test results are read in 48 to 72 hours; in both active and inactive tuberculosis, a positive reaction develops 2 to 10 weeks after infection. However, people with a severe depressed immune system may never develop a positive reaction. (See *Understanding tuberculin skin tests*, page 109.)

The doctor also orders *stains and cultures* of sputum, urine, the fluid that bathes the brain and spinal cord, and drainage from abscesses to check for characteristic findings.

How is it treated?

Daily oral doses of the drugs INH, Rifadin, and Tebrazid (and sometimes Myambutol) for at least 6 months usually cure tuberculosis. After 2 to 4 weeks, the disease generally is no longer infectious. The person can resume a normal lifestyle while taking the medication. People with atypical or drug-resistant tuberculosis may require other drugs, such as Capastat, streptomycin, para-aminosalicylic acid, Seromycin, Amikin, and a quinolone. (See *Coping with tuberculosis*.)

3

NERVOUS SYSTEM DISORDERS

ALZHEIMER'S DISEASE

What do doctors call this condition?
Presenile dementia, primary degenerative dementia

What is this condition?
Alzheimer's disease is a type of dementia — a condition marked by mental deterioration. An estimated 5% of people over age 65 have the severe form of this disease, and an additional 12% suffer from a mild-to-moderate form. A cure has not yet been found for the disorder.

What causes it?
The cause of Alzheimer's disease is unknown. However, several factors are thought to contribute to the condition. These include shortages of certain chemicals in the brain, known as *neurotransmitters,* which allow stimuli to travel from one nerve cell to another; environmental factors, such as dietary intake of manganese; slow-growing viruses in the brain or spinal cord; injuries; and genetic immunologic factors.

What are its symptoms?
Onset of Alzheimer's disease is slow and subtle. At first, the person experiences almost imperceptible changes, such as forgetfulness, inability to recall recent events, difficulty learning and remembering new information, inability to concentrate, and declining personal hygiene and appearance.

Gradually, tasks that require abstract thinking and judgment become more difficult. The person experiences progressive difficulty communicating with others and severe deterioration in memory, language ability, and coordination. The ability to write or speak may be lost. Personality changes and insomnia are common.

Eventually, the person becomes disoriented. His or her emotions may change suddenly. Physical and intellectual functions continue to deteriorate. The person becomes susceptible to infection and accidents. (See *Protecting a person with Alzheimer's disease.*) Usually, death results from infection.

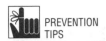
PREVENTION
TIPS

Protecting a person with Alzheimer's disease

A person with Alzheimer's disease needs help to prevent accidents and injuries. You can do two things: Remove potential safety hazards from the surroundings and install assistive devices where needed. The following guidelines will help you provide a safe place to live for a person with Alzheimer's disease.

Remove safety hazards

- Move knives, forks, scissors, and other sharp objects beyond the person's reach.
- Taste the person's food before serving to prevent burns in the mouth or, if an accidental spill occurs, on the body.
- Serve food on unbreakable dishes.
- Remove the knobs from the stove and other potentially hazardous kitchen appliances; put dangerous small appliances, such as food processors and irons, out of reach.
- To prevent accidental burns, adjust your water heater to a lower temperature (no higher than 120° F [49° C]).
- Cover unused electrical outlets, especially those above waist level, with masking tape or safety caps.
- Remove mirrors or install ones with safety glass in rooms used by the person with Alzheimer's.
- Get rid of throw rugs, and cover slippery floors with large area rugs. Place pads under the rugs, and secure them so they don't slide.
- Keep floors and stairways clear of toys, shoes, and other objects that can trip the person.
- Camouflage doors with murals or posters so they don't look like exits, or simply lock them. Install a lock at the base of the door as an extra security measure, or install a childproofing device over the knob.
- Barricade stairways with high gates.
- Remove all breakable wall hangings and pictures, and attach curtains to the wall with Velcro.
- Keep traffic patterns open by moving unsafe furniture to the walls.

- Store all medicines out of the person's reach, preferably in a locked container.

Use assistive devices

You can purchase many assistive devices at large pharmacies that have geriatric departments or from medical supply stores. You can even use childproofing devices, such as safety caps for electrical outlets, soft plastic corners for furniture, and doorknob covers. They're available from catalogs or where baby products are sold. Follow these guidelines:

- Pad sharp furniture corners with masking tape or plastic corners.
- Provide a low bed for the person.
- Keep the house well lit during waking hours. Keep a night-light in the bathroom.
- If the person uses the stairs, mark the edges with strips of yellow or orange tape to compensate for poor depth perception.
- Encourage the person to use the bathroom by making a "path" of colored tape leading in that direction.
- Attach safety rails in the bathtub, near the toilet, and on stairways.
- Glue nonskid strips in the bathtub and by the toilet.
- Provide an identification bracelet, listing the person's name, address, phone number, and medical problems.
- Notify local police about the person's condition. Give them a photograph and physical description, in case they find the person wandering in the neighborhood.

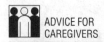
ADVICE FOR
CAREGIVERS

Alzheimer's disease: How you can help

Taking care of a person with Alzheimer's disease requires a great deal of patience and understanding. It also requires you to look at the person's environment with new eyes. That way, you'll learn how to change this environment to help him or her live better and more safely.

Reduce stress

Too much stress can worsen Alzheimer's symptoms. Try to protect the person from these sources of stress:
- a change in routine, caregiver, or environment
- fatigue
- excessive demands
- overwhelming stimuli
- illness and pain
- over-the-counter medications.

Establish a routine

Keep the person's daily routine the same so he or she can respond automatically. Adapting to change may require more thought than the person can handle. Even eating a different food or going to a strange grocery store may prove overwhelming.

Ask yourself: What are the person's daily activities? Then make a schedule:
- List the activities necessary for the person's daily care and include ones that he or she especially enjoys, such as weeding in the garden. Designate a time frame for each activity.
- Establish bedtime routines — especially important to promote relaxation and a good night's sleep for both of you.
- Establish routines for other activities — for example, breakfast first, then dressing. Stick to your schedule as closely as possible so that the person won't be surprised or need to make decisions.

Keep a copy of the person's schedule to give to other caregivers. To help them give better care, include notes and suggestions about techniques that work for you. For instance, tell them to "speak in a quiet voice" or "when helping Mitchell dress or take a bath, take one thing at a time, and wait for him to respond."

Practice reality orientation

In your talks with the person with Alzheimer's, state what day it is and describe the next activity. For instance, say "Today is Tuesday, and we're going to have breakfast now." Do this every day. This keeps the person aware of the surroundings, tells him or her what to expect, and helps reduce his or her frustration about having to remember events.

Simplify the surroundings

A person with Alzheimer's disease will eventually lose the ability to interpret correctly what he or she sees and hears. Protect the person by trying to decrease the noise level in his or her surroundings. Avoid busy areas, such as shopping malls and restaurants.

Does the person mistake pictures or images in the mirror or photos for real people? If so, remove them. Also avoid rooms with busy patterns on wallpaper and carpets because they can overtax the senses.

To avoid confusion and encourage the person's independence, provide cues. For example, hang a picture of a toilet on the bathroom door.

Avoid fatigue

The person will tire easily, so plan important activities for the morning, when energy levels are highest. Plan less demanding activities for later in the day.

Remember to schedule breaks — one in the morning and one in the afternoon. About 15 to 30 minutes of listening to music or just relaxing is sufficient in the early stages of disease.

As the disease progresses, schedule longer, more frequent breaks (perhaps 40 to 90 minutes). If naps are needed during the day, have the person sleep in a reclining chair rather than in a bed to prevent confusion of day and night.

Alzheimer's disease: How you can help *(continued)*

Don't expect too much

Accept the person's limitations. Don't demand too much because this can cause frustration. Offer help when needed, and distract the person if he or she tries too hard. You'll feel less stressed, too.

Prepare for illness

If the person becomes ill, expect behavior to deteriorate and plan accordingly. Expect a low tolerance for pain and discomfort.

Never rely on the person to take medication. He or she may forget to take it or may take too much or too little.

Use the sense of touch

Because sight and hearing are distorted, the person has an increased need for closeness and touching. Remember to approach the person from the front. You don't want to frighten the person or provoke belligerence or aggressiveness.

Respect the person's need for personal space. Limit physical contact to the person's hands and arms at first; then move to more central parts of the body, such as the shoulders or head.

Using long or circular motions, lightly stroke the person to help relieve muscle tension and express your feelings of intimacy and caring.

Allowing the person to touch objects in the environment can help relieve stress by providing information. Let him or her handle, pull, poke, or shake objects — for example, a handbag, a brush, or a comb. Make sure they're unbreakable and can't cause harm.

Handle problem behavior

If the person with Alzheimer's becomes restless or agitated, divert attention with an appropriate activity. Good choices include walking, rocking in a rocking chair, sanding wood, folding laundry, or hoeing the garden. These repetitive activities don't require any special planning. A warm bath, a drink of warm milk, or a back massage can also be calming.

Get additional help

Contact a local Alzheimer's support group. You can also get in touch with the Alzheimer's Disease and Related Diseases Association at 1-800-559-0404.

How is it diagnosed?

Early diagnosis of Alzheimer's disease is difficult because the person's signs and symptoms are obscure. To make a diagnosis, the doctor relies on information provided by a family member, supported by tests of mental status, neurologic examinations, and psychometric testing.

Currently, certain diagnostic tests are performed to rule out other disorders. The diagnosis cannot be confirmed until after death, when an exam of brain tissue shows the disorder's effects.

How is it treated?

Overall treatment is focused on supporting the person's abilities and compensating for those that have been lost. (See *Alzheimer's disease: How you can help*.) The doctor may prescribe a variety of drugs to help a person with Alzheimer's. Some of these drugs help to increase circulation in the brain — for example, Hydergine, Vasodilan, and

Cyclospasmol. The doctor may prescribe other drugs (such as Ritalin) to enhance the person's mood. If depression seems to exacerbate the person's condition, the doctor may prescribe antidepressants. To treat memory deficits, the doctor may prescribe Cognex.

Sometimes, a person with Alzheimer's will undergo hyperbaric (pressurized) oxygen treatment to increase the oxygen supply to the brain. The person is placed inside a special chamber where he or she breathes 100% oxygen.

Additional drugs are being tried to assess their ability to slow the disease process. These include choline salts, lecithin, Antilirium, enkephalins, and Narcan.

BELL'S PALSY

What is this condition?
Bell's palsy is a disease of the seventh (facial) cranial nerve that produces unilateral facial weakness or paralysis. Onset is rapid. Although it affects all age-groups, it occurs most often in persons under age 60. In 80% to 90% of people, it subsides spontaneously, with complete recovery in 1 to 8 weeks; however, recovery may be delayed in elderly people. If recovery is partial, contractures may develop on the paralyzed side of the face. Bell's palsy may occur again, on the same or opposite side of the face.

What causes it?
Bell's palsy blocks the seventh cranial nerve, which is responsible for the nerve supply to the muscles of the face. The nerve gets blocked because of an inflammatory reaction (usually at the internal auditory meatus), which is often associated with infections and can result from internal bleeding, tumor, meningitis, or local trauma.

What are its symptoms?
Bell's palsy usually causes facial weakness on one side, occasionally with aching pain around the angle of the jaw or behind the ear. On the affected side, the mouth droops (causing the person to drool from the corner of the mouth), and taste perception is distorted over the affected front of the tongue. In addition, the forehead appears smooth, and the person's ability to close the eye on the weak side is

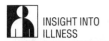

INSIGHT INTO
ILLNESS

Hallmarks of Bell's palsy

Bell's palsy causes paralysis on one side of the face. This produces a distorted appearance, with an inability to wrinkle the forehead, close the eyelid, smile, show the teeth, or puff out the cheek.

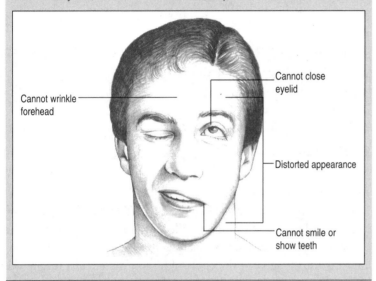

Cannot wrinkle forehead

Cannot close eyelid

Distorted appearance

Cannot smile or show teeth

markedly limited. When attempting to close this eye, it rolls upward (called *Bell's phenomenon*) and shows excessive tearing. Although Bell's phenomenon occurs in normal persons, it's not apparent because the eye closes completely and covers this eye motion. In Bell's palsy, incomplete eye closure makes this upward motion obvious. (See *Hallmarks of Bell's palsy*.)

How is it diagnosed?

Diagnosis depends on clinical presentation: distorted facial appearance and inability to raise the eyebrow, close the eyelid, smile, show the teeth, or puff out the cheek. After 10 days, a test called electromyography helps predict the level of expected recovery by distinguishing a temporary conduction defect from a serious inflammation of nerve fibers.

How is it treated?

Treatment consists of Orasone, an oral corticosteroid that reduces facial nerve swelling and improves nerve conduction and blood flow.

SELF-HELP

Advice for the person with Bell's palsy

Follow these pointers to increase comfort during your recovery:
• To help maintain muscle tone, massage your face with a gentle upward motion two to three times daily for 5 to 10 minutes. When the doctor permits you to do active exercises, grimace in front of a mirror, as instructed.
• To protect your eye, cover it with an eye patch, especially when outdoors. Keep warm and avoid exposure to dust and wind. When exposure is unavoidable, cover your face.
• To cope with difficulty in eating and drinking, chew on the unaffected side of your mouth. Eat a soft, nutritionally balanced diet, avoiding hot foods and fluids.
• Be aware that recovery is likely within 1 to 8 weeks.

After 14 days of Orasone therapy, electrotherapy may help prevent atrophy of facial muscles.

During treatment with Orasone, the person may develop side effects, especially gastrointestinal distress and fluid retention. If gastrointestinal distress occurs, an antacid, taken at the same time, usually provides relief. If the person has diabetes, Orasone must be used cautiously and with frequent monitoring of blood sugar levels. (See *Advice for the person with Bell's palsy*.)

BRAIN ANEURYSM

What do doctors call this condition?
Cerebral aneurysm

What is this condition?
Brain aneurysm is a localized swelling of a cerebral artery that results from a weakness in the arterial wall. Its most common form is the berry aneurysm, a saclike outpouching in a cerebral artery. Brain aneurysms usually arise in the circle of Willis, the circular area at the base of the brain where the major cerebral arteries meet. Brain aneurysms often rupture and cause bleeding in the subarachnoid space (membranes surrounding the brain tissue).

The prognosis is guarded. Probably half the people suffering a subarachnoid hemorrhage die immediately; of those who survive untreated, 40% die from the effects of the hemorrhage; another 20% die later from recurring hemorrhage. With new and better treatment, the prognosis is improving.

What causes it?
Brain aneurysm may result from a congenital defect, a degenerative process, or a combination of both. For example, high blood pressure and atherosclerosis (fatty deposits in the arteries) may disrupt blood flow and exert pressure against a congenitally weak arterial wall, stretching it like an overblown balloon and making it likely to rupture. After such rupture, blood spills into the space normally occupied by cerebrospinal fluid (the fluid that bathes the brain and spinal cord). Sometimes, the blood also spills into the brain tissue and sub-

sequently forms a clot. This may result in potentially fatal increased intracranial pressure and brain damage.

Incidence of brain aneurysm is slightly higher in women than in men, especially those in their late 40s or early-to-middle 50s, but it may occur at any age, in both women and men.

What are its symptoms?

Occasionally, rupture of a brain aneurysm causes warning symptoms that last several days, such as headache; stiff neck, back, and legs; and intermittent nausea. Normally, however, it occurs abruptly and without warning, causing a sudden severe headache, nausea, vomiting and, depending on the severity and location of bleeding, altered consciousness (including deep coma).

Bleeding causes meningeal irritation, resulting in stiff neck, back and leg pain, fever, restlessness, irritability, occasional seizures, and blurred vision. Bleeding into the brain tissues causes slight paralysis and sensory defects on one side, difficulty swallowing, and visual defects. If the aneurysm is near the internal carotid artery, it compresses the oculomotor nerve and causes double vision, drooping eyelid, dilated pupil, and inability to rotate the eye.

The severity of symptoms varies considerably from person to person, depending on the site and amount of bleeding. Generally, brain aneurysm poses three major threats:

- *Death from increased intracranial pressure:* This increased pressure may push the brain downward, impair brain stem function, and cut off blood supply to the part of the brain that supports vital functions.
- *Rebleeding:* Typically, after the initial bleeding episode, a clot forms and seals the rupture, which reinforces the wall of the aneurysm for 7 to 10 days. However, after the 7th day, the clot begins to dissolve, increasing the risk of rebleeding. This rebleeding produces signs and symptoms similar to the initial hemorrhage. Rebleeding episodes during the first 24 hours after the initial hemorrhage are not uncommon, and they contribute to brain aneurysm's high mortality.
- *Vasospasm:* Why this occurs isn't clearly understood. Usually, spasms occur in blood vessels located near the aneurysm, but they may extend to major vessels of the brain, causing decreased blood flow and altered brain function.

How is it diagnosed?

In brain aneurysm, diagnosis is based on the person's history and a neurologic exam; a computed tomography scan (commonly called a

Brain aneurysm poses three major threats: rebleeding, vasospasm, and death from increased intracranial pressure.

CAT scan), which reveals blood in various areas of the brain; and magnetic resonance imaging (commonly called an MRI), or magnetic resonant angiography, which can identify a brain aneurysm as a "flow void" or by computer reconstruction of the involved blood vessels.

Cerebral angiography remains the procedure of choice for diagnosing brain aneurysm. Lumbar puncture may be used to identify blood in cerebrospinal fluid if other studies are negative and the person has no signs of increased intracranial pressure.

Other typical lab tests include blood studies, urinalysis, and electrolyte and sugar levels.

How is it treated?

Treatment aims to reduce the risk of vasospasm and cerebral infarction by repairing the aneurysm. Usually, surgical repair (by clipping, tying off, or wrapping the aneurysm neck with muscle) takes place 7 to 10 days after the initial bleeding; however, surgery performed within 1 to 2 days after hemorrhage has also shown promise in some cases. When surgical correction is risky, when the aneurysm is in a dangerous location, or when surgery is delayed because of vasospasm, treatment includes:

- bed rest in a quiet, darkened room; if immediate surgery isn't possible, bed rest may continue for 4 to 6 weeks
- avoidance of coffee, other stimulants, and aspirin
- codeine sulfate or another analgesic, as needed
- Apresoline or another antihypertensive agent if the person has high blood pressure
- calcium channel blockers to decrease spasm
- corticosteroids to reduce edema
- Dilantin or another antiseizure drug
- Barbita or another sedative
- Amicar, a fibrinolytic inhibitor, to minimize the risk of rebleeding by delaying blood clot lysis. However, this drug's effectiveness is controversial.

After surgical repair, the person's condition depends on the extent of damage from the initial bleeding and the degree of success in treating complications. Surgery cannot improve the person's neurologic condition unless it removes a hematoma or reduces bleeding-related compression effects.

CEREBRAL PALSY

What is this condition?

The most common cause of crippling in children, cerebral palsy comprises a group of neuromuscular disorders resulting from central nervous system damage before, during, or after birth. Although non-progressive, these disorders may become more obvious as an affected infant grows older. Three major types of cerebral palsy occur — *spastic, athetoid,* and *ataxic* — sometimes in mixed forms.

Motor impairment may be minimal (sometimes apparent only during physical activities such as running) or severely disabling. Associated defects, such as seizures, speech disorders, and mental retardation, are common.

Prognosis varies. In mild impairment, proper treatment may make a near-normal life possible.

Cerebral palsy occurs in an estimated 1.5 to 5 per 1,000 live births every year. Incidence is highest in premature infants and in those who are small for their gestational age. Cerebral palsy is slightly more common in boys than in girls and occurs more often in whites. (See *What causes cerebral palsy?*)

What are its symptoms?

The *spastic* form of cerebral palsy is the most common, occurring in about 70% of affected infants. This form is characterized by hyperactive deep tendon reflexes; increased stretch reflexes; rapid, alternating muscle contraction and relaxation; muscle weakness; underdevelopment of affected limbs; muscle contraction in response to manipulation; and a tendency toward contractures. Typically, a child with spastic cerebral palsy walks on the toes with a scissors gait, crossing one foot in front of the other.

In *athetoid cerebral palsy,* which affects about 20% of people, involuntary movements — grimacing, wormlike writhing, irregular muscle movements, and sharp jerks — impair voluntary movement. Usually, these involuntary movements affect the arms more severely than the legs; involuntary facial movements may make speech difficult. These athetoid movements become more severe during stress, decrease with relaxation, and disappear entirely during sleep.

Ataxic cerebral palsy accounts for about 10% of people with cerebral palsy. Its characteristics include disturbed balance, incoordination (especially of the arms), hypoactive reflexes, rapid eyeball movement,

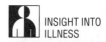

INSIGHT INTO ILLNESS

What causes cerebral palsy?

Prenatal problems
- Anoxia (lack of oxygen delivery to the central nervous system)
- Maternal infection (especially rubella)
- Radiation
- Toxic substances in the blood
- Maternal diabetes
- Abnormal placental attachment
- Malnutrition
- Blood incompatibility between mother and fetus

Difficulties during birth
- Forceps delivery
- Breech presentation
- Placenta previa (a disorder in which the placenta is implanted in the lower uterine segment)
- Placental abruption (premature separation of the placenta from the uterine wall)
- Effects of general or spinal anesthetic on the mother
- Prolapsed cord with delay in delivery of head
- Premature birth
- Prolonged or unusually rapid labor
- Multiple births

Problems in infancy
- Brain infection
- Head trauma
- Prolonged anoxia
- Problems in circulation to the brain
- Release of blood clots or other substances into the circulation

Helping your child with cerebral palsy

You'll need to help your child meet his or her basic needs. Here are some useful tips.

Communicate clearly

Speak slowly and distinctly. Encourage your child to speak. Listen patiently.

Ensure adequate nutrition

■ Provide an adequate diet to meet your child's energy needs.

■ During meals, maintain a quiet, unhurried atmosphere without distractions. Your child may need special utensils and a chair with a solid footrest. Teach your child to place food far back in the mouth to ease swallowing.

■ Encourage your child to chew food thoroughly, drink through a straw, and suck on lollipops to help develop muscle control needed to reduce drooling.

Promote independence

■ Let your child wash and dress independently, assisting only as needed. You may need to have clothing modified.

■ Give all care in an unhurried manner; otherwise, muscle spasticity may increase.

■ Set realistic goals.

■ Plan crafts and other activities for your child.

■ Be aware that your child needs to develop peer relationships. Avoid being overprotective.

muscle weakness, tremor, lack of leg movement during infancy, and a wide gait as the child begins to walk. Uncoordinated muscle movements make sudden or fine movements almost impossible.

How is it diagnosed?

Early diagnosis is essential for effective treatment and requires careful clinical observation during infancy and precise neurologic assessment. The doctor will suspect cerebral palsy whenever an infant:

■ has difficulty sucking or keeping the nipple or food in the mouth

■ seldom moves voluntarily or has arm or leg tremors with voluntary movement

■ crosses legs when lifted from behind rather than pulling them up or "bicycling" like a normal infant

■ has legs that are hard to separate, making diaper changing difficult

■ persistently uses only one hand or, as he or she gets older, uses hands well but not legs.

Infants at particular risk include those with low birth weight, low Apgar scores at 5 minutes (a normal score is expected after 1 minute), seizures, and metabolic disturbances. However, all infants should have a screening test for cerebral palsy as a regular part of their 6-month checkup.

How is it treated?

Cerebral palsy can't be cured, but proper treatment can help affected children reach their full potential within the limits set by this disorder. Such treatment requires a comprehensive and cooperative effort involving doctors; nurses; teachers; psychologists; the child's family; and occupational, physical, and speech therapists. Home care is often possible. (See *Helping your child with cerebral palsy.*) Treatment usually includes:

■ braces or splints and special appliances, such as adapted eating utensils and a low toilet seat with arms, to help these children perform activities independently

■ an artificial urinary sphincter for the incontinent child who can use the hand controls

■ range-of-motion exercises to minimize contractures

■ orthopedic surgery to correct contractures

■ Dilantin, Barbita, or other antiseizure drugs

■ muscle relaxants or neurosurgery, possibly, to decrease spasticity.

Children with milder forms of cerebral palsy should attend a regular school; severely afflicted children need special education classes.

ENCEPHALITIS

What is this condition?

In this disorder, a person develops severe inflammation and swelling of the brain. This disorder may produce only mild effects, or it may be severe, causing permanent neurologic damage and even death.

What causes it?

In rural areas, encephalitis is usually caused by a virus carried by a mosquito or a tick. However, the disorder may be transmitted by other means. For example, a person may get the disorder by accidentally inhaling or ingesting the virus — perhaps by drinking infected goat's milk.

In urban areas, encephalitis is most frequently caused by a group of viruses called *enteroviruses,* which infect the gastrointestinal tract and are discharged in feces. Encephalitis also may be caused by other types of viruses (herpesvirus, mumps virus, HIV, and adenoviruses). It may also result from diseases that destroy the protective sheath surrounding the nerves or spinal cord. Such diseases may occur following measles, chickenpox, rubella, or vaccination.

What are its symptoms?

All forms of encephalitis caused by viruses produce similar signs and symptoms, although certain differences do occur. Usually, the acute illness begins with sudden onset of fever, headache, and vomiting. Later, the person may experience neck and back stiffness. Many symptoms may result from physiologic changes to the brain and nervous system: drowsiness, coma, paralysis, seizures, inability to coordinate voluntary muscular movements and, possibly, psychotic behavior. After the acute phase of illness, coma may persist for days or weeks.

The severity of encephalitis symptoms varies greatly. Encephalitis caused by mosquito- or tick-borne virus may be so mild that it goes unnoticed, or it may be rapidly fatal. Encephalitis caused by herpesvirus also produces effects that range from mild illness to acute and potentially fatal disease. Severe disease may occur suddenly and with great intensity. (See *How to help a person with encephalitis,* page 124.)

How to help a person with encephalitis

If you're taking care of a family member or friend with encephalitis, here are some helpful things you can do.

Keep the surroundings quiet
- Encephalitis causes sensitivity to light and headaches. So, keep the person's room dark and quiet.
- If the person naps during the day and can't sleep at night, plan quiet daytime activities. That way, you'll minimize napping and promote restful sleep at night.

Give emotional support
- Remember, the person is probably frightened by the illness and frequent tests.
- Tell a dazed or confused person where he or she is and who you are. Keep a calendar and clock in the room.
- The effects of encephalitis usually disappear. However, if the person is suffering from the severe form of the disease, the effects can be permanent. If that happens, the person will need to attend a rehabilitation program after the worst phase of illness has passed.

How is it diagnosed?

During an encephalitis epidemic, diagnosis is made based on the person's signs and symptoms and health history. However, sporadic cases are difficult to distinguish from other illnesses that produce fever, such as gastroenteritis or meningitis (inflammation of the spinal cord and membranes). Testing for viral encephalitis includes blood studies, cerebrospinal fluid analysis, and inoculation of mice with a specimen taken from the person.

An electroencephalogram may show abnormalities in the brain's electrical activity. Occasionally, a computed tomography scan (commonly called a CAT scan) may be performed to rule out cerebral hematoma (a localized blood clot in the brain).

How is it treated?

The antiviral drug Avirax is effective in treating encephalitis caused by herpesvirus, but it does not work against encephalitis caused by other viruses. Treatment of all other forms of encephalitis addresses the effects of illness, but does not eliminate the causal viruses. Drug therapy includes antiseizure drugs such as Dilantin, usually administered intravenously; glucocorticoids to reduce cerebral inflammation and swelling; Lasix or Osmitrol to reduce cerebral swelling; sedatives for restlessness; and aspirin or Tylenol (or another drug with acetaminophen) to reduce fever.

Other treatment measures include making sure the person gets enough fluids and electrolytes to prevent dehydration and providing antibiotics to treat any associated infection, such as pneumonia.

EPILEPSY

What do doctors call this condition?
Seizure disorder

What is this condition?

Epilepsy is a brain condition that makes a person susceptible to recurrent seizures, sudden events linked to abnormal electrical discharges of nerve cells. Epilepsy probably affects 1% to 2% of the population. The prognosis is good if the person adheres strictly to the prescribed treatment.

What causes it?

In about half the cases, the cause is unknown. However, some possible causes of epilepsy include:

- birth trauma, such as inadequate oxygen supply to the brain, head injury, blood incompatibility between mother and newborn, or heavy bleeding; or infection shortly before, during, or just after birth
- infectious diseases (such as brain abscess or inflammation of membranes of the brain or spinal cord), inherited disorders (such as phenylketonuria), metabolic disorders (such as low blood sugar or underactive parathyroid glands), or degenerative disease
- ingestion of toxins (such as mercury, lead, or carbon monoxide)
- brain tumors or stroke.

What are its symptoms?

The hallmarks of epilepsy are recurrent seizures, which doctors classify as partial or generalized. Some people may have more than one type of seizure.

Partial seizures

Partial seizures arise from a specific part of the brain, causing distinctive symptoms. (In some people, partial seizure activity may spread to the entire brain, causing a generalized seizure.) Types of partial seizures include jacksonian and complex partial seizures.

A *jacksonian seizure* starts as a localized motor seizure, with abnormal activity spreading to nearby brain regions. Typically, one extremity stiffens or jerks, accompanied by a tingling sensation in the same area. The person seldom loses consciousness. A jacksonian seizure may progress to a generalized tonic-clonic seizure.

Symptoms of a *complex partial seizure* vary but usually include purposeless behavior. This seizure may start with an abnormal sensation, called an *aura,* felt immediately before the seizure. An aura marks the start of abnormal electrical discharges within a specific brain area. It may include an unusual smell or taste, nausea or indigestion, a rising or sinking feeling in the stomach, a dreamy feeling, or a visual disturbance. During the seizure, the person may have a glassy stare, pick at his or her clothes, wander aimlessly, smack his or her lips or make chewing motions, and speak unintelligibly. For several minutes after the seizure, the person may seem confused and appear psychotic or intoxicated with alcohol or drugs.

Epilepsy is a brain condition that makes a person susceptible to recurrent seizures, sudden events linked to abnormal electrical discharges of nerve cells. Epilepsy probably affects 1% to 2% of the population. In about half the cases, the cause is unknown.

How epilepsy can affect your lifestyle

People with epilepsy often have questions about their condition and its effect on their life. Three of their most commonly asked questions are answered below.

How will seizures interfere with my normal activities?
Once your seizures are under control, you'll be able to continue your normal activities — with some safety precautions. Avoid potentially dangerous activities when you're alone — for example, swimming or climbing the ladder to paint the house. If you drive, contact your state's motor vehicle department. Most states won't let you drive until you've been seizure-free for a certain period, possibly up to 1 year.

What will happen if I have a seizure in a public place?
To make sure you're cared for correctly, always wear a medical identification bracelet or necklace stating that you have a seizure disorder. This will alert others to your condition. If you feel a seizure coming on, find a safe spot and lie down. (Of course, you should be aware of your trigger factors and avoid them, if possible.)

Will I lose my job?
You shouldn't lose your job because you have epilepsy. If you're honest with your employer about your disorder, you're protected by the equal opportunity laws. However, keep in mind that your exact job description may change, depending on the position's requirements and on liability considerations.

Generalized seizures

As the name suggests, these seizures result from a generalized electrical abnormality within the brain. They include several distinct types.

Absence (petit mal) seizures are most common in children, although they can affect adults as well. Usually, they begin with a brief alteration of consciousness, indicated by blinking or rolling of the eyes, a blank stare, and slight mouth movements. The person appears frozen in position but, after the seizure ends, continues whatever he or she was doing before the seizure started. Typically, absence seizures last 1 to 10 seconds. If not properly treated, they can recur up to 100 times a day. An absence seizure may progress to a generalized tonic-clonic seizure.

A *generalized tonic-clonic (grand mal) seizure* typically starts with a loud cry as air rushes from the lungs through the vocal cords. The person then falls to the ground, losing consciousness. The body stiffens (*tonic phase*), then alternates between episodes of muscle spasm and relaxation (*clonic phase*). Tongue-biting, loss of bowel or bladder control, labored or absent breathing, and a bluish skin tinge may also occur. The seizure stops after 2 to 5 minutes when abnormal brain activity ends. The person then regains consciousness but is somewhat confused and may have trouble talking. If lucid, the individual may complain of drowsiness, fatigue, headache, muscle soreness, and arm or leg weakness, and then may fall into deep sleep.

In a *myoclonic seizure,* the person has brief, involuntary muscle jerks, which may occur in a rhythmic fashion.

In an *akinetic seizure,* posture becomes slack and the person briefly loses consciousness. This seizure, which occurs in young children, is sometimes called a *drop attack* because it causes the child to fall.

Status epilepticus

This continuous seizure state can occur in all seizure types. The most life-threatening form is generalized tonic-clonic status epilepticus, in which the person remains unconscious throughout. Status epilepticus is accompanied by respiratory distress.

Causes of this condition include abruptly stopping antiseizure drug therapy, brain disorders called *hypoxic* or *metabolic encephalopathy*, acute head trauma, or blood infection caused by inflammation of the brain or its membranes.

How is it diagnosed?

The doctor obtains diagnostic information from the person's history, descriptions of seizure activity, physical and neurologic exams, and the family history. A computed tomography scan (commonly called a CAT scan) or magnetic resonance imaging (commonly called an MRI) can provide density readings of the brain and may show abnormalities in internal structures.

An electroencephalogram (a recording of brain wave activity) can confirm the diagnosis by showing the continuing tendency to have seizures. (But a negative electroencephalogram doesn't rule out epilepsy because the brain wave changes are intermittent.)

Other tests may include blood sugar and blood calcium studies, lumbar puncture (sometimes called a spinal tap), skull X-rays, a brain scan, and cerebral angiography (an X-ray study of the brain's blood vessels).

How is it treated?

Generally, the person receives drug therapy specific to the type of seizure experienced. The most commonly prescribed drugs include Dilantin, Tegretol, Barbita, or Mysoline for generalized tonic-clonic seizures and complex partial seizures. Someone with absence seizures may receive Depakene, Klonopin, or Zarontin. Neurontin is a new antiseizure drug.

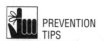 PREVENTION TIPS

Staying seizure-free

To help you avoid seizures, follow these tips.

Take medications
Take the *exact* dose of your anti-seizure medicine at the right times. Missing doses, doubling them, or taking extra ones can cause a seizure.

Eat right
- Eat balanced, regular meals. Low blood sugar levels and inadequate vitamin intake can lead to seizures.
- Check with your doctor to find out whether you may drink any alcohol.

Rest and relax
- Get enough sleep. Excessive fatigue can provoke a seizure.
- Learn to control stress, such as by using deep-breathing exercises and other relaxation techniques.

Control fevers
Treat a fever early during an illness. If you can't lower your fever, call your doctor.

Avoid triggers
Avoid known seizure triggers, such as flashing lights, breathing too quickly, loud noises, and video games. Stay alert for odors that also may trigger a seizure.

Responding to a seizure

Be aware of what to do and what not to do if a person with epilepsy experiences a seizure.

Generalized tonic-clonic seizures

Don't restrain the person. Help him or her to a lying position, loosen any tight clothing, and place something flat and soft (such as a pillow, jacket, or your hand) under the head. Clear the area of hard objects.

Don't force anything into the mouth if teeth are clenched—a tongue blade or spoon could tear the mouth and lips or displace teeth, causing respiratory distress. However, if the person's mouth is open, protect the tongue by placing a soft object (such as a folded cloth) between the teeth. Then turn the head to the side to provide an open airway. After the seizure subsides, provide reassurance, orient to time and place, and inform the person that he or she has had a seizure.

Complex partial seizures

Don't restrain the person during the seizure. Clear the area of hard objects. Prevent injury by gently calling the person's name and directing him or her away from any source of danger. After the seizure passes, provide reassurance as above.

Family members and caregivers must monitor a person taking antiseizure medication for signs of drug toxicity: involuntary eye movements, poor coordination, sluggishness, dizziness, drowsiness, slurred speech, irritability, nausea, and vomiting.

If drug therapy fails, the person may undergo surgery if diagnostic tests show that a specific part of the brain (called a focal lesion) is responsible for the seizures. In any case, family members and caregivers should be ready to respond if the person experiences a seizure. (See *Responding to a seizure.*)

The person with status epilepticus needs emergency treatment, which usually consists of Valium (or Ativan), Dilantin, or Barbita. If the seizures are caused by low blood sugar, the person will also receive dextrose 50% intravenously; if they're caused by chronic alcoholism or withdrawal, he or she will need an intravenous vitamin B_1 preparation.

What can a person with epilepsy do?

- Express your feelings about your condition.
- Be aware that most people with epilepsy can maintain a normal lifestyle, that epilepsy is not contagious, and that it can usually be controlled by following the prescribed drug regimen. (See *How epilepsy can affect your lifestyle,* page 126.)
- Be sure to comply with the prescribed drug regimen. Antiseizure drugs are safe when taken *as directed.* Keep track of the amount of medication left so you don't run out.
- Watch for the side effects of antiseizure drugs, which indicate that your dosage should be adjusted. They include drowsiness, sluggishness, hyperactivity, confusion, and visual and sleep disturbances. Report these side effects immediately.
- If you're taking Dilantin, practice conscientious oral hygiene to manage gum overgrowth.
- Have blood drawn for antiseizure drug levels at regular intervals, even if your seizures are under control.
- Drink alcoholic beverages in moderation or not at all. (See *Staying seizure-free,* page 127.)
- Contact the Epilepsy Foundation of America for general information. Call your state motor vehicle department for information about any driving restrictions.

FLUID IN THE BRAIN

What do doctors call this condition?
Hydrocephalus

What is this condition?
In this disorder, an excessive amount of cerebrospinal fluid — the fluid that bathes the brain and spinal cord — accumulates within the ventricular spaces of the brain. This condition occurs most often in newborns, but it can also occur in adults as a result of injury or disease. In infants, fluid in the brain enlarges the head, and in both infants and adults, the resulting compression can damage brain tissue.

With early detection and surgical intervention, the prognosis improves but remains guarded. Even after surgery, such complications as mental retardation, impaired motor function, and vision loss can persist. Without surgery, the prognosis is poor: death may result from increased intracranial pressure in persons of all ages; infants may also die prematurely of infection and malnutrition.

What causes it?
Fluid in the brain may result from an obstruction in the flow of cerebrospinal fluid (noncommunicating hydrocephalus) or from its faulty absorption (communicating hydrocephalus).

In *noncommunicating hydrocephalus*, the obstruction occurs most frequently between the third and fourth ventricles of the brain. This obstruction may result from faulty fetal development, infection (syphilis, granulomatous diseases, meningitis), a tumor, cerebral aneurysm, or a blood clot (after intracranial hemorrhage).

In *communicating hydrocephalus*, faulty absorption of cerebrospinal fluid may result from surgery to repair a myelomeningocele (protrusion of the spinal cord and its covering through a vertebral defect), adhesions between meninges at the base of the brain, or meningeal hemorrhage.

What are its symptoms?
In infants, the unmistakable sign of fluid in the brain is head enlargement clearly disproportionate to the infant's growth. Other characteristic changes include distended scalp veins; thin, shiny scalp skin;

and underdeveloped neck muscles. In severe cases, the roof of the eye orbit is depressed, the eyes are displaced downward, and the sclera (the white part of the eyes) are prominent. Other signs include a high-pitched, shrill cry; abnormal muscle tone of the legs; irritability; loss of appetite; and projectile vomiting.

In adults and older children, indicators of fluid in the brain include decreased level of consciousness, uncoordinated involuntary movements, incontinence, and impaired intellect.

How is it diagnosed?

In infants, head size that is abnormally large for the child's age strongly suggests fluid in the brain. Skull X-rays show thinning of the skull with separation of the sutures (fibrous joints of the skull) and widening of the fontanelles (soft spots).

Other diagnostic tests for fluid in the brain, including angiography, computed tomography scan (commonly called a CAT scan), and magnetic resonance imaging (commonly called an MRI), can differentiate between fluid in the brain and intracranial lesions.

How is it treated?

Surgical correction is the only treatment for fluid in the brain. Usually, such surgery consists of inserting a shunt (an artificial passage) to transport excess fluid from the lateral ventricle of the brain into the peritoneal cavity of the abdomen. A less common procedure is insertion of a shunt to drain fluid from the brain's lateral ventricle into the right atrium of the heart, which moves the fluid into the venous circulation.

Complications after shunt insertion include shunt infection or infection in the blood, septicemia, adhesions and paralytic ileus, peritonitis, and intestinal perforation.

What can parents of an infant with fluid in the brain do?

- Have your infant's growth and development checked periodically, and set goals consistent with the child's ability and potential. Focus on strengths, not weaknesses.
- Provide sensory stimulation appropriate for your child's age.
- Watch for signs of shunt malfunction, infection, and paralytic ileus. Be aware that a shunt requires periodic surgery to lengthen it as the child grows, to correct malfunctioning, or to treat infection.

GUILLAIN-BARRÉ SYNDROME

What do doctors call this condition?
Infectious polyneuritis, Landry's syndrome

What is this condition?
Guillain-Barré syndrome is an acute, rapidly progressive and potentially fatal form of polyneuritis that causes muscle weakness and mild distal sensory loss. This syndrome can occur at any age but is most common between ages 30 and 50; it affects both sexes equally.

Recovery is spontaneous and complete in about 95% of people, although mild motor or reflex loss in the feet and legs may persist. The prognosis is best when symptoms disappear between 15 and 20 days after onset.

What causes it?
Precisely what causes Guillain-Barré syndrome is unknown, but it may be a cell-mediated immunologic attack on peripheral nerves in response to a virus. This results in deterioration of the myelin sheath that covers the peripheral nerves. Because this syndrome causes inflammation and degenerative changes in both the posterior (sensory) and anterior (motor) nerve roots, signs of sensory and motor losses occur simultaneously. (See *How nerves degenerate in Guillain-Barré syndrome,* page 132.)

What are its symptoms?
About 50% of people with Guillain-Barré syndrome have a history of minor febrile illness, usually an upper respiratory tract infection or, less often, gastroenteritis. When infection occurs first, signs of infection subside before neurologic features appear. Other possible precipitating factors include surgery, rabies or swine influenza vaccination, viral illness, Hodgkin's lymphoma or some other malignant disease, and lupus.

Muscle weakness, the major neurologic sign, usually appears in the legs first (the ascending type), then extends upward to the arms and facial nerves in 24 to 72 hours. Sometimes, muscle weakness develops in the arms first (the descending type), or in the arms and legs simultaneously. In milder forms of this disease, muscle weakness may affect only the cranial nerves or may not occur at all.

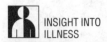

INSIGHT INTO
ILLNESS

How nerves degenerate in Guillain-Barré syndrome

Guillain-Barré syndrome can make you feel numb and weak and also can stop you from moving your arms and legs the way you want. That's because the disorder attacks the peripheral nerves — the nerves outside the brain and spinal cord — and prevents them from sending messages correctly to the brain.

What goes wrong
In Guillain-Barré syndrome, the nerve's covering, a thin myelin sheath, degenerates for unknown reasons. This sheath covers the nerve and conducts nerve impulses along the nerve pathways. With degeneration comes inflammation, swelling, and patchy loss of myelin. As Guillain-Barré syndrome destroys myelin, the nodes of Ranvier (at the junctures of the myelin sheaths) widen. This delays and impedes transmission of nerve impulses, causing tingling, numbness, and weakness.

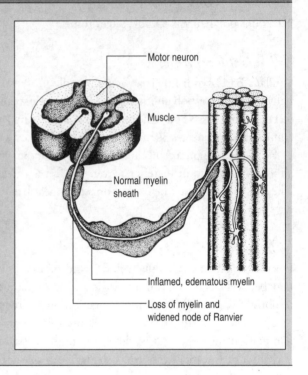

Motor neuron

Muscle

Normal myelin sheath

Inflamed, edematous myelin

Loss of myelin and widened node of Ranvier

Another common neurologic sign is numbness and tingling in the arms or legs, which sometimes precedes muscle weakness but tends to vanish quickly. However, some people with this disorder never develop this symptom. Other clinical features may include facial paralysis (possibly with ocular paralysis), difficulty swallowing or speaking and, less often, weakness of the muscles supplied by the 11th cranial nerve. Muscle weakness develops so quickly that muscle atrophy doesn't occur, but loss of muscle reflexes and tone do. Stiffness and pain in the form of a severe "charley horse" often occurs.

The clinical course of Guillain-Barré syndrome is divided into three phases. The *initial phase* begins when the first definitive symptom develops; it ends 1 to 3 weeks later when no further deterioration is noted. The *plateau phase* lasts several days to 2 weeks and is followed by the *recovery phase*, which is believed to coincide with regeneration of nerve fibers. The recovery phase lasts 4 to 6 months;

people with severe disease may take up to 2 years to recover, which may not be complete.

Significant complications of Guillain-Barré syndrome include respiratory failure, aspiration, pneumonia, sepsis, joint contractures, and deep vein thrombosis. Unexplained autonomic nervous system involvement may cause rapid or slow heart rate, high blood pressure, postural low blood pressure, or loss of bladder and bowel control.

How is it diagnosed?

A history of recent febrile illness (usually a respiratory tract infection) and typical clinical features suggest Guillain-Barré syndrome.

Several days after onset of signs and symptoms, the protein level of the cerebrospinal fluid (the fluid that bathes the brain and spinal cord) begins to rise, peaking in 4 to 6 weeks, probably as a result of widespread inflammatory disease of the nerve roots. The white blood cell count in cerebrospinal fluid remains normal, but, in severe disease, the pressure of this fluid may rise above normal.

Probably because of predisposing infection, a complete blood count initially shows leukocytosis and a shift to immature cell forms early in the illness, but blood studies soon return to normal. Electromyography may show repeated firing of the same motor unit, instead of widespread sectional stimulation. Nerve conduction velocities are slowed soon after paralysis develops. Diagnosis must rule out similar diseases, such as acute poliomyelitis.

How is it treated?

Treatment is primarily supportive, consisting of endotracheal intubation or tracheotomy if the person has difficulty clearing secretions.

Orasone may be tried if the course of the disease is relentlessly progressive. If Orasone produces no noticeable improvement after 7 days, the drug is discontinued. Plasmapheresis (removal and replacement of blood plasma to remove disease elements) is useful during the initial phase but offers no benefit if begun 2 weeks after onset.

What can a person recovering from Guillain-Barré syndrome do?

- Be sure to follow your doctor's instructions on the proper way to move from a bed to a wheelchair and from a wheelchair to a toilet or tub, and on how to walk short distances with a walker or cane.
- Maintain a regular bowel and bladder routine.

HEADACHE

The most common medical complaint, headache is usually a symptom of an underlying disorder. About 90% of headaches result from blood vessel disturbances, tension, or a combination of these factors.

What is this condition?

The most common medical complaint, headache is usually a symptom of an underlying disorder. About 90% of headaches result from vascular (blood vessel) disturbances, tension, or a combination of these factors; 10% result from disorders within the skull, diseases affecting the body as a whole, or psychological disorders.

Migraine headaches, probably the most intensively studied, are throbbing, vascular headaches that usually begin in childhood or adolescence and recur throughout adulthood. Affecting up to 10% of Americans, they're more common in women and tend to run in families.

What causes it?

Typically, a chronic headache results from tension, or muscle contraction, which may be caused by emotional stress, fatigue, menstruation, or environmental stimulation (such as noise, crowds, or bright lights). Other possible causes include glaucoma (elevated pressure in the eye that can lead to blindness); inflammation of the eyes or sinuses; diseases of the scalp, teeth, arteries in the head, or external or middle ear; and muscle spasms of the face, neck, or shoulders. In addition, headaches may be caused by drugs and other agents that dilate blood vessels, such as nitrates, alcohol, and histamine; diseases affecting the entire body; lack of oxygen in the blood, or high blood pressure; head trauma; or bleeding, abscess, aneurysm, and tumors in the brain.

The cause of migraine headache is unknown, but it's linked to constriction and dilation of arteries in the head. Researchers suspect that certain biochemical abnormalities occur during a migraine attack. These include leakage of a vessel-dilating substance called *neurokinin* through the arteries and a drop in the level of a chemical messenger in the brain, called *serotonin*.

Headache pain often arises from outside the skull; from the pain-sensitive structures of the skin, scalp, muscles, arteries, and veins of the head; or from the cranial or cervical nerves.

Within the skull, headache may result from pulling or displacement of arteries or veins, as well as inflammation or compression of the cranial nerves whose pain fibers lead to the brain and spinal cord.

What are its symptoms?

Both tension and vascular headaches may cause a dull, persistent ache; tender spots on the head and neck; and a feeling of tightness around the "hatband" area of the head. The pain is often severe and unrelenting. If caused by bleeding within the skull, the headache does not respond to narcotic pain medications and may progress to nervous system problems such as abnormal sensations and muscle weakness. If the headache results from a brain tumor, pain is most severe on awakening.

At first, migraine headache usually produces one-sided, pulsating pain, which later becomes more generalized. Often, the headache follows a striking visual sensation, or aura, in which a luminous object with zigzag outlines appears before the eyes. During the aura, the person's vision is obscured in half the visual field; the person may also experience abnormal sensations, such as prickling or tingling, on one side of the body, or speech disorders. The person may also experience irritability, appetite loss, nausea, vomiting, and abnormal sensitivity to light.

How is it diagnosed?

The doctor investigates the person's history of recurrent headaches, examines the head and neck, and conducts a complete nervous system exam. If the doctor suspects that the headache may be caused by a systemic disease (such as high blood pressure) or a psychosocial problem, the patient will be evaluated further.

Diagnostic tests may include skull X-rays, electroencephalography (a recording of brain-wave activity), computed tomography scan (commonly called a CAT scan) of the brain, and lumbar puncture (sometimes called a spinal tap).

How is it treated?

Depending on the type of headache, analgesics ranging from aspirin to codeine sulfate or Demerol may relieve symptoms. A tranquilizer such as Valium may help during acute attacks. For vascular headache, the doctor may include dietary instructions (see *Changing your diet to avoid vascular headaches,* page 136). The doctor will also try to identify and eliminate factors that cause headache and may recommend psychotherapy for headaches caused by emotional stress. For chronic tension headaches, muscle relaxants may be prescribed.

For migraine headache, Ergostat or Cafergot may be effective. These drugs and others work best when taken early in the course of

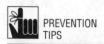

PREVENTION
TIPS

Changing your diet to avoid vascular headaches

By changing your diet, you can help prevent vascular headaches. That's because chemicals in certain foods act directly on blood vessels to trigger your headache. Here's a list to help you decide which foods to avoid and which ones are safe to eat.

For best results, plan a balanced diet from this list. Eat three or more small meals a day, and schedule meals at about the same time each day. Don't skip meals or fast.

FOOD GROUP	FOODS TO AVOID	FOODS TO ENJOY
Bread and cereal	• Hot, fresh homemade yeast bread, yeast coffee cake, sourdough bread, doughnuts • Bread or crackers containing cheese • Baked goods made with chocolate or nuts	• Bagels; crackers; English muffins; French or Italian, rye, white, or whole-wheat bread; melba toast • All cereals
Dairy products	• Cultured dairy products, such as buttermilk and sour cream • Chocolate milk • Bleu, brick, Camembert, cheddar, Gouda, mozzarella, Parmesan, provolone, Romano, Roquefort, Stilton, and Swiss (Emmentaler) cheeses	• Whole milk, 2% and 1% milk, skim milk • American, cottage, cream, farmer, and ricotta cheeses; processed and imitation cheeses • Yogurt (no more than ½ cup per day)
Meat, fish, and poultry	• Aged, canned, cured, or processed meat or fish, such as hot dogs, canned ham, pickled herring, cold cuts, and bacon • Meat prepared with meat tenderizer, soy sauce, or yeast extract	• All fresh or frozen beef, lamb, pork, poultry, and veal • Fresh and frozen fish • Eggs (no more than three per week)
Fruits and vegetables	• Apples, applesauce, apricots, avocados, cherries, figs, fruit cocktail, papaya, passion fruit, peaches, pears, raisins, and red plums • Broad, fava, lima, navy, pinto, or pole beans; garbanzos; lentils; olives; onions (except for seasoning); pickles; sauerkraut; snow peas	• All fruits and vegetables except those listed unless instructed otherwise by the doctor • Citrus fruit (limit to ½ cup per day)
Sweets and desserts	• Mincemeat pie • Cake, candy, cookies, ice cream, or pudding containing carob or chocolate	• Cake and cookies made without chocolate or yeast, gelatin, ice milk • Jam, jelly, hard candy, honey, sugar
Miscellaneous	• Bouillon cubes, canned soup, or soup base with monosodium glutamate (MSG) • Cheese sauce; snack foods and dishes containing cheese • Yeast and yeast extract, brewer's yeast • Meat tenderizer, MSG, seasoned salt, soy sauce (read labels) • Marinated, pickled, or preserved food • Nuts and seeds	• Cream soups made with permissible ingredients, homemade broth • Salt (in moderation), lemon juice • Butter, margarine, cooking oil • Whipped cream • White vinegar, commercial salad dressing in small amounts

an attack. If the person can't take these drugs by mouth because of nausea and vomiting, they may be taken as rectal suppositories.

Many doctors prefer Imitrex to treat acute migraine attacks or cluster headaches. Drugs that can help prevent migraine headache include Inderal, Tenormin, Catapres, and Elavil.

What can a person with a headache do?

Lie down in a dark, quiet room during an attack and place ice packs on your forehead or a cold cloth over your eyes. If you get vascular headaches, follow your doctor's dietary instructions.

If migraine is involved, take the prescribed medication at the *onset* of migraine symptoms. To prevent dehydration, drink plenty of fluids after migraine-related nausea and vomiting subside.

*H*UNTINGTON'S DISEASE

What do doctors call this condition?

Huntington's chorea, hereditary chorea, chronic progressive chorea, adult chorea

What is this condition?

Huntington's disease is a hereditary disease in which degeneration of the cerebral cortex and basal ganglia cause chronic progressive chorea (involuntary movements) and mental deterioration, ending in dementia. Huntington's disease usually strikes persons between ages 25 and 55 (the average age is 35); however, 2% of cases occur in children, and 5% as late as age 60. Death usually results 10 to 15 years after onset, from suicide, congestive heart failure, or pneumonia.

What causes it?

The cause of Huntington's disease is unknown. Because this disease is transmitted as a genetic trait common to men and women, either sex can transmit and inherit it. Each child of a parent with this disease has a 50% chance of inheriting it; however, the child who doesn't inherit it can't pass it on to his or her own children.

Each child of a parent with Huntington's disease has a 50% chance of inheriting the disease. The child who doesn't inherit it cannot pass it on to his or her own children.

Caring for the person with Huntington's disease

If you're taking care of someone with this disorder, here are some things you can do:
- Allow the person extra time to express himself or herself, thereby decreasing frustration.
- If the person has difficulty walking, provide a walker to help maintain balance.
- The disease can cause severe depression. So, stay alert for possible suicide attempts. Control the person's environment to prevent self-inflicted injury.
- If appropriate, seek genetic counseling. Each child of a parent with this disease has a 50% chance of inheriting it. For more information about this degenerative disease, contact the Huntington's Disease Association.

What are its symptoms?

Onset is insidious. The person eventually becomes totally dependent, emotionally and physically, through loss of musculoskeletal control. Gradually, the individual develops progressively severe choreic movements. Such movements are rapid, often violent, and purposeless. Initially, they appear on one side and are more prominent in the face and arms than in the legs. They progress from mild fidgeting to grimacing; tongue smacking; indistinct speech; slow, writhing movements (especially of the hands) related to emotional state; and contracted neck muscles.

Ultimately, the person with Huntington's disease develops dementia, although the dementia doesn't always progress at the same rate as the chorea. Dementia can be mild at first but eventually severely disrupts the personality. Such personality changes include obstinacy, carelessness, untidiness, moodiness, apathy, inappropriate behavior, loss of memory and concentration, and sometimes paranoia.

How is it diagnosed?

Huntington's disease can be detected by positron emission tomography and DNA analysis. Diagnosis is based on a characteristic clinical history: progressive chorea and dementia, onset in early middle age (35 to 40), and confirmation of a genetic link. Computed tomography scan (commonly called a CAT scan) and magnetic resonance imaging (commonly called an MRI) demonstrate brain atrophy. Molecular genetics may detect the gene for Huntington's disease in people at risk while they're still symptom-free.

How is it treated?

Because a cure for Huntington's disease has not yet been found, treatment is supportive, protective, and symptomatic. Tranquilizers, as well as antipsychotics such as Thorazine, Haldol, and Tofranil, help control choreic movements. They also relieve discomfort and depression, making the person easier to manage. However, tranquilizers increase rigidity and can't stop mental deterioration. Institutionalization is often necessary because of mental deterioration. (See *Caring for the person with Huntington's disease.*)

INFLAMMATION OF THE SPINAL CORD

What do doctors call this condition?
Myelitis, acute transverse myelitis

What is this condition?
Inflammation of the spinal cord can result from several diseases. Poliomyelitis, one form of spinal cord inflammation, affects the cord's gray matter and produces motor dysfunction; leukomyelitis affects only the white matter and produces sensory dysfunction.

Acute transverse spinal cord inflammation, which affects the entire thickness of the spinal cord, produces both motor and sensory dysfunctions. This condition develops rapidly and is the most devastating type of spinal cord inflammation.

The prognosis depends on the severity of cord damage and prevention of complications. If spinal cord tissue death occurs, the prognosis for complete recovery is poor. Even without tissue death, residual nervous system deficits usually persist after recovery.

What causes it?
Acute transverse spinal cord inflammation has many causes. It often follows acute infectious diseases, such as measles or pneumonia (the inflammation occurs after the infection has subsided), and primary infections of the spinal cord itself, such as syphilis or acute disseminated encephalomyelitis. Acute transverse spinal cord inflammation can accompany demyelinating diseases, such as acute multiple sclerosis, and inflammatory and necrotizing disorders of the spinal cord, such as hematomyelia.

Certain toxic agents (carbon monoxide, lead, and arsenic) can cause a type of spinal cord inflammation in which acute inflammation (followed by hemorrhage and possible necrosis) destroys the entire circumference of the spinal cord.

Other forms of spinal cord inflammation may result from poliovirus, herpes zoster, herpesvirus B, or rabies virus.

What are its symptoms?
In acute transverse spinal cord inflammation, onset is rapid, with motor and sensory dysfunctions below the level of spinal cord damage appearing in 1 to 2 days.

People with acute transverse spinal cord inflammation develop flaccid paralysis of the legs (sometimes beginning in just one leg) with loss of sensory and sphincter functions. Such sensory loss may follow pain in the legs or trunk. Reflexes disappear in the early stages but may reappear later. The extent of damage depends on the level of the spinal cord affected; transverse spinal cord inflammation rarely involves the arms. If spinal cord damage is severe, it may cause shock.

How is it diagnosed?

Paraplegia (paralysis of both legs) that develops suddenly usually points to acute transverse spinal cord inflammation. In these people, a neurologic exam confirms paraplegia or neurologic deficit below the level of the spinal cord lesion and also shows absent or, later, hyperactive reflexes. Cerebrospinal fluid may be normal or show increased lymphocytes or elevated protein levels.

Diagnostic evaluation must rule out spinal cord tumor and identify the cause of any underlying infection.

How is it treated?

No effective treatment exists for acute transverse spinal cord inflammation. However, this condition requires appropriate treatment of any underlying infection. Some people with postinfectious or multiple sclerosis-induced spinal cord inflammation have received corticosteroid therapy, but its benefits aren't clear.

LOU GEHRIG'S DISEASE

What do doctors call this condition?

Amyotrophic lateral sclerosis, ALS

What is this condition?

Lou Gehrig's disease is the most common of the motor neuron diseases causing muscular atrophy. Other motor neuron diseases include progressive muscular atrophy and progressive bulbar palsy. Onset occurs between ages 40 and 70. A chronic, progressively debilitating disease, Lou Gehrig's disease is rapidly fatal.

More than 30,000 persons have Lou Gehrig's disease; about 5,000 new cases are diagnosed each year, with men affected three times more often than women.

What causes it?

The exact cause of Lou Gehrig's disease is unknown, but about 5% to 10% of cases have a genetic component (an autosomal dominant trait) that affects men and women equally.

Lou Gehrig's disease and other motor neuron diseases may result from a slow-acting virus, nutritional deficiency related to a disturbance in enzyme metabolism, impaired nucleic acid production by the nerve fibers, or autoimmune disorders that affect immune complexes in the kidney's renal glomerulus and basement membrane.

Precipitating factors for acute deterioration include trauma, viral infections, and physical exhaustion.

What are its symptoms?

People with Lou Gehrig's disease develop small muscle contractions accompanied by muscle wasting and weakness, especially in the forearms and the hands. Other signs include impaired speech; difficulty chewing, swallowing, and breathing, particularly if the brain stem is affected; and, occasionally, choking and excessive drooling. Mental deterioration doesn't usually occur, but people may become depressed as a reaction to the disease. Progressive bulbar palsy may cause crying spells or inappropriate laughter.

Lou Gehrig's disease is the most common of the motor neuron diseases causing muscular atrophy. The disease strikes mostly men ages 40 to 70. It's progressively debilitating and rapidly fatal.

How is it diagnosed?

Characteristic signs and symptoms indicate a combination of upper and lower motor neuron involvement without sensory impairment. Electromyography and muscle biopsy help show nerve, rather than muscle, disease. Cerebrospinal fluid protein levels are increased in one-third of affected people, but this finding alone doesn't confirm Lou Gehrig's disease. Diagnosis must rule out multiple sclerosis, spinal cord tumor, polyarteritis, syringomyelia, myasthenia gravis, and progressive muscular dystrophy.

How is it treated?

No effective treatment exists for Lou Gehrig's disease. Management aims to control symptoms and provide emotional, psychological, and physical support. (See *Helping your loved one communicate without speech,* page 142.)

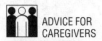

ADVICE FOR
CAREGIVERS

Helping your loved one communicate without speech

As Lou Gehrig's disease progresses, it may cause speech impairment. To prevent your loved one from becoming isolated, you'll need to find new ways to communicate, such as lipreading or using a communication board or a talking computer. Whichever method you choose, start to practice with the person before he or she must rely on it completely.

Lipreading
Although lipreading is one of the most effective ways to communicate without speech, it takes time and effort to learn.

Here are some tips to make lipreading easier:
- Tell your loved one to pause after forming each word with his or her lips. Then repeat the word aloud to make sure you understood it. If you can't make out the word, ask the person to spell it by forming each letter with his or her lips.
- Ask simple questions that require a yes-or-no answer. For example, ask "Would you like to sit outside now?" rather than "What do you feel like doing this afternoon?"
- Try to anticipate your loved one's needs so you can communicate more efficiently. Pay attention to nonverbal cues. For instance, if he or she looks bored or depressed while watching television, suggest a game of cards or visiting with a neighbor to cheer him or her up.

- Don't put words in the person's mouth. Give the person the opportunity to express himself or herself, even if it takes more time.

Communication boards
With a communication board, a person can express himself or herself by pointing to words, letters, pictures, or phrases on the board.

Communication boards come in various forms, including manual versions and ones that operate on a home computer. When using a communication board, remember the following:
- Make sure the person can see it clearly.
- Decide how the person will identify the figure or character on the board. If the person can't lift an arm to point, perhaps you can point. Or think about getting a special pointer that requires only slight hand or arm movement.
- Talk to a speech pathologist, who can help you decide which board best suits the person's needs and teach you how to use it.

Talking computers
If you own or wish to purchase a home computer, you may want to investigate "talking software." These programs provide a mechanical voice for the person with Lou Gehrig's disease, who controls the program through a computer keyboard.

MENINGITIS

What is this condition?
In this disorder, the brain and the spinal cord meninges become inflamed, usually as a result of bacterial infection. Such inflammation may involve all three meningeal membranes: the dura mater, the arachnoid, and the pia mater. The prognosis is good and complications are rare, especially if the disease is recognized early and the in-

fecting organism responds to antibiotics. However, the death rate in untreated disease is 70% to 100%. The prognosis is poorer for infants and elderly people.

What causes it?

Meningitis is almost always a complication of another bacterial infection: bacteremia (especially from pneumonia, pus in a body cavity, osteomyelitis, or endocarditis), sinus or middle ear infection, encephalitis, myelitis, or brain abscess.

This disorder may also follow skull fracture, a penetrating head wound, lumbar puncture, or ventricular shunt insertion. Aseptic inflammation of the brain and spinal cord membranes also may result from a virus or other organism. (See *What is aseptic meningitis?* page 144.) Sometimes, no causative organism can be found. Inflammation of the brain and spinal cord membranes may progress to congestion of adjacent tissues and destroy some nerve cells.

What are its symptoms?

The cardinal signs of this disorder are the same as those of infection (fever, chills, malaise) and of increased intracranial pressure (headache, vomiting and, rarely, swelling of the optic disk). Signs of meningeal irritation include rigidity at the nape of the neck, involuntary knee flexion when the neck is passively flexed, inability to extend the leg completely when sitting, exaggerated and symmetrical deep-tendon reflexes, and backward arching of the back and extremities so that the body rests on the head and heels.

Other symptoms are irregular heartbeats, irritability, extreme sensitivity to light, double vision and other visual problems, and delirium, deep stupor, and coma.

An infant may show signs of infection and is often fretful and refuses to eat. Such an infant may vomit a great deal, leading to dehydration.

As this disease progresses, twitching, seizures (in 30% of infants), or coma may develop. Most older children have the same symptoms as adults. In the subacute form, onset may be gradual.

How is it diagnosed?

A lumbar puncture (spinal tap), showing typical cerebrospinal fluid findings, and certain physical exam findings usually establish this diagnosis. The fluid may appear cloudy or milky white, depending on the number of white blood cells present. Protein levels in cerebrospi-

Meningitis is almost always a complication of another bacterial infection such as bacteremia, sinus or middle ear infection, encephalitis, myelitis, or brain abscess.

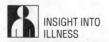
INSIGHT INTO
ILLNESS

What is aseptic meningitis?

This relatively harmless syndrome results from a virus, such as an enterovirus (most common), arbovirus, herpes simplex virus, mumps virus, or lymphocytic choriomeningitis virus.

How the syndrome starts
This syndrome starts suddenly, with a fever of up to 104° F (40° C), drowsiness, confusion, and neck or spine stiffness, which is slight at first. (This stiffness occurs when the person bends forward.) Other symptoms include headache, nausea, vomiting, stomach pain, vague chest pain, and a sore throat.

How the doctor forms a diagnosis
The doctor relies on the person's history of recent illness and knowledge of seasonal epidemics to identi-

fy this syndrome. Negative bacterial cultures and a spinal fluid analysis suggest this diagnosis. To confirm it, however, the doctor must isolate the virus from spinal fluid.

How the syndrome is treated
Treatment includes bed rest, measures to maintain fluid and electrolyte balance, pain-relieving drugs, and exercises to combat residual weakness. To prevent spreading the disease, the person and caregivers must wash their hands thoroughly and often.

nal fluid tend to be high; sugar levels may be low. (In subacute disease, fluid findings may vary.) Cerebrospinal fluid culture and sensitivity tests usually identify the infecting organism unless it's a virus.

To help determine the major sites of infection, the doctor will take cultures of the blood, urine, and nose and throat secretions; a chest X-ray; and an electrocardiogram. An abnormally high level of white blood cells and electrolyte abnormalities also are common. Computed tomography (commonly called a CAT scan) can rule out brain hematoma, hemorrhage, or tumor.

How is it treated?

To treat this disorder, the person receives appropriate antibiotic therapy and vigorous supportive care. Usually, intravenous antibiotics are given for at least 2 weeks, followed by oral antibiotics. Such antibiotics include Bicillin, Omnipen, or Nafcil. However, if the person is allergic to penicillin, Chloromycetin or Kantrex may be given. Other drugs include a cardiac glycoside such as Lanoxin to control irregular heartbeats, Osmitrol to decrease brain swelling, an antiseizure drug (usually given intravenously) or a sedative to reduce restlessness, and aspirin or Tylenol (or another acetaminophen product) to relieve headache and fever.

Supportive measures include bed rest, reduction of body temperature, and measures to prevent dehydration. The person must be isolated if the nasal cultures are positive for certain organisms. Of course, treatment includes appropriate therapy for any coexisting conditions, such as pneumonia.

MULTIPLE SCLEROSIS

What is this condition?

Multiple sclerosis (MS) is a progressive disease caused by demyelination (loss of myelin sheath material, essential in nerve impulse transmission) in the white matter of the brain and the spinal cord. In this disease, sporadic patches of demyelination throughout the central nervous system induce widely disseminated and varied neurologic dysfunction. Characterized by flare-ups and remissions, MS is a major cause of chronic disability in young adults. (See *How MS affects the body,* page 146.)

The prognosis is variable. MS may progress rapidly, disabling the person by early adulthood or causing death within months of onset. However, 70% of people with MS lead active, productive lives with prolonged remissions.

What causes it?

The exact cause of MS is unknown, but current theories suggest a slow-acting or latent viral infection and an autoimmune response. Other theories suggest that environmental and genetic factors may also be linked to MS.

Emotional stress, overwork, fatigue, pregnancy, and acute respiratory infections have been known to precede the onset of this illness. (See *How MS affects childbearing and birth control,* page 147.)

MS usually begins between ages 20 and 40 (the average age of onset is 27). It affects three women for every two men and five whites for every black. Incidence is low in Japan; it is generally higher among urban populations and upper socioeconomic groups. A family history of MS and living in a cold, damp climate increase the risk.

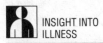

INSIGHT INTO
ILLNESS

How MS affects the body

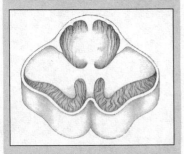

This view of the spine shows a partial loss of myelin, the white matter that covers nerve fibers. Myelin loss, which is characteristic of MS, is called *demyelination.*

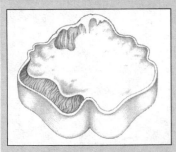

In this illustration, the loss of myelin is nearly complete. Symptoms of MS depend on the extent of demyelination.

What are its symptoms?

Clinical findings in MS depend on the extent and site of myelin destruction, the extent of remyelination, and how well the restored nerves can transmit impulses.

Signs and symptoms in MS may come and go quickly, or they may last for hours or weeks. They may wax and wane with no predictable pattern, vary from day to day, and be bizarre and difficult for the person to describe. In most people, visual problems and sensory impairment, such as numbness and tingling sensations, are the first signs that something may be wrong.

Other characteristic changes include the following:
- *eye disturbances* — inflamed optic nerve, double vision, blurred vision, paralysis of the eye's motor nerves, and rapid eyeball movement
- *muscle dysfunction* — weakness, paralysis of one or more limbs, spasticity, hyperreflexia, tremor, and uncoordinated gait
- *urinary disturbances* — incontinence, frequency, urgency, and frequent infections
- *emotional lability* — mood swings, irritability, euphoria, or depression.

Associated signs and symptoms include poorly articulated or scanning speech and difficulty swallowing. Clinical effects may be so mild that the person is unaware of them or so bizarre that the individual appears hysterical.

How is it diagnosed?

Because early symptoms may be mild, years may elapse between the first signs of MS and its diagnosis. Diagnosis requires evidence of multiple neurologic attacks and characteristic remissions and flare-ups. Magnetic resonance imaging (commonly called an MRI) may detect MS lesions; however, diagnosis remains difficult. Periodic testing and close observation of the person are necessary, perhaps for years, depending on the course of the disease. Diagnosis also may include a psychological evaluation.

Electroencephalograms (recordings of brain-wave activity) are abnormal in one-third of people with MS. Lumbar puncture (spinal tap) shows elevated gamma globulin levels but normal total cerebrospinal fluid proteins. Elevated levels of gamma globulin in cerebrospinal fluid are significant only when contrasted with normal serum gamma globulin levels, and reflects hyperactivity of the immune system from chronic demyelination.

STRAIGHT
TALK

How MS affects childbearing and birth control

People with MS often have questions about sex, birth control, and having children. Here are answers to some common questions.

Will MS keep me from having children?

MS doesn't affect your reproductive capabilities, but before deciding to have children, consider carefully the physical and financial changes MS will make in your life. For example, you may find that emotional, motor, vision, and speech changes dampen your enthusiasm to become a parent. You may also discover that the health care costs accompanying MS limit your financial ability to provide for children.

Now that I have MS, my husband and I have decided not to have children. What birth control method should I use?

The one or ones that suit your physical abilities and personal preferences. For example, if you have little uterine sensation, avoid an intrauterine device because you may not feel the pain or cramping that signal infection or perforation. If your mobility decreases, don't use oral contraceptives because these drugs may increase your risk of blood clots in your veins. If you're positive you don't want children, talk to your doctor about tubal ligation.

Before my fiancé got MS, he used a condom whenever we had sex. Now he says he won't use this method. What can I do?

You could ask your doctor about prescribing oral contraceptives, an intrauterine device, or a diaphragm for you. You might consider using a female condom, contraceptive foams, or jellies. But don't overlook the possibility that your fiancé has diminished hand function and genital sensation that makes it difficult to use a condom. If so, perhaps you could offer to help him apply the device.

Differential diagnosis must rule out spinal cord compression, foramen magnum tumor (may mimic the flare-ups and remissions of MS), multiple small strokes, syphilis or other infection, and psychological disturbances.

How is it treated?

The aim of treatment is to diminish flare-ups and relieve neurologic deficits so that the person can resume a normal lifestyle. Corticotropin (ACTH), Orasone, or Decadron is used to reduce swelling of the myelin sheath during flare-ups. ACTH and corticosteroids may relieve symptoms and hasten remission but don't prevent future flare-ups.

Other drugs used with ACTH and corticosteroids include Librium to minimize mood swings, Lioresal or Dantrium to relieve spasticity, and Urecholine or Ditropan to relieve urine retention and minimize urinary frequency and urgency. Betaseron may be used for ambulatory people with relapsing-remitting MS to reduce the frequency of flare-ups. Immunosuppressants, such as Imuran or Cytoxan, may suppress the immune response. During acute flare-ups, supportive measures include bed rest, massages, avoiding fatigue, preventing pressure ulcers, bowel and bladder training (if necessary), administering antibiotics for bladder infections, physical therapy, and counseling.

What can a person with MS do?

- Avoid stress, fatigue, and exposure to people with infections. Rest often, if necessary, and exercise daily.
- To help maintain your independence, develop new ways to perform daily activities.
- Eat a nutritious, well-balanced, high-fiber diet and drink plenty of fluids to prevent constipation. Use suppositories if necessary.
- Be aware that flare-ups are unpredictable, requiring physical and emotional adjustments in lifestyle.
- For more information, contact the National Multiple Sclerosis Society.

MYASTHENIA GRAVIS

What is this condition?

Myasthenia gravis produces sporadic but progressive weakness and abnormal fatigue of skeletal muscles, which is exacerbated by exercise and repeated movement but improved by anticholinesterase drugs. Usually, this disorder affects muscles controlled by the cranial nerves (face, lips, tongue, neck, and throat), but it can affect any muscle group.

Myasthenia gravis follows an unpredictable course of recurring flare-ups and periodic remissions. There's no known cure. However, drug treatment has improved the prognosis and allows people to lead relatively normal lives except during flare-ups. When the disease involves the respiratory system, it may be life-threatening.

What causes it?

Myasthenia gravis causes a failure in transmission of nerve impulses at the neuromuscular junction. Theoretically, such impairment may result from an autoimmune response, or dysfunctional neurotransmitter activity.

Myasthenia gravis strikes 1 in 25,000 people of all age-groups, but incidence peaks between ages 20 and 40. It is three times more common in women than in men, but after age 40, it appears equally in both sexes. About 20% of infants born to myasthenic mothers have transient (or occasionally persistent) myasthenia. This disease may coexist with immune system and thyroid disorders; about 15% of people with myasthenia gravis have thymoma (a tumor formed by thymus gland tissue). Remissions occur in about 25% of people with this disease.

What are its symptoms?

The dominant symptoms of myasthenia gravis are skeletal muscle weakness and fatigability. In the early stages, easy fatigability of certain muscles may appear with no other findings. Later, it may be severe enough to cause paralysis. Typically, the muscles are strongest in the morning but weaken throughout the day, especially after exercise. Short rest periods temporarily restore muscle function. Muscle weakness is progressive; eventually some muscles may lose function entirely. Resulting symptoms depend on the muscle group affected; they become more intense during menstrual periods and after emotional stress, prolonged exposure to sunlight or cold, or infections.

Onset may be sudden or insidious. In many people, weak eye closure, drooping eyelids, and double vision are the first signs that something is wrong. People with myasthenia gravis usually have blank and expressionless faces and a nasal voice. They experience frequent nasal regurgitation of fluids and have difficulty chewing and swallowing. Because of this, they often worry about choking. They may also have difficulty breathing. (See *Undergoing respiratory function tests*.) Because their eyelids droop, they may have to tilt their heads back to see. Their neck muscles may become too weak to support their heads without bobbing.

People with myasthenic crisis (sudden development of respiratory distress) are predisposed to pneumonia and other respiratory tract infections. This situation may be severe enough to require an emergency airway and mechanical ventilation.

How is it diagnosed?

Muscle fatigue that improves with rest strongly suggests a diagnosis of myasthenia gravis. Tests for this neurologic condition record the effect of exercise and subsequent rest on muscle weakness. Electro-

Undergoing respiratory function tests

Before you take these tests, you should tell the nurse or respiratory therapist whether you feel especially tired or have just eaten or expended energy, because these activities will affect your test results.

Vital capacity test
This test measures lung capacity (the maximum amount of air a person can breathe in and out), allowing the doctor to evaluate muscle effort and expansion. You'll be asked to blow out all the air in your lungs, breathe in as deeply as you can, and then blow out all the air you can.

Tidal volume test
This test measures the volume of air you breathe in and out normally. You'll be asked to breathe normally through a tube. Then the nurse or respiratory therapist will measure the amount of air you breathe in and out with each average, normal breath.

Negative inspiratory force test
This test measures the pressure created when you take a deep breath. You'll be instructed to breathe in through a device as hard as you can.

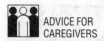
ADVICE FOR
CAREGIVERS

When to get help

For many people with myasthenia gravis, symptoms usually remain under control. Sometimes, though, they may need immediate medical attention if their condition worsens suddenly. Such an episode may involve severe muscle weakness that affects breathing. It's called *myasthenic crisis.*

What can trigger a crisis?

Emotional stress, infection, surgery, or accidental injury can cause a crisis. A change in or an overdose of medicine can also lead to extreme weakness. Then, if the weakness becomes severe enough, the person may experience a crisis that can affect the whole body.

Warning symptoms

If the person in your care has any of the following symptoms — especially if they occur within 1 hour after taking medicine — call the doctor or go to the nearest hospital emergency department at once:

- blurred vision
- difficulty breathing, chewing, or swallowing
- difficulty speaking or pronouncing words
- inability to cough
- increased secretion of saliva
- twitching around the mouth or eyes
- nausea and vomiting
- pounding or fluttering heartbeat
- muscle spasms
- severe stomach cramps or diarrhea
- severe weakness in any muscle
- cold, moist skin and sweating
- extreme restlessness or anxiety
- confusion
- seizures
- fainting.

myography, with repeated nerve stimulation, may help confirm this diagnosis.

The classic proof of myasthenia gravis is improved muscle function after an intravenous injection of Tensilon or Prostigmin. In people with myasthenia gravis, muscle function improves within 30 to 60 seconds after drug administration and lasts up to 30 minutes. However, long-standing eye muscle dysfunction may fail to respond to such testing. This test can differentiate a myasthenic crisis from a cholinergic crisis (caused by acetylcholine overactivity at the neuromuscular junction). Evaluation should rule out thyroid disease and thymoma.

How is it treated?

Treatment aims to minimize symptoms. Anticholinesterase drugs, such as Prostigmin and Mestinon, counteract fatigue and muscle weakness and allow about 80% of normal muscle function. However, these drugs become less effective as the disease worsens. Corticosteroids may relieve symptoms. Plasmapheresis (filtering of disease elements from the plasma) is used in severe flare-ups.

People with thymomas require removal of the thymus gland, which may cause remission in some cases of adult-onset myasthenia gravis. Acute flare-ups that cause severe respiratory distress require emergency treatment. Tracheotomy, positive-pressure ventilation, and vigorous suctioning to remove secretions usually produce improvement in a few days. Because anticholinesterase drugs aren't effective in myasthenic crisis, they're stopped until respiratory function improves. Myasthenic crisis requires immediate hospitalization and vigorous respiratory support. (See *When to get help* and *Coping with myasthenia gravis*.)

PARKINSON'S DISEASE

What do doctors call this condition?

Parkinsonism, paralysis agitans, shaking palsy

What is this condition?

Named for James Parkinson, the English doctor who wrote the first accurate description of the disease in 1817, Parkinson's disease produces progressive muscle rigidity, loss or absence of voluntary motion (akinesia), and involuntary tremors. Deterioration progresses for an average of 10 years, at which time death usually results from aspiration pneumonia or some other infection.

One of the most common crippling diseases in the United States, Parkinson's disease affects men more often than women, and strikes 1 in every 100 people over age 60. Because of increased longevity, this amounts to roughly 60,000 new cases diagnosed annually in the United States alone.

What causes it?

Although the cause of Parkinson's disease is unknown, studies of the brain have established that a deficiency of a neurotransmitter, dopamine, prevents brain cells from performing their normal function within the central nervous system.

 SELF-HELP

Coping with myasthenia gravis

Follow these guidelines to help you cope with your condition.

Balance activity and rest

- Plan daily activities to coincide with your energy peaks. Rest often throughout the day.
- Avoid strenuous exercise, stress, and needless exposure to the sun or cold weather. All of these things may worsen your symptoms.

Spot side effects

Learn to recognize drug side effects: sweating, stomach cramps, nausea, vomiting, diarrhea, and excessive saliva. Call your doctor if any of these symptoms develop.

Compensate for changes

- Expect to have periodic remissions, flare-ups, and day-to-day fluctuations. These are common.
- If you have double vision, wear an eye patch or glasses with one frosted lens.

Look ahead

For more information and an opportunity to meet people with myasthenia gravis who lead full, productive lives, contact the Myasthenia Gravis Foundation.

What are its symptoms?

The cardinal symptoms of Parkinson's disease are muscle rigidity and akinesia and an insidious tremor that begins in the fingers (unilateral "pill-roll" tremor), increases during stress or anxiety, and decreases with purposeful movement and sleep. Muscle rigidity results in resistance to passive muscle stretching, which may be uniform or jerky.

Akinesia causes the person with Parkinson's disease to walk with difficulty, either bent backward or falling forward. (See *Keeping your balance*.)

Akinesia also produces a high-pitched, monotone voice; drooling; a masklike facial expression; loss of posture control; and difficulty swallowing or speaking (or both). Occasionally, the person's eyes are fixed upward, with involuntary tonic movements, or the eyelids are completely closed. Parkinson's disease itself doesn't impair the intellect, but a coexisting disorder, such as arteriosclerosis, may do so.

How is it diagnosed?

Lab tests are not usually helpful in identifying Parkinson's disease, so the diagnosis is based on the person's age and history, and the characteristic clinical picture of the disease. However, a urinalysis may support the diagnosis by revealing decreased dopamine levels. A conclusive diagnosis is possible only after ruling out involutional depression, cerebral arteriosclerosis, other causes of tremor and, in people under age 30, intracranial tumors, Wilson's disease, or toxicity from phenothiazine or other drugs.

How is it treated?

Because there's no cure for Parkinson's disease, the primary aim of treatment is to relieve symptoms and keep the person functional as long as possible. Treatment consists of drugs, physical therapy and, in severe cases unresponsive to drugs, neurosurgery.

Drug therapy usually includes Larodopa, a dopamine replacement that's most effective during early stages of the disease. It's given in increasing doses until symptoms are relieved or side effects appear. Because side effects can be serious, a combination drug — Sinemet—is frequently given. When Larodopa proves unsuitable, alternative drug therapy includes anticholinergics, such as Artane; antihistamines, such as Benadryl; and Symmetrel, an antiviral agent. Eldepryl, an enzyme-inhibiting agent, allows conservation of dopamine and enhances the therapeutic effect of Larodopa.

SELF-HELP

Keeping your balance

If you have Parkinson's disease, walking with a wide-based gait and swinging your arms will help you to maintain balance and keep moving forward. (It helps to look ahead when walking and not at your feet.) Use the following step-by-step guidelines to practice this technique:
- Start by positioning your feet 8 to 10 inches (20 to 25 centimeters) apart. Stand as straight as you can.
- Now lift your foot high with your toes up, taking as large a step as possible.

- As you bring your foot down, place your heel on the ground first and roll onto the ball of your foot and then your toes. Perform the same steps with the other foot, as shown below. Repeat these movements.
- Swing your right arm forward when moving your left leg. Swing your left arm forward when moving your right leg.

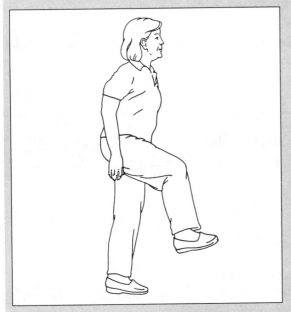
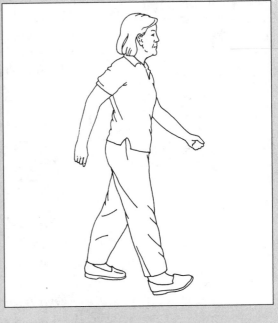

When drug therapy fails, stereotactic neurosurgery may be an alternative. In this procedure, electrical coagulation, freezing, radioactivity, or ultrasound is used to inactivate a small, specific portion of the brain to prevent involuntary movement. This is most effective in young, otherwise healthy people with unilateral tremor or muscle rigidity. However, neurosurgery can only relieve symptoms.

Individually planned physical therapy complements drug treatment and neurosurgery to maintain normal muscle tone and function.

SELF-HELP

Making eating more enjoyable

If you have Parkinson's disease, you may have difficulty eating. To help manage this problem, follow these suggestions:
- Keep your food on a warming tray, especially if you eat slowly.
- Keep an extra supply of napkins on hand during meals to absorb excess saliva.
- Use an arm brace to steady your hand if you have severe tremors.
- Use flexible straws or cups with lid spouts, such as travel cups.
- Use utensils with built-up handles that provide a better grip.

What can a person with Parkinson's disease do?

- If you have difficulty eating, eat frequent small meals to increase your caloric intake. (See *Making eating more enjoyable*.)
- To help establish a regular bowel elimination routine, drink plenty of fluids and eat high-fiber foods.
- If you have trouble moving from a standing to a sitting position, consider installing an elevated toilet seat.
- If you have excessive tremors, you may achieve partial control of your body by sitting on a chair and using its arms to steady yourself.
- Remember that fatigue may cause you to depend more on others.
- As instructed by your doctor, use proper positioning to help prevent bed sores and contractures.
- If you're taking Larodopa, follow your doctor's instructions on which foods to avoid (such as multivitamin preparations and fortified cereals).
- Take household safety measures to prevent accidents.
- For more information, contact the National Parkinson Foundation or the United Parkinson Foundation.

PERIPHERAL NERVE DEGENERATION

What do doctors call this condition?

Multiple neuritis, peripheral neuritis, peripheral neuropathy, polyneuritis

What is this condition?

This disorder involves degeneration of peripheral nerves supplying the distal muscles of the extremities. It results in muscle weakness with sensory loss and atrophy as well as decreased or absent deep tendon reflexes. Although peripheral nerve degeneration can occur at any age, incidence is highest in men between ages 30 and 50. Because onset is usually subtle, a person may compensate by overusing unaffected muscles; however, the disease may begin rapidly with severe infection and chronic alcohol intoxication. If the cause can be identified and eliminated, the prognosis is good.

What causes it?

Causes of peripheral nerve degeneration include:

- chronic intoxication (with ethyl alcohol, arsenic, lead, carbon disulfide, benzene, phosphorus, and sulfonamides)
- infectious diseases (meningitis, diphtheria, syphilis, tuberculosis, pneumonia, and mumps)
- metabolic and inflammatory disorders (gout, diabetes, rheumatoid arthritis, polyarteritis nodosa, and lupus)
- nutritional disorders (beriberi and other vitamin deficiencies, and malnourishment).

What are its symptoms?

The signs and symptoms of peripheral nerve degeneration develop slowly, and the disease usually affects the motor and sensory nerve fibers. The condition typically produces flaccid paralysis, wasting, loss of reflexes, pain of varying intensity, loss of ability to perceive vibratory sensations, and numbness, tingling, increased sensitivity to pain or touch, or anesthesia in the hands and feet. Deep-tendon reflexes are diminished or absent, and atrophied muscles are tender or hypersensitive to pressure or palpation. Footdrop may also be present. Skin manifestations include glossy red skin and decreased sweating. Many people with the disease have a history of clumsiness and complain of frequent vague sensations.

How is it diagnosed?

The person's history and physical exam reveal characteristic distribution of motor and sensory deficits. Electromyography may show a delayed action potential if peripheral nerve degeneration impairs motor nerve function.

How is it treated?

Effective treatment consists of supportive measures to relieve pain, adequate bed rest, and physical therapy, as needed. Most important, however, the underlying cause must be identified and corrected. For instance, it's essential to identify and remove the toxic agent, correct nutritional and vitamin deficiencies (the person needs a high-calorie diet rich in vitamins, especially the B-complex group), or counsel the person to avoid alcohol.

What can a person with peripheral nerve degeneration do?

- Rest frequently and avoid using the affected arm or leg. To avoid bed sores, use a foot cradle. To prevent contractures, use splints, boards, braces, or other orthopedic appliances.
- After the pain subsides, passive range-of-motion exercises or massage may be beneficial. The doctor may recommend electrotherapy for nerve and muscle stimulation.

REYE'S SYNDROME

What is this condition?

Reye's syndrome is an acute childhood illness that causes fatty infiltration of the liver with increased blood ammonia levels, encephalopathy (degenerative disease of the brain), and increased intracranial pressure. In addition, fatty infiltration of the kidneys, brain, and heart muscle may occur.

Reye's syndrome affects children from infancy to adolescence and occurs equally in boys and girls. It affects whites over age 1 more often than blacks.

The prognosis depends on the severity of central nervous system depression. Previously, the mortality rate was as high as 90%. Today, however, early detection and treatment of increased intracranial pressure, along with other treatment measures, have cut mortality to about 20%. Death is usually a result of brain swelling or respiratory arrest. Comatose children who survive may have residual brain damage.

What causes it?

Reye's syndrome almost always follows within 1 to 3 days of an acute viral infection, such as an upper respiratory infection, type B influenza, or chickenpox. Incidence often rises during flu outbreaks and may be linked to aspirin use. (See *Guarding against Reye's syndrome.*)

In this disorder, damaged liver cells disrupt the urea cycle, which normally changes ammonia to urea for its excretion from the body. This results in high blood ammonia and low blood sugar levels and an increase in serum short-chain fatty acids, leading to encephalopathy. Simultaneously, fatty infiltration is found in kidney cells, brain tissue, and muscle tissue, including the heart.

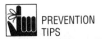

PREVENTION
TIPS

Guarding against Reye's syndrome

Although Reye's syndrome affects fewer than 3 children of every 100,000 who've had the flu, it's extremely serious. Linked to viral illnesses, such as chickenpox, the flu, and measles, and aspirin use in children under age 18, the disorder causes liver changes, brain swelling, heart damage, coma and, sometimes, death.

No cure for Reye's syndrome exists, so early detection and treatment are crucial. Statistics show that the death rate from this condition drops dramatically if treatment starts early.

Avoiding aspirin
To help prevent Reye's syndrome, avoid giving aspirin to your child if he or she has the flu, measles, or chickenpox. Scrutinize the labels of over-the-counter cold or flu remedies to make sure they don't contain aspirin (also known as ASA or acetylsalicylic acid). To control fever or to ease flu-related achiness, give your child an aspirin substitute, such as acetaminophen (Tylenol).

What to watch for
Seek medical attention at once if your child has these warning signs of Reye's syndrome:
- vomiting
- violent headaches
- listlessness
- irritability
- delirium
- disturbed breathing
- stiff arms and legs
- coma.

What are its symptoms?

The severity of the child's signs and symptoms varies with the degree of encephalopathy and brain swelling. In any case, Reye's syndrome develops in five stages: After the initial viral infection, a brief recovery period follows when the child doesn't seem seriously ill. A few days later, he or she develops intractable vomiting; lethargy; rapidly changing mental status (mild to severe agitation, confusion, irritability, delirium); rising blood pressure, respiratory rate, and pulse rate; and hyperactive reflexes.

Reye's syndrome often progresses to coma. As the coma deepens, seizures develop, followed by decreased tendon reflexes and, frequently, respiratory failure.

How is it diagnosed?

A history of a recent viral disorder with typical clinical features strongly suggests Reye's syndrome. An increased blood ammonia level, abnormal clotting studies, and evidence of liver dysfunction confirm it. Testing the serum salicylate level rules out aspirin overdose.

Absence of jaundice despite increased liver transaminase levels rules out acute liver failure and other liver diseases.

How is it treated?

Treatment depends on the disease stage. During the early stages, the child typically receives intravenous fluids and a diuretic to decrease intracranial pressure and brain swelling. He or she may also receive vitamin K or fresh frozen plasma. During the middle stage, typified by coma, the doctor may insert a device into the skull to monitor intracranial pressure, and may also start mechanical ventilation and prescribe intravenous Osmitrol. For deepening coma, some pediatric centers use barbiturate coma, decompressive craniotomy, hypothermia, or exchange transfusion.

To prevent Reye's syndrome, parents should give their children nonsalicylate analgesics and antipyretics, such as Tylenol or other drugs containing acetaminophen, instead of aspirin products.

SPINAL CORD DEFECTS

What do doctors call these conditions?

Spina bifida, meningocele, myelomeningocele

What are these conditions?

Defective neural tube closure in the embryo during the first trimester of pregnancy causes various spinal malformations. Generally, these defects occur in the lumbosacral area, but they are occasionally found in the sacral, thoracic, and cervical areas.

Spina bifida occulta is the most common and least severe spinal cord defect. Although one or more vertebrae fail to close completely, the spinal cord or meninges (membranes covering the brain and spinal cord) do not protrude.

However, in more severe forms of spina bifida, incomplete closure of one or more vertebrae causes the spinal contents to protrude and form an external sac or cystic lesion. In *spina bifida with meningocele,* this sac contains meninges and cerebrospinal fluid. In *spina bifida with myelomeningocele*, this sac contains meninges, cerebrospinal fluid, and a portion of the spinal cord or nerve roots distal to the conus medullaris. (See *Types of spinal cord defects.*)

In the United States, approximately 12,000 infants each year are born with some form of spina bifida.

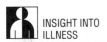
INSIGHT INTO
ILLNESS

Types of spinal cord defects

MENINGOCELE

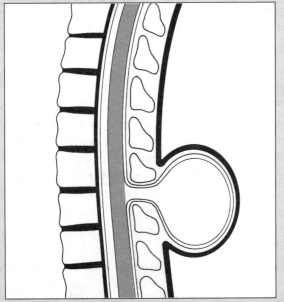

MYELOCELE

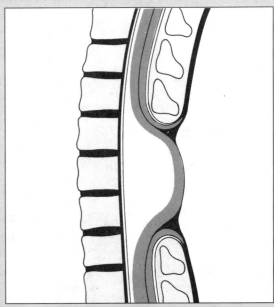

MYELOMENINGOCELE

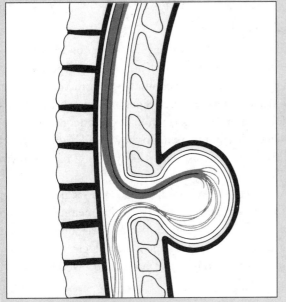

SPINA BIFIDA OCCULTA

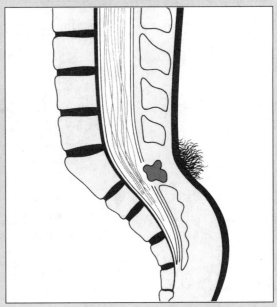

Spina bifida is relatively common, affecting about 5% of the population. In the United States, approximately 12,000 infants each year are born with some form of spina bifida.

The prognosis varies with the degree of accompanying neurologic deficit. It's worst in people with large open lesions, neurogenic bladders (which predispose to infection and kidney failure), or total paralysis of the legs. Because such features are usually absent in spina bifida occulta and meningocele, the prognosis is much better than in myelomeningocele, and many people with these conditions can lead normal lives.

What causes them?

Normally, about 20 days after conception, the embryo develops a neural groove in the dorsal area. This groove rapidly deepens, and the two edges come together to form the neural tube. By about day 23, this tube is completely closed except for an opening at each end. If the posterior portion of the neural tube fails to close by the fourth week of pregnancy, or if it closes but then splits open from a cause such as an abnormal increase in cerebrospinal fluid later in the first trimester, a spinal defect is likely to result.

Viruses, radiation, and other environmental factors may be responsible for such defects. However, spinal cord defects occur more often in offspring of women who have previously had children with similar defects, so genetic factors may contribute.

What are their symptoms?

Spina bifida occulta is often accompanied by skin abnormalities — such as a depression or dimple, tuft of hair, soft fatty deposits, portwine nevi (skin discoloration), or a combination of these — located over the spinal defect; however, such signs may be absent. Spina bifida occulta doesn't usually cause neurologic dysfunction but occasionally is associated with foot weakness or bowel and bladder disturbances. Such disturbances are especially likely during rapid growth phases.

In both meningocele and myelomeningocele, a saclike structure protrudes over the spine. Like spina bifida occulta, meningocele rarely causes neurologic deficits. But myelomeningocele, depending on the level of the defect, causes permanent neurologic dysfunction, such as flaccid or spastic paralysis and bowel and bladder incontinence.

How are they diagnosed?

Spina bifida occulta is often overlooked, although it's occasionally palpable and spinal X-ray can show the bone defect. Myelography can differentiate it from other spinal abnormalities, especially spinal cord tumors.

Meningocele and myelomeningocele are obvious on examination; backlighting the protruding sac can sometimes distinguish between them. (Light typically passes through a meningocele, but not through a myelomeningocele.) In myelomeningocele, a pinprick exam of the legs and trunk shows the level of sensory and motor involvement; skull X-rays, skull measurements, and computed to-mography scan (commonly called a CAT scan) demonstrate associat-ed fluid in the brain. Other appropriate lab tests in people with myelomeningocele include urinalysis, urine cultures, and tests for kidney function — starting in the neonatal period and continuing at regular intervals.

Although amniocentesis can detect only open spinal defects, this procedure is recommended for all pregnant women who have pre-viously had children with spinal cord defects because there is a greater risk of having another child with similar defects. If these defects are present in the fetus, amniocentesis shows increased alpha-fetoprotein levels by the 14th week of pregnancy. Ultrasonography can also de-tect or confirm the presence and extent of neural tube defects.

How are they treated?

Spina bifida occulta usually requires no treatment. Treatment of meningocele consists of surgical closure of the protruding sac and continual assessment of growth and development. Treatment of myelomeningocele requires repair of the sac and supportive measures to promote independence and prevent further complications. Sur-gery doesn't reverse neurologic deficits. A shunt may be inserted to relieve associated fluid in the brain.

Rehabilitation measures may include waist supports, long leg braces, walkers, crutches, and other orthopedic appliances; diet and bowel training to manage fecal incontinence; neurogenic bladder management to reduce urinary stasis; possibly intermittent catheter-ization; and antispasmodics such as Urecholine or Pro-Banthine. In severe cases, insertion of an artificial urinary sphincter is often suc-cessful; urinary diversion is used as a last resort to preserve kidney function. (See *Caring for a child with a spinal cord defect.*)

ADVICE FOR CAREGIVERS

Caring for a child with a spinal cord defect

If your child has a spinal defect, here are some care guidelines.

Avoid complications

- Look for the early signs of complications, such as bed sores and urinary tract infection.
- Increase your child's fluid in-take to prevent urinary tract in-fection. You may need to learn techniques for catheterization if the doctor orders these.

Avoid constipation

- Increase your child's fluid in-take and provide a high-fiber diet. Encourage exercise.
- Administer a stool softener, as directed. If possible, help your child defecate by telling him or her to bear down. Give a glycerin suppository if needed.

Get help for problems

- If your child has learning problems, arrange follow-up IQ assessment to help plan realis-tic educational goals. At home, plan activities appropriate to your child's age and abilities.
- For more help, contact the Spina Bifida Association of America.

STROKE

What do doctors call this condition?
Cerebrovascular accident

What is this condition?
Stroke refers to impaired circulation in one or more of the blood vessels supplying the brain. The brain's oxygen and blood supply is reduced or cut off, which damages or destroys localized areas of brain tissue. The sooner circulation is returned to normal after a stroke, the better the person's chances for complete recovery. However, about half of those who survive a stroke are permanently disabled and experience a recurrence within weeks, months, or years. About 500,000 people have strokes each year. Stroke is the third most common cause of death in the United States.

Classifying strokes
Strokes are classified according to how they progress. The least severe type is the *transient ischemic attack,* or "little stroke," which results from a brief interruption of blood flow. A *progressive stroke, or stroke-in-evolution,* starts with a slight nervous system deficit and worsens in a day or two. In a *completed stroke,* nervous system deficits are greatest right at the start.

What causes it?
The major causes of stroke are thrombosis, embolism, and hemorrhage. *Thrombosis* is the formation of a thrombus, a clotlike substance, in a blood vessel. A stroke occurs when the thrombus blocks the blood vessel, cutting off blood flow to the brain tissue supplied by the vessel and causing congestion and swelling.

A person may develop thrombosis while sleeping or shortly after awakening; it can also occur during surgery or after a heart attack. Thrombosis is the leading cause of stroke in middle-aged and elderly people (these groups are more likely to have hardening of the arteries, diabetes, and high blood pressure). The risk of thrombosis rises with obesity, smoking, and use of oral contraceptives. Cocaine-induced stroke is now being seen in younger people.

Embolism, the second most common cause of stroke, is blockage of a blood vessel by an embolus — a fragmented clot, a tumor, a fatty substance, bacteria, or air. It can occur at any age, especially among people who've undergone open-heart surgery or who have a history of rheumatic heart disease, endocarditis (inflammation of the heart's inner lining), certain types of heart valve disease, or certain types of irregular heartbeats. Embolism usually develops rapidly — in 10 to 20 seconds — and without warning.

Hemorrhage (heavy bleeding), the third most common cause of stroke, may occur suddenly at any age. Hemorrhage results from chronic high blood pressure or aneurysm, which causes a brain artery to suddenly burst; the rupture impedes blood supply to the area served by this artery. Blood also builds up deep within the brain, further compressing brain tissue and causing even more damage.

Risk factors

Factors that increase the risk of stroke include a history of transient ischemic attacks, hardening of the arteries, high blood pressure, irregular heartbeats, electrocardiogram changes, rheumatic heart disease, diabetes, gout, decreased blood pressure when rising to a standing position, an enlarged heart, high serum triglyceride levels, lack of exercise, use of oral contraceptives, cigarette smoking, and a family history of stroke.

What are its symptoms?

Symptoms of a stroke vary with the artery affected, the severity of damage, and the extent of secondary circulation that develops to help the brain compensate for decreased blood supply. If the stroke occurs in the left side of the brain, it produces symptoms on the right side of the body. A stroke in the right side causes symptoms on the left side of the body. (However, a stroke that damages the cranial nerves causes signs of cranial nerve dysfunction on the same side.)

Generalized symptoms of stroke include headache, vomiting, mental impairment, seizures, coma, rigidity at the nape of the neck, fever, and disorientation. Rarely, a person gets warning symptoms before a stroke, such as drowsiness, dizziness, headache, and mental confusion.

How is it diagnosed?

To diagnose a stroke, the doctor evaluates the person's symptoms, performs a physical exam, checks for a history of risk factors, and orders a variety of diagnostic tests.

Computed tomography scan (commonly called a CAT scan) shows signs of hemorrhagic stroke immediately but may not show evidence of thrombotic damage for 48 to 72 hours. Magnetic resonance imaging (commonly called an MRI) or a brain scan may help identify damaged and swollen areas in the brain. Lumbar puncture (sometimes called a spinal tap) reveals bloody cerebrospinal fluid in hemorrhagic stroke. Ophthalmoscopy (eye exam) may show signs of high blood pressure and hardening in the arteries that serve the retina. Angiography (an X-ray study of the brain's blood vessels) outlines vessels and locates sites of narrowing or rupture. Finally, electroencephalography (a recording of brain-wave activity) helps locate damaged brain areas.

Lab studies include urinalysis, blood clotting studies, and a complete blood count.

How is it treated?

A person with a thrombotic or embolic stroke may undergo surgery to improve circulation to the brain. In an operation called *endarterectomy,* the surgeon removes atherosclerotic plaque (obstructing matter) from the artery's inner walls. In a microvascular bypass, the surgeon joins a blood vessel outside the skull to one inside the skull.

Medications useful for treating a person who's had a stroke include:

- Ticlid, which may be more effective than aspirin in preventing stroke and reducing the risk of recurrence
- tissue plasminogen activator (also called t-PA or Activase), which is being used experimentally to dissolve clots
- anticonvulsants, such as Dilantin or Barbita, to treat or prevent seizures
- stool softeners to avoid straining, which increases pressure within the skull
- corticosteroids, such as Decadron, to minimize brain swelling
- analgesics, such as codeine sulfate, to relieve the headache that typically follows hemorrhagic stroke.

What can the family of a person recovering from a stroke do?

- Establish and maintain communication. If the person has a language or speech impairment, set up a simple method for communicating basic needs. Phrase your questions so that the individual will be able to answer using this system. Repeat yourself quietly and calmly (remember, the person isn't deaf), and use gestures if necessary to help with understanding. Even the unresponsive person can hear, so don't say anything in his or her presence that you wouldn't want heard and remembered. Simplify your language, asking yes-or-no

SELF-HELP

Making eating easier

If you've had a stroke, special glasses, cups, plates, and utensils can make eating easier and more enjoyable. Here are some suggestions for using these devices.

Glasses and cups

If you have trouble holding a glass, use an unbreakable plastic tumbler instead. Plastic is lighter and less slippery than glass. Or use terry cloth sleeves over glasses to make them easier to grasp.

You can also choose from many specially designed cups. For instance, you can use a cup with two handles that is easier to keep steady than a cup with one handle. You can try a pedestal cup or a T-handle cup, which is easy to grasp. You can also try a cup with a weighted base that helps prevent spills.

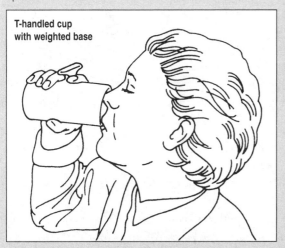

T-handled cup
with weighted base

If you have a stiff neck, use a cup with a V-shaped opening on its rim. You can easily tip this cup to empty it without bending your neck backward.

If your hands are unsteady, you may find it easier to hold a cup with a large handle. Or drink from a lidded cup with a lip to help decrease spills. If you have decreased sensation or feeling in your hands,

use an insulated cup or mug to avoid burning yourself.

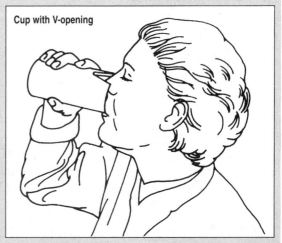

Cup with V-opening

Drinking straws

Flexible or rigid straws, either disposable or reusable, come in several sizes. Some straws are wide enough for you to drink soups and thick liquids through them. To hold the straw in place, use a snap-on plastic lid with a slot for the straw.

Dishes

If possible, try to use only unbreakable dishes. To keep a plate from sliding, place a damp sponge, washcloth, paper towel, or rubber disk under it. Consider using a plate with a nonskid base or place mats made of dimpled rubber or foam. Suction cups attached to the bottom of a plate or bowl also help prevent slipping.

You may want to consider using a plate guard. This device prevents food from falling off the plate so that it can be picked up easily with a fork or spoon. Attach the guard to the side of the plate opposite the hand you use to feed yourself.

A scooper plate has high sides that provide a built-in surface for pushing food onto the utensil.

(continued)

Making eating easier *(continued)*

Eating from a sectioned plate or tray may also be convenient.

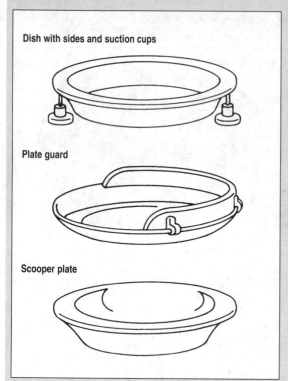

Dish with sides and suction cups

Plate guard

Scooper plate

Flatware

If your hand is weak or your grip is shaky, you may want to try ordinary flatware with ridged wood, plastic, or cork handles — all easier to grasp than smooth metal handles. Or try building up the handles with a bicycle handgrip, a foam curler pad, or tape (this also works for holding pens and pencils, toothbrushes, or razors). You can also try strapping the utensil to your hand.

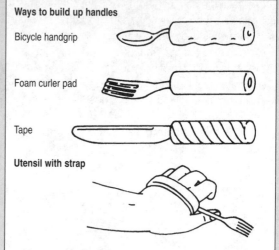

Ways to build up handles

Bicycle handgrip

Foam curler pad

Tape

Utensil with strap

questions whenever possible. Don't correct the person's speech or treat him or her like a child.

■ Encourage the person to use the unaffected side to exercise the affected side.

■ If necessary, teach the person to comb his or her hair, eat, dress, and wash. (See *Making eating easier,* pages 165 and 166.)

■ Ask a physical or an occupational therapist to help you obtain any appliances the person may need during rehabilitation, such as walking frames, hand bars for the toilet, and ramps. (See *Tips for managing daily activities,* page 167.)

■ If speech therapy is needed, encourage the person to start as soon as possible and to follow through with the speech pathologist's suggestions.

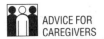

ADVICE FOR
CAREGIVERS

Tips for managing daily activities

As a family member or companion recovers from a stroke, you can use these common sense tips to help the person relearn ways to carry out daily activities.

Help with directions
- To help distinguish left from right, suggest that the person wear a watch or bracelet on the left wrist as a "landmark." Or, mark the left shoe sole with an *L* or tag the inside left trouser leg or sweater sleeve with a colored tape to distinguish left from right.
- If the person has problems with spatial relations, use maps or colored dots to mark a daily route. Keep the environment as uncluttered as possible —

for example, keep only a few items on the nightstand. Also, point to objects to give clues in remarks such as "*in* the wastebasket" or "*under* the desk."
- If the person has trouble dressing, advise buttoning shirts or blouses from the bottom up. Some people find it easier to match buttonholes that way.

Offer praise
Whatever the task, praise your loved one's efforts. Discouragement can be disabling in itself. If the stroke was on the right side of the brain, the person will understand encouraging words. If it was on the left side, the person may respond better to physical encouragement, such as a pat on the back.

- If the doctor prescribes aspirin to reduce the risk of embolic stroke, don't substitute Tylenol instead; it won't produce the desired effect.
- If the person displays or complains of warning signs of a stroke — severe headache, drowsiness, confusion, and dizziness — call the doctor immediately.
- Make sure the person sees the doctor regularly for follow-up visits.

*T*RIGEMINAL NEURALGIA

What is this condition?

Trigeminal neuralgia (also called *tic douloureux*) is a painful disorder of one or more branches of the fifth cranial (trigeminal) nerve that produces sudden attacks of excruciating facial pain when triggered by stimulation of a sensitive zone of the face. It occurs primarily in people over age 40, in women more often than men, and on the right side of the face more often than the left. Trigeminal neuralgia can subside spontaneously and have remissions lasting from several months to years.

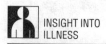

Mapping the trigeminal nerve

In trigeminal neuralgia, the exact location of facial pain depends on which trigeminal nerve branch is involved. With three branches — ophthalmic, maxillary, and mandibular — the trigeminal nerve can distribute pain across several facial areas.

To help visualize where pain travels within a trigger zone, first ask the doctor which nerve branch is producing your pain. Then use the illustration below to follow the nerve's course and the area supplied by that branch.

Pain around the eyes

The *ophthalmic branch* carries sensory fibers to the skin on the forehead, upper eyelids, and parts of the scalp and nose. It also innervates the eyeballs, the cornea, and the mucosa of the frontal and nasal sinuses.

Pain around the temples

The *maxillary branch* carries sensory fibers to the skin on the temples, lower eyelids, upper cheeks and lip, and part of the nose. It also innervates the gums, the molar and premolar canine teeth, and the mucosa of the mouth, nose, and maxillary sinus.

Pain around the cheeks and chin

The *mandibular branch*, the largest of the three, carries both sensory and motor fibers. The motor fibers control the muscles involved in chewing. The sensory fibers innervate the skin on the cheeks, chin, lower jaw, lower teeth and gums, the oral mucosa, and part of the ear.

TRIGEMINAL NERVE

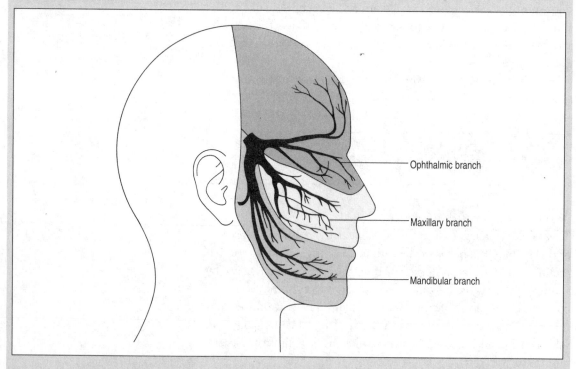

Ophthalmic branch

Maxillary branch

Mandibular branch

What causes it?

Although the cause remains undetermined, trigeminal neuralgia may reflect an afferent reflex phenomenon located centrally in the brain stem or more peripherally in the sensory root of the trigeminal nerve. The facial pain may also be related to compression of the nerve root by posterior fossa tumors, middle fossa tumors, or vascular lesions (subclinical aneurysm), although such lesions usually produce simultaneous loss of sensation. Occasionally, trigeminal neuralgia is a manifestation of multiple sclerosis or herpes zoster (shingles). (See *Mapping the trigeminal nerve*.)

Whatever the cause, the pain of trigeminal neuralgia is probably produced by an interaction or short-circuiting of touch and pain fibers.

What are its symptoms?

Typically, the person reports a searing or burning pain that occurs in lightning-like jabs and lasts from 1 to 15 minutes (usually 1 to 2 minutes) in an area supplied by one of the divisions of the trigeminal nerve. The pain rarely affects more than one of the possible areas and seldom the first division (ophthalmic) or both sides of the face. It affects the second (maxillary) and third (mandibular) divisions of the trigeminal nerve equally.

These attacks characteristically follow stimulation of a trigger zone, usually by a light touch to a hypersensitive area, such as the tip of the nose, the cheeks, or the gums. Although attacks can occur at any time, they may follow a draft of air, exposure to heat or cold, eating, smiling, talking, or drinking hot or cold beverages. The frequency of attacks varies greatly, from many times a day to several times a month or year.

Between attacks, most people are free of pain, although some have a constant, dull ache.

How is it diagnosed?

The person's pain history is the basis for diagnosis because trigeminal neuralgia produces no objective clinical or pathologic changes. A physical exam shows no impairment of sensory or motor function; indeed, sensory impairment implies a space-occupying lesion as the cause of pain.

Observation during the exam shows the person favoring (guarding) the affected area. To ward off a painful attack, the person often holds his or her face immobile when talking and may also leave the affected side of the face unwashed and unshaven or protect it with a coat or shawl. When asked where the pain occurs, the individual points to — but never touches — the affected area. Witnessing a typical attack helps to confirm the diagnosis. Skull X-rays and a computed tomography scan (commonly called a CAT scan) rule out sinus or tooth infections and tumors.

How is it treated?

Oral administration of Tegretol or Dilantin may temporarily relieve or prevent pain. Narcotics may be helpful during the pain episode.

When these medical measures fail or attacks become increasingly frequent or severe, neurosurgery may provide permanent relief. The preferred procedure is electrocoagulation of nerve rootlets through the skin under local anesthesia. New treatments include a percutaneous radio frequency procedure, which causes partial root destruction and relieves pain, and microsurgery for vascular decompression of the trigeminal nerve. (See *Advice for the person with trigeminal neuralgia*, page 169.)

MUSCLE AND BONE DISORDERS

Achilles tendon surgery: Speeding your recovery

Follow these guidelines to ensure lengthening of your Achilles tendon.

Preparing to walk

• Keep your foot raised on pillows to reduce swelling and pressure on blood vessels.
• Get ready to walk again by dangling your foot off the bed for short periods (5 to 15 minutes) to allow a gradual increase of blood in the veins; about 24 hours after surgery, you can use crutches and a non–weight-bearing or touch-down gait.
• Elevate your foot when sitting or any time it throbs or feels swollen.

Caring for the cast

• Keep your cast clean and dry to avoid irritating your skin.
• When you clean the skin around and under the cast, use rubbing alcohol. Don't use oils or powders — they tend to soften and irritate the skin.
• If you used to wear high heels frequently, wear them less after the cast is removed.

Getting exercise

Exercise regularly to stretch the Achilles tendon. Ask the doctor or therapist how much exercise and walking are recommended as you recover.

ACHILLES TENDON CONTRACTURE

What is this condition?

Achilles tendon contracture is a shortening of the heel tendon that causes foot pain and strain and restricts ankle movement.

What causes it?

Achilles tendon contracture may be caused by an inherited structural problem or a muscle's response to chronic poor posture, especially in women who wear high heels or joggers who land on the balls of their feet instead of their heels. Other causes include diseases that paralyze the legs, such as polio or cerebral palsy.

What are its symptoms?

Sharp, spasmodic pain when the person points the toes toward the knee is one sign of the reflex type of Achilles tendon contracture. In this contracture, called *footdrop,* the tight foot muscle prevents placing the heel on the ground.

How is it diagnosed?

The doctor can confirm Achilles tendon contracture by interviewing the person and with a simple test: While the person keeps the knee bent, the doctor flexes the foot upward. As the person straightens the knee, the tightened tendon forces the foot to point down.

How is it treated?

The doctor may use manipulation or a wedged plaster cast to stretch the tendon. The person may be given pain relievers to ease discomfort as stretching begins.

Fixed footdrop may require surgery. Although cutting can weaken the tendon, it allows stretching. After surgery, a short leg cast will hold the foot at a right angle for 6 weeks. Some surgeons allow the person to use a walking cast after 2 weeks. (See *Achilles tendon surgery: Speeding your recovery.*)

What can a person with Achilles tendon contracture do?

If the contracture is caused by something like high heels, gradually lowering the heels of the shoes and performing regular stretching exercises may be effective.

CARPAL TUNNEL SYNDROME

What is this condition?

Carpal tunnel syndrome is a pinched wrist nerve that affects the use of the hand. When the nerve is compressed together with blood vessels and tendons going to the fingers and thumb, it causes numbness and pain. Assembly-line workers and packers, computer users, and persons who use poorly designed tools are most likely to develop this disorder, especially women between ages 30 and 60. Any strenuous use of the hands — repetitive grasping, twisting, or flexing — aggravates the condition and interferes with work and everyday activities.

What causes it?

The carpal tunnel is formed by the wrist bones and the band of ligament that holds them in place. Swelling or abnormal growths on the tendons that pass through the tunnel pinch the nerve. Besides repetitive motions, some familiar medical conditions that can cause the swelling include the following:

- rheumatoid arthritis
- inflammation from rheumatic disease
- pregnancy or menopause
- diabetes
- benign tumors
- a fracture, dislocation, or acute sprain of the wrist.

What are its symptoms?

Carpal tunnel syndrome usually starts with feelings of weakness, pain, burning, numbness, or tingling in one or both hands. The discomfort affects the thumb, forefinger, middle finger, and half of the fourth finger, making it difficult to clench the hand into a fist. Fingernails may look dull; the skin, dry and shiny.

How to relieve symptoms of carpal tunnel syndrome

To get relief and prevent permanent damage, you need to stop or cut back on the activity that produces the strain. If the activities are related to your job or hobbies, the change takes careful planning. Here are some helpful suggestions.

Make changes at work
Modify your work habits and work area. If you work on an assembly line or have a repetitive job, ask your supervisor to help you change or eliminate activities that strain your wrist. Follow these guidelines:
- Make sure your tools fit your hand correctly so you don't need to twist your wrist too much when turning, gripping, or squeezing objects.
- If you must lift and move objects, use both hands rather than the hand with carpal tunnel syndrome.
- Install a padded armrest at your work station to relieve the stress on your hands, wrists, and shoulders.
- Arrange to rotate your duties, or find a different technique that puts less stress on your wrist.
- If you work at a typewriter, computer, or another type of terminal, try lowering your work table to decrease the angle your wrist flexes.
- Raise your chair or sit on a pillow if you can't adjust your work table. Just be sure to support your feet for good posture and good circulation in your lower legs.

Wear a restraining device
Wear a splint or a specially designed glove whenever you perform repetitive activities, or all the time, if your doctor advises. These devices are available by prescription from medical supply stores.

Slow down
Slow down when performing repetitive activities with your hands. For example, if knitting causes symptoms, you can knit at a slower pace. But if you do work that is paced by a machine, discuss the problem with your supervisor or union representative.

Do hand exercises
Your doctor, nurse, or physical therapist can teach you special exercises to strengthen all your hand and wrist muscles. If all your muscles are strong, you'll put less strain on one particular muscle or group of muscles.

Reduce swelling
If fluid retention aggravates your symptoms, ask your doctor about taking diuretics to relieve swelling in the carpal tunnel. Or drink plenty of fluids (coffee and tea are natural diuretics). Elevating your hand may reduce swelling temporarily.

The symptoms are often worse at night or in the morning when circulation slows down. The pain may spread to the forearm and, in severe cases, as far as the shoulder. The person can usually relieve the pain by shaking the hands vigorously or dangling the arms at the sides.

How is it diagnosed?
After people with carpal tunnel syndrome notice a loss of feeling in affected fingers (less reaction to a light touch or pinpricks), about half

of them lose muscle strength as well. Other diagnostic indicators include:

- a tap on the wrist that produces a tingling sensation in the hand
- holding the forearms vertically and allowing both hands to drop down at the wrists for 1 minute, reproducing the symptoms
- a blood pressure cuff, inflated on the forearm for 1 to 2 minutes, causing pain and tingling in the wrist
- electromyography, a test of nerve response that measures an abnormal delay in impulses to the hand.

How is it treated?

The doctor may suggest conservative treatment first, including resting the hands by splinting the wrists in a neutral position for 1 to 2 weeks. If there's a definite link between the syndrome and the person's work, the doctor may suggest that the person modify his or her work or even change jobs. Effective treatment may also require correction of an underlying disorder.

If conservative treatment fails, the alternative is surgery. The most common procedures aim to remove pressure from the nerve by opening the carpal tunnel ligament or by using endoscopic surgical techniques. Neurolysis, the freeing of the nerve fibers by cutting them, may also be necessary.

What can a person with carpal tunnel syndrome do?

Take mild pain relievers and use your hands as much as possible. If the dominant hand is hurt, you may need help with eating and bathing. (See *How to relieve symptoms of carpal tunnel syndrome.*)

After surgery

Learn how to apply a splint and keep it loose enough for comfort. The nurse or therapist will show you how to remove the splint and gently exercise your hand, daily, perhaps while holding it in warm water. If your arm is in a sling, you'll learn to remove it and do exercises for your elbow and shoulder. (See *Exercises for people with carpal tunnel syndrome*, page 176.)

SELF-HELP

Exercises for people with carpal tunnel syndrome

If you limit your hand motions to relieve pain, you'll need daily exercises to maintain muscle tone.

Wrist and hand exercises

Extend your arm — palm down, fingers straight. Keep your palm flat. Slowly raise your fingers as far as they'll comfortably go. Avoid flexing your wrist. Then slowly lower your fingers as far downward as is comfortable.

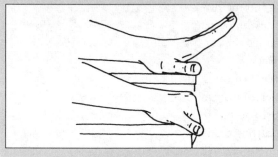

Keeping your arm in the extended position, wave or rock your hand from side to side. Then gently twist your hand from side to side. Next, move it in small circles in one direction and then the other.

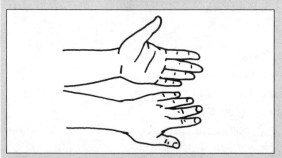

Finger and thumb exercises

With a rubber band around your fingers for mild resistance, spread your fingers as far apart as possible. Then bring them back together. Now make a fist.

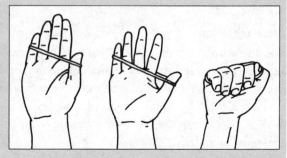

Hold up your hand and touch your little finger and thumb together. Repeat this movement, touching your other three fingers to your thumb.

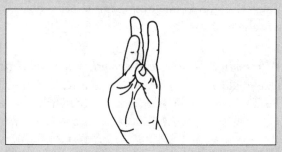

Finally, bend all your fingers up and down, as though waving goodbye.

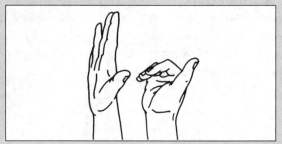

Gout

What is this condition?

Gout is a metabolic disease marked by localized deposits of uric acid salts that are normally excreted through the kidneys. The deposits cause painfully arthritic joints. Gout usually strikes the feet and legs of men over age 30 and women past menopause. In elderly people, it is linked to other diseases.

Though gout may disappear for years between attacks, it can lead to disability or crippling. Fortunately, most people get better with treatment.

What causes it?

Although the exact cause is unknown, gout seems linked to a genetic defect in metabolism, which causes overproduction and retention of uric acid. Too much uric acid leads to urate deposits in the joints or tissues, causing local damage. Secondary gout, linked to other conditions (such as obesity, diabetes, high blood pressure, sickle cell anemia, and kidney disease) or to drug therapy, produces similar harmful substances.

Another condition, called pseudogout, or chondrocalcinosis, causes arthritic pain too, but for different reasons. (See *False gout: How is it different?*)

What are its symptoms?

Gout develops in four stages (asymptomatic, acute, intercritical, and chronic) that produce the following findings:
- In asymptomatic gout, urate levels rise in the blood but produce no symptoms. Later, gout may cause high blood pressure or show up in severe back pain.
- The first acute attack strikes suddenly and peaks quickly, causing extreme pain in one or only a few joints. Affected joints feel hot, tender, inflamed, and look dusky red or bruised. The joint of the big toe usually becomes inflamed first, then the instep, ankle, heel, knee, or wrist joints. Some attacks pass quickly and then come back at irregular intervals. Severe attacks may last for days or weeks.
- Intercritical periods are the symptom-free intervals between gout attacks. Most people have a second attack within 6 months to 2 years, but others are symptom-free for 5 to 10 years. Those delayed attacks

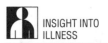

INSIGHT INTO
ILLNESS

False gout: How is it different?

It may feel like gout, but false gout is caused by deposits of calcium-based (instead of urate-based) crystals in the joints and affects primarily elderly people. Without treatment, it permanently damages joints in half the people who get it.

Symptoms

Like gout, false gout causes abrupt joint pain and swelling, usually in the knee, wrist, ankle, hands, or feet. These repeated, short attacks may be triggered by stress, injury, surgery, severe dieting, thiazide therapy, and alcohol abuse.

Diagnosis

Diagnosis depends on analysis of fluid from the joints, which shows calcium crystals. X-rays reveal an accumulation of calcium in the cartilage and markings along bone ends. Blood tests may detect an underlying endocrine or metabolic disorder

Treatment

Effective treatment of false gout may include drawing fluid from the joint to relieve pressure, injection of corticosteroids, use of painkillers or anti-inflammatory drugs and, if appropriate, treatment of the underlying endocrine or metabolic disorder.

SELF-HELP

How to make yourself comfortable

There are many measures you can take to relieve the pain of gout, including the following.

Rest
Get plenty of bed rest, but use a bed cradle to keep bedcovers off your sensitive, inflamed joints.

Control pain
Take your pain medication, as needed, especially during attacks. Apply hot or cold packs to inflamed joints. (If you are taking Benemid or Anturane, avoid aspirin or any other salicylate. Their combined effect causes urate retention.)

Eat and drink smart
▪ Avoid rich foods, such as anchovies, liver, sardines, kidneys, sweetbreads, lentils, and alcoholic beverages — especially beer and wine — that raise the urate level.
▪ If you are obese, follow a gradual weight-reduction diet. Such a diet features foods containing moderate amounts of protein and little fat.
▪ Drink plenty of fluids (up to a half-gallon a day) to prevent formation of kidney stones.

can strike untreated people with longer-lasting, severe pain in several joints, sometimes all at once and sometimes in one joint after another.
▪ Eventually, chronic gout sets in. This final, continuous stage shows up in persistently painful joints, with large urate deposits in the cartilage, membranes between the bones, tendons, and soft tissue. Deposits form primarily in arms and legs and, rarely, in organs, such as the kidneys and heart lining.

The skin over the deposits may develop sores and release a chalky, white material or pus. Chronic inflammation and urate deposition progress to further restrict movement and harm the person's general health, possibly including formation of kidney stones.

How is it diagnosed?

The doctor can find evidence of gout in fluid taken from an inflamed joint or a deposit and by checking the level of uric acid in the blood. In chronic gout, X-rays show damage to the cartilage and bones.

How is it treated?

The doctor first tries to stop the pain and prevent complications by suggesting bed rest and protection for the painful joints. Hot or cold packs and pain relievers may help with mild attacks. For more severe attacks and chronic gout, treatment may include the following:
▪ drugs to reduce inflammation, including Colsalide, Butazolidin, and Indocin, and injections of corticosteroids or corticotropin
▪ slower-acting drugs to reduce the uric acid level in the blood, including Zyloprim, Colsalide, Benemid, and Anturane
▪ diet changes, primarily to avoid alcohol and some rich foods; obese people should try to lose weight because the extra weight puts more stress on painful joints (See How to make yourself comfortable.)
▪ surgery to improve joint function or correct deformities. Deposits must be opened and drained if they become infected or ulcerated. Deposits can also be cut out to prevent ulceration, improve the joint's appearance, or make it easier to wear shoes or gloves.

HAMMER TOE

What is this condition?

In hammer toe, the big toe becomes crooked at the joint where it lines up with the other toes. The end of the bone is enlarged and a bunion (inflamed, thickened toe joint tissues) forms where it rubs the shoes. Hammer toe can cause a callus on the sole of the foot and make walking painful.

What causes it?

Hammer toe may be inherited, but it more often develops in people with degenerative arthritis or in those who place prolonged pressure on the foot, especially from narrow-toed high-heels. That's why hammer toe is more common in women. The condition also can develop in children who rapidly outgrow shoes and socks.

In congenital hammer toe, abnormal alignment of the bones (increased space between joints) causes bunion formation. In acquired hammer toe, the bone alignment is normal before the disorder occurs.

What are its symptoms?

Hammer toe usually begins as a tender bunion covered by deformed, hard skin and a bump that feels distended with fluid. The first indication of hammer toe may be pain over the bunion from shoe pressure. The pain could come from injury-caused arthritis, bursitis, or abnormal stresses on the foot because hammer toe changes the way a person walks. In an advanced stage, the foot may appear flat and spread out, with severely curled toes and a small bunion on the fifth toe.

How is it diagnosed?

A red, tender bunion makes hammer toe obvious. X-rays confirm the diagnosis by showing a crookedness of the big toe.

How is it treated?

Depending on the severity, hammer toe may require the following treatment:
■ In children (and some adults), repeated foot manipulation and splinting may relieve pain and correct hammer toe.

If you have surgery

To speed your recovery after surgery for a bunion, do the following.

Practice walking
Prepare to walk by first dangling your foot over the side of the bed for a short time to allow a gradual increase in blood pressure in your foot. In the hospital, you'll practice using crutches and managing the cast shoe or boot that protects your dressing.

Get rest
Stick to a schedule that allows you to rest frequently, with your feet elevated. When you rest, support your foot with pillows or by raising the foot of the bed. Put your feet up whenever you have pain or swelling, and wear wide-toed shoes and sandals after the dressings are removed.

Care for and exercise the foot
■ Practice proper foot care regarding cleanliness and massage. Cut your toenails straight across to prevent ingrown nails and infection.
■ Exercise at home to strengthen your foot muscles by standing at the edge of a step on your heel, then by raising and pointing up with the top of your foot.
■ Get prompt medical attention for any new bunions, corns, and calluses.

■ If the disease progresses to severe deformity with disabling pain, the person may need surgery to remove the bunion. After surgery, the toe is immobilized in its corrected position with either a soft dressing or a short cast.

■ After surgery, the person may need crutches for 4 to 6 weeks, or may simply learn to walk on his or her heels for a few days. The individual may be taught about physical therapy, such as applying warm compresses and soaks and doing exercises, as well as using drugs to relieve pain and stiffness. (See *If you have surgery.*)

What can a person with hammer toe do?

In the very early stages of acquired hammer toe, good foot care and proper shoes may eliminate the need for further treatment.

A person can use felt pads to protect the bunion, foam pads or other devices to separate the first and second toes at night, and a supportive pad and exercises to strengthen the arch. Early treatment is vital if other foot problems caused by rheumatoid arthritis or diabetes are present.

HERNIATED DISK

What do doctors call this condition?

Herniated nucleus pulposus

What is this condition?

Herniated disk is a back problem that starts when all or part of the soft, central portion of a spinal disk is forced through the disk's weakened or torn outer ring. When this happens, the protruding disk may rub against spinal nerve roots or the spinal cord itself, causing back pain and other signs of pinched nerves. Herniated disks mostly affect men under age 45.

What causes it?

Herniated disks may result from a bad fall or strain, or may be related to joint degeneration. In elderly people, whose disks have begun to degenerate, a minor injury may cause herniation. Most disk damage

STRAIGHT
TALK

How pelvic traction works

If the doctor orders pelvic traction for your disk condition, you'll spend most of your time in this device for about 2 weeks. You'll be allowed out of traction for about 4 hours a day to eat meals, use the bathroom, and perform other necessary activities. Here are common questions about pelvic traction.

What is the traction setup?
A beltlike device will be placed around your hips. Make sure that you have the correct size belt. It should fit snugly. Straps on each side of the belt attach to pulleys, which are attached to weights (8 to 10 pounds [3.7 to 4.5 kilograms] each). Each strap has its own pulley system. Your body weight provides countertraction.

How does traction work?
By pulling on your body, traction aligns the lower spine and reduces pressure on the spinal nerve roots. This helps ease back pain and muscle spasms.

How should I lie while in traction?
The head of your bed will be raised 20 to 30 degrees. The traction will hold your lower legs parallel to the floor. Be sure to lie with your hips and knees flexed 30 degrees so that your back is flat against the mattress. (However, avoid lying totally flat. This stresses the lower spine and may increase your pain.)

What else can I do to stay comfortable?
Most people feel comfortable in pelvic-belt traction. However, if your pain increases, contact the doctor. He or she may stop the traction or have you use it only intermittently.

Because the traction device is attached directly to your skin, skin breakdown can occur. Remember to check your skin at least twice a day for signs of inflammation, such as redness and swelling.

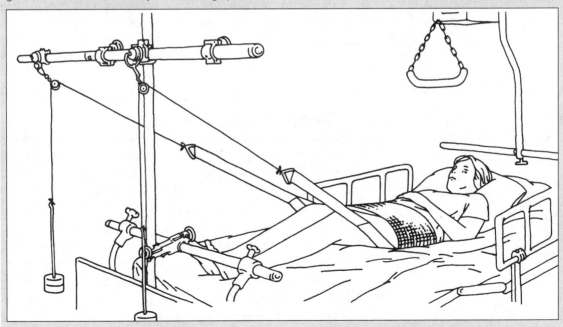

(90%) occurs in the lower back; 8%, in the neck area; and 1% to 2%, at chest level.

A person with this condition who was born with a small lower back spinal canal or who has abnormal vertebral bone formation may be more susceptible to pinched and damaged nerves.

What are its symptoms?

The main symptom of lower-back herniated disk is severe, low back pain, which radiates to the buttocks, legs, and feet, usually on one side. If the disk was hurt in a fall, the pain may begin suddenly, fade in a few days, then recur and intensify. Hip pain follows, beginning as a dull pain in the buttocks. Coughing, sneezing, or bending intensifies the pain and sometimes causes muscle spasms.

Herniated disk may also cause numbness around the pinched spinal nerve and, in later stages, weakness of the leg muscles.

How is it diagnosed?

The doctor will ask for detailed information about what causes pain because that helps pinpoint the damage. The person will be put through several leg-raising and other motion tests to check for evidence of a pinched nerve. A spinal X-ray won't show the damaged disk, but can rule out other causes of leg pain or numbness.

After the physical exam and X-rays, additional scans using a dye or multiple views can show a more exact picture of herniated disk material.

How is it treated?

Treatment depends on the severity of the damage done by the herniated disk and can include the following:

▪ several weeks in bed, possibly in pelvic traction, unless nerve damage progresses rapidly. (See *How pelvic traction works*, page 181.) This conservative treatment progresses to an exercise program. The person may use a hot pad and take aspirin to reduce inflammation and swelling. Sometimes, the doctor prescribes muscle relaxants or, rarely, corticosteroids.

▪ surgery for a herniated disk that fails to respond to conservative treatment. The most common procedure, called *laminectomy*, involves removing a portion of a thin plate of bone and the protruding disk. If surgery doesn't relieve symptoms, a spinal fusion may be necessary to stabilize the spine. (See *How to help someone with a herniated disk.*)

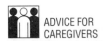

ADVICE FOR
CAREGIVERS

How to help someone with a herniated disk

Taking care of someone with a herniated disk means more than waiting on the person while he or she is bedridden. You can provide emotional support and steady reinforcement during the treatment and the recovery period.

- If the treatment is conservative (bed rest and then exercises), a physical therapist may teach the person some leg- and back-strengthening exercises that are more easily performed with a partner. Try to support the person's regular exercise routine.
- After laminectomy, microsurgery, or spinal fusion, the person may spend most of the day in bed and may need your help to begin walking. The person may need pain relievers before facing the demands of getting out of bed every day.

- You can help with recovery by installing an extra-firm mattress or a bed board at home.
- Other aids are a straight-backed chair for limited sitting and high-topped sneakers to support ankle muscles.
- After spinal fusion, the person may need help to manage a brace as well as larger-sized clothing to fit over it.
- Try to reinforce the person's newly learned body mechanics, such as bending at the knees and hips (never at the waist), standing straight, and carrying heavy objects close to the body. These techniques also are good for you (and other caregivers) when you lift and help your family member.
- Finally, help the person reach or maintain proper weight to prevent swayback caused by obesity.

- instead of laminectomy, injection of an enzyme called Chymodiactin into the herniated disk to dissolve the disk's nucleus, or microsurgery to remove fragments of the damaged disk.

HUMPBACK

What do doctors call this condition?
Kyphosis

What is this condition?
Humpback is a frontward curving of the spine that causes a bowing of the back. A normal spine is slightly curved, but a severe curve, usually at chest level, is harmful. In adults and children, humpback is successfully treated with braces and exercises. It rarely requires surgery.

> *Humpback may be caused by growth retardation, many diseases, congenital malformation, or poor posture.*

What causes it?

Adults and children get humpback for different reasons.

Adolescent humpback

The most common form of adolescent humpback is linked to growth retardation, a blood circulation problem around the spine during periods of rapid growth, or even poor posture. Sometimes, infection, inflammation, and disk degeneration can put vertebrae under stress and produce the curve. Humpback is discovered in more girls than boys and most often between ages 12 and 16.

Adult humpback

Adult humpback may result from aging and related degeneration of disks between the vertebrae or from the collapse of vertebrae. The list of contributing diseases and conditions is long: hyperparathyroidism, Cushing's disease, prolonged corticosteroid therapy, arthritis, Paget's disease, polio, fractured vertebrae, cancers, or tuberculosis. In adults, as well as children, humpback can result from poor posture.

Congenital humpback

This disorder, in which the vertebrae are badly formed, is rare but usually severe enough to press against the lungs.

What are its symptoms?

Development of adolescent humpback is usually subtle, but the clues include:
- curving of the back, often after a history of excessive sports activity
- mild pain at the top of the curve (in about half of affected adolescents)
- fatigue, tenderness, or stiffness in the involved area or along the entire spine
- prominent growths on vertebrae, producing swayback and hamstring tightness
- neurologic damage and spasms (rarely)
- inability to straighten the spines while lying down (reported in adolescents and adults).

Adult humpback produces the characteristic roundback appearance and the following symptoms:
- pain (possibly), weakness of the back, and generalized fatigue
- tenderness (rarely), except when the humpback is linked to osteoporosis or a recent fracture (as in elderly people).

SELF-HELP

How therapy works to correct humpback

If you have humpback, the cure will require patience and hard work. You may need emotional support to deal with frustrations and periods of depression.

This is especially true for a teenager facing the long corrective process. The doctor and the therapist will help with corrective devices and exercises, such as the following.

Exercise routine (in or out of a brace)
- Pelvic tilts stretch back muscles and decrease swayback.
- Hamstring stretches overcome shortened muscles in back of the thigh.
- Working hard to move your shoulders back and your chest up helps to flatten the humpback curve.

Side-view X-rays, taken every 4 months, will show whether the curve is being reduced and (in teenagers) the spine is fully grown. The X-ray results will determine whether you can spend more time outside the brace.

Improved posture
- If you are still growing and poor posture caused your humpback, exercising and practicing basic shoulders-back, buttocks-tucked-under posture is important.
- The doctor and therapist will recommend that you use a firm mattress, preferably with a bed board.

Back brace
If you need a brace, you'll be taught how and when to wear it. Then concentrate on good skin care (no lotions, ointments, or powders where the brace contacts the skin). Remember to have the doctor or orthotist adjust the brace as needed.

How is it diagnosed?

The doctor can see the curvature, and X-rays may show changes in the shape of vertebrae. To confirm adolescent humpback, the doctor will check for tuberculosis and other inflammatory or new-growth-producing diseases. Because these suspected diseases cause severe pain and other definite symptoms or test results, they can be ruled out quickly.

How is it treated?

For humpback caused by poor posture alone, the usual treatment includes:
- bed rest on a firm mattress (with or without traction)
- a brace to straighten the curve until spinal growth is complete
- therapeutic exercises (see *How therapy works to correct humpback*).

If treatment is needed for other diseases that cause humpback, the doctor may fuse the bones in the spine to relieve symptoms. Although rarely necessary, the surgery may be recommended when humpback causes nerve damage, a spinal curve greater than 60 degrees, or stubborn and disabling back pain in an adult.

MUSCULAR DYSTROPHY

What is this condition?

Muscular dystrophy is actually a group of inherited disorders characterized by a progressive, symmetrical wasting away of skeletal muscles that occurs without causing pain or loss of feeling in the limbs. Paradoxically, these damaged muscles tend to enlarge because of connective tissue and fat deposition, giving a false impression of muscle strength.

So far, there is no cure for the condition, but there are four main types of muscular dystrophy, each with a different outcome. *Duchenne type muscular dystrophy* accounts for 50% of all cases. It generally strikes during early childhood and results in death by age 20. *Becker's muscular dystrophy* is slower to develop, and people with it usually live into their 40s. The two last types (*dystrophy of the face, shoulders, and arms* and *limb-girdle dystrophy*) usually don't shorten life expectancy.

What causes it?

Muscular dystrophy is caused by various genes. The Duchenne and Becker types are carried by sex-linked genes affecting only men. Dystrophy of the face, shoulders, and arms and limb-girdle dystrophy are not sex-linked, so affect both sexes about equally.

What are its symptoms?

Each type of muscular dystrophy causes progressive muscle deterioration, but incidence and severity varies in the following ways:

- The Duchenne type begins subtly, between ages 3 and 5. Children with this disorder have a waddling gait and difficulty climbing stairs, fall down often, can't run properly, and their shoulder bones flare out (or "wing") when they raise their arms.

Usually, a child with muscular dystrophy is confined to a wheelchair by ages 9 to 12. Finally, progressive weakening of the heart muscle leads to death from sudden heart failure, respiratory failure, or infection.

Muscular dystrophy is a group of inherited disorders that cause skeletal muscles to waste away without causing pain or loss of feeling in the limbs. Paradoxically, these damaged muscles appear enlarged due to connective tissue and fat deposition.

- Although similar to the Duchenne type, the symptoms of Becker's muscular dystrophy progress more slowly. Symptoms start around age 5, but children can still walk well beyond age 15 — sometimes into their 40s.
- Dystrophy of the face, shoulders, and arms is a slowly progressive and relatively harmless type that commonly occurs before age 10 but may develop during early adolescence. In the early stages, infants may not be able to suckle; children can't pucker their mouths or whistle or raise their arms above their heads. Affected children may have abnormal facial movements and a lack of facial movements when laughing or crying.
- Limb-girdle dystrophy follows a similarly slow course and often causes only slight disability. Usually, it begins between ages 6 and 10, causing muscle weakness first in the upper arm and pelvic muscles; then, the other common symptoms appear.

How is it diagnosed?

The doctor examines the child, asks questions of the family, and orders certain tests. If another family member has muscular dystrophy, that person's symptoms usually tell a lot about the child's future. If no one else has the disorder, tests of nerve activity in the affected muscles can reveal muscular dystrophy, and a muscle biopsy can show cell changes or cell fat and tissue deposits.

Medical centers with the most advanced immunologic and molecular biological techniques can accurately predict muscular dystrophy in the fetus. They can also test parents and relatives who may carry the genes for Duchenne and Becker's muscular dystrophies.

How is it treated?

No treatment has yet been found that can stop the progressive muscle deterioration of muscular dystrophy. However, orthopedic appliances, as well as exercise, physical therapy, and surgery to correct contractures, can help preserve the child or young adult's mobility and independence for a time. (See *Muscular dystrophy: How you can help*, page 188.)

Family members who are carriers of muscular dystrophy should receive genetic counseling regarding the risk of transmitting this disease to their children.

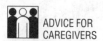
ADVICE FOR CAREGIVERS

Muscular dystrophy: How you can help

Taking care of a child with muscular dystrophy involves learning about the progression of the disease and calling on every available resource to help you deal with this disorder.

Regular activities
- Encourage and help the child with exercises to preserve joint mobility and prevent muscle atrophy.
- Keep a regular schedule with a physical therapist.
- Investigate splints, braces, or surgery to correct contractures.
- Install trapeze bars or overhead slings to help the child in a wheelchair move himself in and out of the chair.
- Use a footboard or high-topped sneakers to increase comfort and support weak ankle muscles.

Lifestyle changes
- To keep the child active, limit TV viewing and other sedentary activities.
- Because inactivity may cause constipation, provide a diet with plenty of fiber and fluids.
- Because a child with muscular dystrophy may be prone to obesity, help him or her maintain a low-calorie, high-protein, high-fiber diet.
- Always allow the child plenty of time to perform even simple physical tasks because the child is likely to need more time.

- Help your child maintain his friendships and grow intellectually by attending regular school as long as possible.
- When the lungs are involved in Duchenne type muscular dystrophy, encourage coughing, deep-breathing exercises, and diaphragmatic breathing. Ask a nurse or therapist how to recognize early signs of respiratory complications.

Emotional help
- Just as your child may need emotional support to deal with continual changes in his or her body, you may need help to sustain your level of caregiving. Ask the nurse or therapist to refer you to someone who can talk about your needs and worries.
- If the person with muscular dystrophy is an adult, and if it seems appropriate, encourage him or her to make use of such services as sexual counseling and vocational rehabilitation. (Contact the Department of Labor and Industry in your state for more information.) For information on social services and financial assistance, contact the Muscular Dystrophy Association.

OSTEOARTHRITIS

What is this condition?

Osteoarthritis, the most common form of arthritis, is an ongoing process that breaks down cartilage around a bone, then causes new bone to grow around and under the affected joint. It usually occurs in the hips and knees. Osteoarthritis is widespread and affects both sexes after age 40. It can be disabling and usually gets worse as the person ages, ranging from minor dysfunction of the fingers to severe hip or knee problems.

STRAIGHT
TALK

Common questions about osteoarthritis

I've been a typist for 30 years. Is that why I have osteoarthritis in my hands?

It's possible. Years of excessive use may trigger osteoarthritis in a joint or group of joints. That's why osteoarthritis typically affects individuals in such fields as typing, construction, and athletics. Other contributors are obesity, a family history of arthritis (especially of hands and fingers), a history of joint injury or inherited abnormality, and certain diseases.

Will the arthritis in my knee spread to my hip?

Probably not. Osteoarthritis typically affects only one joint, usually a weight-bearing joint, such as the knee. In some cases, the disease affects several joints, but it doesn't spread in the usual sense of the word.

Will I eventually be crippled by my osteoarthritis?

Unlike rheumatoid arthritis, osteoarthritis isn't a crippling disease that affects the entire body. Many people with osteoarthritis have only mild symptoms that don't much interfere with their daily activities. By avoiding activities that increase the risk of joint injury and by following your doctor's guidelines on rest and exercise, you can help retard further deterioration of the affected joint.

What causes it?

Osteoarthritis, a normal part of aging, results from many metabolic, genetic, chemical, and mechanical factors. One form of osteoarthritis results from a specific event, such as a fall, an inherited deformity, or obesity that leads to degenerative changes.

What are its symptoms?

The most common symptom of osteoarthritis is deep, aching joint pain, which occurs particularly after exercise or other joint stress. The pain goes away when the person rests. Other symptoms include stiffness in the morning (again, relieved by rest), aching during changes in weather, "grating" of the joint during motion, and tight muscles that hamper movements. These symptoms are worse if the person has poor posture or job stress or is obese. When it affects the hands, osteoarthritis changes the shape of the joints and can eventually make them red, swollen, tender, and numb.

How is it diagnosed?

The doctor can assess obvious changes in the person's joints and use X-rays to see such signs as joint deformity, bony deposits, and joint fusion. There is no lab test specific for osteoarthritis, but tests can rule out other inflammatory joint problems. (See *Common questions about osteoarthritis.*)

How is it treated?

The doctor will prescribe medications to relieve pain and minimize stiffness. Medications include aspirin (or other nonnarcotic pain relievers), Butazolidin, Indocin, Nalfon, Advil or Motrin, or Darvon and, in some cases, injections of corticosteroids. Such injections, given every 4 to 6 months, may delay the development of new deposits in the person's hands. The person will also be taught specific exercises to promote flexibility. (See *How to do range-of-motion exercises.*)

Other treatments

The doctor may put the person in a brace or traction, suggest a cane or crutches for walking, and encourage other supportive measures such as massage, steam baths, paraffin (wax) dips for the hands, and exercise. Surgery is reserved for people who have severe disability or uncontrollable pain.

What can a person with osteoarthritis do?

Pace yourself. Plan rest periods during the day and be protective about getting a good night's sleep. Because osteoarthritis is not a disease of your whole body, concentrate on therapy that improves your flexibility and comfort.

Specific treatments

- Hand: Hot soaks and paraffin dips can relieve pain.
- Lower and middle back: Use a firm mattress (or bed board) to decrease morning pain.
- Neck: Check the tightness of your cervical collar; watch for redness after prolonged use.
- Hip: Use moist heat pads to relieve pain (usually with prescribed antispasmodic drugs) and do stretching and strengthening exercises. You may need to inspect your braces or a walker for proper fit.
- Knee: Regularly exercise to maintain flexibility, muscle tone, and strength. Consider a brace or an elastic wrap for support.

More good moves

- Take your medication exactly as prescribed, and report side effects immediately.
- Avoid overexertion, and learn to stand and walk without stressing joints. Be especially careful when stooping or picking up objects.
- Wear well-fitting supportive shoes; don't allow the heels to become too worn down.

SELF-HELP

How to do range-of-motion exercises

Review the following guidelines before you begin doing active range-of-motion exercises:

- Do your exercises daily to steadily gain from them.
- Repeat each exercise three to five times or as often as your doctor recommends. (As you get stronger, he or she may tell you to increase your activity.)
- Do your routine in a specific order. If you're exercising all your major joints, begin at your neck; then work toward your toes.
- Move slowly and gently so that you don't injure yourself. If an exercise hurts, stop doing it. Then ask your doctor about changing your routine.
- Take a break and rest after an exercise that's especially tiring.
- Consider spacing your exercises over the day if you prefer not doing them in a single session.

Neck exercise
Slowly tilt your head as far back as possible. Next, move it to the right, toward your shoulder.

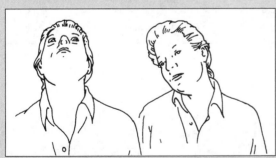

Still with your head to the right, lower your chin as far as it will go toward your chest. Then move your head toward your left shoulder. Complete a full circle by moving your head back to its usual upright position.

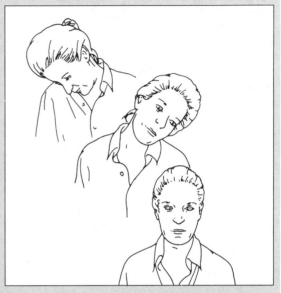

After you do the recommended number of counterclockwise circles, do an equal number of clockwise circles.

Shoulder exercise
Raise your shoulders as if you were going to shrug. Next, move them forward, down, then up, in a single circular motion.

Now move them backward, down, then up again in a single circular motion.

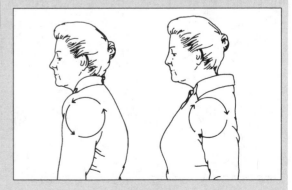

(continued)

How to do range-of-motion exercises *(continued)*

Continue to alternate forward and backward shoulder circles throughout the exercise.

Elbow exercise
Extend your arm straight out to your side. Open your hand, palm up, as if to catch a raindrop. Now, slowly reach back with your forearm so that you touch your shoulder with your fingers. Then slowly return your arm to its straight position. Now repeat with your other arm.

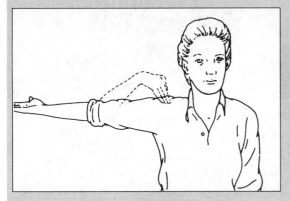

Continue to alternate arms throughout the exercise.

Wrist and hand exercise
Extend your arms, palms down and fingers straight. Keeping your palms flat, slowly raise your fingers and point them back toward you. Then slowly lower your fingers and point them as far downward as you comfortably can.

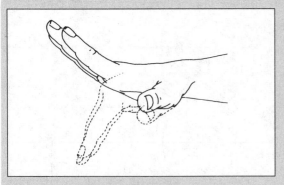

Finger exercise
Spread the fingers and thumb on each hand as wide apart as possible without causing discomfort. Then bring the fingers back together into a fist.

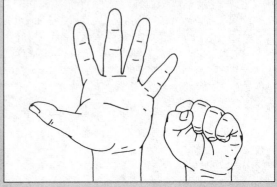

Leg and knee exercise
Lie on your bed or on the floor. Bend one leg so the knee is straight up and the foot is flat on the bed or floor.

Now, bend the other leg, raise your foot, and slowly bring your knee as far toward your chest as you can without discomfort.

Then straighten this leg slowly while you lower it.

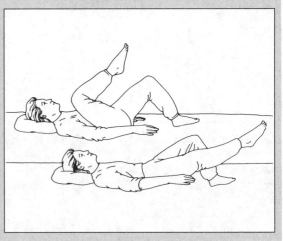

Repeat this exercise with your other leg.

How to do range-of-motion exercises *(continued)*

Ankle and foot exercise

Raise one foot and point your toes away from you. Move this foot in a circular motion—first to the right, then to the left.

Point your toes back toward you. With your foot in this position, make a circle with it, first right, then left.

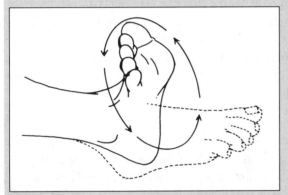

Now do the same exercise with your other foot.

Toe exercise

Sit in a chair or lie on your bed. Stretch your legs out in front of you with your heels resting on the floor or the bed. Slowly bend your toes down and away from you. Next, bend your toes up and back toward you. Finally, spread out your toes so that they're totally separated. Then squeeze your toes together.

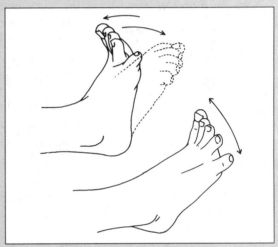

- Install safety devices at home, such as hand rails in the bathroom.
- Maintain your proper weight to lessen stress on joints.

OSTEOMYELITIS

What is this condition?

Osteomyelitis is a pus-producing bone infection that can be acute or chronic. Although osteomyelitis often remains in one location, it can spread through the bone marrow and the membrane that covers the bones. Acute osteomyelitis is usually carried in the bloodstream. The condition most often affects rapidly growing children.

Osteomyelitis is declining, except in drug abusers. With prompt treatment, the form that strikes children is curable. For the adult chronic type, the prognosis is poor.

What causes it?

The disease usually starts with a small bruise that is affected by a major bacterial infection somewhere else in the body. The most common bacterium involved in osteomyelitis is *Staphylococcus aureus*, commonly called *staph*. Osteomyelitis strikes more children than adults, particularly boys who have a serious infection. The most common sites in children are the lower end of the thigh bone (femur), the upper end of the shin bone (tibia), the upper arm bone (humerus), and the forearm bone on the side of the thumb (radius). In adults, the most common sites are the pelvis and backbone, generally the result of contamination associated with surgery or injury.

Both forms of osteomyelitis are declining, except in drug abusers. With prompt treatment, the osteomyelitis that strikes children is curable. For the adult chronic type, the prognosis is still poor.

How it develops

Once *Staphylococcus* or a similar bacteria finds some damaged tissue, it multiplies and spreads directly to the bone. As the infection grows and produces pus within the bone, it cuts off the bone's blood supply, forms abscesses, and may kill the tissue. Tissue death stimulates the bone to create new abscesses and drainage, and the osteomyelitis may become chronic.

What are its symptoms?

Acute osteomyelitis starts abruptly, with sudden pain in the affected bone and tenderness, heat, swelling, and restricted movement over it. Other symptoms include irregular heartbeat, sudden fever, nausea, and general discomfort. Generally, chronic and acute osteomyelitis look the same, except that the chronic infection can recede and then flare up after a minor injury.

How is it diagnosed?

The doctor examines the person, asks about symptoms, and then orders blood tests to confirm osteomyelitis. X-rays may not show bone damage until the disease has been active for about 2 to 3 weeks. Bone scans can detect early infection. The diagnosis must rule out poliomyelitis, rheumatic fever, myositis, and bone fractures.

How is it treated?

The doctor usually starts antibiotic treatment for acute osteomyelitis even before the diagnosis is confirmed, and may prescribe large doses of intravenous penicillin, such as Nafcil or Bactocill.

Other treatments

If an abscess forms, treatment includes incision and drainage, culture of the drainage, and antibiotics. The drugs may be given orally, washed over the infected bone with a blood drainage system, or applied with antibiotic-soaked dressings.

Chronic osteomyelitis usually requires surgery to remove dead bone and to promote drainage. Even after surgery, the prognosis is poor, leaving the person in great pain or perhaps even needing amputation. Some doctors use hyperbaric oxygen to help the blood fight the infection and plastic surgery to repair damaged areas and increase blood supply.

What can a person with osteomyelitis do?

A person who is discharged from the hospital can carefully follow instructions related to wound care and must report signs of recurrent infection (increased temperature, redness, localized warmth, and swelling.) The person must also seek prompt treatment for possible sources of recurrent disease, such as boils, styes, blisters, and impetigo.

OSTEOPOROSIS

What is this condition?

In osteoporosis, bones deteriorate faster than the body can replace them. The bones lose calcium and phosphate salts and become porous, brittle, and prone to fracture. Typically, osteoporosis is simply age-related or linked to an underlying disease. The disease is often called *senile* or *postmenopausal osteoporosis* because it develops mostly in elderly women.

What causes it?

The cause of osteoporosis is unknown. However, a mild but prolonged deficiency in calcium, resulting from a calcium-poor diet, may be an important contributing factor. Other suspected causes are

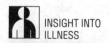

INSIGHT INTO
ILLNESS

Who gets osteoporosis?

Everyone loses some bone tissue with age. However, some circumstances and behavior cause more bone loss than average. The following factors affect a person's risk for osteoporosis:
- sex—osteoporosis affects four times as many women as men
- age—after age 50 the osteoporosis risk increases
- race—Whites and Asians are at greater risk than Blacks
- body frame—osteoporosis affects more petite, small-boned persons than average-sized, large-boned persons
- onset of menopause in women—the earlier the onset (whether natural or by hysterectomy), the higher the risk

- calcium-deficient diet
- sedentary lifestyle
- family history of osteoporosis
- regular alcohol and tobacco use or excessive caffeine consumption
- long-term corticosteroid, heparin, or certain antibiotic and antiseizure drug use
- medical conditions, such as chronic kidney failure and Cushing's syndrome; eating disorders, such as anorexia; hyperparathyroidism; hyperthyroidism; intestinal absorption disorders requiring special therapy, such as intestinal bypass or gastrectomy; liver disease or rheumatoid arthritis.

the decline of gonadal or adrenal gland function, faulty protein metabolism due to estrogen deficiency, and a sedentary lifestyle.

Osteoporosis is also caused by prolonged therapy with steroids or heparin, total immobilization or disuse of a bone, alcoholism, malnutrition, malabsorption, scurvy, lactose intolerance, and overactive thyroid gland. (See *Who gets osteoporosis?*)

What are its symptoms?

Osteoporosis is usually discovered when an elderly person bends to lift something, hears a snapping sound, and then feels a sudden pain in the lower back. The collapse of vertebrae, producing a backache with pain that radiates around the trunk, is the most common symptom. Any movement or jarring aggravates the backache.

Sometimes, osteoporosis can develop subtly, with increasing deformity, hunchback, loss of height, and a markedly aged appearance. As the bones in the back weaken, falls and fractures become common. However, the disorder rarely affects other bones as severely.

How is it diagnosed?

If the person's history suggests osteoporosis, the doctor will try to rule out other causes of bone-depleting disease, especially those affecting the spine. The doctor can also use other methods, including:

- X-rays to show typical degeneration in the lower-back vertebrae
- measurement of bone mass to check arms, legs, hips, and spine
- blood tests, which may show elevated parathyroid hormone levels
- bone biopsy to look for thin, porous, but otherwise normal-looking bone.

How is it treated?

Treatment aims to prevent additional fractures and control pain. The doctor may recommend a physical therapy program, emphasizing gentle exercise and activity. Estrogen, started within 3 years after menopause, may be given to decrease the rate of bone-mass loss. Other supplements include sodium fluoride to stimulate bone formation and calcium and vitamin D to support normal bone metabolism. However, drug therapy merely slows down osteoporosis and doesn't cure it.

Other treatments

A back brace may be necessary to support weakened vertebrae and surgery can correct some fractures. Changes in the person's diet and activity can help avoid more fractures. (See *Common questions about a calcium-rich diet*, page 198.) Hormonal and fluoride treatments may help. Osteoporosis caused by other diseases can be prevented through effective treatment of the underlying disease, as well as by corticosteroid therapy, early mobilization after surgery or injury, decreased alcohol consumption, and prompt treatment of an overactive thyroid.

Osteoporosis causes bones to deteriorate faster than the body can replace them. The bones lose calcium and phosphate, becoming porous, brittle, and easily broken.

What can a person with osteoporosis do?

- Be careful to avoid twisting movements and prolonged bending, and to stoop before lifting any objects. Call the doctor right away if new sites of pain develop.
- If you're taking estrogen, examine your breasts monthly for lumps or other abnormalities. Also, report any abnormal bleeding.
- Sleep on a firm mattress but avoid excessive bed rest.

Common questions about a calcium-rich diet

Your body needs calcium for strong bones and teeth. Eating calcium-rich foods is one way to make sure your body gets enough of this vital mineral. Here are some common questions about calcium.

My diet is very well balanced, but how do I know if I'm getting enough calcium?

Your calcium requirements change throughout your lifetime. For example, teenagers need extra calcium to meet the needs of their rapidly growing bones. Women need more calcium after menopause, as well as during pregnancy and while breast-feeding. Ask your nurse or doctor to help you determine exactly how much calcium you need each day.

What foods are the best sources of calcium?

Dairy products (milk, cheese, yogurt, and ice cream) are excellent calcium sources. If you're avoiding cholesterol or fat, you can still have skim or powdered milk and low-fat yogurt.

I don't like milk and it doesn't like me. Now what?

If you have trouble digesting milk, you may still be able to eat yogurt, hard cheeses, acidophilus milk, or lactose-reduced milk. (Ask your grocery store manager to order products such as Lactaid if they're not on the shelf.) Or ask your pharmacist about adding *Lactobacillus acidophilus* to regular milk. Also called Bacid and Lactinex, this substance makes milk easier to digest.

That's still too much dairy for me. Anything else?

Certain vegetables, such as collard or turnip greens and broccoli, are high in calcium, as are oysters, salmon, sardines, and tofu.

Other tips

Some foods, especially very fibrous foods, can interfere with your body's uptake of calcium. So, to get the most calcium from the foods you eat, avoid eating calcium- and fiber-rich foods at the same meal. Also, eat less red meat, chocolate, peanut butter, rhubarb, sweet potatoes, and fatty foods. Cut down also on caffeine-containing drinks, such as coffee, tea, and colas.

Calcium is most effective when your body has enough vitamin D. Spending just 15 minutes in sunshine every day will fill your daily requirement. Besides, most manufacturers add vitamin D to milk and cereals. Egg yolks, saltwater fish, and liver also have this vitamin.

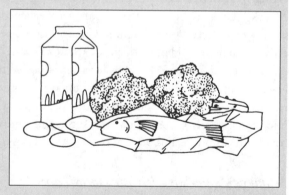

Avoid taking a vitamin D supplement, however, unless your doctor specifically tells you to do so. Too much vitamin D can do more harm than good.

PAGET'S DISEASE

What do doctors call this condition?
Osteitis deformans

What is this condition?
Paget's disease is a slow-paced metabolic bone disease characterized by replacement of sound bone with excessive amounts of abnormal bone. The altered bone is fragile and weak, causing painful deformities of both outside shape and internal structure. Paget's disease usually settles in one or several areas of the skeleton (most frequently the lower torso), but occasionally affects many parts of the body.

The disease can be fatal, especially when associated with congestive heart failure (widespread disease creates a continuous need for high cardiac output), bone cancer, or giant cell tumors.

What causes it?
Although the exact cause is unknown, one theory is that an early viral infection (possibly mumps) leaves behind a dormant skeletal infection that erupts many years later as Paget's disease. In the United States, Paget's disease affects approximately 2.5 million people over age 40 (mostly men). In 5% of cases, the involved bone experiences malignant changes.

What are its symptoms?
There may be no symptoms in early stages of the disease. But when pain does develop, it's usually severe and persistent and may limit the person's movement because new bone growth is rubbing on the spinal cord or sensory nerve root. The pain intensifies with exertion.

The list of potential effects includes enlarged forehead, headaches, hunchback, barrel-shaped chest, and bowed legs and other changes in gait. The affected areas are warm and tender, susceptible to breaks, and slow to heal. The disease progresses to add bone growth that interferes with sight, hearing, and balance; complications such as hypertension, gout, and congestive heart failure may develop.

How is it diagnosed?
X-rays, taken even before symptoms appear, can show increased bone expansion and density. A bone scan, which is more sensitive than

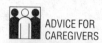

ADVICE FOR
CAREGIVERS

Paget's disease: How you can help

The person with Paget's disease must deal with constant pain and restricted movements. Here are some changes you can make to promote independence and comfort.

Teach the patient

• To expedite lifestyle changes imposed by this disease, teach the person how to pace activities; if necessary, provide instruction with crutches, a walker, or other devices.

• Encourage the person to follow a recommended exercise program, avoiding both immobilization and excessive activity.

• Encourage a schedule of regular checkups, including eye and ear exams.

Increase comfort

• Get the person a firm mattress or a bed board to minimize spinal deformities.

• To prevent falls at home, remove throw rugs and other small obstacles.

Get more help

• Help your family members make use of community support resources, such as a visiting nurse or home health agency.

• For more information, contact the Paget's Disease Foundation.

X-rays, clearly shows early so-called *pagetic lesions*. Bone biopsy reveals a characteristic mosaic pattern. Blood tests and other laboratory tests aid early diagnosis.

How is it treated?

Primary treatment consists of drug therapy and includes one of the following:

• Cibacalcin, a hormone, given by injection, and Didronel to retard bone resorption (which relieves bone lesions). Although Cibacalcin requires long-term maintenance therapy, there is noticeable improvement after the first few weeks of treatment. Didronel produces improvement after 1 to 3 months.

• Mithracin, an antibiotic that produces remission of symptoms within 2 weeks and biochemical improvement within 1 to 2 months. However, the drug may destroy blood cells or harm kidney function. Self-administration of Cibacalcin and Didronel helps people with Paget's disease lead near-normal lives. Still, they may need surgery to reduce or prevent fractures, correct secondary deformities, and relieve pinched nerves. Aspirin, Indocin, or Advil or Motrin usually controls pain. (See *Paget's disease: How you can help.*)

SCOLIOSIS

What is this condition?

Scoliosis is a sideways curvature of the spine that may affect any segment of the spine. The curve may be convex to the right (more common in chest-level curves) or to the left (more common in lower back curves). The spine may be rotated around its axis, deforming the rib cage. Scoliosis is often associated with humpback and swayback.

What causes it?

The deformity of scoliosis may be *structural*, in which the spinal curvature is fixed, or *functional*, in which the spine is temporarily deformed from poor posture or uneven leg heights.

Structural scoliosis may result from an inherited defect, such as wedge-shaped vertebrae, fused ribs or vertebrae, or partial vertebrae. It may be paralytic or musculoskeletal, developing several months after a one-sided paralysis of the trunk muscles due to polio, cerebral

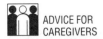

ADVICE FOR
CAREGIVERS

Scoliosis: How to detect it

To check your child for an abnormal curvature of the spine, perform this simple test. First, have your child remove her shirt and stand up straight. Then look at her back, and answer these questions:

- Is one shoulder higher than the other, or is one shoulder blade more prominent?
- When the child's arms hang loosely at her sides, does one arm swing away from the body more than the other?
- Is one hip higher or more prominent than the other?
- Does the child seem to tilt to one side?

Then, ask your child to bend forward, with arms hanging down and palms together at knee level.

- Can you see a hump on the back at the ribs or near the waist?

If your answer to any of these questions is "yes," notify your doctor. Your child needs careful evaluation for scoliosis.

The person shown at right demonstrates the obvious effects of scoliosis: Her body tilts to one side; her left hip is higher than her right hip; and her right shoulder is higher than her left shoulder.

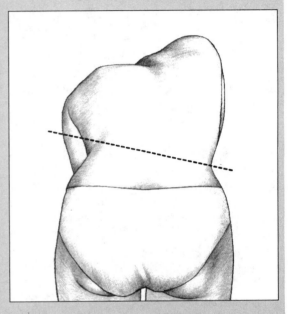

palsy, or muscular dystrophy. Or it may be idiopathic (the most common form), which may be acquired through several genetic traits. This form of scoliosis appears in a previously straight spine during the growth years.

Idiopathic scoliosis can be infantile (affecting mostly male infants between birth and age 3), juvenile (affecting both sexes between ages 4 and 10), or adolescent (usually affecting girls between age 10 and maturity).

What are its symptoms?

The most common deformity in either functional or structural scoliosis begins at chest level and creates an S curve in an attempt to balance the body. Scoliosis rarely produces discomfort until it's well established, when backache, fatigue, and difficulty breathing are among the symptoms.

How to adjust to your brace

Now that you have a brace to help control scoliosis, here are some tips to help you wear it more comfortably and effectively.

How to get used to your brace
Adjusting to your brace may take about 2 weeks. Don't be discouraged if it feels awkward at first. As you gradually build up to wearing the brace full time (the time your doctor recommends), it will feel more natural.

How to care for your skin
- Wear your brace the way your nurse and doctor taught you. If you wear it incorrectly, it can irritate your skin. Always wear a soft, snug undershirt between your brace and your skin. A loose one can wrinkle under the brace and irritate your skin.
- Change your undershirt at least once a day and more often if you perspire. This will help you avoid skin irritation or acne.
- Check your skin for red marks or other irritation whenever you remove your brace. Especially check the skin under the brace pads and over your hip bones. Apply rubbing alcohol to these areas regularly to toughen your skin and help prevent blisters

and skin breakdown. Don't use lotions or powders on the skin under your brace.
- Wash your brace with mild soap and water every few days. And make sure it's dry before you put it back on.

Dressing to cover the brace
- If your usual clothing doesn't fit over the brace, look for looser-fitting clothing.
- If your brace's metal hardware tears your clothing, cover the metal parts with moleskin (available at drugstores).

Resuming activities
After your brace feels more comfortable, you can resume most of your former activities. If you're a student, the doctor may let you remove your brace for gym class or special occasions. And the doctor won't recommend wearing the brace for vigorous activities that require a lot of flexibility, like gymnastics.

Your special exercises
Do the special exercises your physical therapist taught you. These exercises will promote muscle tone and flexibility. Be sure to do them as often as recommended. And always practice standing tall.

Because many teenagers are shy about their bodies, a parent may only eventually notice uneven hemlines, pantlegs that appear unequal in length, or subtle physical signs such as one hip appearing higher than the other. Untreated scoliosis can cause decreased lung capacity, back pain, degenerative spinal arthritis, disk disease, and pain in the hips and thighs. (See *Scoliosis: How to detect it*, page 201.)

How is it diagnosed?
The doctor can see a change in the curvature and flexibility of the young person's spine, uneven shoulder height, and asymmetrical

musculature. A series of spinal X-rays will confirm the scoliosis and tell how far it has gone.

How is it treated?

Treatment is guided by the severity of the deformity and potential spine growth. To be most effective, treatment should begin early when the curvature is still mild.

Here are some of the methods the doctor will use:

■ A curve of less than 25 degrees is mild and monitored by X-rays and an exam every 3 months. An exercise program that includes sit-up pelvic tilts, spine stretching, push-ups, and breathing exercises may strengthen torso muscles and stop the curve's progression. A heel lift in the shoe also may help.

■ A curve of 30 to 50 degrees requires management with spinal exercises and a brace. Stimulation with a mild electrical current may be an alternative. A brace stops progression in most children but doesn't reverse an established curvature. Braces passively strengthen the spine by applying asymmetrical pressure to the skin, muscles, and ribs, and can be adjusted as the child grows and completes bone growth. (See *How to adjust to your brace.*)

■ A curve of 40 degrees or more requires surgery (spinal fusion) because a lateral curve continues to progress at the rate of 1 degree a year even after skeletal maturity. Some surgeons prescribe a belt-pulley-weight system of traction and an exercise program for 7 to 10 days before surgery. The surgery often involves fusing part of the spine and implanting a metal rod as an internal splint to straighten the curve.

*T*ENDINITIS AND BURSITIS

What are these conditions?

Tendinitis is a painful inflammation of tendons and of tendon-muscle attachments to bone, usually in the shoulders, hips, Achilles tendons, or hamstrings. Bursitis is a painful inflammation of one or more of the fluid-filled sacs that cover and cushion the ends of bones. Bursitis usually occurs under the shoulder muscles, at the elbows, the hip sockets, heel bones, or kneecaps.

What causes them?

Tendinitis commonly results from injury (such as strain during sports activity), another musculoskeletal disorder (rheumatic diseases, congenital defects), poor posture, abnormal body development, or loose tendons.

Bursitis usually occurs in middle age from repeated injury to a joint or from an inflammatory joint disease (rheumatoid arthritis, gout). Chronic bursitis follows attacks of acute bursitis or repeated injury and infection. Infectious bursitis may result from wound infection or from bacterial invasion of skin over the bursa.

What are their symptoms?

With tendinitis of the shoulder, rotation of the arm is difficult and painful. The pain is usually worse at night, interfering with sleep. Pain typically extends from the top of the shoulder to a point under the large shoulder muscle in the back. Fluid accumulation causes swelling; in some cases, calcium deposits in the tendon cause weakness. These deposits may spread into nearby joints and bursae, aggravating the condition.

In bursitis, fluid accumulation in the bursae causes irritation, inflammation, and sudden or gradual pain, and limits movement. Other symptoms vary according to the affected site. Shoulder bursitis interferes with arm movement. Kneecap bursitis (housemaid's knee) produces pain when the person climbs stairs. Hip bursitis makes it painful to cross the legs.

How are they diagnosed?

In tendinitis, X-rays may be normal at first but later show bony fragments, changes in the bone, or calcium deposits. Diagnosis of tendinitis must rule out other causes of shoulder pain, such as blocked arteries and tendon injury. Characteristically, heat treatment aggravates the shoulder pain of tendinitis, in contrast to other painful joint disorders, in which heat is palliative.

Localized pain and inflammation and a history of unusual strain or injury 2 to 3 days before pain begins indicate bursitis. During its early stages X-rays may appear normal except in calcific bursitis, in which X-rays may show calcium deposits.

How are they treated?

Treatment to relieve pain includes resting the joint (by immobilizing it with a sling, splint, or cast), pain medication, applying cold or heat,

SELF-HELP

Exercises to ease your aching shoulder

These exercises can help you keep your shoulder relaxed so that it doesn't stiffen. Try to do your exercises once a day or as often as your doctor or physical therapist directs.

Arm circling

- Stand sideways next to a table or the back of a chair. Hold on with your unaffected arm for support. Now, bend forward at the waist. Let your sore arm hang down like a pendulum.
- Make slow circles with your sore arm. Gradually increase the size of the circles until you can swing your arm in large clockwise circles in front of you. Then reverse the direction and make counterclockwise circles.
- As your shoulder inflammation subsides, the doctor may ask you to increase the number of times you do this exercise. Ask him or the physical therapist if you should use weights while you do this exercise.

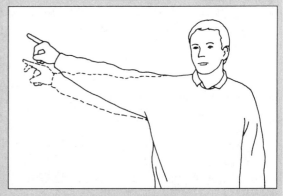

- Next, stand sideways with your sore shoulder facing the wall about an arm's length away. Repeat the previous exercise. As your fingers climb higher, sidestep closer to the wall to allow your shoulder the maximum range of motion.
- Each day, try to reach a higher point on the wall.

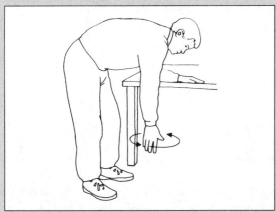

Finger climbing

- Stand facing a wall, an arm's length away. Place the hand of your sore arm on the wall and slowly walk your index and middle fingers up the wall as high as you can without discomfort. Hold this position for a few seconds; then walk your fingers down again. Repeat as often as your doctor instructs.

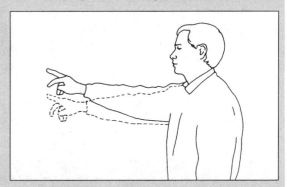

Arm lifting with a pulley

- Drape a bath towel over a secure shower rod, or attach a pulley and rope in an open doorway. Grab an end of the towel or rope with each hand. Using your unaffected arm, gently pull on the towel or rope, lifting your sore arm upward.
- When you've raised your sore arm as high as you can without discomfort, hold the position for a few seconds. Then let your arm drop slowly.

(continued)

Exercises to ease your aching shoulder *(continued)*

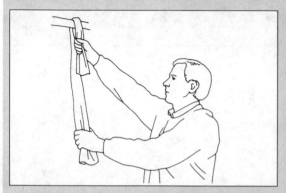

Extending the arm with a broomstick
- Grasp a broomstick (or cane or yardstick) with both hands at hip level and raise it up over your head.
- Lower it behind your head to the back of your neck. Hold the position for as long as you comfortably can; then reverse the procedure.
- Each day, try to hold the broom behind your head a little longer, until you can hold the position for several minutes.

Elbow raising
- Place the hand of your sore arm on the opposite shoulder. Using your unaffected hand, gently push the elbow of your sore arm straight up as far as you can without discomfort.
- Lower your elbow to the starting position.
- Each day, try to hold your elbow up a little longer, until you can hold the position for a few minutes.

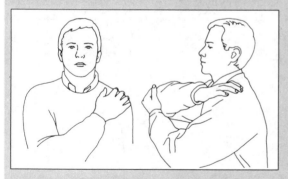

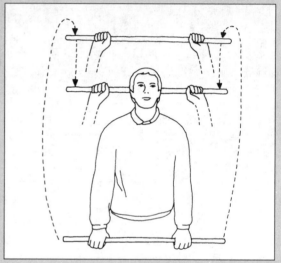

ultrasound therapy, or local injection of an anesthetic and corticosteroids to reduce inflammation. A mixture of a corticosteroid and an anesthetic, such as Xylocaine, generally provides immediate pain relief. Extended-release injections of corticosteroids offer longer pain relief.

Treatment also includes oral anti-inflammatory agents, such as Clinoril and Indocin, and other pain relievers, until the person is free of pain and able to perform range-of-motion exercises easily. (See *Exercises to ease your aching shoulder*, pages 205 and 206.)

Other treatments

Other treatments include fluid aspiration (removal through a needle), physical therapy to preserve motion and prevent frozen joints (usually effective in 1 to 4 weeks), and heat therapy; and ice packs for calcific tendinitis. Rarely, calcific tendinitis requires surgical removal of the calcium deposits. Long-term control of chronic bursitis and tendinitis may require changes in the person's activities to prevent more joint irritation.

TENNIS ELBOW

What do doctors call this condition?

Epicondylitis, epitrochlear bursitis

What is this condition?

Tennis elbow is a painful inflammation of the forearm extensor tendon fibers at the point where they attach to the upper arm (humerus) adjacent to the elbow joint.

What causes it?

Tennis elbow probably begins as a partial tear on the involved tendon and is common among tennis players and other persons whose activities require a forceful grasp, wrist extension against resistance, or frequent rotation of the forearm. Left untreated, the condition can become disabling.

What are its symptoms?

The first symptom is elbow pain that gradually worsens and often radiates to the forearm and back of the hand whenever the person grasps an object or twists his or her elbow. Other symptoms are tenderness over the joint and a weak grasp. In rare instances, tennis elbow may cause local heat, swelling, or restricted range of motion.

How is it diagnosed?

Because X-rays are almost always negative, the doctor depends on the person's reports of pain while playing tennis or a similar activity. The

 SELF-HELP

How to deal with your tennis elbow

Here are some tips to relieve the pain and speed the recovery of tennis elbow:
- Take your anti-inflammatory drugs with food to avoid stomach irritation.
- Rest the elbow until inflammation subsides.
- If you are wearing a support, remove it daily, and gently move the arm to prevent stiffness and contracture.
- Follow the prescribed exercise program. For example, you can stretch your arm and flex your wrist to the maximum; then, press the back of your hand against a wall until you can feel a pull in your forearm. Hold this position for 1 minute.
- Warm up for 15 to 20 minutes before beginning any sports activity.
- Wear an elastic support or splint during any activity that stresses the forearm or elbow.

pain can be reproduced by having the person move his or her wrist in a manner similar to that used when swinging a racket.

How is it treated?

Treatment aims to relieve pain, usually by local injection of corticosteroid and a local anesthetic and by taking aspirin or Indocin. Supportive treatment includes an immobilizing splint from the forearm to the elbow, which generally relieves pain in 2 to 3 weeks. Some doctors use heat therapy, such as warm compresses and ultrasound, and physical therapy, such as manipulation and massage. (See *How to deal with your tennis elbow*, page 207.)

A "tennis elbow strap" has helped many people. This strap, which is wrapped snugly around the forearm, helps relieve the strain on affected forearm muscles and tendons. If these measures prove ineffective, surgical release of the tendon at the hand may be necessary.

DIGESTIVE DISORDERS

ANAL FISSURE

What is this condition?

An anal fissure is a cut or crack in the lining of the anus that extends to the sphincter muscle. A fissure at the back of the anus, the most common injury, occurs equally in males and females. A fissure in the front of the anus, the rarer type, is 10 times more common in females. The chance for cure is very good, especially with surgery and good anal hygiene.

What causes it?

A fissure at the back of the anus results from passage of large, hard stools that stretch the rectal lining beyond its limits. A fissure at the front usually results from strain on the perineum during childbirth and, rarely, from scar tissue that narrows the passage. Occasionally, the fissure is caused by inflammation, anal tuberculosis, or cancer.

What are its symptoms?

An acute anal fissure starts with tearing, cutting, or burning pain during or immediately after a bowel movement. A few drops of blood may streak toilet paper or underclothes. Swelling at the lower end of the fissure, called a *sentinel pile*, can cause painful spasms. A fissure may heal spontaneously and completely, or it may partially heal and break open again. Repeated fissures leave scar tissue that hampers normal bowel movement.

How is it diagnosed?

The doctor can use a scope to see the tear. Probing the area will cause pain and bleeding. The doctor may also pull back the skin to expose the swelling at the end of the fissure.

How is it treated?

If the tear is superficial and no hemorrhoids have developed, the doctor may numb the area with a local anesthetic and stretch the sphincter muscle with his or her fingers. If the fissure has caused complications, it may require surgery to remove some tissue and loosen the muscle. (See *After surgery for a fissure.*)

ANAL ITCHING AND BURNING

What do doctors call this condition?
Pruritis ani

What causes it?
Anal itching and burning is more common in men than in women. It can be caused by poor hygiene or overly intense cleaning of the area. Medications, therapies, and dietary changes used to treat anal disorders also may cause anal itching and burning.

What are its symptoms?
Anal itching and burning usually happens after a bowel movement, during stress, or at night. If it is severe, scratching produces reddened skin and weeping sores. With chronic itching, the skin becomes thick, leathery, and discolored.

How is it diagnosed?
The doctor asks for a detailed history of the symptoms and then examines the anal area to rule out fissures (cracks or cuts) and fistulas (abnormal, tubelike passages from one body cavity to another). The person may be tested for allergies or have a biopsy taken to rule out cancer.

How is it treated?
First, the condition or activity causing the discomfort is eliminated. Then the doctor or nurse will suggest proper ways to keep the anal area clean, such as wiping the area with witch hazel pads and tucking cotton balls between the buttocks to absorb moisture. (See *Preventing anal itching*.)

SELF-HELP

Preventing anal itching

Proper anal hygiene is the most effective way to avoid anal itching. If the itching and burning are associated with another health problem, get treatment for the underlying cause of the discomfort.

Conditions requiring treatment
- Minor injury caused by straining to move bowels
- Small skin growths in the anal area
- Diseases, such as diabetes and liver disorders
- Localized problems such as hemorrhoids, a fistula, or fissure
- Skin diseases, such as dermatitis or psoriasis
- Skin conditions, such as some cancers, syphilis, and tuberculosis
- Fungi or parasites, such as pinworms, itch mites (scabies), and lice
- Food allergies

Possible aggravating factors
- Too much cleaning of the area with harsh soap and scrubbing with a washcloth or toilet paper
- Antibiotics, such as E-Mycin, Lincocin, and Achromycin
- Antihypertensives or antacids that cause diarrhea
- Anxiety
- Conditions that cause excessive sweating in the groin area, such as tight clothing, hot climates, or obesity
- Spicy foods, coffee, alcohol, or food preservatives
- Self-prescribed creams or powders, perfumed soaps, perfumed or colored toilet paper, detergents, or certain fabrics that may be irritating

ANORECTAL ABSCESS

What is this condition?

Anorectal abscess is a localized accumulation of pus that results from inflamed tissues near the rectum or anus. Inflammation may produce a fistula — an abnormal tubelike passage in the skin — that opens into the rectum. This condition is far more common in men than in women, possibly because men wear coarser clothing, which may irritate the skin and interfere with air circulation.

What causes it?

Inflammation and the resulting abscess typically begin with a scrape or tear in the lining of the anal canal, rectum, or skin that later becomes infected. It may be caused by an injection for treatment of internal hemorrhoids; an enema tip; internal puncture wound from undigested sharp objects such as eggshells or fishbones; or by insertion of a foreign object. Muscle strains or an illness may start the abscess, but many abscesses develop without an obvious cause.

As pus develops, a fistula may form in the soft tissue beneath the muscle fibers of the sphincters (especially the external sphincter).

What are its symptoms?

The person with an abscess feels a throbbing pain and tenderness at the infection site. A hard, painful lump develops on one side that makes sitting uncomfortable.

How is it diagnosed?

The doctor can find the abscess with his or her fingers and by a visual exam. Usually it appears as a red, tender, oval swelling close to the anus. Sitting or coughing increases pain, and pus may drain from the abscess. Less often, the abscess covers a large area and the doctor can see a hard mass that bulges into the anal canal. An abscess higher in the canal may produce a dull, aching pain in the rectum, tenderness and, occasionally, a swelling and hardness the doctor can find with his or her finger.

An abscess high in the pelvis is rare, but it may be heralded by a fever and a tender mass. Sometimes the doctor will insert a scope to examine the area or order barium enema X-rays to rule out other problems.

How the abscess drains

If the abscess drains by forming a fistula, the pain usually goes away. The doctor sees the drainage and irritated skin where the fistula opens. If the infection is severe, the person may have chills, fever, nausea, vomiting, and feel generally uncomfortable.

How is it treated?

Anorectal abscesses require surgery, with a local anesthetic, to drain the pus. If the abscess has formed a fistula, that must also be removed and then a drain inserted for 48 hours.

What can a person with an anorectal abscess do?

After surgery, the person receives medication for pain relief and begins a recovery that takes 4 to 5 weeks for a common abscess and 12 to 16 weeks it it's more involved. Cleaning the area regularly and gently will avoid another infection. The person also may need a stool-softening laxative, such as Hydrocil Instant or Metamucil, to avoid constipation, which might stress the incision.

APPENDICITIS

What is this condition?

Appendicitis is a medical emergency in which the appendix is inflamed due to obstruction and may rupture and spread infection. This is the most common major surgical emergency, affecting men and women equally. Left untreated, appendicitis is fatal, but surgery is an effective cure. Also, the use of antibiotics has helped reduced the number of cases and, thus, the death rate.

What causes it?

Appendicitis is probably the result of an obstruction in the tube that passes through the appendix from the intestine. This blockage may be caused by a bit of stool, constriction of the tube, or a viral infection. The obstruction causes inflammation, which may lead to infection, a clot, tissue decay, and perforation. If the appendix ruptures or perforates, the infection spills into the abdominal cavity, causing the most common and dangerous complication of appendicitis — peritonitis. (See *If you suspect appendicitis.*)

What are its symptoms?

Symptoms usually occur in the following sequence:
- pain in or around the upper right abdomen
- loss of appetite, nausea, and vomiting
- pain concentrated in the lower right abdomen, with a "boardlike" abdominal rigidity
- increasing tenderness, increasingly severe abdominal spasms and, almost always, soreness to the touch
- lower left side too tender to touch, suggesting the lining of abdomen is inflamed
- constipation (possibly diarrhea), slight fever, and rapid heartbeat
- abdominal pain that ends suddenly (usually means that the appendix has perforated or burst).

How is it diagnosed?

Your doctor will ask about symptoms, check for tenderness, and look for a mild fever and a moderately high white blood cell count. The physical exam and blood test rule out many illnesses with similar symptoms.

 SELF-HELP

If you suspect appendicitis

Because the start of appendicitis can feel like the flu or another sort of stomach ache, some people treat themselves with home remedies. That's a mistake. If you have appendicitis symptoms, you need emergency treatment immediately.

Avoid home remedies
Some home remedies may be harmful. For instance:
- Never take a laxative or an enema.
- Never apply heat to your lower right side. It may cause your appendix to rupture.
- Don't take pain-relief medication because it may mask your symptoms.

Colitis complications

Colitis may lead to complications that affect other areas of the body, including:
- anemia from iron deficiency, clotting defects due to vitamin K deficiency
- red bumps on the face and arms, sores on the legs and ankles
- eye inflammation
- liver thickening, cirrhosis, possibly cancer
- arthritis, stiff back, loss of muscle mass
- narrowing, growths, infection of the stomach and intestine.

How is it treated?

Appendectomy, surgery to remove the appendix, is the only effective treatment. Laparoscopic appendectomies, performed through very small incisions, shorten the recovery time.

If the infection has spread and peritonitis develops, the doctor will use antibiotics to fight it and tubes to drain the abdominal cavity.

COLITIS

What do doctors call this condition?

Ulcerative colitis

What is this condition?

Colitis is an inflammatory, often chronic disease that affects the lining of the lower intestine. It starts in the lowest section and often extends upward into the colon, producing swelling and open sores. The small intestine is rarely involved. Most cases are mild and localized; however, prompt medical attention is necessary because the disorder can progress rapidly and may cause a perforated colon and potentially fatal infection of the abdominal lining.

People with colitis run a higher than average risk of developing colon cancer, especially if the disease begins before age 15 or persists for longer than 10 years.

What causes it?

The exact cause of colitis is not known. One theory links it to abnormal immune response in the stomach and intestine, possibly associated with food or bacteria. Stress, once suspected of causing colitis, has been shown merely to worsen it. It is most common in young adults, especially women, and symptoms seems to peak between ages 15 and 20, with another peak between ages 55 and 60.

What are its symptoms?

The primary symptoms of colitis are repeated attacks of pain accompanied by bloody diarrhea, often containing pus. The intensity of the attacks varies with the extent of inflammation. Other symptoms include spastic rectum and anus, abdominal pain, weakness, irritability, loss of appetite, weight loss, nausea, and vomiting. (See *Colitis complications*.)

How is it diagnosed?

The doctor can use a scope to see changes in the mucous lining of the lower intestine and detect thick pus. He or she may also obtain a specimen for study to confirm the condition and use a deeper scope to check how far the disease extends and what harm it's done. A barium enema X-ray can show the extent of the disease and detect complications, such as narrowed passages and cancer. Lab tests and blood tests reveal the severity of the attack.

How is it treated?

Severe colitis requires hospitalization. Drugs are used to treat inflammation, nutrition is monitored, and dehydration due to excessive diarrhea is corrected. Intravenous feeding helps the intestinal tract to rest, decreases stool volume, and restores positive nitrogen balance. Blood transfusions or iron supplements may be needed to correct anemia.

Surgery is a last resort and is performed only if other measures fail or the symptoms become unbearable. The most common surgical procedure simply removes the diseased section of intestine. Another type of surgery creates a reservoir, known as a *Kock pouch*, from a loop of small intestine that empties through a tube opening just above the pubic hairline. (See *What to expect after Kock-pouch surgery*.)

CROHN'S DISEASE

What do doctors call this condition?

Regional enteritis, granulomatous colitis

What is this condition?

Crohn's disease is an inflammation of any part of the digestive tract. The inflammation extends through the intestinal wall. Swelling caused by a blockage in the intestinal wall leads to inflammation, sores, narrowing of passages and, possibly, abscesses and fistulas (abnormal passages between body cavities).

The most common site is the end of the small intestine. It may affect nearby lymph nodes as well as the membrane that holds the small intestines. Mild cases are relieved by changes in diet and lifestyle.

What causes it?

Crohn's disease is most common in adults ages 20 to 40 and may run in families. Its exact cause is unknown. Some experts suspect allergies and other immune disorders or infection; others are investigating possible genetic links.

What are its symptoms?

Symptoms depend on the location and size of the inflammation. The mild, yet persistent symptoms of chronic Crohn's disease are most common and include diarrhea, pain in the lower right abdomen, excessive fat in the stools, weight loss, occasionally fatigue and, rarely, clubbing of the fingers. In a flare-up of Crohn's disease, symptoms mimic those of appendicitis: steady, colicky, pain in the lower right abdomen, cramping, tenderness, release of gas, nausea, fever, diarrhea and, possibly, bloody stools. Complications can include intestinal obstruction, bowel-bladder fistulas, abscesses in the abdomen and around the anus or rectum, and perforation.

How is it diagnosed?

Lab tests will show an increase in white blood cells and other imbalances. A barium enema X-ray and other X-ray studies may be used to check changes in the shape of the bowel. Also, the doctor may use a special scope to inspect for patchy areas of inflammation to rule out ulcerative colitis. However, biopsy (obtaining a tissue specimen for study) is the only way to confirm a diagnosis.

How is it treated?

Initial treatment involves easing symptoms. For example, if the person is very sick, the doctor will order intravenous liquids and nutrients to rest the gastrointestinal tract and prescribe drugs to reduce inflammation, subdue the body's immune system, and fight bacterial infection. Serious side effects may necessitate surgery to correct bowel perforation or massive bleeding. Only in the most severe cases is the diseased colon surgically removed.

Crohn's disease is most common in adults ages 20 to 40 and may run in families. Its exact cause is unknown. Possible factors include allergies, other immune disorders, infection, or genetic predisposition.

What can a person with Crohn's disease do?

The most helpful steps you can take involve making lifestyle changes: get more rest, restrict dietary fiber (no fruit or vegetables), and eliminate dairy products (for lactose intolerance). If stress is clearly an aggravating factor, consider getting counseling.

DAMAGED ESOPHAGUS

What do doctors call this condition?

Corrosive esophagitis and stricture

What is this condition?

Damaged esophagus refers to the inflammation and injury to the throat after someone swallows a caustic chemical. Similar to a burn, this injury may be temporary or lead to permanent narrowing that requires surgery. If severe, the injury can quickly cause inflammation, perforation, and death from infection, shock, and bleeding (if perforation involves the nearby aorta).

What causes it?

The most common cause is swallowing lye or another strong alkali; less often, a strong acid. After exposure to the toxic chemical, tissue becomes swollen and inflamed, sores form and dead tissue sloughs off, leaving scars. Damage may be limited to the mucous lining or it may affect all layers of the esophagus. In children, damaged esophagus usually results from accidentally swallowing household chemicals; in adults, it usually accompanies attempted suicide.

What are its symptoms?

Symptoms range from none at all to intense pain in the mouth and chest, excessive salivation, inability to swallow, and rapid breathing. Bloody vomit that contains pieces of tissue signals severe damage. A rattling sound may mean that the esophagus has been destroyed. If the person can't speak, the voice box may be damaged. The first 3 to 4 days afterward are critical. During this time, the person will be unable to eat. Fever may mean the wound is infected. In rare cases, scar tissue may make swallowing difficult — even years later.

ADVICE FOR CAREGIVERS

Damaged esophagus: How you can help

If you discover someone has swallowed a caustic chemical, here are some important suggestions.

Act at the scene
- Don't try to make the person vomit or try to rinse his or her throat because doing so may injure the esophagus again.
- Don't let the person swallow anything because the corrosive chemical may cause further damage to the mucous membrane lining of the stomach.
- If necessary, be prepared to give CPR.

Get immediate help
- Get the person to a doctor as fast as possible.
- Take the container that held the chemical with you to help the doctor identify it.

Following up
- Because the adult who has swallowed a corrosive chemical is usually attempting suicide, help and encourage him or her to seek psychological counseling.
- If a child has swallowed a chemical, check the home environment and take preventive measures, such as locking cabinets and keeping all household chemicals out of his reach.

How is it diagnosed?

The doctor will ask about the type and amount of chemical the person has swallowed and will inspect the throat for burns, white membranes, or swelling. He or she may use a scope or order a barium swallow X-ray and other X-ray studies to measure the injury and its progress over several weeks. (See *Damaged esophagus: How you can help.*)

How is it treated?

Conservative treatment includes drugs to control inflammation and inhibit scarring, and an antibiotic to prevent infection. The doctor may use a thin, flexible, instrument called a *bougie* to dilate the person's esophagus and, thereby, minimize narrowing. Some doctors begin this treatment immediately and continue it regularly; others delay starting for a week to avoid the risk of perforating the esophagus. Intravenous fluids and nutrients are administered while the person can't swallow. Clear liquids and then soft foods are added to the diet as recovery progresses.

Perforation of the esophagus requires immediate surgery. Also, surgery may be used to correct a narrowing that can't be treated with a bougie. This procedure usually involves transplanting a piece of the colon to the damaged esophagus. However, even after surgery, closing may recur at the site of the damage.

DIVERTICULOSIS

What do doctors call this condition?

Diverticular disease, diverticulitis

What is this condition?

In diverticulosis, bulging pouches (called diverticula) in the stomach or intestinal wall push through the surrounding muscle. Usually, the pouches are in the lower intestine, but they may develop anywhere, from the top of the stomach (rare) to the anus. An inherited form, called Meckel's diverticulum, is the most common genetic disorder of the intestinal tract.

Diverticulosis takes two forms. In one, the pouches are present but don't cause symptoms. In the other, the pouches are inflamed and may cause potentially fatal intestinal blockage, infection, or bleeding.

What causes it?

Diverticulosis is most common in men over age 40. In these individuals, pouches probably result from straining, which pushes the intestines against weak spots in the gastrointestinal wall.

Lack of dietary fiber may be a contributing factor. Without adequate fiber, fecal matter solidifies and the bowel tunnel narrows, requiring higher abdominal pressure during bowel movements. This theory is supported by the fact that diverticulosis is most prevalent in industrialized nations, where processing removes much of the fiber from foods.

How the pouches become inflamed

Undigested food mixed with bacteria accumulates in these intestinal pouches and forms a hard mass. This condition restricts blood flow to the thin walls of the pouches, making them more susceptible to attack by the bacteria in the colon. Inflammation follows, possibly leading to perforation, abscess, peritonitis, obstruction, or bleeding. Occasionally, the inflamed segment may produce a fistula, or tunnel, by sticking to the bladder or other organs. (See *How diverticula form*.)

What are its symptoms?

Usually, diverticulosis produces no symptoms; however it may cause recurrent pain in the lower left abdomen that disappears after bowel movements or passing gas. The person may have alternating constipation and diarrhea and symptoms similar to those of irritable bowel syndrome — or may have both disorders at once. In rare cases, some elderly people develop bleeding in uninfected pouches, but this is easily controlled with medication.

A mildly infected pouch produces some pain in the lower left abdomen, mild nausea, gas, irregular bowel movements, and a low-grade fever. A severely infected pouch can rupture and produce abscesses or infection in the abdominal cavity. Rupture, which occurs in about 20% of all cases, constitutes a medical emergency. The individual typically feels abdominal rigidity and pain in the lower left abdomen. Other symptoms of rupture include fever, chills, low blood pressure and, possibly, internal bleeding. Chronically infected pouches may cause growths and adhesions that narrow or obstruct the bowel. Symptoms of incomplete obstruction are constipation,

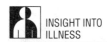
INSIGHT INTO ILLNESS

How diverticula form

Diverticula are small pouches that form along the colon wall. They develop from a buildup of pressure that pushes the mucous layer out through a weakness in the muscular layer.

As this close-up shows, a narrow neck connects a diverticulum to the interior space of the intestine. Fecal matter may accumulate within this pouch, cutting off its blood supply and leading to infection and inflammation.

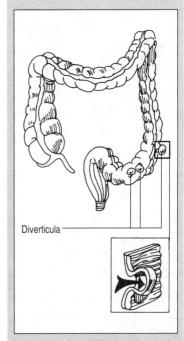

Diverticula

SELF-HELP

How to deal with diverticulosis

If you have uncomplicated diverticulosis, you can probably avoid future digestive tract problems by following these suggestions.

Adjust your diet
- Be aware that lack of roughage in the diet helps to encourage undigested food to collect in pouches on the intestine and risks serious infection.
- Learn how to change your diet to avoid the harmful effects of constipation and straining to move your bowels.
- Increase your intake of foods high in roughage (undigestible fiber), including fresh fruits and vegetables, whole grain bread, and wheat or bran cereals.

Avoid discomfort
- Be prepared for the diet change to temporarily cause gas and discomfort.
- You can relieve constipation with stool softeners or bulk-forming laxatives, but take them with plenty of water. Swallowed dry, they may absorb enough moisture in the mouth and throat to swell and choke you.

ribbonlike stools, intermittent diarrhea, and abdominal distention. Increasing obstruction causes abdominal rigidity and pain, nausea, and vomiting.

How is it diagnosed?

Because it rarely produces symptoms, diverticular disease is often discovered coincidentally during a physical exam that includes an upper GI barium X-ray series. These X-rays show or rule out diverticulosis of the esophagus and upper bowel. A barium enema X-ray confirms or rules out diverticulosis of the lower bowel. A biopsy (tissue specimen obtained for study) can rule out cancer.

How is it treated?

Diverticulosis without symptoms generally doesn't need treatment. For pain, mild gastric distress, constipation, or difficult bowel movements, the doctor may prescribe a liquid or bland diet, stool softeners, and occasional doses of mineral oil to relieve symptoms and reduce the risk of severe disease. After the pain subsides, most people also benefit from a high-fiber diet, perhaps supplemented with a bulk medication such as Metamucil.

Treating infected pouches when there are no signs of perforation involves preventing constipation and combating infection. This typically includes rest, a liquid diet, stool softeners, a broad-spectrum antibiotic, and medication to control pain, relax smooth muscles, and control muscle spasms. (See *How to deal with diverticulosis.*)

Additional treatments

If the infected pouches fail to respond to other treatment, surgery is used to remove the involved segment. Perforation, peritonitis, obstruction, or fistulae that develop from untreated pouches may require a temporary colostomy to drain abscesses and rest the colon. This procedure is later followed by reconstructive surgery.

People who hemorrhage need blood replacement and careful monitoring of fluid and electrolyte balance. The bleeding usually stops spontaneously. If it continues, the surgeon can insert a tube to deliver medication into the bleeding vessel.

GASTROENTERITIS

What do most people call this condition?
Viral enteritis, intestinal flu, traveler's diarrhea, food poisoning

What is this condition?
Gastroenteritis is a severe stomach upset marked by diarrhea, nausea, vomiting, and abdominal cramping. It affects people of all ages and is a major health threat in underdeveloped nations. In North America, gastroenteritis ranks second to the common cold as a cause of lost work time and fifth as the cause of death among young children. It can be life-threatening in elderly people and those weakened by other conditions. Most adults, however, recover without incident.

What causes it?
Gastroenteritis has many possible causes, including acute food poisoning by bacteria, such as *Salmonella, Clostridium botulinum,* and *Escherichia coli*; amoebae and other parasites; viruses; swallowed toxins (such as plant parts or toadstools); drug reactions (antibiotics); enzyme deficiencies; and food allergies.

What are its symptoms?
Reactions can be mild or severe, depending on the strength of the toxin and how far it spreads. Symptoms include diarrhea, abdominal discomfort, nausea, and vomiting. Other possible symptoms include fever, general discomfort, and rumbling bowels.

How is it diagnosed?
The doctor will ask about symptoms or order a lab exam of stool or blood samples for bacteria or parasites that cause gastroenteritis.

How is it treated?
The doctor will advise rest and an increase in fluids. For a child, older person, or someone in poor health, the doctor may recommend hospitalization and prescribe an antiemetic, specific antibiotics, and intravenous replacement of fluids and electrolytes.

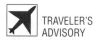
TRAVELER'S ADVISORY

How to avoid traveler's diarrhea

If you travel, here are tips to help reduce your chances of getting traveler's diarrhea.

Fluid precautions
- Drink water (and brush your teeth with water) only if it's chlorinated. Chlorination protects the water supply from such bacterial contaminants as *Escherichia coli.*
- Avoid beverages in glasses that may have been washed in contaminated water.
- Don't use ice cubes made from possibly impure water.
- Ask for drinks made with boiled water, such as coffee or tea, or beverages contained in bottles and cans.
- Sanitize impure water by adding 2% tincture of iodine (5 drops per quart [liter] of clear water; 10 drops per quart of cloudy water) or by adding liquid laundry bleach (2 drops per quart of clear water; 4 drops per quart of cloudy water).

Food precautions
- Avoid uncooked vegetables, fresh fruits with no peel, salads, unpasteurized milk, and other dairy products.
- Beware of foods offered by street vendors in developing nations.

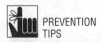

How to avoid food poisoning

Most kinds of food poisoning are caused by bacteria that live in food, on utensils and cutting boards, or on your hands. Once bacteria get into food, they grow and thrive at room temperature. You can protect yourself by following a few simple precautions when you handle, store, and prepare food.

When handling food
- Wash your hands *thoroughly* before you start.
- Avoid using your hands to mix foods.
- Wear plastic gloves if you have a cut or an infection on your hands.
- Wash the tops of cans before you open them.
- Wash all dishes, surfaces, and utensils used to prepare raw meat or poultry with hot, soapy water *before and after* you use them. Also, don't let uncooked foods such as salads touch these utensils or surfaces.

When shopping and storing food
- Make food shopping your last errand; then get it home and into your refrigerator promptly to minimize the time food bacteria remain at room temperature.
- Select meats, frozen foods, and dairy products last. Don't buy partially defrosted foods or foods in cracked or torn packages.
- Buy perishable foods in small amounts.
- Don't leave poultry or meat in their original wrappings for more than 1 or 2 days. Instead, rewrap them loosely in waxed paper or plastic wrap. When freezing, wrap items tightly and date them. Then use the older items first.
- Trust your eyes and nose: If it looks or smells bad, toss it.

When preparing food
- Thaw frozen foods in the refrigerator. If you're in a hurry, submerge them in warm water, use a microwave oven, or begin cooking them partially frozen. *Never* defrost food on the counter.
- Clean poultry thoroughly. If you're making stuffing, add it just before cooking and pack it loosely so heat can penetrate (the stuffing must reach 165° F [73.9° C]).
- Heat food thoroughly to kill bacteria — especially when cooking milk products, eggs, meat, poultry, fish, and shellfish. Don't guess; use a meat thermometer to verify internal temperature.
- Serve hot foods hot and cold foods cold.
- Store leftovers in the refrigerator promptly — don't let hot foods cool on the stove or counter. Remember to reheat leftovers thoroughly.
- Avoid raw fish, meats, and raw (unpasteurized) milk, unless you know that it was handled hygienically.

What can a person with gastroenteritis do?
- Follow medication directions carefully to get maximum relief from your symptoms (for example, take antiemetics 30 to 60 minutes before meals, to avoid vomiting).
- If you can eat, replace lost fluids and electrolytes with broth, ginger ale, and lemonade.
- Vary your diet to make it more enjoyable, but avoid milk and milk products, which may start the infection over again.
- Take precautions when traveling and preparing food (see *How to avoid traveler's diarrhea*, page 223) and proper food handling (see *How to avoid food poisoning*) to prevent another bout of illness.

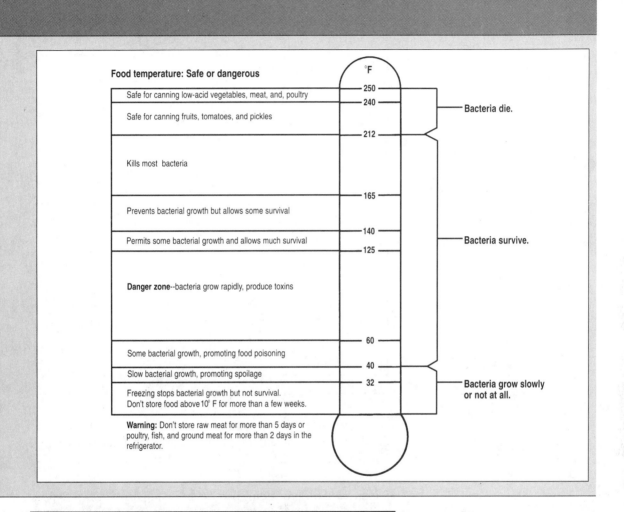

Food temperature: Safe or dangerous

	°F	
Safe for canning low-acid vegetables, meat, and, poultry	250	Bacteria die.
	240	
Safe for canning fruits, tomatoes, and pickles		
	212	
Kills most bacteria		
	165	
Prevents bacterial growth but allows some survival		Bacteria survive.
	140	
Permits some bacterial growth and allows much survival	125	
Danger zone--bacteria grow rapidly, produce toxins		
	60	
Some bacterial growth, promoting food poisoning		
	40	Bacteria grow slowly or not at all.
Slow bacterial growth, promoting spoilage	32	
Freezing stops bacterial growth but not survival. Don't store food above 10° F for more than a few weeks.		

Warning: Don't store raw meat for more than 5 days or poultry, fish, and ground meat for more than 2 days in the refrigerator.

GROIN HERNIA

What do doctors call this condition?
Inguinal hernia

What is this condition?
An inguinal, or groin, hernia occurs when part of an organ — typically the large or small intestine, abdominal lining, or bladder — pokes through an abnormal opening in the body cavity. The herniat-

Common hernia sites

The illustration below shows the sites in the body where hernias commonly occur.

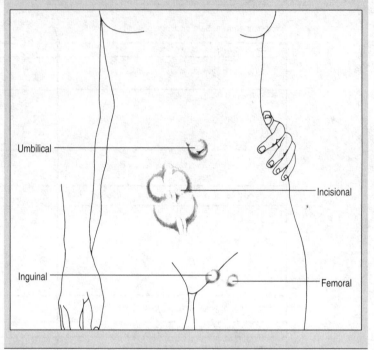

Umbilical

Incisional

Inguinal

Femoral

ed structure may follow the path of the spermatic cord (men) or the round ligament (women) into the scrotum or labia, respectively. (See *Common hernia sites*.)

Hernias are classified as:

- *Reducible* if the protruding part can be manipulated back into place with relative ease
- *Incarcerated* if it can't be pushed back because parts have grown together
- *Strangulated* if part of the herniated intestine becomes twisted or swollen, seriously interfering with normal blood flow and muscle action and possibly leading to intestinal obstruction and tissue decay.

What causes it?

Hernias in men and women can result from weak abdominal muscles caused by congenital malformation, injury, or aging or from increased abdominal pressure caused by heavy lifting, pregnancy

STRAIGHT
TALK

Common questions about a child's hernia

Parents of a child about to undergo surgery to repair a hernia ask themselves many questions. Here are the most frequently asked questions about the condition and the procedure — and the answers.

Did we do something to give our son this hernia?
No. In most cases this type of hernia occurs as the child develops in the womb. The peritoneal sac fails to close properly after the testicle descends, allowing the intestine to slip through the opening.

How does the doctor know for sure it's a hernia?
Diagnosing a hernia in a child can be difficult. Other conditions can mimic a hernia or occur simultaneously. To be sure, your doctor will have your child perform a task that makes the hernia more prominent and detectable, such as jumping up and down or blowing up a balloon.

Can my child outgrow this problem?
No, surgery is the only real cure. Although some hernias may become less prominent and easier to re-pair as the child grows, they do not go away. If your child is an infant, surgery may be delayed until he or she weighs 10 pounds (4.5 kilograms) or is about 2 months old.

Is the surgery dangerous?
Surgery to repair a hernia in an infant or child is usually uneventful. The procedure takes about 30 minutes, and the child typically returns to school in 2 or 3 days. Strenuous activities and sports, however, are off limits until the doctor says it's okay.

Are there complications to worry about?
Occasionally, a water-filled sac develops after surgery. This condition usually goes away on its own within 6 months and rarely requires additional surgery.

(women), obesity, or straining. A groin hernia, which is three times more common in men than women, can develop at any age but is most prevalent in infants. In infants, groin hernia often coexists with an undescended testicle or a collection of water in the scrotum. (See *Common questions about a child's hernia*.)

What are its symptoms?
When the person stands or strains, a lump usually appears over the herniated area and then disappears when the person lies down. Pushing on the lump may cause a sharp, steady pain in the groin, which fades if the hernia can be pushed back inside the muscle wall. Serious hernias produce severe pain and may lead to partial or complete bowel obstruction and life-threatening complications involving shock, high fever, and bloody stools.

SELF-HELP

Recovery after surgery for a hernia

If you've recently had this surgery, here are some helpful suggestions.

Promote comfort
- If your doctor prescribes a truss, put it on in the morning before you get out of bed.
- Prevent skin irritation from the truss by taking a daily bath and liberally applying cornstarch or baby powder.
- To reduce scrotal swelling, support the scrotum with a rolled towel and apply an ice bag.
- Increase your fluid intake to prevent constipation.
- Use the techniques for protecting the incision when coughing and doing the deep-breathing exercises you learned in the hospital. At home, avoid lifting or straining.

Be alert for problems
Keep the incision clean and covered until sutures are removed and watch for signs of infection (oozing, tenderness, warmth, redness). Watch for signs of incarceration or strangulation. If they appear, call the doctor immediately.

How is it diagnosed?

If the hernia is large, the doctor can see an obvious swelling or lump in the groin. If the hernia is small, the area may just seem full and the doctor may be able to feel the hernia when the person moves. To detect a hernia in a man, the doctor can insert a finger into the scrotum, ask him to cough, and determine the hernia's location by pressure on the finger.

If the person reports a sharp or "catching" pain when lifting or straining, that helps confirm the diagnosis. Suspected bowel obstruction requires X-rays and a blood test for confirmation.

How is it treated?

If the hernia can be pushed back into place, the pain may be temporarily relieved. A truss may keep the abdominal contents in place, but it is not a cure. This option may help those who are poor candidates for surgery, for example, older individuals and people with generally poor health.

For most individuals, surgery is the preferred treatment. During the procedure, the surgeon returns the herniated structure to its proper place and then closes the opening, occasionally reinforcing the weakened area. Normally, this procedure requires only one overnight in the hospital.

How a complicated hernia is treated

A strangulated or decaying hernia requires removal of part of the bowel; rare cases require a temporary colostomy. A complicated hernia involves a longer hospital stay and treatment with antibiotics and fluids. (See *Recovery after surgery for a hernia*.)

HEARTBURN

What do doctors call this condition?

Gastroesophageal reflux

What is this condition?

Heartburn — a burning sensation in the throat or chest — is caused by a backflow of stomach or upper intestinal contents, or both, into the esophagus. Even without belching or vomiting, stomach acid can reflux into the esophagus. Mild cases, which produce few or no lasting symptoms or effects, can be remedied with an antacid or a change in diet. However, persistent heartburn can lead to esophagitis (inflammation of the throat lining).

What causes it?

Normally, constrictive pressure in the lower esophageal sphincter prevents stomach acid from flowing into the esophagus. If this pressure is weak, stomach acid can flow back into the esophagus. Unfortunately, a person with heartburn can't swallow often enough to clear stomach acid from the lower esophagus and acid can remain in the esophagus for prolonged periods. (See *Understanding the cause of heartburn.*)

The following conditions increase your likelihood of experiencing heartburn:

- surgery on the pylorus (the valve at the bottom of the stomach)
- a hospital stay of 4 or 5 days with tubes running through the nose to the stomach
- diet and drugs that decrease lower esophageal sphincter pressure
- hiatal hernia (especially in children)
- any condition or position that increases abdominal pressure.

What are its symptoms?

Heartburn may worsen with vigorous exercise, bending, or lying down, and may be relieved by antacids or sitting upright. Sometimes heartburn is accompanied by painful swallowing followed by a dull chest ache. Occasionally, throat pain and spasms develop. If they become chronic, they may mimic symptoms of angina in the neck, jaws, and arms.

If inhaled, the stomach acid can cause respiratory problems such as chronic pulmonary disease, nighttime wheezing, bronchitis, asthma, morning hoarseness, or chronic cough. In children, severe symptoms can include slow development, forceful vomiting, or aspiration pneumonia.

How is it diagnosed?

After asking about symptoms, the doctor will visually inspect the throat lining for problems, often using a special scope. If further in-

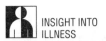 INSIGHT INTO ILLNESS

Understanding the cause of heartburn

If the food goes down...
Normally, the food and beverages you swallow are moved down the esophagus by wave-like involuntary muscle contractions called peristalsis. A small ring of muscle at the lower end of the esophagus (called the lower esophageal sphincter) opens to let food pass into your stomach. Normally, the sphincter closes to keep the food in the stomach.

It may come back up...
In the process that produces heartburn, the sphincter can't stay closed. As a result, your stomach's acidic contents wash back up the esophagus, causing heartburn and other symptoms.

How to relieve heartburn with diet

A change in the timing, size, and content of your meals can help relieve the backup of stomach acid and heartburn symptoms. Getting back to your normal weight helps too because the extra fat pushes upward when you sit, lie down, or bend over. Here are some helpful suggestions.

Change eating habits
- Eat small, frequent meals — four to six small meals daily. Eating frequently prevents the stomach from becoming totally empty, thereby reducing the acid it secretes during digestion. Eating small meals reduces stomach bulk, which also helps relieve your symptoms.
- Eat slowly to reduce stomach secretions. And sit up while you're eating so that gravity can help drain acid back into the stomach if it begins to come up.
- To decrease nighttime distress, eat your evening meal (a small one) at least 3 hours before bedtime. Also drink water after eating to clean the esophagus.
- Keep track of what you eat. Then avoid the foods that seem to cause discomfort.

Choose food and beverages carefully
- Avoid beverages that may intensify your symptoms, such as acidic juice (for example, orange juice), caffeinated coffee or tea, alcohol, and carbonated beverages.

- Eliminate raw fruits and highly seasoned foods (such as chili) from your diet. Also avoid foods high in fat (such as fatty meats, eggs, and potato chips) or high in carbohydrates (such as beans). Instead, consume easily digested foods, such as skim milk rather than whole milk, or broiled chicken with the skin removed instead of fried chicken.
- Stay away from extremely hot or cold foods and drinks because they can cause gas.

Go on a sensible diet
- Lose weight (if you need to) using the weight-loss program your doctor recommends. If a special diet is not recommended, ask your doctor's opinion of the 1,400-calorie American Diabetic Association food plan used by Weight Watchers. Food exchanges provide for more balanced meals than calorie counting.
- If you've ever been on a diet before, consider what strategies worked best (or worst) for you. Losing weight isn't easy, but it's worth the effort to avoid hernia symptoms.

formation is needed, a barium swallow X-ray may be ordered. In children, X-rays can detect the backup.

How is it treated?

The doctor will suggest positions, especially for sleeping, that help keep stomach acid out of the esophagus and may prescribe drugs to strengthen the lower esophageal sphincter, neutralize stomach acid, and reduce abdominal pressure. Often, simply staying upright and taking antacids is enough to resolve mild cases of heartburn. (See *How to relieve heartburn with diet* and *Avoiding heartburn*.)

Surgery may be necessary to address serious, recurrent conditions such as inhaling stomach acid, bleeding, obstruction, severe pain, perforation, incompetent esophageal sphincter, or hiatal hernia caused by the backup.

HEMORRHOIDS

What do doctors call this condition?

Varicosities in the venous plexus

What is this condition?

Hemorrhoids are painful, enlarged, bleeding veins in the region of the anus. They can be inside or protrude from the rectum. (See *Types of hemorrhoids*, page 232.) This condition is most common in adults between the ages of 20 and 50.

What causes it?

Hemorrhoids probably result from increased pressure in the veins around the anus. Conditions that often coexist with hemorrhoids include:
- jobs requiring prolonged standing or sitting
- straining due to constipation, diarrhea, coughing, sneezing, or vomiting
- heart failure
- liver disease (such as cirrhosis, amebic abscesses, or hepatitis)
- alcoholism
- anal or rectal infection
- loss of muscle tone due to old age, rectal surgery, pregnancy, or episiotomy (with childbirth)
- anal intercourse.

What are the symptoms?

Hemorrhoids usually cause painless, intermittent bleeding that can be seen in bowel movements. Bright-red blood appears on the stool or on toilet paper when the fragile covering of the hemorrhoid is broken. First-degree hemorrhoids may cause itching. Second-degree hemorrhoids, which bulge out of the rectum during bowel move-

Avoiding heartburn

Most people can eliminate heartburn — even people with insufficient lower esophageal sphincter pressure — if they follow these tips.

Avoid strain
- Avoid circumstances that increase abdominal pressure (such as bending, coughing, vigorous exercise, tight clothing, constipation, and obesity).
- During the day, rest in an upright position.
- Elevate the head of your bed to reduce abdominal pressure while you sleep.

Watch drugs, stimulants
- Take antacids on the schedule set by your doctor (usually 1 hour and 3 hours after meals and at bedtime).
- Avoid substances that reduce sphincter control, such as cigarettes, alcohol, and certain drugs (check with your doctor).

Watch diet
- Eat small, frequent meals.
- Avoid highly seasoned food, acidic juices, and foods high in fat or carbohydrates.
- Eat 2 to 3 hours before bedtime (no bedtime snacks).

Types of hemorrhoids

INTERNAL HEMORRHOIDS

Covered by mucosa, internal hemorrhoids bulge into the rectal lumen and may prolapse during bowel movements.

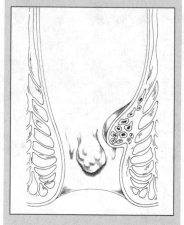

EXTERNAL HEMORRHOIDS

Covered by skin, external hemorrhoids protrude from the rectum and are more likely to thrombose than internal hemorrhoids.

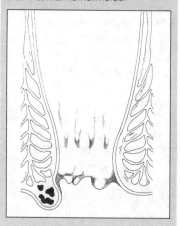

ments and then return, are usually painless. Third-degree hemorrhoids cause constant discomfort. They bulge larger with any abdominal pressure and must be pushed back by hand.

How are they diagnosed?

External hemorrhoids are visible around the anus. Your doctor will use a scope to identify internal hemorrhoids and rule out rectal polyps.

How are they treated?

Treatment depends on the person's general health and the severity of the condition. Generally, treatment involves easing pain, reducing swelling and congestion, and regulating bowel habits. Other nonsurgical treatments include reducing hemorrhoids by hand or with a laser, or injecting a solution to produce scar tissue that keeps hemorrhoids from bulging. *Hemorrhoidectomy* is the surgical procedure used to treat more serious hemorrhoids — for example, those causing bleeding, intolerable pain, or infection.

What can a person with hemorrhoids do?

- Relieve constipation by adding more raw vegetables, fruit, and whole grain cereal to your diet. If your doctor agrees, use a stool softener.
- Spend less time sitting on the toilet to reduce pressure in the veins around the anus.
- Use local anesthetics (lotions, creams, suppositories) to reduce the swelling and pain of hemorrhoids. Astringents and a cold compress followed by a warm sitz bath or thermal pack are also helpful. (See *How to take a sitz bath.*)
- If your doctor prescribes a bulk medication, such as Metamucil, take it about 1 hour after the evening meal, to ensure a daily bowel movement.
- If you have surgery, keep the wound clean to prevent infection and irritation. Be gentle when washing the wound and avoid harsh soaps. Use white toilet paper (chemicals in colored paper can irritate the skin).
- Don't use stool softeners after surgery. A firm stool is a natural dilator and will help prevent scar tissue from tightening the canal.

SELF-HELP

How to take a sitz bath

A warm-water sitz bath can decrease pain and swelling in the rectal area. What's more, a sitz bath can ease discomfort and promote healing after surgery. Take three or four sitz baths a day, especially after bowel movements and before bedtime. Continue the baths until your symptoms disappear.

If you've just had surgery, the hospital may give you a sitz bath kit, or you can buy one at a drugstore. The kit contains a plastic pan and a plastic bag with attached tubing. To take a sitz bath, follow these steps:

- Raise the toilet seat and fit the plastic pan over the toilet bowl. Be sure the drainage holes are in back and the single slot is in front.
- Close the clamp on the plastic bag's tubing and fill the bag with warm water. If the doctor ordered medication for the bath water, add it to the bag now.
- Insert the free end of the tubing into the slot at the front of the pan. Then hang the bag on a doorknob or towel bar, keeping the bag higher than the toilet.
- Sit in the pan and open the clamp on the tubing. The warm water will flow from the bag and fill the pan. The excess water will flow out the drainage holes. Continue to sit in the pan until the water begins to cool.

Afterward, dry yourself completely and apply an ointment or dressing if the doctor orders it.

HIATAL HERNIA

What do doctors call this condition?
Hiatus hernia

What is this condition?
Hiatal hernia is a defect in the diaphragm that permits a portion of the stomach to pass through the diaphragm's opening into the chest. The three types of hiatal hernia are:

- *sliding hernia* — both the stomach and its connection with the esophagus slip up into the chest
- *paraesophageal* or *"rolling" hernia* — a part of the big curve of the stomach rolls through the defect in the diaphragm
- *mixed hernia* — includes features of both of the above.

Sliding hernias are by far the most common type. The risk of developing a hiatal hernia of any type increases with age and women have a higher risk than men.

What causes it?

Hiatal hernia is usually caused by weakened esophageal muscles due to old age or cancer, injury, certain surgical procedures or, possibly, an inherited flaw in the diaphragm. The weakened muscles allow parts of the esophagus and stomach to rise when abdominal pressure is increased. Normal pressure increases occur during bending, straining, coughing, extreme physical exertion, and when you wear tight clothing. Conditions that cause increased pressure include fluid accumulation, pregnancy, and obesity.

What are its symptoms?

A sliding hernia may not produce any symptoms and, consequently, doesn't require treatment. When symptoms occur, they typically reflect acid backup and include:

- heartburn from 1 to 4 hours after eating that is aggravated by reclining, belching, and abdominal pressure, and may be accompanied by regurgitation or vomiting
- high-chest pain due to backup of stomach acid, stomach distention, and spasm that is aggravated by reclining, belching, and abdominal pressure (more common after meals or at bedtime).

Symptoms that may reflect possible complications include:
- difficulty swallowing due to acid backup into the esophagus, especially after consuming very hot or cold foods, alcoholic beverages, or a large meal
- bleeding (mild or massive) caused by damage to the esophagus or stomach
- severe pain and shock resulting from a trapped hernia (a large part of the stomach is caught above the diaphragm), which may perforate the stomach and requires immediate surgery.

Paraesophageal hernia rarely causes a backflow of stomach acid and therefore usually does not produce symptoms. Often, it is discovered during a barium swallow X-ray ordered for some other reason. Symptoms, when present, are subtle displacement or stretching of the stomach that may give the person a feeling of stomach or chest fullness that mimics angina. Although it has few symptoms, this type of hernia requires surgical treatment because it has a high risk of strangulation. (See *What happens in hiatal hernia.*)

How is it diagnosed?

The doctor will use a scope to inspect the esophagus and its muscles for abnormalities and may take a specimen to rule out cancer or other

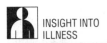

What happens in hiatal hernia

Hiatal hernia includes two classic types: sliding and rolling (or paraesophageal) or a combination of both.

Two types

In *sliding hernia* (over 90% of adult hernias), the stomach slips upward into the chest cavity, displacing organs and causing the esophagus to spasm when you lie down, bend over, or sneeze. When you stand, the stomach usually slides back into the abdomen. In *rolling hernia,* the stomach opening remains below the diaphragm, but part of the stomach rolls up beside the esophagus when abdominal pressure rises or you lie down.

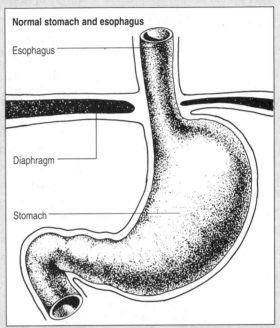

Normal stomach and esophagus

Esophagus

Diaphragm

Stomach

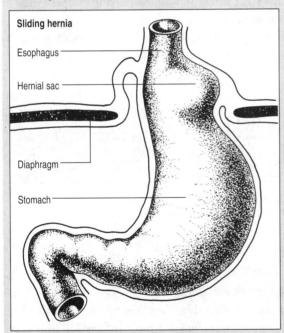

Sliding hernia

Esophagus

Hernial sac

Diaphragm

Stomach

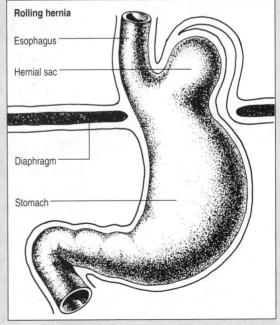

Rolling hernia

Esophagus

Hernial sac

Diaphragm

Stomach

growths. Lab studies and procedures provide more information. For example, chest X-ray can reveal a large hernia, and a barium study may show the hernia as a pouch at the lower end of the esophagus. Other lab tests can confirm stomach acid reflux, bleeding, anemia, or blood in stools.

How is it treated?

Initial treatment focuses on relieving symptoms and preventing complications. The doctor will recommend changes in diet, prescribe drugs to strengthen the lower esophageal sphincter, and explain how positioning can ease discomfort. Also the person will be provided with a list of things to avoid, such as abdominal pressure (coughing, straining, bending), constrictive clothing, and smoking (stimulates gastric acid production). Other suggested treatments include using antiemetics, antacids, cough suppressants, and stool softeners, and losing any extra weight.

If these therapies fail or complications develop, surgery may be required. Most surgeons create an artificial closing mechanism at the end of the esophagus to create a barrier between the stomach and the chest.

INFLAMMATION OF THE STOMACH LINING

What do doctors call this condition?
Gastritis

What is this condition?
Inflammation of the stomach lining is an irritation or infection that leaves the lining red, swollen, bleeding, and scarred. It can be an acute attack or a chronic problem. Chronic inflammation is common among elderly persons and persons with pernicious anemia. It's often found to inflame all the stomach lining layers. Acute or chronic, the inflammation can affect people of any age.

What causes it?

Acute inflammation has many possible causes, including:

- irritating foods, such as hot peppers or alcohol (or an allergic reaction to them)
- drugs such as aspirin (large doses), caffeine, corticosteroids, antimetabolites, Butazolidin, and Indocin
- swallowing corrosives or a poison such as DDT, ammonia, mercury, or carbon tetrachloride
- bacterial infection
- other acute illnesses, especially following a serious injury, burn, severe infection, or surgery.

Chronic inflammation of the stomach lining may be linked to conditions that back up bile and other acids into the stomach, bacterial infections, anemia, kidney disease, diabetes, and a list of irritating substances: drugs, alcohol, cigarette smoke, environmental chemicals.

What are its symptoms?

A person experiencing acute inflammation typically reports a rush of symptoms: stomach discomfort, indigestion, cramping, loss of appetite, nausea, vomiting, or vomiting blood. Symptoms may last from a few hours to a few days.

A person with chronic inflammation may have similar symptoms or only mild discomfort. Often symptoms are vague, such as an intolerance for spicy or fatty foods or slight pain relieved by eating.

How is it diagnosed?

The doctor may order lab tests to detect traces of blood in vomit or stools (or both) if stomach bleeding is suspected. Also, blood tests may help distinguish anemia from bleeding. The doctor may use a scope to check for inflammation and obtain a specimen for study.

How is it treated?

Inflammation cause by bacteria is treated with antibiotics and swallowed poisons are neutralized with the appropriate antidote.

Simply avoiding aspirin and spicy foods may relieve chronic inflammation of the stomach lining. If symptoms develop or persist, the person may take antacids. If other serious illnesses are the cause, drug therapy may relieve symptoms, but a total cure is difficult. (See *Coping with inflammation of the stomach lining*.)

 SELF-HELP

Coping with inflammation of the stomach lining

If your doctor says you have this condition, these tips can help:

- Change to a bland diet; avoid foods known to cause an upset stomach.
- Eat small, frequent meals.
- Take antacids and other medications according to your doctor's orders; avoid compounds that contain aspirin.
- If your appetite is dulled by pain or nausea, ask your doctor about prescribing an analgesic or antiemetic.
- Avoid alcohol, caffeine, and smoking.
- If symptoms such as nausea and vomiting become recurrent, call your doctor.

INTESTINAL OBSTRUCTION

What is this condition?

Intestinal obstruction is a partial or complete blockage of the small or large bowel. Small-bowel obstruction is far more common (90% of cases) and usually more serious because it progresses quickly. Complete blockage is a life-threatening condition that must be treated within hours. An obstruction is most likely to occur after abdominal surgery or in persons with congenital bowel deformities.

What causes it?

Bowel sections that grow together and pockets of trapped wastes usually cause small-bowel obstruction. Cancer is a major cause of large-bowel obstruction. Other causes are foreign bodies (fruit pits, gallstones, worms) or compression of the bowel wall due to stiffening, twisting, or tumors. Illness, infection, and nerve disorders can trigger an obstruction too.

Intestinal obstruction develops in three stages:
- simple — blockage prevents intestinal contents from passing, with no other complications
- strangulated — blood supply to part or all of the obstructed section is cut off, in addition to blockage of the tube
- close-looped — both ends of a bowel section are plugged, isolating it from the rest of the intestine.

In all three forms, fluid, air, and gas collect near the blockage. Muscle action increases temporarily, as the bowel tries to force its contents through the obstruction, injuring the bowel lining and bulging the blocked section. The bulge blocks blood flow in the surrounding veins, stops the normal absorption of wastes, and forms a pool of water and salts. Because the body can't process food or liquid, the person becomes dehydrated and feels extremely ill.

What are its symptoms?

Colicky pain, nausea, vomiting, constipation, and abdominal bulging characterize small-bowel obstruction. It may also cause drowsiness, intense thirst, general discomfort, dry mouth, and aching. The doctor may be able to hear the agitated bowel, even without a stethoscope, and find tenderness when pushing on the abdomen. The higher the obstruction, the earlier and more severe the vomiting.

Complete intestinal blockage is a life-threatening condition that must be treated within hours.

Symptoms of large-bowel obstruction develop more slowly, because the colon can absorb fluid from its contents and stretch well beyond its normal size. Constipation may be the only effect for days; then abdominal pain may appear suddenly, producing short spasms that occur every few minutes. Continuous pain and nausea may develop and bulges in the abdominal wall may be visible.

How is it diagnosed?
The doctor will ask about the person's abdominal pain and confirm the cause of any bulge with X-rays and lab tests.

How is it treated?
First, the doctor will correct the person's fluid and electrolyte imbalances with intravenous liquids. Then to relieve the abdominal pressure, a tube will be put down the person's throat to bring up the trapped material. The long, weighted tube usually works, especially in small-bowel obstruction.

If the tube isn't effective, surgery is necessary. In large-bowel obstruction, surgical removal of the damaged portion of intestine usually follows decompression with a tube. Then the person may need treatment for nutrition deficits or infection. Drug therapy includes analgesics, sedatives, and antibiotics.

IRRITABLE BOWEL SYNDROME

What do some people call this condition?
Spastic colon, spastic colitis

What is this condition?
Irritable bowel syndrome is a common condition marked by chronic or occasional diarrhea, alternating with constipation and accompanied by straining and abdominal cramps. Most people can control or eliminate this condition by avoiding the foods and activities that cause it.

What causes it?
This problem with the way the digestive tract works is often linked to psychological stress. However, irritable bowel may be caused by dis-

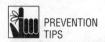

How to manage your irritable bowel syndrome with diet

Your condition is one that you can reduce or eliminate by changing what you eat and drink. Follow these suggestions.

To reduce upper digestive tract symptoms
- Follow a low-fat diet. Fats reduce the useful pressure where your esophagus meets your stomach. So does alcohol. This reduced pressure permits a backup of acid into your throat.
- Avoid substances that irritate the lining of your throat and stomach, including alcohol, caffeinated beverages, chocolate, peppermint, tomatoes, and orange juice.

To stop diarrhea
- One by one, eliminate citrus fruits, coffee, corn, dairy products, tea, and wheat. Testing your reaction to those foods will show which ones you can't tolerate. Caffeine, for instance, may disrupt your stomach and intestine muscles.
- Avoid sorbitol, an artificial sweetener, that may cause diarrhea.

- Eat more products that contain bran. Adding dietary fiber increases the time the stool remains in the bowel, allowing it time to form correctly.

To reduce abdominal fullness and bloating
Avoid lactose- and sorbitol-containing foods and carbohydrates, such as beans and cabbage. These foods produce gas. For instance, if you lack a digestive enzyme called lactase, your body can't digest lactose-containing foods. Unabsorbed lactose causes excessive hydrogen and other gases.

To stop constipation and abdominal pain
- Increase your dietary fiber by 15 to 20 grams daily, using such sources as wheat bran, oatmeal, oat bran, rye cereals, prunes, dried apricots, and figs. The added bulk provided by fiber increases stool weight and may minimize the effect of useless intestinal contractions that may trap waste or slow its passage and cause pain.
- Unless the doctor says you have a problem with fluids, drink eight glasses of water daily.

ease, abuse of laxatives, food poisoning, colon cancer or, most probably, eating and drinking things that a person can't tolerate. (See *How to manage your irritable bowel syndrome with diet.*)

What are its symptoms?
Irritable bowel syndrome usually produces lower abdominal pain (often relieved by a bowel movement or passage of gas) and diarrhea during the day. These symptoms alternate with constipation or normal bowel function. Stools are often small and contain visible mucus. The person may have indigestion and bloating too.

How is it diagnosed?
The doctor will ask about recent events in the person's life, such as a stressful change that may interfere with his or her digestion. The doctor will also rule out other disorders, such as infections, colon cancer,

and lactose intolerance. The exam may include using a scope to see into the intestine, a barium enema X-ray, rectal biopsy, and stool analysis for blood, parasites, and bacteria.

How is it treated?

The doctor may recommend counseling if the person needs to learn about the relationship between stress and illness. Strict dietary restrictions aren't necessary, but the person can pinpoint foods that are irritating and avoid them.

Rest and heat applied to the abdomen are helpful, as is judicious use of sedatives, such as Barbita, and antispasmodics. However, with continued use, a person could become dependent on these drugs. If the cause of irritable bowel syndrome is chronic laxative abuse, the individual can learn other methods to achieve regularity.

What can a person with irritable bowel syndrome do?

While you work on discovering what foods to avoid, investigate the value of increased bulk in your diet to avoid laxatives. Getting help with the stress in your life may be the best way to avoid dependence on sedatives or antispasmodics.

Finally, even though you may solve your immediate problem, get regular checkups because irritable bowel syndrome is associated with a higher-than-normal chance of diverticulitis and colon cancer. If you are over age 40, get an annual sigmoidoscopy and rectal exam to be safe.

*O*RAL INFECTIONS

What do doctors call these conditions?

Stomatitis, gingivitis, periodontitis, Vincent's angina

What are these conditions?

Stomatitis in an inflammation of the oral tissues that may include the inside of the cheeks, lips, and palate. It is a common infection that can be part of some other disease. There are two main types, called *acute herpetic stomatitis* and *aphthous stomatitis*. Acute herpetic stomatitis is usually self-limiting, but it can be severe. In newborns, the infection can spread and is potentially fatal. Aphthous stomatitis usually heals spontaneously, without a scar, in 10 to 14 days. Other oral infections include gingivitis, periodontitis, and Vincent's angina. (See *More about oral infections*.)

What causes them?

Acute herpetic stomatitis is caused by the herpes simplex virus. It's a common cause of stomatitis in children between ages 1 and 3.

Aphthous stomatitis is common in girls and female adolescents, especially if they suffer from stress, fatigue, anxiety, frequent fevers, injury, and excessive exposure to sun.

What are their symptoms?

Acute herpetic stomatitis begins suddenly with mouth pain, general discomfort, lethargy, loss of appetite, irritability, and fever, which may persist for 1 to 2 weeks. The person's gums are swollen and bleed easily, and the mouth is extremely tender. The person may get sores in the mouth and throat that eventually become blisterlike lesions with reddened edges. Pain usually disappears from 2 to 4 days before the sores heal completely. If a child with stomatitis sucks his or her thumb, the sores spread to the hands.

A person with aphthous stomatitis will typically report burning, tingling, and slight swelling in the mouth. Single or multiple shallow sores appear with whitish centers and red borders. They appear at one site but recur at another.

How are they diagnosed?

The doctor can diagnose most oral infections by sight. If Vincent's angina is suspected, a sample of pus from a sore will be examined to identify the organism that caused the infection.

How are they treated?

For acute herpetic stomatitis, the doctor will use conservative treatment, giving warm-water mouth rinses (antiseptic mouthwashes are not used because they are irritating) and a painted-on anesthetic to relieve mouth-sore pain. The doctor will recommend a bland or liquid diet and, in severe cases, intravenous fluids and bed rest.

For aphthous stomatitis, the doctor first applies a topical anesthetic, but a long-term cure requires eliminating the causes of the oral infection.

Stomatitis is an inflammation of the oral tissues that may include the inside of the cheeks, lips, and palate. The infection commonly accompanies some other disease. In newborns, the infection can spread and is potentially fatal.

More about oral infections

This list of oral infections is a quick reference to help you identify conditions, their causes, and treatment.

Gingivitis

Gingivitis in an inflammation of the gums that's linked to vitamin deficiency, diabetes, and blood disorders. Sometimes it's related to oral contraceptive use.
- Symptoms are inflammation with painless swelling, redness, change in normal contours, bleeding, and periodontal pockets (gum detachment from the teeth).
- Treatment focuses on removal of irritating factors (plaque along the gums, faulty dentures) plus good oral hygiene, regular dental checkups, and vigorous chewing. Sometimes oral or topical corticosteroids are prescribed.

Periodontitis

Periodontitis is the next step beyond gingivitis, with more severe inflammation of the gums, and it's the major cause of tooth loss after middle-age. It's also linked to vitamin deficiency, diabetes, blood disorders and, occasionally, oral contraceptives.
- Symptoms are bright red gum inflammation, painless swelling around the teeth, and bleeding. Sometimes the teeth loosen and bone loss and severe infection with fever and chills occur.
- Treatment includes scaling, root planing, and removal of gum tissue for infection control. Periodontitis may require surgery to prevent recurrence, followed by improved oral hygiene, regular dental checkups, and vigorous chewing.

Vincent's angina

Vincent's angina, also called *trench mouth,* refers to sores on the gums caused by an infection. It strikes people suffering from stress, bad nutrition, and insufficient rest and those who smoke.
- Symptoms are painful, superficial, bleeding gum sores covered with a gray-white membrane. The sores become blisterlike after slight pressure or irritation. The infected person may have a mild fever, excessive salivation, bad breath, pain on swallowing or talking, and enlarged lymph nodes in the jaw.
- Treatment includes removal of damaged tissue and administration of antibiotics (penicillin or E-Mycin) for infection.

Glossitis

Glossitis is an inflammation of the tongue brought on by a strep infection. It's related to irritation or injury by jagged teeth, ill-fitting dentures, biting during seizures, alcohol, spicy foods, smoking, and sensitivity to toothpaste or mouthwash. Glossitis can be linked to vitamin B deficiency, anemia, and some skin conditions.
- Symptoms are a reddened, sore-covered or swollen tongue that causes painful chewing and swallowing, even difficulty in speaking. It may obstruct the airway.
- Treatment aims to eliminate the causes. Use of an anesthetic mouthwash or pain killers (aspirin or Tylenol) for painful sores is recommended. The person should follow good oral hygiene with regular dental checkups and avoid hot, cold, or spicy foods, and alcohol.

PANCREATITIS

What is this condition?

Pancreatitis is inflammation of the pancreas that can start with a stomachache and progress to swelling and tissue damage or bleeding. In men, this disease is commonly linked to alcoholism. In women, it's linked to bile tract disease. The chance of recovery is good when it follows bile tube disease, but poor with alcoholism. The death rate is as high as 60% when the pancreas is damaged and bleeding.

What causes it?

Beside the common causes, pancreatitis can also be caused by pancreatic cancer, injury, peptic ulcers, or certain drugs. Some people get pancreatitis as a complication of mumps or exposure to freezing temperatures. A combination of diabetes and pancreatic insufficiency and calcification occurs in young persons, probably from malnutrition and alcoholism, leading to pancreatic damage. Regardless of the cause, in pancreatitis, the organ harms itself — enzymes normally excreted by the pancreas digest the pancreatic tissue instead.

What are its symptoms?

In many people, the first and only symptom of mild pancreatitis is steady stomach pain centered close to the navel and radiating out. Though it may feel like flu, vomiting doesn't help.

A severe attack of pancreatitis causes extreme pain, persistent vomiting, abdominal rigidity, diminished bowel activity (suggesting peritonitis), and the doctor can hear crackles in the person's lungs. In addition, the person feels extreme discomfort and restlessness, with mottled skin; irregular heartbeat; a low-grade fever; and cold, sweaty arms and legs. In the worst case, pancreatitis causes massive bleeding that leads to shock or coma.

How is it diagnosed?

The doctor will ask about symptoms and diet, especially alcohol consumption, and examine the person. However, blood tests and analysis of urine and other fluids is necessary to distinguish pancreatitis from other disorders, such as a perforated peptic ulcer, appendicitis, and bowel obstruction. The doctor may use an electrocardiogram to spot chemical imbalances caused by pancreatitis, X-rays to see calcification of the pancreas or changes in the lungs, tests to measure pressure in the stomach, or ultrasonography to see how far damage to the pancreas has gone.

How is it treated?

The doctor will work to maintain the person's circulation and fluid volume. Treatment measures must also relieve pain and decrease pancreatic secretions. If the pancreatic attack is an emergency, the doctor will use intravenous replacement of electrolytes and proteins to treat

In pancreatitis, inflammation of the pancreas can progress to tissue damage or bleeding. In men, this disease is commonly linked to alcoholism, in which the chance of recovery is poor.

SELF-HELP

How to combat pancreatitis with a low-fat diet

If you have chronic pancreatitis, your best defense is to eat less fat. You should eat no more than 2 teaspoons of fat daily, including the fat used in cooking. And you should avoid fatty foods, such as nuts, cream sauces, gravy, peanut butter, french fries, and potato chips. The preferred low-fat diet is high in protein and carbohydrate.

Normally, the pancreas secretes enzymes into the digestive tract, where they help to break down food. In chronic pancreatitis, the duct through which these enzymes leave the pancreas is blocked. As a result, the digestive system has trouble changing food into the nutrients and energy your body needs. By following the list of foods to eat or avoid, you may find relief from your symptoms.

Fruits and vegetables
- Eat most fruits and fruit juices, white or sweet potatoes, and all other vegetables that don't cause discomfort.
- Avoid avocado (unless well tolerated), apples, melon, broccoli, brussel sprouts, cabbage, cauliflower, cucumbers, garlic, dried peas or beans, onions, green peppers, rutabaga, sauerkraut, turnips.

High-protein foods, such as meat
- Eat about 6 ounces daily of lean meat, fish, poultry (baked, broiled, roasted, or stewed); fat-free, broth-based soups (such as chicken noodle) or soups made with skim milk.

- Avoid highly seasoned or fatty meats, such as ham, hot dogs, sausage, bacon, cold cuts, corned beef, goose, duck, poultry skin, spareribs, regular ground beef, tuna packed in oil, all cheeses not made from skim milk, commercial soups or any soup made with milk or cream.

Milk and dairy products
- Eat skim milk, buttermilk made from skim milk, one whole egg daily (including that used in cooking), egg whites (prepared without fat), low-fat cottage cheese or cheese made from skim milk.
- Avoid ice cream, whole milk, 2% milk, beverages made from cream.

Grains and cereals
- Eat pasta, rice, enriched white and whole-grain bread, graham crackers, saltines, cereals.
- Avoid quick breads, muffins, biscuits, high-fat or sweet breads and rolls, party crackers, 100% bran cereal (unless well tolerated).

Sweets and beverages
- Eat angel food cake, sherbet, gelatin desserts, fruit whips, sugar, honey, jam, jelly, syrup, molasses, desserts made from skim milk or egg whites.
- Avoid candy; commercial desserts; desserts made with nuts, chocolate, cream, coconut, or lots of fat; alcoholic beverages; caffeine-containing drinks, such as coffee, tea, breakfast cocoa, and regular colas.

the person in shock. Drug treatment may include MS Contin for pain, Valium for restlessness and agitation, and antibiotics for bacterial infection.

After the emergency phase, the person may still need intravenous therapy for 5 to 7 days. If the person is not ready to eat by then, a feeding tube may be necessary. In extreme cases, the person may need surgery to drain the pancreas or to remove part of the organ. For long-term recovery, the doctor will recommend changes in diet and alcohol consumption. (See *How to combat pancreatitis with a low-fat diet*, page 245.)

PEPTIC ULCER

What is this condition?

Peptic ulcers are sores that develop in the mucous lining of the lower esophagus, stomach, and sections of the intestine called pylorus, duodenum, and jejunum. They are most common in the following circumstances:

- About 80% of all peptic ulcers are duodenal ulcers, which affect part of the small intestine and most often strike men between ages 20 and 50.
- Gastric ulcers, which affect the stomach lining, are most common in middle-aged and elderly men, especially in chronic users of some anti-inflammatory drugs or alcohol.
- Duodenal ulcers usually follow a chronic course, with remissions and flare-ups, but 5% to 10% of sufferers develop complications that require surgery.

What causes it?

Though the precise cause is not known, peptic ulcers are thought to develop when the mucous lining becomes weakened, gets inadequate blood flow, or is defective. Recent research findings include the following:

- Stress may stimulate long-term overproduction of gastric secretions that can erode the stomach, duodenum, or esophagus.
- Backup of stomach acid through a lining damaged by chronic gastritis or irritants, such as aspirin or alcohol, is a likely cause of gastric ulcers.
- In elderly people, the pylorus begins to malfunction, permitting bile to back up into the stomach — a common cause of gastric ulcers in this age-group. For unknown reasons, these ulcers often strike people with type A blood and become malignant more often than duodenal ulcers.
- Too much acid secretion, possibly caused by an overactive vagus nerve, contributes to the formation of duodenal ulcers. These ulcers

STRAIGHT
TALK

Commonly asked questions about ulcers

Should I drink milk to heal my ulcer?
Maybe yes, maybe no. Milk's role in ulcer therapy remains controversial, so your best bet is to consume milk in moderation, unless your doctor recommends otherwise. Here's why. In the past, milk was the mainstay of an ulcer diet. Then, a few years ago, experts found that although milk relieves pain, it stimulates acid production. The latest findings show that milk neutralizes acidity and contains substances (prostaglandins and growth factors) that protect the stomach lining.

My doctor says smoking will aggravate my ulcer. Why?
Smoking irritates the stomach lining and the duodenum by altering pancreatic secretions that help neutralize stomach acid. Smoking also increases gastric motility, making food pass more quickly into the duo-

denum. When that happens, excessive (and irritating) gastric acid passes too. Both of these effects can delay ulcer healing.

I know that my high-pressure job isn't good for my ulcer, but I can't quit. Does this mean I'll have an ulcer forever?
Try to modify your routine to diminish stress. Start by trying to reduce your workload. Failing that, plan your work schedule more realistically. If your workplace is noisy, listen to soothing music through earplugs. Install soft lighting or rearrange your workspace to provide more privacy. If possible, take short breaks.
   At night, get enough sleep to refresh you for the next day. Engage in relaxing activities and exercise moderately (avoid strenuous activity because it increases acid secretion). Possibly, consult a therapist or attend a stress-management workshop.

tend to afflict people with type O blood. Duodenal ulcers may persist for life. If they do heal, they usually leave scars that can later break down and ulcerate again.

What are its symptoms?

Heartburn and indigestion usually signal the start of a gastric ulcer attack. Eating a large meal can stretch the person's stomach, causing pain and a feeling of fullness and bloating. Other typical effects include weight loss and repeated episodes of digestive tract bleeding.

   Duodenal ulcers produce heartburn and pain in the middle of the stomach that is relieved by food. The person gains weight (eating to relieve discomfort) and feels a peculiar sensation of hot water bubbling in the back of the throat. Attacks usually occur about 2 hours after meals, whenever the stomach is empty, after taking aspirin, or after drinking orange juice, coffee, or alcohol. Attacks recur several times a year. Vomiting and other digestive disturbances are rare.

SELF-HELP

Easing discomfort

Follow these guidelines to reduce symptoms of your ulcer.

Watch drugs and stimulants
- Take antacids 1 hour after meals. Use low-sodium antacids if your doctor recommends them.
- Avoid aspirin-containing drugs, Reserpine, Indocin, and Butazolidin. Also cut down on alcohol and coffee, and avoid stress during flare-ups. All of these can irritate the stomach lining.
- Don't smoke: It stimulates gastric secretion.

After gastric surgery
For comfort, lie down after meals, drink fluids between meals rather than with meals, avoid eating large amounts of carbohydrates, and eat four to six small, high-protein, low-carbohydrate meals during the day.

Other symptoms and complications

Any of these ulcers may be symptom-free or may penetrate the pancreas and cause severe back pain. Other complications of peptic ulcers include perforation, hemorrhage, and obstruction of the opening between the stomach and the small intestine.

How is it diagnosed?

Upper digestive tract X-rays show abnormalities in the mucous lining. The doctor can analyze stomach secretions for evidence or use a scope to see the ulcers. Stools may test positive for traces of blood.

How is it treated?

If you have a peptic ulcer, the doctor will probably treat you with an antibiotic at least once to wipe out a bacterium called *Helicobacter pylori* because it can infect ulcers even with other causes. He or she may prescribe a familiar drug such as Achromycin or Amoxil. People who take anti-inflammatory drugs may use a drug called Cytotec to reduce ulceration. A coating agent also may be administered to a person with duodenal ulcers. Mostly, the doctor treats your symptoms with drug therapy and rest, starting with antacids. (See *Commonly asked questions about ulcers,* page 247.)

If you have a bleeding ulcer, the doctor begins emergency treatment with insertion of a nasal tube to bathe the ulcer with iced salt water, possibly containing norepinephrine. A scope can be used to see the bleeding site and a laser or cautery to control bleeding. If the ulcer perforates or persists, or if malignancy is suspected, surgery will be recommended. (See *Easing discomfort.*)

PERITONITIS

What is this condition?

Peritonitis is an acute or chronic inflammation of the peritoneum, the membrane that lines the abdominal cavity and covers the abdominal organs. The inflammation may extend throughout the peritoneum or may create an abscess in one spot.

Peritonitis commonly decreases the intestine's action and causes it to bulge with gas. The death rate is 10%. Mortality was much higher before the advent of antibiotics.

What causes it?

In peritonitis, bacteria invade the peritoneal membrane. The bacteria typically come from the digestive tract during traumatic disorders such as appendicitis, diverticulitis, peptic ulcer, ulcerative colitis, volvulus, strangulated bowel obstruction, an abdominal tumor, or a stab wound. Peritonitis can also be a chemical inflammation. This can follow rupture of a fallopian tube, ovarian tube, or the bladder. Other possible causes include perforation of a gastric ulcer or release of pancreatic enzymes. In both types of inflammation, accumulated fluids containing proteins and electrolytes make the normally transparent peritoneum red, inflamed, and swollen.

What are its symptoms?

The person with peritonitis feels sudden, severe, and widespread abdominal pain that tends to intensify and localize in the area of the underlying infection. For instance, if appendicitis causes the rupture, pain focuses in the lower right abdomen.

The person is often weak, pale, sweating, and has cold skin due to excessive loss of fluid, electrolytes, and protein into the abdominal cavity. Intestinal muscles stop working and the resulting obstruction causes nausea, vomiting, and abdominal rigidity.

Other symptoms include light-headedness, irregular heartbeat, signs of dehydration (thirst, dry swollen tongue, pinched skin), acutely tender abdomen, and a fever. Inflammation of the peritoneum around the diaphragm may cause shoulder pain and hiccups. Abdominal pressure can interfere with breathing. Typically, the person with peritonitis tends to breathe shallowly and move as little as possible to minimize pain.

How is it diagnosed?

Severe abdominal pain in a person with tenderness suggests peritonitis. The doctor will use abdominal X-rays to confirm that the small and large bowels are distended. If the person has perforation of a visceral organ, the X-ray shows air in the abdominal cavity. Other tests that may provide information include chest X-ray, blood studies, paracentesis, and laparotomy.

How is it treated?

The doctor will try to treat any digestive tract inflammations early enough to prevent peritonitis. After peritonitis develops, however,

Peritonitis commonly decreases the intestine's action and causes it to bulge with gas. The death rate is 10%. Mortality was much higher before the advent of antibiotics.

the doctor will take emergency measures to combat infection, restore intestinal activity, and replace fluids and electrolytes.

Massive antibiotic therapy usually includes administration of Mefoxin with an aminoglycoside or Bicillin L-A and Cleocin with an aminoglycoside, depending on the infecting organisms. To decrease muscle movement and prevent perforation, the person should receive nothing by mouth, but should receive supportive fluids and electrolytes intravenously.

Surgical treatment

When peritonitis is caused by perforation, surgery is necessary as soon as the person's condition is stable enough to tolerate it. To prepare the person for surgery, the doctor will give pain relievers and use a nasal tube to relieve pressure in the bowel and, possibly, a rectal tube to help the person pass gas.

The surgeon's job is to eliminate the source of infection by evacuating the spilled contents and inserting drains. Occasionally, a tube is used to remove accumulated fluid. Irrigation of the abdominal cavity with antibiotic solutions during surgery may be appropriate in some cases.

PILONIDAL DISEASE

What is this condition?

Pilonidal disease is an infected cyst over the small triangular bone at the bottom of the spine. It usually contains hair and becomes an abscess, a draining sinus (channel), or a fistula (abnormal tubelike passage). The people who most often get pilonidal disease are hairy men ages 18 to 30.

What causes it?

Pilonidal disease may be linked to a person's tendency to be hairy, or it may be caused by stretching or irritating the base of the spine (intergluteal fold) with rough exercise (such as horseback riding), heat, excessive perspiration, or constricting clothing.

What are its symptoms?

Generally, a pilonidal cyst produces no symptoms until it becomes infected, causing local pain, tenderness, swelling, or heat. The cyst may drain and the person may have chills, fever, headache, and general discomfort.

How is it diagnosed?

The doctor can see the cyst and may find a series of openings along the midline, with thin, brown, foul-smelling drainage or a protruding tuft of hair. Pressure may produce pus, but there is no perforation to the intestines (a common concern).

How is it treated?

The doctor may take a conservative approach by making an incision to drain the abscesses and suggesting regular extraction of protruding hairs and sitz baths (four to six times daily). However, persistent infections may require surgery to remove the entire affected area. After removal of a pilonidal abscess, the person requires regular follow-up visits to check on the healing wound.

The surgeon may periodically probe the wound during healing with a cotton-tipped applicator, wipe away excess scabbing, and extract loose hairs to promote healing from the inside out and to prevent dead cells from collecting in the wound. Complete healing may take several months.

What can a person with pilonidal disease do?

If you have surgery, you'll be encouraged to walk within 24 hours and follow these guidelines to care for your incision:

- Wear a gauze sponge over the wound site after the dressing is removed, to allow ventilation and prevent friction from clothing.
- Take sitz baths. After your bath, air-dry the area instead of using a towel.
- After the wound is healed, you should briskly wash the area daily with a washcloth to remove loose hairs.

PSEUDOMEMBRANOUS ENTEROCOLITIS

What is this condition?

Pseudomembranous enterocolitis is an acute inflammation that damages the tissue of the small and large intestines. It usually affects the mucus coating but may extend into submucosa and, rarely, other layers of the intestine. Marked by severe diarrhea, this rare condition is generally fatal in 1 to 7 days from severe dehydration and from toxicity, peritonitis, or perforation.

What causes it?

The exact cause of pseudomembranous enterocolitis is unknown, but *Clostridium difficile* may produce a toxin that may play a role in its development. It typically strikes people weakened by abdominal surgery or those receiving broad-spectrum antibiotics. The infection begins suddenly with lots of watery or bloody diarrhea, abdominal pain, and fever. Serious complications may follow this disorder, including severe dehydration, electrolyte imbalance, hypotension, shock, and perforated colon.

This disease is one of the hardest to spot because it comes on so fast. Fortunately, it's also one of the rarest.

How is it diagnosed?

The doctor may have difficulty making a diagnosis because onset of enterocolitis is sudden and creates an emergency situation. The doctor needs to know the patient's history, but uses a rectal biopsy to confirm pseudomembranous enterocolitis. Stool cultures can identify *C. difficile*.

How is it treated?

A person who is receiving broad-spectrum antibiotic therapy must immediately stop. The doctor usually prescribes orally administered Flagyl. Oral Vancocin is typically given for severe or resistant cases. A person with mild pseudomembranous enterocolitis may take anion exchange resins, such as Questran, to bind the toxin produced by *C. difficile*. The person must be protected from dehydration, hypotension, and shock.

RECTAL POLYPS

What is this condition?

Rectal polyps are masses of tissue that erupt through the mucous membrane of the colon and rectum and protrude into the digestive tract. Types of polyps include common polypoid adenomas, villous adenomas, hereditary polyposis, focal polypoid hyperplasia, and juvenile polyps (hamartomas). Most rectal polyps are benign. However, villous and hereditary polyps are likely to become malignant.

What causes it?

Formation of polyps results from unrestrained cell growth in the upper layer of the intestinal wall. Predisposing factors include heredity, age, infection, and diet. Men over age 55 are the most likely to develop villous adenomas. Women between ages 45 and 60 develop common polypoid adenomas. The incidence of rectal polyps rises in both sexes after age 70. Juvenile polyps occur most frequently among children under age 10.

What are its symptoms?

Because rectal polyps don't generally cause symptoms, they're usually discovered incidentally during a digital exam or a colonoscopic exam. Rectal bleeding is a common sign, and can vary according to the lesion's location in the colon or rectum. High rectal polyps leave a streak of blood on stools. Low rectal polyps bleed more freely. Villous adenomas may grow large and cause painful bowel movements, but, because they are soft, they rarely cause an obstruction. Hereditary polyposis can cause diarrhea, bloody stools, and secondary anemia. In people with this type, a change in bowel habits with abdominal pain usually signals rectosigmoid cancer.

Juvenile polyps are large, inflammatory lesions, often without an epithelial covering, and focal polypoid hyperplasia produces small grainy growths.

How is it diagnosed?

To get a firm diagnosis of rectal polyps, the doctor will identify them by looking through a colonoscope or similar instrument and by analyzing a biopsy specimen. A barium enema test can help identify polyps that are located high in the colon. Supportive lab findings

Most rectal polyps are benign. However, villous and hereditary polyps are likely to become malignant.

include traces of blood in the stools, blood studies showing low hemoglobin and hematocrit (with anemia) and, possibly, electrolyte imbalances in people with villous adenomas.

How is it treated?

Treatment varies according to the type and size of the polyps and their location in the colon or rectum. Common polypoid adenomas less than ½ inch (1 centimeter) in diameter require removal, frequently by fulguration (destruction by high-frequency electricity). For common polypoid adenomas over 1½ inches (4 centimeters) in diameter and all invasive villous adenomas, the surgeon will remove part of the intestine.

Focal polypoid hyperplasia can be removed by biopsy. Depending on digestive tract involvement, hereditary polyps require total removal of the affected section. Juvenile polyps are prone to shearing off on their own. If that doesn't happen, removal with a snare during colonoscopy is the treatment of choice.

RECTAL PROLAPSE

What is this condition?

In rectal prolapse, one or more layers of the mucous membrane bulge from the circumference of the anus. Prolapse may be complete (procidentia), with all layers of the rectum protruding, or partial. A child may outgrow the condition, and drugs or surgery will help an adult.

What causes it?

Rectal prolapse usually affects men under age 40, women around age 45 (three times more often than men), and children ages 1 to 3 (especially those with cystic fibrosis). The list of related conditions includes increased abdominal pressure (especially with strained bowel movements); conditions that affect the pelvic floor or rectum (weak sphincters or weak muscles due to neurologic disorders); nutritional disorders; injury; tumors; aging; and chronic wasting diseases, such as tuberculosis, cystic fibrosis, or whooping cough.

What are its symptoms?

In rectal prolapse, tissue may bulge from the rectum during bowel movements or while walking. The person may have other symptoms, including persistent sensation of rectal fullness, bloody diarrhea, and pain in the lower abdomen caused by ulceration. Hemorrhoids or rectal polyps may coexist with a prolapse.

How is it diagnosed?

The doctor will ask about symptoms and examine the person's anus. In complete prolapse, exam reveals the full thickness of the bowel wall and, possibly, the sphincter muscle protruding, and mucosa collapsing into bulky, concentric folds. In partial prolapse, the doctor finds partially protruding mucosa and a smaller mass. He or she may ask the person with rectal prolapse to strain during the exam to show the full extent of prolapse. (See *Two kinds of rectal prolapse.*)

How is it treated?

Treatment varies according to the underlying cause. Sometimes eliminating the cause (straining, coughing, nutritional disorders) is the only treatment necessary. In a child, prolapsed tissue usually diminishes as the child grows. In an older person, an injection (to cause a fibrotic reaction) fixes the rectum in place. Severe or chronic prolapse requires surgery to strengthen or tighten the sphincters with wire or to cut away some of the prolapsed tissue.

What can a person with rectal prolapse do?

If you have rectal prolapse, here are some helpful suggestions:
- Change your diet to prevent constipation. Ask your nurse or a dietitian about the correct diet and stool-softening routine.
- If you have severe prolapse and incontinence, wear a perineal pad while you recover.
- Ask your doctor or nurse about perineal-strengthening exercises.

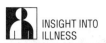

INSIGHT INTO ILLNESS

Two kinds of rectal prolapse

Partial rectal prolapse involves only the mucosa and a small mass of radial mucosal folds. However, in complete rectal prolapse, the full rectal wall, sphincter muscle, and a large mass of concentric mucosal folds protrude. Ulceration is possible after complete prolapse.

PARTIAL PROLAPSE

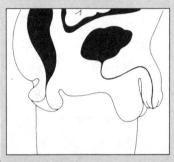

COMPLETE PROLAPSE

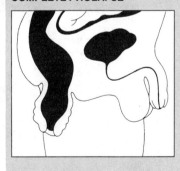

VOLVULUS

What is this condition?

Volvulus is a 180-degree or more twist of the intestine. The twist pinches blood vessels and cuts off the blood supply to that section of the bowel.

What causes it?

The twist may be caused by an unusual curve in the intestine, something swallowed, or an adhesion. In some cases, however, the cause is unknown. The most common site, especially in adults, is the S-shaped section of the intestine before it reaches the rectum. In children, volvulus usually occurs in the small bowel.

What are its symptoms?

The person has vomiting and rapid, marked abdominal distention following the sudden onset of severe abdominal pain. Without immediate treatment, volvulus can lead to strangulation of the twisted bowel loop, loss of blood supply, deterioration, perforation, and fatal peritonitis when the bowel material infects the abdominal cavity.

How is it diagnosed?

The doctor will recognize the person's description of sudden, severe abdominal pain and can probably feel the bulge of the intestine. Other special tests include the following:
- Abdominal and chest X-rays may show the obstruction and abnormal air-fluid levels in the bowels.
- Barium enema X-ray shows typical volvulus shapes.
- The person's white blood cell count will be higher than normal.

How is it treated?

Surgery is recommended for children with midgut volvulus. For adults with lower colon volvulus, the doctor will use a scope to check for packed feces. If possible, the doctor removes the blockage by inserting a scope or a long rectal tube to deflate the bowel.

If surgery is required and the bowel is distended but healthy, the surgeon will untwist the bowel. If there's tissue damage, the damaged part will be cut away and the healthy intestine reconnected.

Without immediate treatment, volvulus can lead to strangulation of the twisted bowel loop, with loss of blood supply, perforation, and fatal peritonitis when the bowel material infects the abdominal cavity.

6

LIVER AND GALLBLADDER DISORDERS

CIRRHOSIS OF THE LIVER

What is this condition?

Cirrhosis is a chronic liver disease marked by the widespread destruction of liver cells and their replacement by fibrous cells. This disease alters the liver's structure and its blood vessels. The fibrous cells interfere with blood and lymph flow and ultimately cause liver failure.

Cirrhosis is twice as common in men as in women and is especially prevalent among malnourished, chronic alcoholics over age 50. The death rate is high: Many persons die within 5 years of its start. A person with the first signs of cirrhosis will benefit from diet and lifestyle changes. (See *How to fight cirrhosis by eating better.*)

What causes it?

There are many types of cirrhosis, linked to various causes:

- Portal, nutritional, or alcoholic cirrhosis, called *Laënnec's cirrhosis,* is the most common type. It affects 30% to 50% of people with the disorder, and 90% of them have a history of alcoholism. Liver damage results from malnutrition, a lack of dietary protein, and heavy drinking for a long period.
- Biliary cirrhosis (15% to 20% of cases) is caused by bile duct diseases that suppress bile flow.
- Postnecrotic cirrhosis (10% to 30% of cases) is caused by various types of hepatitis.
- Pigment cirrhosis (5% to 10% of cases) may be caused by disorders such as abnormal iron metabolism.
- In about 10% of people with cirrhosis, there is no known cause.

What are its symptoms?

The symptoms are similar for all types, regardless of the cause. At first, symptoms are vague, but the person with cirrhosis usually has stomach troubles, including loss of appetite, indigestion, nausea, vomiting, constipation or diarrhea, and a dull ache in the abdomen. Additional symptoms develop as the liver deteriorates:

- fluid in the lungs, reduced chest expansion, and light-headedness
- lethargy, mental changes, slurred speech, a flapping tremor, neuritis, paranoia, hallucinations, and coma
- nosebleeds, easy bruising, bleeding gums, and anemia

SELF-HELP

How to fight cirrhosis by eating better

Because you have cirrhosis, you need to pay special attention to your diet. Healthful eating habits will help damaged liver cells grow back and protect your healthy cells. Here are some helpful suggestions.

How to eat better
- Ask your doctor, nurse, or dietitian for information. They can tell you how many calories you need and how to best meet your nutritional requirements. If you're used to eating fast foods, they can help you choose the most nutritious ones on a fast-food menu.
- Eat small, frequent meals. Instead of the traditional three square meals, try eating five or six lighter ones to relieve the bloated or sick feeling that cirrhosis can cause.
- Keep a food diary. After each meal, jot down the foods you ate, the time of day, and how you feel.
- After a week, study your food diary for patterns. For example, did certain foods disagree with you? If so, avoid them. What time of day were you hungriest? Plan to eat your biggest meal then. Use the diary to make smarter choices about what and when to eat.

- Weigh yourself daily, and keep a chart. If your weight goes up more than 5 pounds (about 2 kilograms), call your doctor — you may be retaining fluid.
- Set an attractive table. To perk up your appetite, use nice tableware, add a colorful garnish to your plate, and set an appropriate mood with relaxing music or conversation.

What to avoid
- Avoid drinking alcoholic beverages, even occasionally. Alcohol destroys liver cells, so abstain completely.
- Stay away from coffee or tea. Avoid all caffeine-containing beverages and foods, which can cause indigestion.
- Steer clear of spicy foods, which may upset your stomach.
- Eliminate salt in your cooking, and don't salt your food heavily. Too much salt may make you retain fluid. Ask your doctor if you should follow a special salt-restricted diet.
- Don't go on a quick weight-loss diet. If you've gained weight because of fluid buildup in your body, eating less won't help you.

- testicular atrophy and chest-hair loss in men and menstrual irregularities in women
- severe itching, extreme dryness, patches on the skin and, possibly, jaundice
- fluid accumulation in the stomach, swollen legs, and other symptoms of full-fledged cirrhosis
- musty breath odor, loss of muscle from disuse, a fever, stomach pain that worsens when the person sits up or leans forward, bleeding from the throat, and an enlarged liver or spleen.

How is it diagnosed?

The doctor will perform a liver biopsy (obtain a tissue specimen for study) to confirm cirrhosis and may order X-ray scans to check the gallbladder and bile duct for gallstones. To learn more about the ex-

Common questions about cirrhosis

How did alcohol damage my liver?

Heavy drinking for a long period eventually kills liver cells. Scar tissue then forms and impairs blood flow to the liver, thereby damaging remaining healthy cells. Many persons with drinking problems are malnourished, which also harms the liver.

Will my liver ever recover?

Damaged liver cells can recover if given the chance. Be sure to get adequate rest, eat properly, avoid alcohol, and try to prevent infection. Your liver will improve in about 3 weeks and regain normal function in 4 months. However, dead liver cells aren't replaced. That puts a greater burden on healthy ones.

Why is my skin itchy, yellow, and dry? And what can I do about it?

A healthy liver processes and excretes bilirubin, a pigment found in bile. With liver damage, it accumulates in the body and in the skin, causing itching and yellowing. As your liver heals, skin symptoms should disappear (in 4 to 6 months). Meanwhile, to relieve itching, finish your shower or bath with a cool rinse; then pat (don't rub) dry. While your skin is still moist, apply an oil-based moisturizer.

tent of the cirrhosis and its complications, the doctor may order lab tests of blood, feces, and urine.

How is it treated?

Treatment aims to remove or alleviate the cause of cirrhosis, prevent further liver damage, and prevent or treat complications. Salt and fluids are usually restricted. The person may benefit from a high-calorie and moderate- to high-protein diet (unless he or she also has hepatic encephalopathy, a condition that requires less protein).

If the person's condition continues to deteriorate, he or she may need tube feedings or vitamin supplements. Recovery depends on a regimen of rest, moderate exercise, and avoidance of infections and whatever substances caused the disorder.

Drugs must be given cautiously, because the diseased liver can't detoxify harmful substances efficiently. If possible, the doctor will avoid prescribing sedatives but may prescribe an antiemetic for nausea, a vasoconstrictor to stop disease-related bleeding in the throat and, possibly, diuretics to reduce swelling.

The doctor may recommend surgery to repair disease-related bleeding in the throat and to remove portions of damaged organs such as the spleen. Finally, prevention and control of cirrhosis depends on the person avoiding alcohol. (See *Common questions about cirrhosis*.)

FATTY LIVER

What do doctors call this condition?
Steatosis

What is this condition?

Fatty liver is a common problem in which triglycerides and other fats accumulate in liver cells. In severe fatty liver, fat makes up as much as 40% of the liver's weight (as opposed to 5% in a normal liver), and the weight of the liver may increase from slightly over 3 pounds (1.5 kilograms) to as much as 11 pounds (5 kilograms). A mild case may be temporary and cause no pain. A severe case may cause pain, permanently impaired liver function, or even death. However, fatty liver usually can be reversed if the person follows a strict therapy program and especially avoids alcohol.

What causes it?

Fatty liver is common in alcoholics. Its severity is directly related to the amount of alcohol consumed over time.

Other causes include malnutrition (especially protein deficiency), obesity, diabetes, Cushing's syndrome, Reye's syndrome, pregnancy, bypass surgery, large doses of certain drugs, prolonged intravenous feeding, and pesticide poisoning.

What are its symptoms?

Symptoms vary with the degree of fat accumulation. Many persons in initial stages of fatty liver have no symptoms. For others, the most typical sign is a large, tender liver. Common symptoms include pain in the upper right abdomen (with rapid or massive fat infiltration), swelling (see *Swollen stomach*), and fever — all with liver damage or decreased bile function. Nausea, vomiting, and appetite loss are less common. A large, tender spleen usually accompanies cirrhosis.

How is it diagnosed?

The doctor can see the symptoms in most people — especially if they're alcoholic, obese, malnourished, or severely diabetic. He or she can use a biopsy (tissue specimen obtained for study) to confirm excessive fat in the liver. Diagnosis is supported by blood tests.

How is it treated?

The doctor will help you work to ease or eliminate the cause of fatty liver. For instance, when fatty liver results from intravenous feeding, decreasing the rate of carbohydrate infusion may correct the disease. In alcoholic fatty liver, proper diet and staying away from alcohol can begin to correct liver changes within 4 weeks. If a chronic illness is causing malnutrition, you may need a special diet, especially if you have protein deficiency.

What can a person with fatty liver do?

The best news is that fatty liver is reversible if you strictly follow the therapeutic program. You can avoid permanent liver damage. Here are some helpful suggestions:

- If alcohol is causing your problem, get help from one of the many available support groups for you and your family.

Swollen stomach

A possible effect of fatty liver is a massively swollen stomach. In this complication, a large amount of fluid accumulates in the person's abdomen. The person's arms and chest become withered.

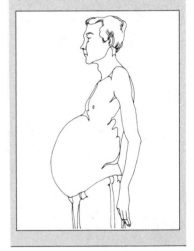

- Persons with diabetes and their families can learn about proper care, such as the purpose of insulin injections, diet, and exercise. A visiting nurse or group classes can help with instruction.
- If obesity is the problem, you should avoid fad diets that may be nutritionally inadequate. For people more than 20% overweight, a doctor-supervised diet is recommended. For others, group diet and exercise programs may help.

GALLSTONES

What do doctors call this condition?
Cholelithiasis, choledocholithiasis, cholecystitis, cholesterolosis, biliary cirrhosis, gallstone ileus

What is this condition?
Gallstones and other diseases of the gallbladder and bile duct are common, often painful conditions that usually require surgery to remove grainy deposits in the gallbladder and relieve inflammation. Gallstones may be life-threatening.

What causes it?
Gallstones are caused by changes in the chemistry of the person's bile, a greenish fluid secreted by the liver that aids in the absorption of fats. The stones are made of cholesterol, a mixture of calcium and bilirubin compounds, or a mixture of cholesterol and bilirubin pigment. Stones form when the gallbladder is sluggish because of pregnancy, oral contraceptive use, diabetes, celiac disease, cirrhosis of the liver, or pancreatitis.

Gallstones are the fifth leading cause of hospitalization among adults, accounting for 90% of all gallbladder and duct diseases. Most people recover with treatment unless they develop an infection, when recovery depends on its severity and how it responds to antibiotics.

Most gallbladder and bile duct diseases strike people between ages 20 and 50. The diseases are 6 times more common in women until after age 50, when they appear in both sexes about equally. The risk of getting these diseases increases with each succeeding decade. Each disorder can produce its own complications, the worst of which are perforations and infections in the abdominal cavity, which can lead to shock and death.

Types of gallstones

Gallstone and bile duct diseases have a variety of sources and possible outcomes:

■ One out of every ten people with gallstones develops choledocholithiasis, or gallstones in the common bile duct (sometimes called *common-duct stones*). Stones that have passed out of the gallbladder lodge in the liver and common bile ducts and block the flow of bile into the stomach. Most people recover with treatment unless infection occurs.

■ Cholecystitis, acute or chronic inflammation of the gallbladder, is usually associated with a gallstone stuck in the cystic duct, causing painful distention of the gallbladder. Cholecystitis accounts for 10% to 25% of all people requiring gallbladder surgery. The acute form is most common during middle age; the chronic form, among elderly people. Most people recover with treatment.

■ Cholesterolosis (cholesterol polyps or cholesterol crystal deposits in the gallbladder's lining) may be caused by high cholesterol and low bile salts in bile secretions. The chance for cure is good with surgery.

■ Biliary cirrhosis sometimes follows viral destruction of liver and duct cells, but the primary cause is unknown. This condition usually leads to obstructive jaundice. It strikes women ages 40 to 60 nine times more often than men. The chance of a cure is poor without a liver transplant.

■ Gallstone ileus is caused by a gallstone that has lodged at the opening to the large intestine. This condition is more common in elderly people, and the chance of cure is good with surgery.

■ Leftover gallstones or stricture of the common bile duct may occur in 1% to 5% of all people whose gallbladders have been surgically removed and may produce abdominal pain, colic, fatty food intolerance, and indigestion. The chance of a cure is good with selected radiologic procedures, endoscopic procedures, or more surgery.

What are the symptoms?

Although gallbladder diseases may produce no symptoms, most, at their worst, produce the symptoms of a classic gallbladder attack. The attacks often follow meals rich in fats or may occur at night, suddenly awakening the person. They begin with acute, upper right abdominal pain that may radiate to the back, between the shoulders, or to the front of the chest. The pain may be so severe that the person

Recovering from a laparoscopy

After a laparoscopy, you'll be discharged from the hospital on the same day or within 48 hours. Within 24 hours, you should have minimal pain, be able to tolerate a regular diet, and return to normal activity within a few days to a week. Here are some helpful suggestions for your recovery.

Before you're discharged

• The nurse or therapist will encourage you to walk soon after the procedure and to practice deep breathing and leg exercises every hour. For the latter, use elastic stockings to support your leg muscles, promote blood flow, and reduce the risk of clot formation.

• The doctor may prescribe pain relievers to help you perform your deep breathing and leg exercises. You may have an upset stomach until you have a bowel movement, which relieves the discomfort.

After you're discharged

• Don't lift heavy objects or do physical activities that cause you to strain. However, you should walk daily.

• No food restrictions are normally required unless you have an allergy or other underlying condition (such as diabetes or high blood pressure).

goes to a hospital emergency department for help. Other signs of gallbladder disease may include recurring fat intolerance, colic, belching, flatulence, indigestion, sweating, nausea, vomiting, chills, low-grade fever, jaundice (if a stone obstructs the common bile duct), and clay-colored stools.

How is it diagnosed?

Ultrasound and other tests can detect gallstones. Specific procedures include the following:

• Ultrasound detects stones in the gallbladder with 96% accuracy.

• Fluoroscopy distinguishes between gallbladder or bile duct disease and cancer of the pancreas in persons with jaundice.

• An endoscopy with a special dye is used to examine the common bile and pancreatic ducts. An endoscopy done through the mouth or rectum may also reveal stones.

• An injected radioisotope (HIDA) scan of the gallbladder detects obstruction of the cystic duct.

• Computed tomography (CAT) scan, although not used routinely, helps distinguish between jaundice with and without obstruction.

• A flat plate X-ray of the abdomen identifies calcified, but not cholesterol, stones with 15% accuracy.

• Blood tests help distinguish gallstone-related diseases from other diseases with some of the same symptoms, such as heart attack, ulcers, and hernia.

How is it treated?

Treatment during an acute attack may include insertion of a nasogastric tube, an intravenous line and, possibly, antibiotics. Surgery, usually elective, is the doctor's first recommendation for gallbladder and bile duct diseases. Surgery may be performed using an open procedure or a laparoscopic (using a small incision and a long tube) procedure to remove stones; the bile duct may also be explored. (For home care after laparoscopic surgery, see *Recovering from a laparoscopy.*)

Other approaches

Other treatment includes a low-fat diet to prevent attacks and vitamin K for itching, jaundice, and bleeding tendencies. (See *Common questions about treating gallstones.*)

In a recently developed nonsurgical treatment for choledocholithiasis, the surgeon inserts a flexible catheter into the common bile duct and, guided by fluoroscopy, moves the catheter toward the

STRAIGHT
TALK

Common questions about treating gallstones

I just found out that I have gallstones. Will a fat-free diet cure me?

No, this is a common misconception. Your gallstones weren't caused by fatty foods, and a special diet won't make them go away. Stones develop when the liver secretes bile that's supersaturated with cholesterol. When the bile reaches the gallbladder — where it's stored — the cholesterol hardens, forming stones.

Fatty foods can cause a gallbladder attack in a person who already has gallstones. That's because dietary fat triggers a hormone that stimulates gallbladder contractions, forcing stored bile into the duodenum, the opening to the small intestine. If stones block the bile flow, you may experience sudden, severe abdominal pain, nausea, and vomiting.

Suppose the doctor wants to remove my gallbladder. How can I get along without it if it stores bile?

The gallbladder functions to store bile until it's needed in the small intestine to help digest fats. After gallbladder removal, the liver delivers bile directly to the small intestine. So the gallbladder is one of the few organs you can live without.

Once my gallbladder is removed, can I eat what I like, even french fries?

Yes. But not too many fats at first. Follow a low-fat diet for the first few weeks after surgery; then, increase fats gradually up to 30% of your daily caloric intake. As your body adjusts to not having a gallbladder and as bile flow to the intestine increases, so will your ability to digest fats.

---

stone. A "Dormia" basket is threaded through the catheter, opened, twirled to entrap the stone, closed, and withdrawn through the catheter.

Chenodiol, a drug that dissolves certain kinds of stones, may be given to persons who are either too weak for surgery or who refuse it. The drug has some drawbacks, however: It requires a prolonged course of treatment and causes serious side effects. What's more, gallstones may recur after the drug is stopped.

HEPATIC COMA

What do doctors call this condition?

Hepatic encephalopathy

What is this condition?

Hepatic coma develops as a complication of chronic liver disease. Most common in people with cirrhosis, this syndrome is caused by the accumulation of ammonia in the brain. It may be acute and self-limiting, or be chronic and progressive.

The person with hepatic coma may receive treatment to lower blood ammonia levels, but then the initial cause of the problem must be corrected. If the syndrome is advanced, the person's chances for recovery are extremely poor despite vigorous treatment.

What causes it?

Normally, the ammonia in the body is converted to another chemical, urea, in the liver. If the liver can't convert the ammonia because of cirrhosis or another problem, the ammonia circulates through the bloodstream and reaches the brain, where it causes damage. People who are already extremely ill or affected by infection, sedatives, narcotics, and general anesthetics are vulnerable to hepatic coma.

What are its symptoms?

Early symptoms are often overlooked because they're so subtle: slight personality changes (disorientation, forgetfulness, and slurred speech) and a slight tremor. Each successive stage of the syndrome worsens the person's control over emotions and limb movements. A flapping of the hands, called *liver flap* or *flapping tremor,* is the hallmark of hepatic coma. The person may fall into a stupor and then a coma.

How is it diagnosed?

The doctor may check for a history of liver disease and test the person's blood for high ammonia levels to confirm hepatic coma. Slowed brain activity indicated by an electroencephalogram supports the diagnosis.

How is it treated?

The doctor may use drugs to reduce blood ammonia levels and stop progression of the coma. The drugs include Mycifradin to suppress bacterial actions and Cholac to trap ammonia in the bowel and speed its removal.

Treatment may also include potassium supplements to correct alkalosis (from increased ammonia levels), especially if the person is taking diuretics. Sometimes, dialysis can temporarily clear the blood of toxic substances, and blood transfusions may provide dramatic but temporary improvement.

If the liver can't convert ammonia, the ammonia circulates through the bloodstream and reaches the brain, where it causes damage.

LIVER ABSCESS

What is this condition?

A liver abscess occurs when bacteria or protozoa destroy liver tissue, producing a cavity that fills with infectious organisms, liquefied liver cells, and white blood cells. Dead tissue then seals off the cavity from the rest of the liver.

Although liver abscess is relatively uncommon, its death rate is 30% to 50%. The death rate soars to more than 80% with multiple abscesses, and to more than 90% with complications, such as a rupture into another body cavity. About 70% of pus-filled liver abscesses affect men, usually between ages 20 and 30.

What causes it?

Pus-filled liver abscesses commonly result from infection by such bacteria as *Escherichia coli, Klebsiella, Enterobacter, Salmonella, Staphylococcus,* and *Enterococcus.* These bacteria may invade the liver through a liver wound, or spread from the lungs, skin, or other organs through the liver's artery, veins, or bile duct. More than one abscess is usually present, and they often follow cholecystitis, peritonitis, pneumonia, and bacterial endocarditis.

An amebic abscess is caused by infection with the protozoa *Entamoeba histolytica,* the same organism that causes dysentery. There's usually one amebic abscess, which occurs in the right lobe of the liver.

What are its symptoms?

Some people with liver abscess are acutely ill. In others, the abscess is recognized only at autopsy after death from another illness. Symptoms of a pus-filled abscess come on suddenly. An amebic abscess is more subtle. Common signs include right abdominal and shoulder pain, weight loss, fever, chills, perspiration, nausea, vomiting, and anemia. If the abscess extends through the diaphragm, there will be signs in the lungs. Abscess-related liver damage may cause jaundice.

How is it diagnosed?

After reviewing the person's history, the doctor can use a liver scan to check for filling defects at the area of the abscess. A liver ultrasound may also indicate abscesses but is less definitive than a liver scan. A computed tomography scan (commonly called a CAT scan) confirms the diagno-

Liver abscess may follow other diseases and has a death rate of 30% to 50%. With complications, the death rate can reach 90%.

sis. Lab tests provide additional detail. For example, a blood culture can identify the causative organism in a pus abscess. Stool culture and blood tests can isolate the suspected protozoan in amebic abscesses.

How is it treated?

If the doctor hasn't isolated the causal organism, he or she will start antibiotic therapy immediately. If cultures show that the infection is caused by *Escherichia coli*, treatment includes the drug ampicillin. If the doctor finds *Entamoeba histolytica*, treatment includes Aralen or Flagyl. The therapy continues for 2 to 4 months. An abscess that fails to respond is surgically removed.

NONVIRAL HEPATITIS

What is this condition?

Nonviral hepatitis, also called *toxic* or *drug-induced hepatitis*, is a form of liver inflammation that usually is caused by exposure to certain drugs and chemicals, including household cleaning products. Most people recover from this illness, although some develop rapidly progressing hepatitis or cirrhosis.

What causes it?

Various substances — carbon tetrachloride, vinyl chloride, trichloroethylene, poisonous mushrooms, and overdoses of Tylenol (or other acetaminophen-containing drugs) — can cause the toxic form of this disease. Liver damage usually occurs within 48 hours after exposure to these substances, depending on the size of the dose. Factors that increase the risk of damage from some of these chemicals include alcohol consumption, oxygen deficiency, and liver disease.

Toxic hepatitis appears to strike indiscriminately. Drug-induced hepatitis may affect only certain sensitive people. Among the drugs that may cause this type of hepatitis are Nia-Bid, Fluothane, Thorazine, INH, Aldomet, and others.

What are its symptoms?

In most people, the symptoms resemble viral hepatitis: loss of appetite, nausea, vomiting, jaundice, dark urine, possible abdominal pain, and stools that are clay-colored or contain pus. Some chemicals cause additional symptoms. For example, carbon tetrachloride poisoning also produces headache, dizziness, drowsiness, and circulation problems. Thorazine produces abrupt fever, rash, aches, and abdominal pain.

How is it diagnosed?

The doctor will ask about the person's symptoms and can order blood tests to detect liver inflammation. He or she may use a liver biopsy (tissue specimen obtained for study) to identify the underlying cause.

How is it treated?

The doctor will first remove the harmful substance by flushing out the stomach, inducing vomiting or hyperventilation, to clear the substance out of the person's system. The doctor can prescribe an antidote for Tylenol overdoses. There's no antidote for drug-induced hepatitis caused by other substances. A person with drug-induced hepatitis may be treated with corticosteroids. Thioctic acid, an investigational drug, may successfully treat mushroom poisoning.

What can a person with nonviral hepatitis do?

The person should learn about the proper use of drugs and the proper handling of cleaning agents and solvents to avoid future poisoning.

VIRAL HEPATITIS

What is this condition?

Viral hepatitis is a fairly common infection that destroys liver cells. It leads to appetite loss and yellow skin and eyes. In most people, liver cells grow back with little residual damage, but it can take months of rest and good diet. Elderly people and those with other serious diseases are at increased risk for complications.

There are five types of hepatitis:

- Type A (infectious or short-incubation hepatitis) is increasing among homosexuals and in people with HIV infection.

- Type B (serum or long-incubation hepatitis) also is increasing among people who are HIV-positive. Routine blood screening has reduced transfusion-related cases, but transmission through needle-sharing among drug abusers is a major problem.
- Type C accounts for about 20% of all viral hepatitis cases and for most transfusion-related cases.
- Type D (delta hepatitis) is responsible for about 50% of all cases of sudden and severe hepatitis, which has a high death rate. In the United States, 1% of persons with Type D hepatitis die of liver failure within 2 weeks, and the infection mostly strikes intravenous drug users and hemophiliacs.
- Type E most often strikes people who have recently returned from endemic areas (India, Africa, Asia, or Central America). It's more common in young adults and more severe in pregnant women.

What causes it?

The five major types are caused by specific viruses: A, B, C, D, or E.
- Type A hepatitis is highly contagious and is usually transmitted when the virus contaminates food or water. (See *How to prevent the spread of hepatitis A.*)
- Type B hepatitis, once thought to be transmitted only by the direct exchange of contaminated blood, is now linked to transmission by human secretions and feces. (See *How to prevent the spread of hepatitis B, C, or D*, page 272.)
- Although Type C hepatitis viruses have been isolated, only a few people have tested positive for them. Doctors trace this type of hepatitis to blood transfusions from donors who don't have symptoms.
- Type D hepatitis is found only in people who have hepatitis B.
- Type E hepatitis is transmitted much like type A. Because this virus is inconsistently spread by feces, detection is difficult.

What are its symptoms?

The doctor will find similar symptoms in all the different types of hepatitis. Symptoms usually progress in the following stages:
- At first, the person tires easily and loses his or her appetite (possibly with mild weight loss). General discomfort, depression, headache, weakness, aches and pains, sensitivity to light, and vomiting also occur.
- The person with hepatitis may have a fever early on. Then, usually 1 to 5 days before jaundice sets in, the person will have dark urine and clay-colored stools.

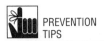
PREVENTION
TIPS

How to prevent the spread of hepatitis A

If the doctor says you have hepatitis A, follow these directions to avoid spreading the infection to others.

How you got hepatitis A

This type of hepatitis is spread when feces from an infected person contaminates food or water. It happens, for instance, when an infected person handles food after using the bathroom and not washing his hands. Or it can happen when raw sewage contaminates food or the water used to prepare it.

Common sources of such contamination include infected restaurant workers, sewage leaks into a water supply, or raw shellfish from polluted waters. Contaminated shellfish carry hepatitis A because they concentrate the virus in their bodies.

Precautions in the hospital

While you're in the hospital, you'll be placed on *Enteric Precautions*. This means you'll have a warning sign on your door, which alerts health care workers to wear gowns and gloves when they handle items that your stools may have soiled, such as hospital gowns or bed linens.

Precautions at home

When you go home from the hospital, observe the following precautions:
- Wash your hands thoroughly after every bowel movement.
- Wash your hands before handling food or preparing meals.
- Don't share food, eating utensils, or toothbrushes.

When you're no longer contagious

Once you develop jaundice — yellowish discoloration of the skin and the whites of the eyes — you're no longer contagious. If hepatitis develops in family members or friends after this stage, they probably didn't get it from you. Instead, both of you may have been exposed to the same virus source.

Preventing hepatitis A after exposure

Family members and others with whom you have close physical contact (such as sexual partners) may already be infected with the virus by the time your hepatitis is diagnosed. These people should see a doctor to receive immunoglobulin G. This drug may prevent hepatitis A. Or, if an attack of hepatitis A occurs, it may make the attack milder.

- During the jaundice stage, which lasts 1 to 2 weeks, the person may have rashes or hives, especially with hepatitis B or C. The doctor may detect a tender abdomen and an enlarged and tender liver.
- During the recovery stage, most symptoms abate or disappear and the doctor may find that liver enlargement is decreased. This stage usually lasts 2 to 12 weeks.

How is it diagnosed?

The doctor will ask about symptoms and, if he or she suspects viral hepatitis, will use blood tests to confirm the diagnosis and determine the specific virus. If the doctor suspects chronic hepatitis, a liver biopsy may be performed.

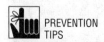
PREVENTION
TIPS

How to prevent the spread of hepatitis B, C, or D

If you're diagnosed with hepatitis B, C, or D, follow these suggestions to avoid spreading the infection to others.

How you got hepatitis
These forms of hepatitis are spread by contact with the blood of an infected person.

How you can infect others
This hepatitis virus is present in your blood and in any of your body fluids that contain visible blood. If any of your blood enters another person's blood-stream (during a blood transfusion, for example), that person can catch hepatitis from you.

If your blood or body fluids come in contact with the insides of another person's mouth, vagina, or rectum, that person can catch hepatitis from you. If your blood or body fluids come in contact with a break in another person's skin, such as a cut or rash, that person also can be infected.

What you should and shouldn't do
- Wash your hands thoroughly and frequently.
- Don't share food, eating utensils, or toothbrushes.
- If you inject drugs, don't share the needle with anyone.
- Because skin forms a natural barrier against the hepatitis virus, try not to cut or injure yourself.
- Don't have sex with anyone.
- Don't donate blood.

When you're no longer contagious
If you have hepatitis, observe all of the precautions above until the doctor determines that you're no long-er contagious. If you have hepatitis C, you may need to do this for as long as 6 months after infection.

Preventing hepatitis after exposure
Anyone who may have been exposed to your blood or body fluids should receive medication or vaccine. This includes sexual partners and anyone who has shared a needle with you.

How is it treated?

Hepatitis C has been treated somewhat successfully with a drug called Alferon N. There's no drug therapy for the other types. (However, vaccines are available to prevent hepatitis A and B.) Instead, the doctor will advise the person to rest in the early stages of the illness and to combat appetite loss by eating small, high-calorie, high-protein meals. Large meals are usually better tolerated in the morning because the person may become nauseated late in the day.

What can a person with viral hepatitis do?

After you recover, you should have regular checkups for at least one year. During that period, you should avoid alcohol and over-the-counter drugs and be alert for signs of reinfection.

NUTRITIONAL AND METABOLIC DISORDERS

CALCIUM IMBALANCES

What do doctors call these conditions?
Hypocalcemia, hypercalcemia

What are these conditions?
Calcium imbalance results from too much or too little calcium in the blood. Too little calcium is called *hypocalcemia*; too much calcium, *hypercalcemia*. Altered calcium levels may interfere with how the body's cells do their job as well as the formation of bones and teeth, blood clotting, transmission of nerve impulses, and normal muscle contraction.

Nearly all (99%) of the body's calcium is found in the bones; the remaining 1% exists in the blood. The body's nervous system relies on this blood-borne calcium supply to function properly. The parathyroid glands (four small glands located in the neck) regulate blood calcium by controlling how much of it is taken up by bone, absorbed from the digestive system, and excreted in urine and feces.

What causes calcium deficiency?
Causes of low calcium levels include:
- too little parathyroid hormone secretion, caused by injury, disease, or surgery
- poor absorption or loss of calcium from the digestive tract, caused by severe diarrhea or laxative abuse — or, sometimes, from lack of vitamin D or parathyroid hormone, or too little acid in the stomach
- consuming too little calcium and vitamin D
- severe infections or burns
- overcorrection of another imbalance called acidosis
- a poorly functioning pancreas
- kidney failure
- too little magnesium.

What causes calcium excess?
Causes of excessive calcium include the following:
- overactive parathyroid glands
- too much vitamin D
- tumors that put calcium into the blood
- multiple fractures and prolonged inactivity
- bone cancers.

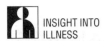
INSIGHT INTO
ILLNESS

How calcium imbalances affect the body

BODY SYSTEM	TOO LITTLE CALCIUM	TOO MUCH CALCIUM
Nervous system	▪ Anxiety, irritability, twitching around mouth, spasm in the larynx, and seizures	▪ Drowsiness, lethargy, headaches, depression or apathy, irritability, and confusion
Muscles and bones	▪ Tingling and numbness of the fingers, tetany or painful tonic muscle spasms, facial spasms, and stomach and muscle cramps	▪ Weakness, muscle flaccidity, bone pain, and pathologic fractures
Heart and blood vessels	▪ Irregular heart rhythm and low blood pressure	▪ Signs of heart block, cardiac arrest, and high blood pressure
Digestive system	▪ Diarrhea	▪ Loss of appetite, nausea, vomiting, constipation, dehydration, and excessive thirst

What are the symptoms of calcium deficiency?

Because too little calcium causes irritated nerves and muscle spasms, the person may feel a tingling around the mouth, twitching, wrist spasm, seizures and, possibly, irregular heartbeats. (See *How calcium imbalances affect the body*.)

When examining a person, a doctor or nurse will look for two reliable signs of calcium deficit:
▪ Chvostek's sign — a tap on the facial nerve by the earlobe that causes the person's upper lip to twitch
▪ Trousseau's sign — a blood pressure cuff applied around the arm and inflated, causing the person's thumb and fingers to twitch.

What are the symptoms of calcium excess?

The person may develop weakness, decreased muscle tone, lethargy, loss of appetite, constipation, nausea, vomiting, dehydration, extreme thirst, and frequent urination. A severe condition may lead to irregular heartbeats and, eventually, coma.

How are they diagnosed?

The doctor will order blood tests and urine tests to measure calcium levels and determine if symptoms are related to a calcium imbalance. The doctor will perform an electrocardiogram to determine the effects of the imbalance on the person's heart.

SELF-HELP

Advice for people with a calcium imbalance

If you have too little
• Be sure the doctor knows of any other medications you may be taking that could interact with large oral calcium doses. For example, if you're receiving Crystodigin or Lanoxin, you should watch for signs of digitalis toxicity (loss of appetite, nausea, vomiting, yellow vision, and irregular heartbeats).
• Take your calcium supplements 1 to 2 hours after meals or with milk.
• To prevent a calcium deficiency, especially if you are an elderly person, eat foods rich in calcium, vitamin D, and protein, such as fortified milk and cheese.
• Don't overuse laxatives or antacids, because they may aggravate your condition.

If you have too much
• The doctor will recommend acid-ash drinks, such as cranberry or prune juice, because calcium salts are more soluble in acid than in alkali.
• Try to walk as soon as possible. Remember that your bone calcium is depleted, so guard against falls and possible fractures.
• To avoid another attack, maintain a low-calcium diet, with increased fluid intake.

How is calcium deficiency treated?

If calcium deficiency is mild, treatment may simply be a change in diet. The doctor may suggest a diet that includes more calcium, vitamin D (found in most multivitamins), and protein, possibly with oral calcium supplements.

If calcium deficiency is severe, the doctor may prescribe intravenous administration of calcium gluconate or calcium chloride. A chronic problem also requires vitamin D supplements to induce the digestive system to absorb the calcium.

How is calcium excess treated?

Treatment primarily involves getting rid of the excess calcium by giving intravenous fluids, which promote calcium excretion in urine. The doctor may also prescribe diuretics to aid excretion of calcium and other drugs if there are complications, such as excessive vitamin D or certain tumors. (See *Advice for people with a calcium imbalance.*)

CHLORIDE IMBALANCES

What do doctors call these conditions?

Hypochloremia, hyperchloremia

What are these conditions?

Chloride imbalance refers to too little or too much chloride in the blood. Too little chloride is called *hypochloremia*; too much, *hyperchloremia.*

Chloride is secreted by the stomach lining as hydrochloric acid to help with digestion and to activate needed enzymes. Chloride also helps the body maintain its chemical (acid-base) balance and body water balance and plays a role in the exchange of oxygen and carbon dioxide in red blood cells. It also helps activate chemicals in the saliva, which in turn starts the digestive process.

What causes chloride deficiency?

Too little chloride may be caused by:
• poorly absorbed or insufficient sodium in the person's diet, potassium deficiency, or metabolic alkalosis (an imbalance caused by too little acid)

- prolonged use of certain diuretics
- intravenous administration of dextrose without electrolytes (chlorides or other dissolved salts)
- excessive chloride loss, which is caused by prolonged diarrhea or sweating
- loss of chloride in stomach acid through vomiting, gastric suctioning, or gastric surgery.

What causes chloride excess?

Too much chloride may be caused by:

- eating or absorbing too much ammonium chloride, or the bowel's reabsorbing too much chloride
- dehydration, which raises the proportion of chloride to other fluids in the blood
- the body's compensating for other metabolic abnormalities.

What are the symptoms of chloride deficiency?

The person with a chloride deficit usually has muscle weakness and twitching, which is also characteristic of sodium imbalance. However, if the deficit results from loss of stomach acids (and sodium imbalance isn't part of the problem), typical symptoms are muscle tension or spasm and shallow, depressed breathing.

What are the symptoms of chloride excess?

Too much chloride usually causes agitation, fluid volume excess, rapid heartbeat, high blood pressure, swelling, and difficulty breathing. If excessive chloride comes from metabolic acidosis, the symptoms are deep, rapid breathing; weakness; confusion; and, ultimately, coma.

How are they diagnosed?

The doctor may check chloride levels through blood tests to confirm chloride imbalances.

How is chloride deficiency treated?

In chloride deficit, the doctor will try to correct the cause and give an oral chloride replacement, such as salty broth. If the person can't drink or eat or if the imbalance causes an emergency, the doctor may prescribe normal saline solution intravenously. The doctor may also prescribe chloride-containing drugs, such as ammonium chloride to increase blood chloride levels and potassium chloride to treat metabolic alkalosis.

How is chloride excess treated?

For severe hyperchloremic acidosis, the doctor will prescribe intravenous sodium bicarbonate to aid chloride excretion. In either kind of chloride imbalance, treatment must correct the underlying disorder.

GALACTOSEMIA

What is this condition?

Galactosemia is the name for any disorder that interferes with the body's ability to metabolize galactose, the sugar found in milk. This disorder produces symptoms ranging from cataracts and liver damage to mental retardation. It occurs in two forms: *classic galactosemia* and *galactokinase-deficiency galactosemia.*

Although a galactose-free diet relieves most symptoms, galactosemia-induced mental impairment is irreversible, and the person may have some vision loss. Caught early, the condition can be stopped by changing from milk-based to meat- or soy-based formulas.

What causes it?

Both forms of galactosemia are inherited as recessive traits and occur in about 1 in 60,000 births in North America. However, up to 1.25% of the population has the gene that may lead to classic galactosemia. The second form, galactokinase-deficiency galactosemia, is rarer. In both forms, inability to normally metabolize the sugar causes galactose accumulation and damage. The mechanism of this defect is still unknown.

What are its symptoms?

Children who inherit the classic galactosemia gene show symptoms at birth or a few days after they start nursing. The symptoms are a failure to thrive, vomiting, and diarrhea. Other effects include yellow skin and eyes, protein in the urine, and cataracts.

If the child continues to drink milk or eat galactose-containing foods, he or she may develop mental retardation, malnourishment,

Children who inherit the classic galactosemia gene show symptoms at birth or a few days after they start nursing.

and progressive liver failure and may eventually die. Although treatment may prevent mental impairment, the condition can produce a short attention span, cataracts, difficulty with spatial and mathematical relationships, and apathetic, withdrawn behavior.

How is it diagnosed?

The doctor will order blood tests and urine tests to check for evidence of both types of galactosemia, but the measurements must be precise. Some infants who consume large amounts of milk have elevated blood galactose levels but don't have the condition. Also, newborns excrete galactose in their urine for about a week after birth; premature infants, even longer. Other tests include biopsy of liver tissue samples and enzyme tests. Amniocentesis, the sampling of the amniotic fluid that's done before the infant is born, is recommended when parents are known to have the gene.

How is it treated?

If galactose and lactose are eliminated from the infant's diet, most of the symptoms disappear. The infant gains weight and the cataracts shrink. If a child has the disorder, the doctor will advise replacing cow's milk formula or breast milk with a meat-based or soy-based formula. As the child grows, a balanced, galactose-free diet must be maintained. (See *Providing the right diet for a child with galactosemia.*)

A pregnant woman who carries the gene should also follow a galactose-restricted diet. Such a diet supports normal growth and development and may delay symptoms in the infant. If the parents of a child with galactosemia want to have another child, the doctor will recommend genetic counseling. In some states, screening of all newborns for galactosemia is required by law.

ADVICE FOR CAREGIVERS

Providing the right diet for a child with galactosemia

If your child has galactosemia, make sure he or she follows a diet free of galactose and lactose.

Foods to allow

A child with galactosemia may eat:

- fish and animal products (except brains and mussels)
- fresh fruits and vegetables (except peas and lima beans)
- bread and rolls, only if they're made from cracked wheat.

Foods to avoid

A child with galactosemia should avoid:

- dairy products
- puddings, cookies, cakes, and pies
- food coloring
- instant potatoes
- canned and frozen foods, if lactose is listed as an ingredient
- medications with lactose on the label as a filler.

HYPERLIPOPROTEINEMIA

What is this condition?

Hyperlipoproteinemia is the name for five distinct metabolic disorders, all of which may be inherited. This condition interferes with how the blood carries fats. Some forms are mild, producing symptoms that can be cured by diet, while others are potentially fatal.

What causes it?

About one in five people with blood tests that show high lipid and lipoprotein levels has hyperlipoproteinemia. The disorder may also be linked to other conditions, such as diabetes, kidney disease, or disorders of the pancreas or thyroid gland.

What are its symptoms and how is it diagnosed?

Each type of hyperlipoproteinemia has distinctive symptoms:

- Type I causes attacks of severe abdominal pain which usually occur when the person eats fatty foods. It may also cause general discomfort, loss of appetite, and a fever. The doctor checks for a rigid or tender abdomen, tenderness around the liver or spleen, and eruptions of pinkish yellow deposits on the skin. He or she also looks for reddish white blood vessels in the retinas of the eyes.

- Type II causes firm masses on the person's Achilles tendons and the tendons of the hands and feet. The doctor checks for yellow patches or nodules on the skin, an opaque ring surrounding the cornea in the eye, and premature coronary artery disease.

- Type III can produce soft, inflamed sores over the elbows and knees. The doctor checks for vascular disease, yellow patches and nodules on the person's skin (especially the hands), and premature clogging of the arteries.

- Type IV is linked to overeating, obesity, and diabetes. The doctor checks for high blood pressure, signs of early coronary artery disease, and clogged arteries.

- Type V causes abdominal pain (most common), yellow nodules on the skin, and reddish white blood vessels in the retinas of the eyes. The doctor checks for an inflamed pancreas, nerve damage, yellow nodules on the arms and legs, and liver problems.

How is it treated?

In this condition, the doctor tries to identify and treat any underlying problem, such as diabetes. If there is no contributing problem, the primary treatment for Types II, III, and IV is dietary management — namely, restricting cholesterol intake. If diet alone isn't effective, it may be supplemented by drug therapy. Other treatments depend on the type of hyperlipoproteinemia. (See *Treating hyperlipoproteinemia.*)

Treating hyperlipoproteinemia

Type I
This type of hyperlipoproteinemia requires long-term weight reduction with fat intake restricted to less than 20 grams per day. A special diet may be necessary to supplement caloric intake, and alcohol must be avoided. The chance of a cure is good with treatment. Without treatment, pancreatitis can cause death.

Type II
Treating this type of hyperlipoproteinemia requires a special diet to restore normal fat levels and decrease the risk of atherosclerosis. With this type, you cut cholesterol intake but eat a diet high in polyunsaturated fats (vegetable oils). If you have inherited the disorder, nicotinic acid together with a bile acid usually normalizes low-density lipoprotein levels.

For severely affected children, a surgical procedure called a *portacaval shunt* can reduce cholesterol levels. The chance of a cure is poor, regardless of treatment. Some people die of a heart attack before age 30.

Type III
Treating this type of hyperlipoproteinemia requires a diet that restricts cholesterol and carbohydrates but increases consumption of polyunsaturated fats. Drugs may be prescribed to help lower blood fat levels. Weight loss also is helpful. With strict adherence to the prescribed diet, the chance for a cure is good.

Type IV
This type of hyperlipoproteinemia may respond to weight reduction without additional treatment. Long-term dietary management includes restricted cholesterol, increased polyunsaturated fats, and avoidance of alcohol. Drugs may lower blood fat levels, but the cure is uncertain because the risk of premature coronary artery disease is high.

Type V
The most effective treatment for this type of hyperlipoproteinemia is weight reduction and long-term maintenance of a low-fat diet. Alcoholic beverages must be avoided. Drugs and a special diet may help, but the chance of a cure is uncertain because the person with Type V risks developing pancreatitis. Increased fat intake may cause recurrent bouts of illness, possibly leading to the formation of cysts, hemorrhage, and death.

HYPOGLYCEMIA

What is this condition?
Hypoglycemia is an abnormally low sugar level in the bloodstream. It occurs when sugar burns up too rapidly, when the sugar release rate falls behind what the body demands, or when too much insulin enters the bloodstream.

Hypoglycemia is classified as one of two types — reactive hypoglycemia or fasting hypoglycemia:

- *Reactive hypoglycemia* is caused by the body's reaction to the timing of meals or the administration of too much insulin.
- *Fasting hypoglycemia* causes discomfort during long periods without food — for example, in the early morning hours before breakfast.

Symptoms of hypoglycemia are often vague and depend on how quickly the person's sugar levels drop. Left uncorrected, hypoglycemia can cause coma and irreversible brain damage.

What causes it?

The two forms of hypoglycemia have different causes.

Reactive hypoglycemia

In a person with diabetes, reactive hypoglycemia may be caused by too much insulin or too much medication. In a person with mild diabetes, it may be caused by excessive insulin production after the person consumes carbohydrates.

A nondiabetic person may suffer reactive hypoglycemia from a sharp increase in insulin output after a meal, but it typically disappears when the person eats something sweet. In some persons, reactive hypoglycemia may have no known cause or may be linked to intravenous feedings.

Fasting hypoglycemia

This condition usually is caused by excess insulin or an insulin-like substance. It can be brought on by alcohol or drug ingestion, or it may be linked to other illnesses, especially tumors and liver disease. (See *How to prevent a hypoglycemic episode*, opposite, and *How to manage a hypoglycemic episode*, page 284.)

What are its symptoms?

The person with reactive hypoglycemia will complain of fatigue, general discomfort, nervousness, irritability, trembling, tension, headache, hunger, cold sweats, and rapid heart rate. These same symptoms occur with fasting hypoglycemia. In addition, fasting hypoglycemia may also cause blurry or double vision, confusion, weakness, seizures, or coma.

In infants and children, the symptoms are vague. A newborn's refusal to feed may be the primary clue to underlying hypoglycemia. The newborn may develop tremors, twitching, weak or high-pitched cry, sweating, limpness, seizures, and coma.

How is it diagnosed?

If the doctor suspects hypoglycemia, he can order a blood test to check the person's sugar level and confirm it. In addition, he may request glucose tests to determine whether the person has reactive hypoglycemia that occurs when meals are too far apart.

SELF-HELP

How to prevent a hypoglycemic episode

Although hypoglycemia (low blood sugar) is a chronic disorder, you can keep it under control and prevent most hypoglycemic episodes. Just follow these simple guidelines.

Stick to your diet
Eat all your meals and snacks at the prescribed time and in the prescribed amounts.
   Also avoid alcohol and caffeine — they can cause your blood sugar level to drop.

Take your medicine
If the doctor prescribes medicine to control your hypoglycemia, strictly follow your dosage and schedule.
   Always check with your doctor before you take any over-the-counter medicine or any other prescribed medicine. Also tell your doctor about any new treatments you're having for another condition.

Control stress
Reduce stress by practicing relaxation techniques, such as deep breathing and guided imagery. Change your lifestyle, if possible: Work less and take more time for hobbies, traveling, and other leisure activities.

Exercise
Take care when you exercise, and don't exercise alone. Do eat extra calories to make up for those burned, and don't exercise when your blood sugar level is likely to drop — for example:

- If you have fasting hypoglycemia, your blood sugar level is likely to drop 5 hours or more after a meal.
- If you have reactive hypoglycemia, your blood sugar level will fall 2 to 4 hours after a meal.
- If you have hypoglycemia linked to other drug treatment, ask your doctor for guidelines.
- If you are diabetic, don't inject your insulin into a part of your body that you'll be exercising during the next few hours.

Carry carbohydrates
Carry a source of fast-acting carbohydrate, such as hard candy or sugar packets, with you at all times.

Know the warning signs
Note what symptoms you typically have before an episode of hypoglycemia. Make certain that your family, friends, and coworkers know the warning signs. Catching hypoglycemia early can prevent an acute episode.

Alert others
Wear a Medic Alert bracelet or carry a medical identification card that describes your condition and what emergency actions to take.

How is it treated?

The treatment varies for the two types of hypoglycemia and for infants.

Reactive hypoglycemia

To treat reactive hypoglycemia, the doctor will advise the person to adjust his or her diet to maintain steady glucose intake. Usually, this means small, frequent meals of complex carbohydrates, fiber, and fat. Simple sugars, alcohol, and fruit drinks should be avoided. The doctor may also prescribe drugs to slow stomach emptying and intestinal motility and to inhibit insulin release.

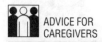

How to manage a hypoglycemic episode

A sudden hypoglycemic (low blood sugar) episode may make it hard for the person in your care to recognize his own symptoms and take care of himself.

It will be up to you to manage the crisis for him or her and raise blood sugar levels immediately to prevent permanent brain damage and even death. Be sure you have sources of sugar available. If the person is conscious, give him or her any of the following.

Foods and fluids

- Apple juice, orange juice, or ginger ale — 4 to 6 ounces
- Regular cola or other soft drink — 4 to 6 ounces
- Corn syrup, honey, or grape jelly — 1 tablespoon
- Hard candy — 5 to 6 pieces
- Jelly beans — 6
- Gumdrops — 10

Glucagon injection

If the person is unconscious or has trouble swallowing, give a subcutaneous injection of glucagon. Be sure to check the expiration date on the glucagon kit frequently and replenish your supply as needed. Here's how to give a glucagon injection:

- Prepare the glucagon following the manufacturer's instructions included in the kit.
- Select an appropriate injection site as the nurse taught you.
- Pull the skin taut; then clean it with an alcohol pad.
- Using your thumb and forefinger, pinch the skin at the injection site; then quickly plunge the needle into the skin fold at a 90-degree angle, up to the needle hub.
- Push the plunger down to quickly inject the glucagon.
- Withdraw the needle, and rub the site with an alcohol pad.
- Turn the person onto his or her side. Because glucagon may cause vomiting, this position reduces the possibility of choking.
- If the person doesn't wake up in 5 to 20 minutes, give a second dose of glucagon and seek emergency help. If the person wakes up and can swallow, give some sugar immediately. (See the list in the first column.) Give sugar because glucagon isn't effective for more than about 90 minutes. Then call the doctor.

Fasting hypoglycemia

In fasting hypoglycemia, surgery and drug therapy are usually required. If the problem is caused by a tumor, the doctor will recommend surgery. The doctor may prescribe drugs to inhibit insulin secretion, plus hormones and long-acting glycogen.

In infants

If a newborn infant has hypoglycemia or is at risk of developing it, the doctor will use preventive measures. The doctor can give the infant dextrose intravenously to correct a severe hypoglycemic state. To reduce the chance of hypoglycemia in high-risk infants, the doctor will recommend feedings — either breast milk or a solution of 5% to 10% glucose and water — as soon after birth as possible.

IODINE DEFICIENCY

What is this condition?

Iodine deficiency occurs when a person lacks sufficient iodine to satisfy the body's daily requirements. Because the thyroid gland uses most of the body's iodine supply, iodine deficiency is apt to cause low thyroid activity and goiter.

Other effects of iodine deficiency range from dental cavities to cretinism in infants born to iodine-deficient mothers. Iodine deficiency is most common in pregnant or nursing women because of their increased metabolic need for this element. Iodine deficiency is quickly reversed with iodine supplements.

What causes it?

Iodine deficiency is usually caused by not eating enough foods containing iodine, such as iodized table salt, seafood, and dark green, leafy vegetables.

Iodine deficiency may also be caused by increased metabolic demands during pregnancy, breast-feeding, and adolescence.

What are its symptoms?

The symptoms of iodine deficiency depend on the degree of hypothyroidism that develops (in addition to the development of a goiter). The person with a mild deficiency may have only mild, vague symptoms, such as fatigue and loss of energy.

In a severe case, the features of hypothyroidism are plainly visible. These features include abnormally slow heartbeat and decreased pulse pressure and heart output. A long list of skin, muscle, and mental problems occur, too. For example, a person may develop hoarseness; dry, flaky, inelastic skin; puffy face; thick tongue; poor memory; hearing loss; chills; and loss of appetite. In women, iodine deficiency may also reduce or stop menstruation.

In infants

In an infant, cretinism (hypothyroidism that develops in the womb) is marked by failure to thrive, jaundice, and a dangerously low body temperature. By ages 3 to 6 months, the infant may have spasms and symptoms similar to those seen in infants with Down syndrome.

Suffering from a mild iodine deficiency? Use iodized table salt and eat lots of seafood and green, leafy vegetables.

How is it diagnosed?

If the doctor suspects iodine deficiency, he can verify it with urine tests and X-rays of the thyroid gland, which require special dyes.

How is it treated?

In severe iodine deficiency, the doctor will prescribe iodine supplements. A mild deficiency may be corrected by increasing iodine in the diet, perhaps by using iodized table salt and eating iodine-rich foods (seafood and green, leafy vegetables).

Iodine supplements should be mixed with milk or juice to reduce stomach irritation and to mask the metallic taste. To prevent tooth discoloration, the supplement should be drunk through a straw. Iodine solutions should be stored in a light-resistant container.

MAGNESIUM IMBALANCES

What do doctors call these conditions?

Hypomagnesemia, hypermagnesemia

What are these conditions?

Too little magnesium in the blood is called *hypomagnesemia*; too much, *hypermagnesemia*. Magnesium imbalance can affect many of the body's functions because magnesium is found in the fluid that surrounds all the body's cells. Its major role is to keep nerves and muscles functioning properly.

Magnesium also stimulates the parathyroid glands, four tiny glands in the neck, to secrete parathyroid hormone. If these glands don't produce sufficient hormones, the level of calcium in the blood will fall.

Magnesium also activates many enzymes that help the body extract nutrients from foods and carry them to the body's organs.

Who suffers from a magnesium imbalance?

Because many common foods contain magnesium, a dietary deficiency is rare. Magnesium deficiency primarily strikes people who have been receiving intravenous feedings or who have other imbalances, especially low calcium and potassium levels. Magnesium excess is common in people with kidney failure and in those who take too many magnesium-containing antacids.

What causes magnesium deficiency?

Low magnesium levels are usually linked to poor absorption of magnesium in the intestines or excessive excretion in the urine or stools. Possible causes include:
- poor absorption because of chronic diarrhea or complications after bowel surgery, chronic alcoholism, prolonged diuretic therapy, suctioning of the stomach by a nasal tube, starvation, or malnutrition
- excessive loss of magnesium due to severe dehydration and diabetic acidosis or imbalances in iodine, calcium, and other elements and hormones.

What causes magnesium excess?

High magnesium levels result from the kidneys' inability to excrete magnesium that was either absorbed from the intestines or taken as medication. Common causes include:
- chronic kidney insufficiency
- use of laxatives (magnesium sulfate, milk of magnesia, and magnesium citrate solutions), especially with kidney insufficiency
- overuse of magnesium-containing antacids
- severe dehydration
- overcorrection of low magnesium levels.

What are the symptoms of magnesium deficiency?

Too little magnesium causes neuromuscular irritability and irregular heartbeats. A person may experience confusion, emotional instability, or even delusions or hallucinations. He or she also may develop nausea, vomiting, loss of appetite, high blood pressure, and a rapid heart rate. (See *How magnesium imbalances affect the body,* page 288.)

What are the symptoms of magnesium excess?

Too much magnesium depresses the nervous system and breathing and produces neuromuscular and heart effects. The person may experience flushing, profuse sweating, muscle weakness, visual disturbances, sluggishness, drowsiness, or even coma. He or she may have low blood pressure and a slow heart rate.

How are they diagnosed?

After asking about symptoms, the doctor will order blood tests to check the level of magnesium in the person's system. The doctor will

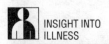
INSIGHT INTO
ILLNESS

How magnesium imbalances affect the body

BODY SYSTEM	TOO LITTLE MAGNESIUM	TOO MUCH MAGNESIUM
Muscles	• Hyperirritability, tetany, and leg and foot cramps	• Diminished reflexes, muscle weakness, flaccid paralysis, and respiratory muscle paralysis that may cause breathing difficulty
Nervous system	• Confusion, delusions, hallucinations, and seizures	• Drowsiness, flushing, lethargy, confusion, and diminished awareness
Heart and blood vessels	• Irregular heartbeats, changes in blood vessels that may lead to low blood pressure and, occasionally, high blood pressure	• Slow heart rate, weak pulse, low blood pressure, heart block, and cardiac arrest

also look for other irregularities, such as low or high levels of potassium and calcium in the blood.

How are they treated?

To treat magnesium imbalance, the doctor will try to identify and correct the underlying cause. For mild low magnesium, the doctor may prescribe an oral form or intramuscular injections of magnesium supplements. For a severe case, the magnesium is given intravenously.

For high magnesium, the doctor will try to flush out excess magnesium by giving diuretics and having the person drink more fluids. For temporary relief of symptoms in an emergency, the doctor may recommend peritoneal dialysis or hemodialysis, especially if kidney function is poor or if excess magnesium can't be eliminated.

METABOLIC ACIDOSIS

What is this condition?

Metabolic acidosis is a combination of excess acid accumulation and insufficient base compounds in the person's system. This acid-base imbalance is usually brought on by a medical disorder.

This imbalance of body chemicals depresses the central nervous system. Left untreated, metabolic acidosis can lead to dangerous changes in heart rate and rhythm, cardiac arrest, and coma. The prognosis improves if the underlying cause is identified quickly and the body's normal acid-base balance is promptly restored.

Metabolic acidosis is more common in children than in adults.

What causes it?

Metabolic acidosis is commonly caused by excessive burning of fats in the absence of usable carbohydrates. This can be caused by diabetes, chronic alcoholism, malnutrition, or a low-carbohydrate, high-fat diet — all of which produce more acids than the body can handle. Other causes include:

- too little oxygen to burn carbohydrates (as occurs after a heart attack) and a corresponding rise in lactic acid level
- kidney insufficiency and failure (the kidneys may fail to secrete sufficient acid)
- diarrhea and intestinal malabsorption, which cause loss of sodium bicarbonate
- aspirin overdose (less frequently) or some other poisoning
- Addison's disease.

What are its symptoms?

Metabolic acidosis typically causes a headache and lethargy, progressing to drowsiness, central nervous system depression, and rapid breathing (as the lungs try to compensate by "blowing off" carbon dioxide), and stupor. If the condition is severe and goes untreated, the person may suffer a coma and die.

The person usually has stomach problems that produce appetite loss, as well as nausea, vomiting, and diarrhea, which may lead to dehydration. If the person has diabetes, he or she may have fruity-smelling breath.

How is it diagnosed?

After he asks about symptoms, the doctor will order blood tests to confirm metabolic acidosis and determine its severity. The key test for detecting metabolic acidosis is called *arterial blood gas analysis.*

How is it treated?

If severe metabolic acidosis is diagnosed, treatment begins with intravenous sodium bicarbonate, which helps to neutralize body acids. The doctor evaluates and corrects other electrolyte imbalances — for example, a person with metabolic acidosis may also need treatment for excessive potassium.

Other treatments may include mechanical ventilation to ensure adequate breathing, replacement of fluids, and antibiotics to treat infection. Ultimately, the doctor must correct the underlying cause. For example, in diabetic ketoacidosis, a low-dose continuous, intravenous infusion of insulin is recommended.

METABOLIC ALKALOSIS

What is this condition?

Metabolic alkalosis is an acid-base imbalance in the body fluids caused by too little acid or too much of a base compound called *bicarbonate*. Metabolic acidosis is always brought on by some other illness. This imbalance causes metabolic, respiratory, and kidney effects and, especially, depressed breathing.

With early diagnosis and prompt treatment, the chance of correcting this chemical imbalance is good. However, untreated metabolic alkalosis may lead to coma and death.

What causes it?

Metabolic alkalosis is caused by loss of acid compounds or retention of base compounds in body fluids due to various disorders or drug actions. The body fluids become more alkaline than acid.

Acid loss

Causes of critical acid loss include vomiting, excessive suctioning of the stomach with a tube, abnormal openings in the stomach (such as perforation caused by ulcers), and the use of certain drugs, including corticosteroids and diuretics. Diseases that cause acid loss include hyperadrenocorticism, Cushing's disease, hyperaldosteronism, and Bartter's syndrome.

Base retention

Causes of base retention include excessive intake of bicarbonate of soda or other antacids (usually for treatment of gastritis or peptic ulcer), too much alkali (as in milk-alkali syndrome with peptic ulcers), or too much intravenous fluid containing bicarbonate.

What are its symptoms?

Symptoms begin when the person's body tries to correct the acid-base imbalance, primarily through hypoventilation, which causes slow, shallow respirations. The person also may feel irritable, pick at his bedclothes, twitch, act confused, and complain of nausea, vomiting, and diarrhea. Because the heart, circulation, and breathing are all disturbed, the person with uncorrected alkalosis may have seizures and fall into a coma.

How is it diagnosed?

Because the person is often in the hospital for another disorder, the doctor can observe his or her symptoms and then confirm metabolic alkalosis with blood tests and urine tests. The most important test for detecting metabolic alkalosis is called *arterial blood gas analysis*. The doctor may also use an electrocardiogram to determine the effects of this imbalance on the heart's function.

How is it treated?

The doctor tries to correct the underlying cause of metabolic alkalosis — for example, by discontinuing the use of drugs such as diuretics or stopping stomach suctioning. Fluids and elements such as potassium may need to be replaced. For the person with severe alkalosis, the doctor may prescribe intravenous ammonium chloride or other solutions to restore the person's chemical balance.

*O*BESITY

What is this condition?

Obesity is an excess of body fat, typically 20% above ideal body weight. For most people who are obese, losing weight is difficult. Fewer than 30% of obese persons succeed in losing 20 pounds (9 kilograms), and only half of these maintain the loss for a long time.

What causes it?

Traditionally, people have attributed obesity to a combination of too many calories and too little exercise. More recently, scientific research points to possible physiologic causes. For example, scientists recently

SELF-HELP

How to control overeating

To diet successfully, you must focus as much on changing your eating habits as on what you eat. These tips can help you modify behaviors that cause overeating:

- To avoid the temptation to munch on leftover food, clear the table immediately after eating.
- Create obstacles to eating between meals. For example, disguise tempting foods by wrapping them in foil or storing them in the back of the refrigerator.
- Never shop for groceries when you're hungry.
- Make small amounts of food look large by serving portions on small plates or spreading food out on larger plates.
- Eat slowly. To stretch out meal times, put down your fork and knife after each bite. Then chew your food thoroughly.

- Plan menus ahead and eat regularly. Don't skip meals.

Change your eating environment
Limit all your eating to one place at home and at work. This eliminates environmental cues that trigger overeating. For example, avoid snacking while watching TV by confining eating to the kitchen (for this to work, you must keep the TV out of the kitchen).

Set the table completely — with flowers, tablecloth, and full place settings — before eating any meal or snack. By providing a feast for your other senses, you may enjoy your food more and feel satisfied with less of it. Also, whenever possible, try to enjoy conversation with meals.

discovered a gene in obese people that seems to send a faulty signal to the part of the brain that controls feelings of satiety. This gene seems to prevent obese people from developing an appropriate feeling of fullness. Some experts believe that psychological factors may also contribute to obesity.

How is it diagnosed?
Comparison of the person's height and weight to a standard table determines obesity. Caliper measurements of subcutaneous fat folds estimate the person's total body fat.

Because obesity may lead to serious health problems, such as respiratory difficulties, high blood pressure, heart disease, diabetes, kidney disease, gallbladder disease, and social difficulties, it's considered a serious disorder.

How is it treated?
If the doctor diagnoses obesity, he or she will try to decrease the person's daily calorie intake while increasing activity levels. The cure is based on a balanced, low-calorie diet that eliminates foods high in fat and sugar. To achieve long-term benefits, these new eating and exer-

Options in weight loss

Fad diets

The popular low-carbohydrate diets (such as the Atkins and Scarsdale diets) offer no long-term benefit. Rapid early weight reduction is due to loss of water, not fat. The major drawback of these and other crash diets is that they don't teach you new eating patterns and often lead to the yo-yo syndrome, episodes of repeated weight loss followed by weight gain.

Fasting

Total fasting is an effective method of rapid weight loss, but you must be closely monitored and supervised to minimize the risk of problems like ketonemia, electrolyte imbalance, low blood pressure, and loss of muscle. Prolonged fasting or extremely low-calorie diets have resulted in sudden death, possibly by causing irregular heartbeats. These methods also don't change your eating patterns to maintain weight control.

Behavior modification

Some people try hypnosis and behavior modification techniques, which may help you make fundamental changes in your eating habits and activity patterns. Psychotherapy also may help because weight reduction may lead to depression or even psychosis.

Appetite suppressants

Amphetamines and similar drugs may help you diet by temporarily suppressing your appetite and creating a feeling of well-being. However, because their value in long-term weight control is questionable and they pose a significant risk of leading to dependence and abuse, most doctors avoid them. If these drugs are used at all, your doctor will prescribe them for short-term therapy only and will monitor you carefully while you use them.

Surgery

As a last resort, morbid obesity (body weight greater than 200% of standard) may be treated surgically with gastroplasty (stomach stapling). Gastroplasty decreases the volume of food that the stomach can hold and makes you feel full with a small meal.

cise patterns must be maintained for life. (See *How to control overeating*. For information on other treatments for obesity, see *Options in weight loss*.)

PHOSPHORUS IMBALANCES

What do doctors call these conditions?
Hypophosphatemia, hyperphosphatemia

What are these conditions?
Insufficient phosphorus in the blood is called *hypophosphatemia*; too much phosphorus, *hyperphosphatemia*. Because phosphorus is im-

portant to many of the body's processes, an imbalance of this element can be harmful.

In the body, phosphorus is found primarily in combination with calcium in teeth and bones. In the body's fluids, the phosphate ion helps a person maintain a long list of functions: utilization of B vitamins, acid-base balance, bone formation, nerve and muscle activity, cell division, transmission of hereditary traits, and metabolism of carbohydrates, proteins, and fats. In the kidneys, reabsorption of phosphate is linked to calcium levels — too much phosphorus causes low calcium levels.

A lack of phosphorus is usually linked to another medical condition. Excess phosphorus usually occurs in children, who tend to consume more phosphorus-rich foods and beverages than adults. It also strikes children and adults with kidney problems. The prognosis for both types of phosphorus imbalance depends on the underlying cause.

What causes phosphorus deficiency?

Too little phosphorus in the diet is often related to malnutrition resulting from a prolonged illness or chronic alcoholism. It may also be linked to imbalances of calcium or magnesium or a deficiency of vitamin D, essential for intestinal phosphorus absorption.

The condition may also be related to long-term use of antacids containing aluminum hydroxide, intravenous feedings with inadequate phosphate content, kidney defects, tissue damage (phosphorus may be released by injured cells), and diabetic acidosis.

What causes phosphorus excess?

Too much phosphorus usually occurs when a person gets too little calcium or too much vitamin D, or has an underactive thyroid or kidney failure (often due to stress or injury). It may also be caused by overuse of phosphate enemas or laxatives with phosphates.

What are the symptoms of phosphorus deficiency?

Not enough phosphorus causes a loss of appetite, weakness, tremors, tingling skin and, when it continues, bone pain.

What are the symptoms of phosphorus excess?

Too much phosphorus usually doesn't produce symptoms unless it leads to low calcium, which may cause seizures.

SELF-HELP

Foods high in phosphorus

FOOD	PORTION	MILLIGRAMS OF PHOSPHORUS
Almonds	⅔ cup	475
Beef liver (fried)	3½ ounces	476
Broccoli (cooked)	⅔ cup	62
Carbonated beverage	12 ounces	up to 500
Milk (whole)	8 ounces	93
Turkey (roasted)	3½ ounces	251

How are they diagnosed?

If the doctor suspects a phosphorus imbalance, he can order blood tests and urine tests to confirm exactly what is wrong.

How is phosphorus deficiency treated?

The doctor will try to correct the underlying cause of phosphorus imbalance. Until that problem is solved, the person with too little phosphorus will be given phosphorus supplements, with a high-phosphorus diet and phosphate salt tablets or capsules. If he has a severely low phosphorus level, the doctor may give an intravenous infusion of potassium phosphate.

How is phosphorus excess treated?

If the person has severe hyperphosphatemia, he may require peritoneal dialysis or hemodialysis to lower the blood's phosphorus level.

What can a person with a phosphorus imbalance do?

To prevent the return of a low-phosphorus condition, you should follow a high-phosphorus diet, including milk and milk products, liver, turkey, and dried fruits. (See *Foods high in phosphorus.*)

To prevent the return of a high-phosphorus condition, you should eat foods with a low phosphorus content, such as vegetables (other than broccoli). If the condition results from chronic kidney insufficiency, you may need to learn more from a dietitian.

POTASSIUM IMBALANCES

What do doctors call these conditions?
Hypokalemia, hyperkalemia

What are these conditions?
Potassium imbalance occurs when the potassium in the blood deviates slightly from the ideal proportion. Potassium deficiency is called *hypokalemia*; potassium excess, *hyperkalemia*.

Potassium is important to many of the body's functions, including contraction of muscles, including the heart; nerve impulse conduction; acid-base balance; enzyme action (enzymes facilitate chemical reactions in the body); and cell membrane function.

Because the correct potassium level in the blood has such a narrow range, a slight change in either direction can make a person ill. Both conditions interfere with nerve impulse conduction; they also diminish nerve impulses in the heart muscle, which may lead to heart failure.

What causes potassium deficiency?
Because many foods contain potassium, a deficiency rarely is caused by a poor diet. Instead, potassium loss is caused by:
- excessive gastrointestinal or urinary losses, which may be related to vomiting, gastric suction, diarrhea, dehydration, loss of appetite, or chronic laxative abuse
- injury, burns, or surgery, in which damaged cells release potassium, which enters blood or extracellular fluid and is excreted in the urine
- chronic kidney disease, with tubular potassium-wasting
- certain drugs, especially potassium-wasting diuretics, corticosteroids, and certain sodium-containing antibiotics (such as Geocillin)
- acid-base imbalances
- prolonged potassium-free intravenous infusion
- other diseases and disorders that remove potassium
- eating too much licorice candy.

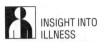
INSIGHT INTO
ILLNESS

How potassium imbalances affect the body

When your body has too much or too little potassium, many of its functions are disrupted.

BODY SYSTEM	TOO LITTLE POTASSIUM	TOO MUCH POTASSIUM
Nervous system	• Malaise, irritability, confusion, depression, speech changes, decreased reflexes, and respiratory paralysis	• Exaggerated reflexes, progressing to weakness, numbness, tingling, and flaccid paralysis
Heart and blood vessels	• Dizziness, low blood pressure, irregular heartbeats, cardiac arrest (with extremely low blood potassium levels)	• Rapid heart rate and later a slow heart rate, irregular heartbeats, and cardiac arrest (with extremely high blood potassium levels)
Digestive system	• Nausea and vomiting, loss of appetite, diarrhea, abdominal distention, and paralytic ileus or decreased peristalsis	• Nausea, diarrhea, and abdominal cramps
Muscles	• Weakness, fatigue, and leg cramps	• Weakness and flaccid paralysis
Urinary system	• Excessive urination	• Decreased or absent urination
Acid-base balance	• Metabolic alkalosis	• Metabolic acidosis

What causes potassium excess?

The body accumulates too much potassium when the kidneys can't excrete excessive amounts of potassium given to the person intravenously or orally. Other causes include:

- decreased urine output
- kidney dysfunction or failure
- the use of potassium-sparing diuretics, such as Dyrenium, by people with kidney disease
- any injuries or conditions that release cellular potassium or promote its retention, such as burns, crushing injuries, failing kidney function, adrenal gland insufficiency, dehydration, or diabetic acidosis.

What are the symptoms?

For information on the effects of potassium imbalance, see *How potassium imbalances affect the body.*

How are they diagnosed?

If the doctor suspects a potassium imbalance, blood tests confirm whether the person has too much or too little of the element. Additional tests may be necessary to find the underlying cause of the imbalance.

How is potassium deficiency treated?

To treat a potassium deficiency, the doctor will start replacement therapy with oral or intravenous potassium chloride. If you need diuretics, the doctor will prescribe the type that minimizes potassium loss.

How is potassium excess treated?

If your problem is too much potassium, the doctor will prescribe intravenous 10% calcium gluconate to protect the heart and then try to eliminate excessive potassium from your blood.

In an emergency, you may need intravenous administration of sodium bicarbonate or a mixture of insulin and glucose. Hemodialysis or peritoneal dialysis also helps remove excess potassium.

PROTEIN-CALORIE MALNUTRITION

What do doctors call this condition?

Marasmus (protein-calorie malnutrition), kwashiorkor (protein-only malnutrition)

What is this condition?

Protein-calorie malnutrition is one of the most prevalent and serious body-depletion disorders. It may occur as protein-calorie deficiency, marked by stunted growth and wasting away, or as protein deficiency, marked by tissue swelling and damage. Both forms vary from mild to severe and may be fatal, depending on whether the person has other problems (particularly infection or injury) and how long he has been malnourished. Protein-calorie malnutrition increases the risk of death from pneumonia, chickenpox, or measles.

What causes it?

Both kinds of malnutrition are common in any geographic area where the diet lacks enough protein to support growth requirements. Protein deficiency typically occurs at about age 1, after infants are weaned from breast milk to a protein-deficient diet. But it can develop at any time during the formative years. Protein-calorie deficiency affects infants age 6 to 18 months as a result of breast-feeding failure or a weakening condition, such as chronic diarrhea.

When diet isn't the problem, protein-calorie malnutrition may be linked to diseases that decrease protein and calorie intake or absorption, or to an injury that increases protein and calorie requirements. In the United States, protein-calorie malnutrition is estimated to affect, to some degree, 50% of surgical patients and 48% of medical patients in hospitals because they are not allowed anything by mouth for an extended period.

What are its symptoms?

Children with chronic protein-calorie malnutrition are small for their age and tend to be physically inactive, mentally apathetic, and susceptible to frequent infections. Loss of appetite and diarrhea are common. In acute protein-calorie malnutrition, children are small, gaunt, and emaciated, with no fat tissue. Their skin is dry and "baggy," and their hair is sparse and dull brown or reddish yellow. They will be weak, irritable, and usually hungry, although they may have loss of appetite, with nausea and vomiting. They also may have a low body temperature and slow pulse and breathing rates.

Unlike protein-calorie deficiency, chronic protein deficiency allows the child to grow in height, but forces his or her body to burn fat tissue for energy. The swelling of edema often masks severe muscle wasting. Dry, peeling skin is common.

How is it diagnosed?

The doctor confirms the condition by looking at the person and learning about his or her diet. If a hospitalized person does not suffer from fluid retention, his or her weight change over time is the best indicator. The doctor will also check other factors, including:
- height and weight less than 80% of standard for the person's age and sex, and below-standard arm circumference and triceps skin folds
- blood tests and urinalysis
- skin tests to check the person's immune status
- moderate anemia.

How is it treated?

The doctor will treat malnutrition by prescribing sufficient proteins, calories, and other nutrients for nutritional rehabilitation and maintenance. If the condition is severe, the doctor may use intravenous infusions or tube feeding to restore fluid and electrolyte balance. The best treatment is oral feeding of high-quality protein foods, especially milk, and protein-calorie supplements. However, the doctor will take care to prevent complications from overloading a person's weakened metabolic system with too much food to process.

SODIUM IMBALANCES

What do doctors call these conditions?

Hyponatremia, hypernatremia

What are these conditions?

Too little sodium is called *hyponatremia;* too much sodium, *hypernatremia.* The sodium level affects the balance and concentration of body fluid, acid-base balance, nerve and muscle function, glandular secretion, and water balance. A disruption in sodium balance affects the way the body transports chemicals between the cells and the fluid surrounding them.

Although the body requires only 2 to 4 grams of sodium daily, most Americans consume 6 to 10 grams daily (mostly in the form of table salt), excreting the excess sodium through the kidneys and skin.

Most Americans consume much more sodium than they need — up to five times the body's requirements.

What causes sodium deficiency?

Causes include the following:
- a low-salt diet or overuse of diuretics
- excessive loss of electrolytes from vomiting, suctioning, or diarrhea
- excessive perspiration or fever
- use of potent diuretics or tap-water enemas
- excessive drinking of water, malnutrition or starvation, and a low-sodium diet — usually in combination with one of the other causes
- injury, surgery (wound drainage), or burns, which cause sodium to shift into damaged cells
- adrenal gland disorders or cirrhosis of the liver

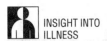

INSIGHT INTO
ILLNESS

How sodium imbalances affect the body

BODY SYSTEM	TOO LITTLE SODIUM	TOO MUCH SODIUM
Breathing and lungs	▪ Bluish skin discoloration with severe deficiency	▪ Shortness of breath, respiratory arrest, and death
Digestive system	▪ Nausea, vomiting, and abdominal cramps	▪ Rough, dry tongue and intense thirst
Heart and blood vessels	▪ Low blood pressure; fast heart rate; with severe deficit, vascular collapse and thready pulse	▪ High blood pressure, fast heart rate, pitting edema, and excessive weight gain
Nervous system	▪ Anxiety, headaches, muscle twitching and weakness, and seizures	▪ Fever, agitation, restlessness, and seizures
Skin	▪ Cold, clammy skin and decreased skin elasticity	▪ Flushed skin and dry, sticky mucous membranes
Urinary system	▪ Diminished or absent urination	▪ Diminished urination

▪ syndrome of inappropriate antidiuretic hormone secretion (marked by excessive release of antidiuretic hormone and causing fluid and electrolyte imbalances, including sodium deficiency); it may be caused by brain tumor, stroke, lung disease, or tumors; certain drugs may produce a condition similar to this syndrome.

What causes sodium excess?

Causes include the following:
▪ decreased water intake (when severe vomiting and diarrhea cause water loss that exceeds sodium loss)
▪ excessive adrenal gland hormones (as in Cushing's syndrome)
▪ diabetes
▪ salt intoxication (less common), which may be caused by eating too much table salt.

What are their symptoms?

Sodium imbalance has major effects and can cause severe abnormalities of the nervous and digestive systems, the heart, and the blood vessels. For example, too little sodium may cause kidney dysfunction or, if sodium loss is abrupt or severe, may cause the person to have seizures. Too much sodium can produce too much fluid in the lungs, circulatory disorders, and decreased level of consciousness. (See *How sodium imbalances affect the body.*)

How are they diagnosed?

The doctor orders blood tests to detect too little or too much sodium in the person's system. However, additional lab studies are necessary to learn the cause and to differentiate between a true deficit and a shift linked to some other problem, such as shock.

How is sodium deficiency treated?

If the doctor says you have mild sodium deficiency, he'll restrict your water intake. If that isn't enough, he can prescribe drugs to promote water excretion.

How is sodium excess treated?

If you have too much sodium in your blood, the usual treatment is intravenous administration of a salt-free solution (such as sugar water) to return your blood levels to normal, followed by intravenous administration of sodium chloride to prevent the other extreme. The doctor may also recommend a low-salt diet and stop any drugs that promote sodium retention.

VITAMIN A DEFICIENCY

What is this condition?

Lack of sufficient vitamin A is a dietary problem that can lead to impaired vision. A fat-soluble vitamin absorbed in the digestive tract, vitamin A maintains function in the retina as well as the tissues that cover the body's surfaces and organs. That's why vitamin A deficiency can cause night blindness, decreased color adjustment, rough skin, and poor bone growth.

Healthy adults have vitamin A reserves to last up to a year; children often do not. Many disadvantaged children have substandard levels of vitamin A, and each year 80,000 people, mostly children, lose their sight from this condition. With therapy, the chance of reversing symptoms of night blindness and milder eye changes is excellent. If the person's cornea (the transparent covering of the eye) becomes damaged, emergency treatment is necessary.

What causes it?

Vitamin A deficiency usually is caused by eating too few foods high in vitamin A (liver, kidneys, butter, milk, cream, cheese, and fortified margarine) or eating too little carotene, a vitamin A compound found in dark green leafy vegetables and yellow or orange fruits.

Less common causes are poor absorption due to disease or habitual use of mineral oil as a laxative. Some people excrete vitamin A in urine or can't store it because of diseases such as cancer, pneumonia, tuberculosis, urinary tract infection, or liver disease.

What are its symptoms?

Typically, the first symptom of vitamin A deficiency is night blindness, which the person discovers when he or she enters a dark place or is caught in the glare of oncoming headlights. As it gets worse, the person's eyes get dry and develop gray spots. Eventually, the eyes become scarred and the person may become blind.

Other symptoms are dry, scaly skin and shrinking and hardening of the mucous membranes, possibly leading to infections of the eyes and the respiratory or genitourinary systems. An infant with severe vitamin A deficiency shows signs of failure to thrive and apathy, along with dry skin and corneal changes, which can lead to ulceration and rapid destruction of the cornea.

How is it diagnosed?

If the doctor sees changes in the eyes and learns the person has had a poor diet, he or she will suspect vitamin A deficiency and order a blood test to check.

How is it treated?

If you have mild eye changes or night blindness, the doctor will suggest vitamin A replacement in the form of cod liver oil or halibut liver oil. If it's an acute deficiency, he'll prescribe vitamin A solution injections, especially when corneal changes have occurred. If you have dry skin, petroleum-based or cream salves will help.

If you have disease-related problems in absorbing vitamin A, the doctor will try to prevent the deficiency by giving you intravenous supplements or oral supplements mixed in water.

VITAMIN B DEFICIENCIES

What are these conditions?

Vitamin B deficiencies are dietary problems linked to a group of water-soluble vitamins called *B complex vitamins*. The B vitamins are essential to normal metabolism, cell growth, and blood formation. The most common deficiencies involve thiamine (B_1), riboflavin (B_2), niacin, pyridoxine (B_6), and cobalamin (B_{12}).

What causes them?

Each type of vitamin B deficiency results from a different combination of causes. (For more information, see *Understanding vitamin B deficiencies*.)

What are their symptoms?

Symptoms of vitamin B deficiencies are specific to the underlying causes.

- *Thiamine deficiency* (beriberi) causes inflammation of nerves and, possibly, brain disturbances known as Wernicke's encephalopathy and Korsakoff's psychosis. In infants (infantile beriberi), this deficiency produces swelling, irritability, abdominal pain, pallor, vomiting, loss of voice and, possibly, seizures. In heart beriberi, which is associated with congestive heart failure, severe swelling starts in the legs and moves up through the body. Dry beriberi, another form, causes numerous neurologic symptoms and an emaciated appearance.

    Thiamine deficiency may also cause heart palpitations, rapid heartbeat, difficulty breathing, and circulatory collapse. Constipation and indigestion are common.
- *Riboflavin deficiency* usually causes cracking of the lips and corners of the mouth, sore throat, and an inflamed tongue. The person may have itchy skin and burning, bloodshot eyes. Late-stage riboflavin deficiency causes nerve damage, mild anemia and, in children, growth retardation.
- *Niacin deficiency* first causes fatigue, loss of appetite, muscle weakness, headache, indigestion, mild skin eruptions, weight loss, and backache. In advanced stages (pellagra), it produces what doctors call the *3-D syndrome* — dementia, dermatitis, and diarrhea. If not reversed by therapeutic doses of niacin, pellagra can be fatal.

At first, niacin deficiency causes fatigue. Eventually, it can give you what doctors call the 3-D syndrome — dementia, dermatitis, and diarrhea.

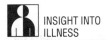
INSIGHT INTO
ILLNESS

Understanding vitamin B deficiencies

Thiamine deficiency
This type of deficiency, rare in the United States, is caused by poor absorption or insufficient intake of vitamin B_1. Beriberi, a serious thiamine deficiency, mostly affects people who subsist on diets of un-enriched rice and wheat. Alcoholics may develop beriberi, which leads to congestive heart failure, nerve damage, and brain disturbances. In times of stress (pregnancy, for example), malnourished young adults may develop beriberi. Infants on low-protein diets and those who are breast-fed by thiamine-deficient mothers may also develop it.

Riboflavin deficiency
This problem is caused by a diet deficient in milk, meat, fish, green leafy vegetables, and legumes. Chronic alcoholism or prolonged diarrhea may also cause it.

Niacin deficiency
In its advanced form, niacin deficiency produces pellagra, which affects the skin, central nervous system, and gastrointestinal tract. It affects persons who eat mainly corn and is rare in the United States. Niacin deficiency can also be linked to some benign tumors and to Hartnup disease.

Pyridoxine deficiency
This deficiency is usually is caused by destruction of pyridoxine by boiling infant formulas. It's uncommon in adults.

Cobalamin deficiency
Most commonly, cobalamin deficiency is caused by a deficiency in the person's gastric secretions or poor absorption because of illness. It may also result from a diet low in animal protein.

- *Pyridoxine deficiency* in infants causes a wide range of symptoms, from skin problems to abdominal pain, vomiting, loss of muscle control, and seizures. This deficiency can also lead to central nervous system disturbances, particularly in infants.
- *Cobalamin deficiency* causes pernicious anemia, which produces loss of appetite and weight loss, abdominal discomfort, constipation, diarrhea, and a swollen tongue. The person may lose muscle control.

How are they diagnosed?
If the doctor suspects a vitamin B deficiency, urine specimens (sometimes over a 24-hour period) can distinguish which of the B vitamins is deficient. The pyridoxine and cobalamin deficiencies are checked with blood tests, and more lab studies may be needed to discover the causes.

How are they treated?

If you have one of the vitamin B deficiencies, the doctor will recommend a new diet and supplementary vitamins to prevent or correct the condition, including the following:

- *Thiamine deficiency* is treated with a high-protein diet with adequate calorie intake, possibly supplemented by B-complex vitamins for early symptoms. Thiamine-rich foods include pork, peas, wheat bran, oatmeal, and liver.
- *Riboflavin deficiency* is treated with supplemental riboflavin for people with intractable diarrhea or those who need it because they're growing, pregnant, nursing mothers, or recovering from a wound. Good sources of riboflavin are meats, enriched flour, milk and dairy foods, green leafy vegetables, eggs, and cereal.
- *Niacin deficiency* is treated with supplemental B-complex vitamins and dietary enrichment for people at risk because of poor diets or alcoholism. Meats, fish, peanuts, brewer's yeast, enriched breads, and cereals are rich in niacin. Someone with a confirmed niacin deficiency needs daily doses of a niacin solution by mouth or intravenously.
- *Pyridoxine deficiency* is treated with preventive doses of pyridoxine for infants and epileptic children. A person with loss of appetite or malabsorption, or one who is taking certain drugs (INH or Cuprimine), may need supplemental B-complex vitamins. Some women who take oral contraceptives may have to supplement their diets with pyridoxine. Confirmed pyridoxine deficiency requires oral or intravenous pyridoxine.
- *Cobalamin deficiency* is treated with intravenous cobalamin solution for severe cases and people with reduced gastric secretion of hydrochloric acid, some malabsorption syndromes, or intestine surgery. Strict vegetarians may have to supplement their diets with oral vitamin B_{12}.

VITAMIN C DEFICIENCY

What is this condition?

Vitamin C deficiency leads to a condition called *scurvy*, or inadequate production of collagen, a substance that binds the cells of the teeth, bones, and capillaries. Scurvy used to strike sailors and others who had no fresh fruits and vegetables for long periods. Now, vitamin C (ascorbic acid) deficiency is rare in North America, except in alcoholics, people on low-fiber diets, and infants weaned from breast milk to cow's milk without a vitamin C supplement.

What causes it?

The primary cause is a diet lacking foods rich in vitamin C, such as citrus fruits, tomatoes, cabbage, broccoli, spinach, and berries. Because the body can't store this water-soluble vitamin in large amounts, the supply needs to be replenished daily. Other causes of vitamin C deficiency include:

- destruction of vitamin C in foods by overexposure to air or by overcooking
- excessive ingestion of vitamin C during pregnancy, which causes the newborn to require large amounts of the vitamin after birth
- low intake of vitamin C during periods of stress — caused by infectious disease, for example — which can deplete vitamin C.

What are its symptoms?

Symptoms appear as the blood capillaries become increasingly fragile. In an adult, vitamin C deficiency produces skin eruptions, the appearance of bruises, anemia, loss of appetite, limb and joint pain (especially in the knees), pallor, weakness, swollen or bleeding gums, loose teeth, lethargy, insomnia, poor wound healing, and bloodshot eyes. Vitamin C deficiency can also cause psychological disturbances, such as irritability, depression, and hysteria.

In a child, vitamin C deficiency produces tender, painful swelling in the legs, causing the child to lie with his legs partially flexed. Other symptoms include fever, diarrhea, and vomiting.

How is it diagnosed?

The doctor will ask about the person's diet. He or she can confirm vitamin C deficiency with a test for ascorbic acid levels in the blood.

How is it treated?

Because scurvy is potentially fatal, the doctor will try to immediately restore adequate vitamin C intake by giving daily doses of 100 to 200 milligrams of vitamin C in synthetic form or in orange juice. If the deficiency is severe, the doctor will double the dose. The person's symptoms usually subside in 2 to 3 days; hemorrhages and bone disorders, in 2 to 3 weeks.

With proper treatment — which may include lots of orange juice — most symptoms of vitamin C deficiency disappear within 2 to 3 days.

To prevent vitamin C deficiency, people who are unable or unwilling to eat foods rich in vitamin C or those facing surgery should take daily supplements of ascorbic acid. Vitamin C supplements may also prevent this deficiency in recently weaned infants or those drinking formula not fortified with vitamin C.

A final note: There *is* such a thing as too much vitamin C. The doctor's recommended dosage should not be exceeded because excessive doses of ascorbic acid may cause nausea, diarrhea, and kidney stone formation and also may interfere with anticoagulant therapy.

VITAMIN D DEFICIENCY

What is this condition?

Vitamin D deficiency causes failure of normal bone growth (called *calcification*), which results in rickets in infants and young children and osteomalacia (a condition marked by softening of the bones) in adults. With treatment, most people are cured. In osteomalacia, deformities may disappear, but the deformities of rickets do not.

What causes it?

Vitamin D deficiency is caused by eating too little of the foods that contain vitamin D, poor absorption of vitamin D, or too little sunlight. Specific causes include the following:

- insufficient vitamin D intake in breast-fed infants or use of a non-fortified milk-based formula in other infants
- poor diets and lack of exposure to sunlight in overcrowded urban areas
- an all-cereal diet (rare in the United States)
- an inherited kidney flaw that keeps the person from absorbing nutrients and can cause vitamin D-resistant rickets
- conditions that lower absorption of fat-soluble vitamin D, such as chronic pancreatitis, celiac disease, Crohn's disease, cystic fibrosis, gastric or small-bowel surgery, colitis, and bile duct obstruction
- liver or kidney diseases, which interfere with the intestine's absorption of vitamin D
- malfunctioning parathyroid glands.

One possible cause of vitamin D deficiency is too little sunlight.

What are its symptoms?

The person with vitamin D deficiency first notices profuse sweating, restlessness, and irritability. In a chronic deficiency, the person will develop bone malformations due to softening of the bones: bowlegs, knock-knees, rachitic rosary (beading of ends of ribs), enlargement of wrists and ankles, pigeon breast, softening of the skull, and bulging of the forehead.

A child may have poorly developed muscles (potbelly), delayed closing of the bones in the skull, and stiff muscles. Bone deformities may make it hard for the person to walk or climb stairs and cause spontaneous multiple fractures and pain in the legs and lower back.

How is it diagnosed?

The doctor will ask about diet, examine the person, and order appropriate lab tests and X-rays that show characteristic bone deformities.

How is it treated?

If you are diagnosed with osteomalacia or your child has rickets, the doctor will order massive oral doses of vitamin D or cod liver oil. The exception is when the deficiency is caused by poor absorption. For rickets resistant to vitamin D or rickets accompanied by liver or kidney disease, the doctor will prescribe other drugs or a synthetic analog of active vitamin D.

What can a person with vitamin D deficiency do?

- Consume foods and beverages high in vitamin D, such as fortified milk, fish liver oils, herring, liver, and egg yolks, and get some sun.
- If you must take vitamin D for a long period, watch for signs of vitamin D toxicity, including headache, nausea, constipation and, after prolonged use, kidney stones.

VITAMIN E DEFICIENCY

What is this condition?

Vitamin E deficiency is a dietary problem that leaves the person unable to properly process fats in his food. It usually affects newborns. It may cause a form of anemia in low-birth-weight or premature infants. With treatment, the child can develop normally.

What causes it?

Vitamin E deficiency in infants is usually caused by formulas high in polyunsaturated fatty acids that are fortified with iron but not vitamin E. A newborn hasn't stored much vitamin E to begin with, because only a small amount passes through the placenta, and the mother retains most of it.

Because vitamin E is a fat-soluble vitamin, deficiency may develop in children with conditions associated with poor fat absorption, such as kwashiorkor, celiac disease, or cystic fibrosis. These conditions may lead to anemia and amino acids in the urine, both of which are reversible if the child is given doses of vitamin E.

Deficiency in adults

Vitamin E deficiency is uncommon in adults but may occur in people whose diets are high in polyunsaturated fatty acids, which increase vitamin E requirements, and in people with poor vitamin E absorption, which hurts red blood cell survival.

What are its symptoms?

Vitamin E deficiency is difficult to recognize. In infants, its early signs include swelling and skin lesions. It adults, it may cause muscle weakness or intermittent claudication.

In premature infants, vitamin E deficiency produces hemolytic anemia, thrombocythemia, and erythematous papular skin eruptions, followed by desquamation.

How is it diagnosed?

The doctor will ask about the person's diet and medical history and then order blood and urine tests to confirm the diagnosis.

How is it treated?

The doctor will prescribe either oral or intravenous vitamin E to cure the deficiency. To prevent the disorder, the doctor may prescribe vitamin E supplements for low-birth-weight infants who are given formulas not fortified with vitamin E. These supplements also work for adults with poor vitamin E absorption. Many commercial multivitamin supplements are easily absorbed by people with this condition.

> *Vitamin E deficiency in infants is usually caused by formulas that are not supplemented with vitamin E. Breast-fed infants get enough of this vitamin.*

What can a person with vitamin E deficiency do?

- New mothers who plan to breast-feed can be assured that human milk provides adequate vitamin E.
- Adults should eat foods high in vitamin E. Good sources include vegetable oils (corn, safflower, soybean, cottonseed), whole grains, dark green leafy vegetables, nuts, and legumes. Also, eating lots of polyunsaturated fats increases the need for vitamin E.

VITAMIN K DEFICIENCY

What is this condition?

Vitamin K is an element required by the liver to form substances that clot the blood. Deficiency of this vitamin causes abnormal bleeding. If the deficiency is corrected, the chance for a cure is excellent.

What causes it?

Vitamin K deficiency is common among newborns in the first few days of life because of poor placental transfer of vitamin K and poor production of vitamin K-producing intestinal flora. This condition may also be caused by:

- prolonged use of drugs that destroy normal intestinal bacteria, such as anticoagulants and antibiotics
- decreased flow of bile to the small intestine because of an obstructed bile duct or bile leakage
- poor absorption of vitamin K due to other vitamin deficiencies (such as pellagra), bowel surgery, or ulcerative colitis
- chronic liver disease
- cystic fibrosis.

What are its symptoms?

The person with vitamin K deficiency always has abnormal bleeding and slow clotting. Administration of vitamin K cures these symptoms. Without treatment, bleeding may be severe and possibly fatal.

How is it diagnosed?

The doctor will check to see how long it takes the person's blood to clot. A wait of 25% longer than the normal range of 10 to 20 seconds confirms the diagnosis of vitamin K deficiency after other causes of delayed clotting (such as anticoagulant therapy or liver disease) have been ruled out. The doctor will repeat the test in 24 hours (and regularly during treatment) to monitor the success of therapy.

How is it treated?

If you have the deficiency, taking vitamin K corrects the abnormal bleeding. To prevent vitamin K deficiency, the doctor will give vitamin K to newborns and people with poor fat absorption or with prolonged diarrhea resulting from intestinal problems or long-term antibiotic drug therapy.

If the deficiency has a dietary cause, a doctor or nutritionist can help you plan a diet that includes important sources of vitamin K, such as green leafy vegetables, cauliflower, tomatoes, cheese, egg yolks, and liver.

8

KIDNEY AND URINARY DISORDERS

STRAIGHT
TALK

Common questions about acute glomerulonephritis

The doctor says I have something called glomerulonephritis. How can one disease cause so many symptoms?

This disease is caused by the antigen-antibody activity when your body fights another infection. The leftover cells from that battle settle in the kidney and interfere with its function, which triggers a long list of problems.

How can a kidney infection give me high blood pressure?

The kidney gets clogged enough that its blood flow is slowed, which reduces urine production and elevates your blood pressure. Because the cells in the kidney can't do their job, water and salts shift around and swell the kidney, causing it to produce hormones that contribute to high blood pressure.

Why is the doctor watching for uremic poisoning?

Leftover cells from the battle against infection cause the kidney's capillaries to weaken, allowing protein to escape into the bowel where it breaks down and passes into your blood. The chemicals produced by the breakdown of protein, which normally are excreted in urine, enter the blood and become toxic. This is called *uremic poisoning*.

ACUTE GLOMERULONEPHRITIS

What do doctors call this condition?

Acute poststreptococcal glomerulonephritis

What is this condition?

Acute glomerulonephritis is a relatively common inflammation of the glomeruli — tiny masses of capillary blood vessels that function to filter waste products from the blood. It affects people who have had a streptococcal infection of the respiratory tract or, less often, a skin infection such as impetigo.

Acute glomerulonephritis is most common in boys ages 3 to 7, but anyone can get it. Up to 95% of children and up to 70% of adults with acute glomerulonephritis recover fully. The rest may have serious complications, such as chronic kidney failure, within months.

What causes it?

Acute glomerulonephritis is caused by an abnormal immune reaction, which produces clusters of antigen-antibody cells. The cell clusters become trapped in the glomeruli, inflaming them and interfering with their function. Sometimes this allows red blood cells and proteins to filter through, which can lead to uremic poisoning. (See *Common questions about acute glomerulonephritis.*)

What are its symptoms?

Acute glomerulonephritis begins within 1 to 3 weeks after the person has had an untreated sore throat. Symptoms include mild to moderate swelling, decreased urination, bloody urine, and fatigue. The person may have high blood pressure from sodium or water retention due to impaired kidney function. Symptoms may progress to congestive heart failure and fluid in the lungs.

How is it diagnosed?

The doctor will ask about symptoms and any recent illness, then order lab tests, including urinalysis to assess kidney filtration, throat culture to check for *Streptococcus*, renal ultrasound to check for kidney enlargement, and biopsy of kidney tissue to confirm the diagnosis in a person with acute glomerulonephritis or assess the kidney's status.

How hemodialysis works

If the doctor orders hemodialysis for you, the nurse or technician will use a dialyzer (pictured below) to do your kidneys' job. By filtering the blood through its internal membranes, a dialyzer removes extra fluids and impurities and returns purified blood to the body.

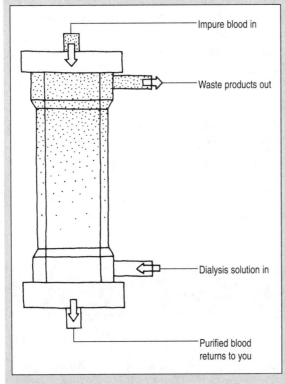

Impure blood in

Waste products out

Dialysis solution in

Purified blood returns to you

Before dialysis

The nurse or technician will weigh you and take your blood pressure once while you're lying down and again while you're standing. Then, the doctor will cut a small opening in your collarbone or groin area. First,

the doctor will make the area numb with an anesthetic so that you're not uncomfortable, then will put a thin, hollow tube called a *catheter* into the opening. Stitches will keep the catheter in place. It will then be used to transfer some of your blood to the dialyzer.

During dialysis

Next, the nurse will attach the dialyzer to your catheter and turn the machine on to begin the treatment. The nurse will check the dialyzer and all the connections frequently. During hemodialysis, your blood flow will gradually increase, so the nurse will check your blood pressure every half hour or so.

The nurse will also collect blood samples every so often during hemodialysis and when it ends. The blood samples will be tested to see how well hemodialysis is working for you.

You provide the feedback

Be sure to tell the doctor or nurse how you feel, especially if you experience a headache, backache, nausea, vomiting, muscle twitching, difficulty breathing, or pain.

When hemodialysis is over, the nurse will disconnect the catheter from the dialyzer.

After dialysis

When you go home, remember to keep the skin around the catheter clean and dry. If the nurse has taught you how, you may clean it with hydrogen peroxide solution daily until the wound is healed and the stitches are removed.

Call your doctor if you have pain, swelling, redness, or drainage in the catheter area.

How is it treated?

Treatment aims to relieve the person's symptoms and prevent complications. The doctor will urge bed rest, fluid and dietary sodium restrictions, and correction of electrolyte imbalances (possibly with dialysis, although this is rarely necessary). The person may be given diuretics, such as Diulo or Lasix, to reduce fluid overload and blood pressure medicine, such as Alazine.

What can a person with acute glomerulonephritis do?

If you are diagnosed with this serious kidney infection, your recovery, in the hospital and at home, will pass through several slow stages. It's important to follow the doctor's directions:

- Follow a diet high in calories and low in protein, sodium, potassium, and fluids.
- Stay in bed during the acute phase; then gradually resume normal activities as your symptoms subside.
- If you must have dialysis, become familiar with the procedure. (See *How hemodialysis works*, page 315.)
- If you have a history of chronic upper respiratory tract infections, immediately tell the doctor about any signs of infection (fever, sore throat).
- Follow-up examinations are necessary to detect chronic kidney failure, especially if you are pregnant. To avoid complications, your blood pressure, urine protein level, and kidney function must be monitored for several months to detect any return of the disease. Your urine will need to be tested periodically. Other viral infections may cause bloody urine and the results of other urine tests may be abnormal for years to come.

ACUTE KIDNEY FAILURE

What do doctors call this condition?

Acute renal failure

What is this condition?

Acute kidney failure is the sudden interruption of kidney function due to an obstruction, reduced circulation, or kidney disease. It's usually reversible with medical treatment, but can be fatal without it.

What causes it?

Doctors divide the causes of acute kidney failure into three groups, according to where the problem starts: prerenal, intrinsic, and postrenal.

Prerenal failure is caused by any condition (hypovolemia, shock, embolism, blood loss, infection, pooling of fluid in sores or burns, heart disorders) that reduces blood flow to the kidneys.

Intrinsic renal failure is caused by damage to the kidneys themselves, such as infections and blood clots. Postrenal failure is caused by any condition (kidney stones, blood clots, tumors, or swelling from catheterization) that blocks urine flow from both kidneys.

What are its symptoms?

The most common early sign is greatly decreased urination. Electrolyte imbalance and other severe effects follow, as kidney dysfunction disrupts other body systems. Specific symptoms include:

- Digestive system: loss of appetite, nausea, vomiting, diarrhea or constipation, inflamed mouth, bleeding, dry mucous membranes, bad breath
- Central nervous system: headache, drowsiness, irritability, confusion, convulsions, coma
- Skin: dry skin, itchiness, paleness, bruises
- Heart and circulation: low blood pressure (early in the disease); later, high blood pressure, irregular heartbeat, fluid overload, congestive heart failure, swelling, anemia, altered blood clotting
- Breathing: fluid in the lungs.

Fever and chills indicate infection, a common complication.

How is it diagnosed?

The doctor will ask about previous disorders that might cause kidney failure, then will order blood and urine tests to look for specific evidence. Other studies include ultrasound and X-ray studies of the kidneys, ureter, and bladder.

How is it treated?

If you have acute kidney failure, the doctor will first start you on a diet high in calories and low in protein, sodium, and potassium, with supplemental vitamins and restricted fluids. The doctor will watch your body fluids carefully for an excessive amount of potassium, a condition called *hyperkalemia*. If hyperkalemia occurs, acute therapy may include dialysis, glucose and insulin infusions, and sodium bicarbonate — all administered intravenously — and Kayexalate, possibly by enema, to remove potassium from the body.

Acute kidney failure: With treatment it's usually reversible; without treatment it may be fatal.

How peritoneal dialysis works

If your doctor orders peritoneal dialysis for you, the procedure can remove impurities from your blood when your kidneys aren't working properly.

Before dialysis
- The nurse will take your blood pressure twice, once while you're standing and once while you're lying down. To make you more comfortable and to protect your bladder, the nurse will also weigh you and ask you to urinate.
- Next, the doctor will create an opening in your peritoneal cavity, which is near your stomach. (First, the doctor will numb the area with an anesthetic.) The doctor will insert a slender tube called a *catheter* into the opening. The catheter is used to transfer a special warmed solution into your peritoneal cavity. The solution collects impurities that cross through your peritoneum (a membrane that acts like a filter). After a specified time, the solution is drained from your body.
- Both you and the nurse (or the dialysis technician) will wear masks during dialysis to prevent possible infection. The nurse hangs the solution bag above you on a bedside pole and the drainage bag below your bed.

During dialysis
- To start dialysis, the nurse will open a clamp to allow the solution to flow into your peritoneal cavity, where it will remain for a prescribed time. Then, it will drain into the collection bag. The procedure will be repeated for the prescribed number of cycles.
- To ensure your progress, the nurse will take your blood pressure, check your breathing, examine the tubing, and change your catheter dressing whenever it's soiled or wet.

After dialysis
- The nurse will disconnect the tubing and cover the catheter with a sterile, protective cap, then will apply ointment to the catheter site and bandage it.
- Call your doctor if you notice any signs of infection (such as redness or swelling) or fluid imbalance (such as a sudden weight gain or swollen arms or legs). As the nurse has taught you, take your vital signs regularly and change the catheter dressing. And be sure to keep all your follow-up appointments.

If these measures fail to control your symptoms, hemodialysis or peritoneal dialysis may be necessary. (See *How hemodialysis works*, page 315, and *How peritoneal dialysis works*.)

*A*CUTE PYELONEPHRITIS

What is this condition?
Acute pyelonephritis is a sudden inflammation of kidney tissues and is one of the most common kidney diseases. With treatment and continued follow-up care, most people get well, and extensive permanent tissue damage is rare.

What causes it?

Acute pyelonephritis is caused by bacterial infection of the kidneys. Those bacteria usually are normal intestinal and bowel organisms that grow readily in urine. The most common of them is *Escherichia coli*, but *Pseudomonas aeruginosa, Staphylococcus aureus*, and *Streptococcus faecalis* may also cause such infections.

In most people, the infection spreads from the bladder to the kidneys, where it can create colonies of infection within 24 to 48 hours. Infection may also be spread by hospital procedures such as catheterization, cystoscopy, or urologic surgery. The disorder may also result from blood-borne and lymphatic infections, as well as several kinds of urinary obstructions that make it difficult for the person to urinate.

Who gets the infection?

Pyelonephritis occurs more often in women, probably because the urethra is shorter in women than in men, and because the urinary tract lies close to the vagina and the rectum. This allows bacteria to reach the bladder more easily. Women also lack certain antibacterial secretions men produce in this body region. Incidence increases with age and is higher in sexually active or pregnant women and in people with other kidney diseases or diabetes.

What are its symptoms?

The doctor will ask about such things as urgent, frequent or burning urination. The person's urine may appear cloudy and have a fishy odor. Other common symptoms include a temperature of 102° F (38.8° C) or higher, shaking chills, flank pain, poor appetite, and general fatigue.

These symptoms can develop rapidly over a few hours or a few days. Although the symptoms may disappear within days, even without treatment, residual bacterial infection is likely and may cause symptoms to recur.

How is it diagnosed?

After learning about the person's symptoms, the doctor will order a urinalysis. Typical findings include pus cells and, possibly, some red blood cells; significant numbers of bacteria; and a slightly alkaline urine pH.

In pyelonephritis, bacteria spread from the bladder to the kidneys, where they can create colonies of infection within 24 to 48 hours.

PREVENTION
TIPS

Preventing acute pyelonephritis

To avoid this hazardous infection, follow the guidelines below.

Watch for signs of infection
These include cloudy urine, burning urination, and urinary urgency and frequency, especially when accompanied by a low-grade fever.

If you have a history of urinary tract infections, get routine checkups.

If using a urinary catheter
Observe strict sterile technique during catheter insertion and care.

Especially for women
Prevent bacterial contamination by wiping from front to back after a bowel movement.

A plain X-ray film of the kidneys, ureters, and bladder may reveal stones, tumors, or cysts in the kidneys and the urinary tract. X-rays with contrast dyes may reveal asymmetrical kidneys.

How is it treated?

The doctor will choose an antibiotic specifically designed to fight the person's infection. For example, *E. coli* may be treated with Gantrisin, NegGram, and Macrodantin or Furadantin. If the infecting organism can't be identified, the doctor will prescribe a broad-spectrum antibiotic, such as Amcill. If the person is pregnant, the doctor will prescribe antibiotics with caution or urinary analgesics such as Phenazodine.

The person's symptoms may disappear after several days of antibiotic therapy. Usually, the person takes antibiotics for 10 to 14 days. Follow-up testing includes a new urine culture 1 week after drug therapy stops, then periodically for the next year to catch any remaining infection.

Most people with uncomplicated infections respond well to therapy and don't suffer reinfection. In infections resulting from an obstruction, antibiotics may be less effective, and the doctor may recommend corrective surgery. People who have a high risk of recurring urinary tract and kidney infections, such as those undergoing prolonged catheterization or maintenance antibiotic therapy, require long-term follow-up.

What can a person with acute pyelonephritis do?

If you are diagnosed with this kidney infection, here are some helpful suggestions:
- Drink plenty of fluids to help empty your bladder of contaminated urine. However, don't drink more than 3 quarts (3 liters) a day because this may reduce the effectiveness of the antibiotics you're taking.
- Follow the diet you are given to prevent kidney stone formation.
- Complete prescribed antibiotic therapy, even after symptoms go away. Get long-term follow-up care if the doctor says you are at high-risk for more infections. (See *Preventing acute pyelonephritis*.)

CHRONIC GLOMERULONEPHRITIS

What is this condition?

Chronic glomerulonephritis is a slowly progressive disease, marked by inflammation of the kidneys. The inflammation leads to hardening and scarring of tissue and eventual kidney failure.

People with this condition usually don't develop symptoms until the disease is advanced. By this time, the person with chronic glomerulonephritis usually cannot be cured and must rely on dialysis or a kidney transplant.

What causes it?

Common causes of chronic glomerulonephritis include a long list of preexisting kidney disorders, and it may be linked to some other diseases such as strep, lupus, and Goodpasture's syndrome.

What are its symptoms?

Since it develops slowly and silently, people with chronic glomerulonephritis may not have symptoms for many years. At any time, however, it may suddenly worsen, producing high blood pressure and protein and blood in the urine, possibly followed by symptoms of uremic poisoning, such as nausea, vomiting, itchy skin, difficult breathing, and fatigue. Mild to severe swelling and anemia may accompany these symptoms. When the disease involves the heart or leads to kidney failure, the person will require dialysis or a kidney transplant.

How is it diagnosed?

Because the doctor usually can't detect glomerulonephritis with a physical exam or questions, he or she will order urinalysis, which may show blood, protein, and debris from the damaged kidneys. The doctor may use blood tests and X-ray or ultrasound to learn more, and then a kidney biopsy to identify the exact cause and gather data to plan the person's therapy.

How is it treated?

The doctor first works to reduce the person's symptoms and to control high blood pressure with drugs and a low-potassium diet. (See *How to choose low-potassium foods*.)

 SELF-HELP

How to choose low-potassium foods

Because sodium-laden foods usually taste salty, you can easily recognize and avoid them. But avoiding high-potassium foods, which lack a telltale taste, is trickier. Use the guidelines below when choosing meals and snacks.

Avoid these high-potassium foods
- Fruits: all dried fruits, apricot juice, bananas, cantaloupe, grapefruit, honeydew melon, and oranges
- Vegetables: all raw vegetables, leafy green vegetables, legumes, potatoes, and winter squash
- Other: molasses, nuts, and whole grains

Choose these low-potassium foods
- Fruits: apples, cranberries, grapes, and pears (fresh, canned, or juice)
- Vegetables: canned carrots, corn, green beans, or peas; and fresh summer squash (*Note:* Choose canned goods without added salt if your diet also limits sodium.)
- Other: honey, noodles, rice, and white enriched bread

PREVENTION
TIPS

How to reduce the risk of kidney damage from drugs

If you are diagnosed with chronic glomerulonephritis, you have an increased risk of toxic effects from drugs. In fact, any kidney problem means certain drugs must be taken with extra care.

List all your drugs

To establish a safe drug regimen, make a list of all your current medications, both prescription and nonprescription. Also tell your doctor or nurse about any other conditions for which you take medications.

Special alert

Although many drugs can disrupt kidney function, most problems are caused by three major groups:

- antibiotics, such as penicillamine (Cuprimine or Depen)
- nonsteroidal anti-inflammatory drugs (such as Ansaid, Advil, or Motrin)
- contrast dyes used in diagnostic X-ray tests.

The doctor may restrict and guide the person's fluid consumption and prescribe diuretics to prevent congestive heart failure. (See *How to reduce the risk of kidney damage from drugs*.) Treatment may also include antibiotics (for urinary tract infections) and, eventually, dialysis or transplantation. (See *How hemodialysis works*, page 315.)

CHRONIC KIDNEY FAILURE

What is this condition?

Chronic kidney failure usually results from a gradual loss of kidney function. Occasionally it follows rapid loss of kidney function. Few symptoms develop until after more than 75% of the kidney's function is lost.

Without treatment, unfiltered toxins in the blood damage all the person's major organs. If he or she can tolerate it, the person with chronic kidney failure will receive dialysis or a kidney transplant.

What causes it?

Chronic kidney failure can follow a long list of diseases described in other parts of this chapter:

- chronic kidney tissue disease, such as glomerulonephritis (see "Chronic Glomerulonephritis" on page 321)
- chronic infections, such as pyelonephritis (see "Acute Pyelonephritis" on page 318) or tuberculosis
- inherited defects, such as cyst-filled kidneys (see "Polycystic Kidney Disease" on page 344)
- vascular diseases, such as nephrosclerosis or high blood pressure (see "Renal Hypertension" on page 346)
- obstructions, such as kidney stones
- connective-tissue diseases, such as lupus
- drugs that affect the kidneys, such as long-term aminoglycoside therapy
- endocrine diseases, such as complications of diabetes.

All of these factors gradually destroy the kidney's tissue and cause the organ to fail. If the person has acute kidney failure that does not respond to treatment, chronic kidney failure develops. (See *Complications of chronic kidney failure*.)

Complications of chronic kidney failure

If you are diagnosed with chronic kidney failure, sticking to the diet, prescribed medications, and other treatments your doctor recommends will have major benefits. You can help reduce or avoid some of the following complications.

Short-term complications

These include anemia, excessive potassium, high blood pressure, fluid overload, and pericarditis.

- Anemia causes fatigue, decreased tolerance for exercise, and pallor. It's caused by your kidney's inability to produce a hormone that stimulates the bone marrow to produce red blood cells. In addition, these red blood cells have a shortened life span related to uremia, and they're lost because of easy bruising, clotting abnormalities, and the frequent blood studies required to treat your condition.
- Hyperkalemia (excessive potassium) occurs when potassium — normally excreted by the kidneys — accumulates in the blood. This electrolyte imbalance can lead to heart attack, so you should report the weakness, discomfort, and abdominal cramps that signal hyperkalemia.
- High blood pressure is a common complication that can lead to heart disease, stroke, and more kidney damage.
- Fluid overload can be caused by the diseased kidney's inability to remove excess fluid. If you don't manage it with fluid restriction, you may have swelling in your arms and legs, high blood pressure, congestive heart failure, and even fluid in the lungs.
- Pericarditis — an inflammation of the sac that surrounds the heart — can interfere with the heart's normal pumping action. It most commonly occurs with end-stage kidney failure. If you have any sudden chest pain or trouble breathing, report it to the doctor immediately. It may be pericarditis.

Long-term complications

These include bone and coronary artery disease.

- Bone disease is a risk of chronic kidney failure, which depresses calcium levels in the blood and increases phosphorus levels (the failing kidney doesn't excrete phosphorus). The body compensates by reabsorbing calcium from bones. Aluminum hydroxide gels, given to reduce phosphate, also contribute to bone disease.
- You can reduce your risk of coronary artery disease by following a low-fat diet and by avoiding smoking.

What are its symptoms?

Chronic kidney failure produces major changes in all of the person's body systems:

- Kidney and urinary system: Initial changes include low blood pressure, dry mouth, loss of skin tone, listlessness, fatigue, and nausea; later, confusion. As the kidney loses its capacity to excrete sodium, the person suffers sodium retention and overload, with muscle irritation then weakness. The person's urine output decreases, and the urine's chemical composition is altered.
- Heart and circulation: Kidney failure leads to high blood pressure, irregular heartbeat (including life-threatening fast heartbeat or fibrillation), swelling, and congestive heart failure.

- Respiratory: Lung changes include susceptibility to infection, accumulation of fluid, pain, pneumonia, and difficult breathing due to congestive heart failure.
- Gastrointestinal tract: Inflammation and ulceration affect many parts of this system. Obvious symptoms include a metallic taste in the mouth, ammonia on the breath, poor appetite, nausea, and vomiting.
- Skin: Typically, the person's skin is pale, yellowish bronze, dry, and scaly. Fingernails may be thin and brittle with lines, and hair may be dry and brittle, change color, and fall out easily.
- Nervous system: Restless leg syndrome, one of the first signs of nerve damage, causes pain, burning, and itching in the legs and feet. It may be relieved by voluntarily shaking or rocking them. The person also may experience muscle cramping and twitching, shortened memory and attention span, apathy, drowsiness, irritability, confusion, coma, and seizures. The doctor may check for brain wave changes indicating damage.
- Endocrine: Chronic kidney failure can cause stunted growth patterns in children, infertility and reduced sexual drive in both sexes, reduced or stopped menstruation, impotence and decreased sperm production, and increased blood glucose levels similar to diabetes.
- Blood changes: These include anemia, decreased red blood cell survival time, blood loss from dialysis and gastrointestinal bleeding, and mild clotting problems that can get worse.
- Skeletal: Mineral and hormone imbalances cause muscle and bone pain, bone loss, fractures, and calcium deposits in the brain, eyes, gums, joints, heart lining, and blood vessels. Arterial calcification may produce coronary artery disease. In a child, kidney-related rickets may develop.

How is it diagnosed?

The doctor will ask about symptoms of worsening kidney function and order a lab test called the *creatinine clearance test* to assess kidney function. Then, the doctor will order a variety of lab tests to pinpoint the specific problems. Blood and urine samples, X-ray studies, and kidney biopsy may be used to determine the source of the problem.

How is it treated?

The doctor may use dietary therapy to correct the person's specific symptoms. A low-protein diet reduces the production of materials that the kidneys can't excrete. (However, a person receiving continu-

SELF-HELP

How to moderate kidney disease with diet

By following a new diet, you can significantly slow the progress of kidney disease. These restrictions will change, depending on the stage of your disease and whether you're undergoing dialysis. The best results require a fine balance of foods and liquids. There are three main goals:
- regulation of fluid and sodium (salt) intake to control fluid balance
- protein restriction to prevent complications from accumulated wastes
- potassium restriction to prevent weakness and heart abnormalities.

Fluids and sodium
Because your kidney may not be able to concentrate urine, you may be losing sodium. As a result, sodium and fluid restrictions could be harmful, resulting in dehydration and more damage. If you are taking diuretics, that can increase sodium loss, too. Your sodium intake should equal what you lose in the urine (as much as 4 grams daily), and you should drink plenty of fluids.

If your kidney disease progresses, you have to restrict sodium (cut your intake in half, to about 2 grams) to prevent fluid retention, and restrict your fluids to 1 to 1½ quarts (liters). Learn to avoid processed foods, such as canned foods and frozen dinners. The restrictions prevent excessive fluid accumulation between hemodialysis treatments. The restrictions usually aren't required for peritoneal dialysis.

Protein
Protein restriction may start early in kidney disease. To ensure that you have an adequate protein intake, the diet will allow a certain amount of meat, fish, eggs, and dairy products. Correct protein intake can delay the start of uremic poisoning. In nephrotic syndrome, you need more protein to replace protein lost in the urine.

After hemodialysis or peritoneal dialysis begins, you can relax a bit and increase your protein intake because dialysis removes waste products. However, too much protein can worsen your symptoms. In all cases, you need adequate calories from fats or carbohydrates so that your body can use the proteins for tissue growth and repair.

Potassium
Because your kidneys regulate potassium, restrictions are necessary when you've lost more than 90% of kidney function. At this point, potassium accumulation can cause weakness and heart abnormalities. Foods high in potassium include many fruits, vegetables, and high-protein foods, so your potassium levels will be monitored carefully. Remember that salt substitutes often include potassium.

If you're receiving hemodialysis, potassium restrictions should continue because overload can happen between treatments. During peritoneal dialysis, restrictions usually aren't needed.

ous peritoneal dialysis will be given a high-protein diet.) A high-calorie diet prevents mineral imbalances that cause tissue damage. The prescribed diet also restricts sodium and potassium. (See *How to moderate kidney disease with diet*.)

The doctor may work to correct the person's fluid balance with fluid restriction and drugs that control blood pressure, swelling, nausea and vomiting, stomach irritation or constipation, and itching skin. The person may benefit from supplementary vitamins, especially B, D, and essential amino acids.

If the person's gastrointestinal tract is affected, he or she may need regular stool analysis to detect blood and cleansing enemas to remove the blood. Anemia calls for iron and folate supplements, and severe anemia may require transfusions, though they provide only temporary help. The person may be given hormone therapy to increase red blood cell production.

The person with chronic kidney failure in its severe stage may be given either hemodialysis or peritoneal dialysis to help control most of the symptoms. (See *How hemodialysis works*, page 315, and *How peritoneal dialysis works*, page 318.) But anemia, nerve damage, and other complications may persist. Finally, maintenance dialysis itself can produce complications. A kidney transplant may be needed for someone with end-stage kidney disease.

ENLARGED PROSTATE

What do doctors call this condition?
Benign prostatic hypertrophy or hyperplasia

Most men over age 50 experience some prostate enlargement without noticeable symptoms.

What is this condition?
This condition is an overgrowth of the small glands, found in men, that surround the urethra at the point where it leaves the bladder. An enlarged prostate may become large enough to press on the urethra and interfere with urination. Most men over age 50 have some enlargement without noticeable symptoms. Depending on the degree of enlargement, the age and health of the man, and the extent of the obstruction, an enlarged prostate is treated with antibiotics or surgery.

What causes it?
Experts think there is a link between enlarged prostate and complex age-related hormonal changes. Other postulated causes include tumors, clogged arteries, inflammation, and metabolic or nutritional disturbances.

Whatever the cause, the disorder begins with changes in the gland's tissue. As the prostate enlarges, it may press into the bladder and obstruct the flow of urine by compressing or distorting the nearby urethra. An enlarged prostate may also cause a pouch to form in the bladder that retains urine when the rest of the bladder empties. This retained urine may form stones or cysts.

What are its symptoms?

Usually, a person with an enlarged prostate first feels a group of symptoms known as "prostatism" that interfere with urination. (See *How to recognize an enlarged prostate*.)

As his obstruction worsens, urination becomes more frequent, causing incontinence, waking in the night to urinate, and possibly blood in the urine. The doctor may be able to see a bulge that indicates an incompletely emptied bladder and, by inserting a finger in the rectum, can feel the enlarged prostate. The person may also be anemic and have poor kidney function because of the obstruction.

Complications

If the person has an infection or takes decongestants, tranquilizers, antidepressants, certain other drugs, or alcohol, his urine production may shut down. At its worst, an enlarged prostate can lead to infection, poor kidney function, hemorrhage, and shock.

How is it diagnosed?

The doctor can ask about symptoms of an enlarged prostate and feel the gland with a rectal exam, then may use tests and laboratory findings to confirm it, including:

- fluoroscopy with dye to find blockage in the urinary tract and pouches in the bladder
- blood tests that suggest poor kidney function
- urinalysis and urine culture to identify bacteria causing a urinary tract infection
- in severe cases, a cystourethroscopy (visual exam of the bladder and urethra) is definitive, but this test is performed only immediately before surgery to help determine the best procedure. It can show prostate enlargement, bladder wall changes, and a raised bladder. (See *How an enlarged prostate blocks urine flow*, page 328.)

How is it treated?

If you are diagnosed with an enlarged prostate, the doctor may suggest conservative therapy first, including prostate massages, sitz baths, fluid restriction for bladder distention, and antibiotics for infection. Regular ejaculation may help relieve prostate congestion. The doctor may prescribe drugs to relieve bladder outlet obstruction.

 SELF-HELP

How to recognize an enlarged prostate

If you have enlarged prostate, the sooner you recognize it and get treatment, the better. Here are some of the symptoms:

- urgent desire to urinate
- frequent urination (day and night)
- difficulty starting the urine stream
- decreased size and force of the urine stream
- dribbling urine
- incontinence
- incomplete bladder emptying
- urinary tract infection
- acute urine retention.

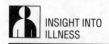

INSIGHT INTO
ILLNESS

How an enlarged prostate blocks urine flow

This illustration shows how the prostrate gland is affected when enlargement narrows the urethra, interfering with urine flow. This may result in urine retention and eventually damage the kidneys.

NORMAL PROSTATE GLAND

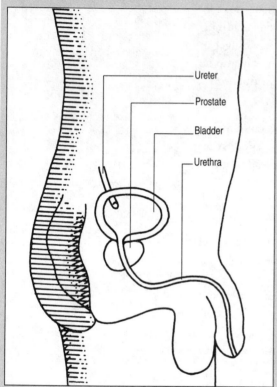

- Ureter
- Prostate
- Bladder
- Urethra

ENLARGED PROSTATE GLAND

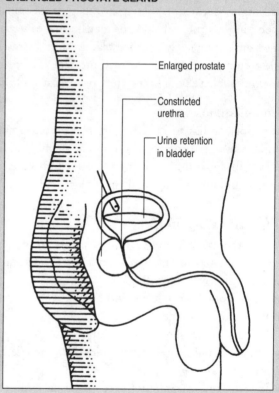

- Enlarged prostate
- Constricted urethra
- Urine retention in bladder

A new drug therapy with Proscar, which may reduce the size of the prostate in some people, is under investigation.

If you need surgery

Surgery is the only effective way to relieve severe urine retention problems, repeated infections, and other intolerable symptoms. The surgeon may use a scope to remove prostate tissue and, if necessary, insert a catheter to drain urine. Another approach — using a balloon to dilate the prostate — is still experimental.

*I*NFLAMMATION OF THE EPIDIDYMIS

What do doctors call this condition?
Epididymitis

What is this condition?
Inflammation of the epididymis is an infection of the long, coiled duct where sperm develops in the testicles. The tube carries sperm from the testicle to the urethra. It is most common in men ages 18 to 40 and usually affects only one side of the reproductive system. If the infection is on both sides or spreads into the testicles, it can lead to sterility. (See *How epididymitis can affect fertility,* page 330.)

What causes it?
Inflammation of the epididymis is most often caused by pus-generating bacteria such as staphylococci, *Escherichia coli,* or streptococci. Usually, these organisms spread from an established urinary tract or prostate infection through the vas deferens to the epididymis.

The inflammation may also be caused by gonorrhea, syphilis, or *Chlamydia* infection. Or it may follow prostate surgery or urinary catheterization.

Chemical inflammation of the epididymis (from nonbacterial causes) is brought on by injury to the tubes or irritation from urine backing up into the vas deferens. This form of inflammation is common in military recruits who may exercise for long periods with a full bladder, which causes the urine backup.

What are its symptoms?
The person with inflammation of the epididymis may feel sudden scrotal pain and see redness and swelling. He may have extreme tenderness of the scrotum and groin (from enlarged lymph nodes in the spermatic cord), fever, chills, and general discomfort. The discomfort may cause him to waddle when he walks, in an attempt to protect the groin area.

Complications
Untreated inflammation of the epididymis can cause sterility. An infection that spreads to one or both testicles can cause a condition

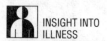

INSIGHT INTO
ILLNESS

How epididymitis can affect fertility

The diagram below shows how sperm normally develop and what can go wrong if you have inflammation of the epididymis.

The male reproductive cells, called *spermatozoa* (sperm), are produced in the testicles — a complex system of coiled tubes. The immature sperm swim out of the testicles into a long, coiled duct, called the *epididymis*, where the maturing process continues. From there, they pass into the vas deferens, where they become fully mature. The vas deferens ends in the prostatic urethra. Finally, the sperm leave the body through the penile urethra when ejaculation occurs.

What goes wrong

The epididymis can become inflamed when bacteria from other parts of the urogenital system, such as the urethra, travel backward through the reproductive tract to invade the epididymis. Once there, these infecting organisms can interfere with sperm development, decreasing your fertility.

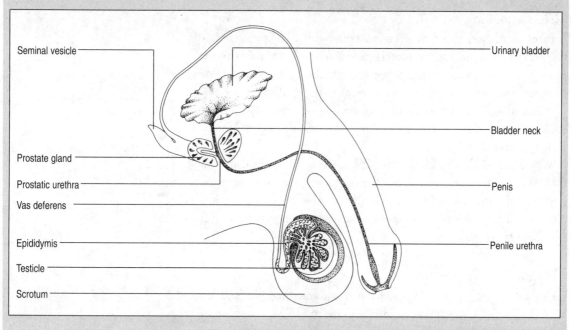

called *orchitis* that affects the testicles and decreases sperm production. (See *Common questions about orchitis.*)

How is it diagnosed?

The doctor may tentatively diagnose inflamed epididymis from the person's medical history, a physical exam, and his description of symptoms. Then the doctor will order tests to confirm the diagnosis, including a white blood cell count, a urinalysis, a urine culture and sensitivity test, urethral discharge and prostatic secretion cultures, and, possibly, segmented bacteriologic localization cultures.

How is it treated?

If you have inflammation of the epididymis, the doctor will work to combat the infection and relieve your symptoms. Treatment must begin immediately (particularly if you have inflammation in both testicles) because sterility is always a threat. Treatment includes antibiotics and analgesics, bed rest with scrotal elevation and ice packs, and sometimes surgery.

What can a person with inflammation of the epididymis do?

First, take the antibiotic exactly as the doctor prescribed it, even if you feel better. Otherwise, the infection could return.

Before the antibiotics reduce the inflammation, you should remain in bed to reduce swelling and relieve pain. Use a towel-wrapped ice bag to elevate your scrotum and relieve swelling, but remove it for several minutes every hour to avoid a burn. Don't take sitz baths or apply heat, because heat destroys sperm cells. You can start walking when your pain and swelling subside, and you should wear an athletic supporter. Avoid vigorous activity until all your symptoms disappear.

Help for severe pain

If you have severe inflammation, the doctor may inject the spermatic cord just above the testicle with an anesthetic, such as Xylocaine, to relieve pain. If you have a fever, consult your doctor before taking aspirin or Tylenol, because they may interfere with your therapy.

If you have surgery

Two surgical procedures are used to treat epididymitis. Both are performed with local anesthetic and do not require a hospital stay. Both procedures also cause sterility. An epididymectomy is performed when antibiotic therapy fails, and a bilateral vasectomy is occasionally performed in men with chronic epididymitis or in elderly persons undergoing open prostate surgery.

- *Epididymectomy:* In an epididymectomy, the surgeon makes a small incision in the scrotum and removes the inflamed portion of the epididymis. Bed rest and ice packs and sitz baths for minor pain and swelling may help promote recovery from surgery. You should abstain from sexual intercourse until the doctor directs otherwise, and

STRAIGHT TALK

Common questions about orchitis

The doctor says that if my inflamed testicles don't get better, I can get orchitis. What is orchitis?

Orchitis is a severe complication — an infected testicle. It can cause permanent sterility.

How can I tell if I have orchitis?

If you have it, you'll notice tenderness, redness, and warmth in one or both testicles, swelling of the scrotum and testicles, gradual increase in pain, and nausea and vomiting. If the pain suddenly stops, you may have an interruption of blood flow to one or both testicles, which can cause permanent damage.

What can the doctor do?

If you're diagnosed with orchitis, the doctor will give you antibiotics immediately. Corticosteroids have also been tried, but their use is still experimental.

In severe cases, a surgeon may make an incision to open and drain the infected duct and to improve blood circulation in the testicles. Otherwise, treatment is similar to that for epididymitis.

you should avoid strenuous activity or heavy lifting for a week or until the doctor advises more activity. Also, you should notify the doctor if you develop fever, persistent abdominal or scrotal pain, or bleeding at the incision.

• *Vasectomy:* In a vasectomy, the surgeon makes a small incision in the scrotum and ties off the vas deferens so that fluid and organisms can no longer pass to the epididymis.

INFLAMMATION OF THE PROSTATE

What do doctors call this condition?
Prostatitis

What is this condition?
Inflammation of the prostate gland may be sudden and acute or chronic. Acute inflammation most often is caused by a specific kind of bacteria and is easy to recognize and treat. But, if the inflammation is chronic, the cause is less easy to recognize. As many as 35% of men over age 50 have chronic inflammation of the prostate gland. It's the most common cause of repeated urinary tract infection in men. Both conditions can usually be cured with antibiotics in a few weeks.

Chronic inflammation of the prostate gland is the most common cause of repeated urinary tract infection in men.

What causes it?
About 80% of men with bacterial inflammation of the prostate are infected by *Escherichia coli.* The rest are infected by other bacteria such as *Klebsiella, Enterobacter, Proteus, Pseudomonas, Streptococcus,* or *Staphylococcus.* These bacteria typically spread to the prostate in the bloodstream or by moving up from the urethra, from the rectum, or in a backup of infected bladder urine in the prostate ducts. Less commonly, the bacteria are spread by sexual intercourse or medical procedures such as cystoscopy or catheterization. Chronic inflammation is usually caused by a bacterial invasion from the urethra.

What are its symptoms?
The person with an acute inflammation of the prostate gland gets fever, chills, low back pain, muscle pain, fullness in the groin, and

joint pain. Urination is frequent and urgent, and he may have painful urination or obstruction. His urine may appear cloudy.

By inserting a finger in the rectum, the doctor can feel that the prostate is tender, hardened, swollen, firm, and warm.

If this condition is chronic, some men may be asymptomatic. Others will have the symptoms described above, but to a lesser degree. Urinary tract infection is a common complication. Some men have painful ejaculation, blood in the sperm, persistent urethral discharge, and sexual dysfunction.

How is it diagnosed?

The doctor will use a urine culture to identify the bacteria and can feel the swelling through the man's rectum. To be sure, the doctor uses a four-stage specimen — three samples taken as the person urinates and then one secretion pressed from the prostate gland. A significantly increased bacteria count in the prostatic specimen confirms inflammation of the prostate.

How is it treated?

The doctor will start drug therapy with an antibiotic, usually Bactrim, given orally. If it kills the bacteria, the drug will be continued for about 30 days.

If there is a likelihood of blood poisoning, the doctor may give Bactrim intravenously along with Amcill, until sensitivity test results are known. If the drug is working, intravenous therapy continues for 48 hours to 1 week; then the person takes an oral form of the prescribed drug for 30 more days. In chronic inflammation caused by *E. coli*, Bactrim is usually given for at least 6 weeks.

While he is recovering, the person will need bed rest and liquids. He may be given pain relievers, something to cool his fever, sitz baths, and stool softeners. If he has chronic inflammation of the prostate with symptoms, regular massage of the prostate is most effective and regular ejaculation may help promote drainage of prostatic secretions.

In some cases where drug therapy is unsuccessful, the doctor may recommend surgery to remove all infected tissue. However, this procedure is usually not performed on young adults because it may cause ejaculation problems and sterility. Removing the prostate is curative, but may cause impotence and incontinence.

KIDNEY STONES

What do doctors call this condition?
Renal calculi

What is this condition?
Kidney stones may form anywhere in the urinary tract but usually develop in two sections of the kidneys, the renal pelvis or the calyces. The stones are formed from calcium, phosphate, or urate compounds that are normally dissolved in the urine.

Kidney stones vary in size and may be single or multiple. They may remain in the renal pelvis or enter the ureter and may damage renal tissue. Large stones damage the tissue with pressure or cause an obstruction that backs up fluids. Most people have repeat attacks. (See *Where kidney stones form.*)

What causes it?
Kidney stones develop in 1 in 1,000 persons, and are more common in men (especially those ages 30 to 50) than in women. They're more common in certain geographic areas, such as the southeastern United States. Although the exact cause of kidney stones is unknown, possible contributing factors include decreased urine production; infection; urinary obstruction; excessive secretion of parathyroid hormone, renal tubular acidosis, elevated uric acid (usually with gout), defects in the body's metabolism of certain substances, and excessive intake of vitamin D or dietary calcium.

What are its symptoms?
Though it varies with the stone's size and location, pain — caused by obstruction — is the key symptom. Large, rough stones plug the opening to the ureter and increase the frequency and force of automatic contractions.

The pain usually moves from the lower back to the flank, to the pubic region, and to the genitalia. The intensity of this pain fluctuates and may be excruciating at its peak. If stones are in the renal pelvis and calyces, pain may be more constant and dull. Back pain (from stones that produce an obstruction within a kidney) and

Although kidney stones typically form in the kidneys, they may form anywhere in the urinary tract. Severe pain is the hallmark symptom.

Where kidney stones form

Kidney stones (calculi) may form at other sites in the urinary tract, including the ureters and bladder.

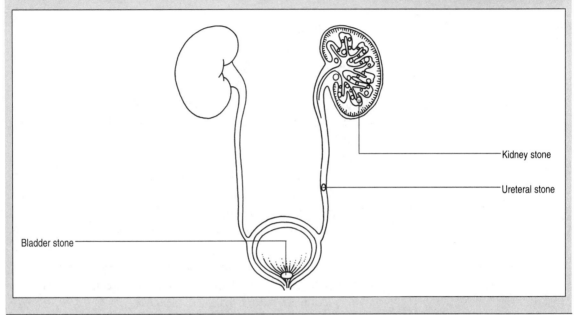

Kidney stone

Ureteral stone

Bladder stone

severe abdominal pain (from stones traveling down a ureter) may also occur. Nausea and vomiting usually accompany severe pain.

The person with kidney stones may also have fever, chills, blood in the urine (when stones injure a ureter), abdominal distention, pus in the urine, and, rarely, retained urine from a blockage.

How is it diagnosed?

The doctor will ask about symptoms, and then will use the following tests:

- Kidney-ureter-bladder X-rays reveal most kidney stones.
- Kidney ultrasound, an easily performed noninvasive test that uses high-frequency sound waves, detects obstructions and changes.
- Intravenous dye and a scan confirms the diagnosis and determines size and location of stones.
- Stone analysis shows their mineral content.
- Urine culture of midstream sample may indicate urinary tract infection.
- Urinalysis may be normal, or may show evidence of different types of stone formation.

- A 24-hour urine collection may be evaluated to determine calcium, phosphorus, and uric acid excretion levels.
- Blood tests may show other imbalances and may indicate gout as the cause.

How is it treated?

Because 90% of kidney stones are smaller than 5 millimeters in diameter, the doctor usually works to promote their natural passage. Along with extra fluids, he or she may prescribe antibiotics to fight the infection found in tests and may prescribe pain relievers and diuretics to prevent urine from staying in the kidney forming more stones.

If the stones are too large for natural passage, they may require surgical removal. When a stone is in the ureter, a cystoscope may be inserted through the urethra and the stone manipulated with catheters or retrieval instruments. Extraction of stones from other areas (kidney calyx or pelvis) may require surgery of the side or lower abdomen.

Procedures called *percutaneous ultrasonic lithotripsy* and *extracorporeal shock wave lithotripsy* shatter the stones into fragments for removal by suction or natural passage. (See *How shock wave lithotripsy removes kidney stones.*)

To prevent stone formation, the doctor may prescribe a low-calcium diet, drugs to prevent uric acid stones, and vitamin C to acidify the urine. If the thyroid is involved, he or she may recommend parathyroidectomy (removal of the parathyroid gland).

What can a person with kidney stones do?

If the doctor suspects you have kidney stones, he or she may ask you to provide urine samples for 24 hours to monitor urine pH. You may also be asked to strain all your urine through gauze or a tea strainer and save any recovered solid material for analysis. To help the stones pass, you should walk, if possible. Also drink plenty of fluids. To help acidify your urine, drink fruit juices, particularly cranberry juice.

You can avoid forming more stones by following the drug regimen and diet your doctor recommends.

If you have surgery

If surgery is necessary, and if your condition requires removal of a kidney, remember that your body can adapt well to one kidney. After surgery, you will probably have an indwelling catheter or a nephrostomy tube inserted for drainage.

How shock wave lithotripsy removes kidney stones

Your doctor will perform a special procedure called *extracorporeal shock wave lithotripsy* to get rid of your stones. During the procedure, a machine will direct shock waves through water or a water-filled cushion and send them into your body, where they will crush the stones. Keep in mind that the energy from these shock waves is targeted at the stones and shouldn't damage your body tissues. Here's what to expect.

Before the procedure
On the night before the procedure, don't eat or drink anything after midnight. The next day when you arrive at the hospital, a nurse will take blood and urine samples and may also perform an electrocardiogram to evaluate your heart function.

Then a nurse will start an intravenous line in your arm or hand so that you can receive fluids and drugs. A doctor will give you an anesthetic to prevent pain and help you remain still during the procedure. And a technician will X-ray your kidneys, ureters, and bladder to find out the size and location of your stones.

During the procedure
You'll sit in a special chair and be secured with a belt. A thin catheter, called a *J-stent*, may be placed in your urinary tract to help remove the stone fragments after the stones have been crushed. The J-stent will remain in place for several days.

Next, you'll be lowered into a tub filled with water up to your shoulders. If necessary, you'll be shifted in the chair so that you're in the best position for the treatment. Or you may lie on a stretcher that's positioned over a water-filled cushion to receive your treatment. Throughout the procedure, you'll be asleep or feel drowsy.

After the procedure
You're usually allowed to go home right after the procedure, unless a fever or other complications develop. Expect the doctor to give you prescriptions for medication to relieve pain and prevent possible infection.

Because internal bleeding is possible, don't take any aspirin or other anti-inflammatory medicines for 7 to 10 days after the procedure. These drugs could worsen any bleeding.

What to do at home
Expect blood-tinged urine and bruising for several days, especially on your back. If these signs continue longer or if you experience fever or excessive pain, call the doctor immediately.

For several days afterward, strain all your urine and save the stone fragments for your doctor to see. If you have a J-stent catheter in place, make an appointment for the doctor to remove it. Also, make an appointment for follow-up X-rays and blood tests.

LOWER URINARY TRACT INFECTIONS

What do doctors call these conditions?
Cystitis and urethritis

What are these conditions?
Lower urinary tract infections (UTIs) are bacterial infections that are nearly 10 times more common in women than in men. Approxi-

mately 10% to 20% of all women get a UTI at least once. Lower UTIs also affect many children, mostly girls. In men and children, the infection is often linked to physical abnormalities.

Urinary tract infections are often easy to cure, but reinfection and resistant bacterial flare-up during treatment are possible.

What causes them?

Most lower UTIs are caused by infection with *Escherichia coli, Klebsiella, Proteus, Enterobacter, Pseudomonas,* or *Serratia.* However, if the person has some other bladder problem, such as neurogenic bladder, a catheter, or an abnormal opening (fistula) between the intestine and bladder, lower UTI may be caused by a mixture of organisms. Experts believe that the person is infected when the bladder's disease resistance breaks down and the bacteria invade and multiply. These bacteria cannot be washed out by normal urination.

Women get the most UTIs, probably because the female urethra is short and bacteria can easily travel from the vagina, rectum, pudendal and perineal skin, or a sexual partner. Men are less vulnerable because their urethras are longer and their prostatic fluid serves as an antibacterial shield. In both men and women, infection usually moves up from the urethra into the bladder.

What are their symptoms?

Lower UTIs usually produce urgent, frequent, or painful urination with cramps or bladder spasms. A person may experience itching or a feeling of warmth during urination. Men may develop urethral discharge. Inflammation of the bladder wall also causes bloody urine and fever. Some people have low back pain, general discomfort, nausea, vomiting, abdominal pain or tenderness over the bladder area, chills, and flank pain.

How are they diagnosed?

The doctor will recognize the symptoms and use a microscope to see red blood cells and white blood cells in the person's urine. A urine specimen with a high bacterial count will confirm the diagnosis. The doctor can take another urine sample after the person starts antibiotic treatment to be sure the drug is working. Sometimes the doctor may do a test to rule out venereal disease or use a scan with dye to check for congenital abnormalities that contribute to repeated infections.

Lower urinary tract infections are nearly 10 times more common in women than in men — most likely because a woman's urethra is more vulnerable to bacterial contamination.

SELF-HELP

How to manage a urinary tract infection

Here's some advice to help you treat your urinary tract infection and prevent it from occurring again.

Treatment guidelines

It's important to take your prescribed medicine exactly as your doctor directs. Don't stop taking your medicine just because you feel better. Finish the prescription to kill all the infection-causing bacteria. Otherwise, you run the risk of getting the infection again.

Lay a warm heating pad on your abdomen and sides to soothe any pain and burning sensations you may have. Try a warm sitz bath, or ask your doctor to prescribe a pain reliever.

Diet tips

What you eat and drink affects your recovery. The following advice can help:

- To increase your urine flow and flush out bacteria, drink 10 to 14 glasses ($2\frac{1}{2}$ to $3\frac{1}{2}$ quarts or liters) of fluid a day.
- Eat foods and drink fluids with a high acid content, such as meats, nuts, plums, prunes, whole-grain breads and cereals, and cranberry and other fruit juices. Acid urine inhibits urinary tract bacteria.
- Here's a note of caution: If you're taking a sulfonamide drug (such as Gantrisin or Gantanol) to treat your infection, avoid cranberry juice because its high acid content can interfere with the action of the drug.
- Limit your intake of milk and other products with a high calcium content.
- Avoid caffeine, carbonated beverages, and alcohol because these substances irritate the bladder.

Prevention tips

- Practice sensible hygiene. For example, wipe from front to back each time you go to the bathroom. This reduces the chance that bacteria from the rectum will enter your urinary tract.
- Change your underpants daily.
- Wear cotton undergarments because cotton "breathes," and ventilation slows bacteria growth.
- Avoid tight slacks that prevent air circulation. Inadequate ventilation encourages bacteria to multiply and grow.
- Take showers instead of baths because bacteria in bath water can enter your urinary tract.
- Avoid bubble baths, bath oils, perfumed vaginal sprays, and strong bleaches and cleaning powders in the laundry. These products can irritate groin skin, which may trigger bacteria growth and infection.
- Urinate frequently (every 3 hours) to completely empty your bladder.
- Use the bathroom as soon as you sense you need to. Delayed urination is a major cause of urinary tract infection.
- Urinate after sexual intercourse. This will help rid your urinary tract of any bacteria.

When to call the doctor

- Call your doctor right away if you suspect you have a new or repeated urinary tract infection.
- Also call the doctor if you notice such symptoms as an increased urge to urinate, increased urination (especially at night), pain when you urinate, or bloody or cloudy urine.

How are they treated?

The doctor will prescribe a specific antibiotic to fight the person's infection. A 7- to 10-day course of antibiotic therapy is standard, but recent studies suggest that a single dose of an antibiotic or a 3- to 5-day antibiotic regimen may be sufficient kill all the bacteria. After 3 days of antibiotic therapy, a urine culture should show no organisms. If the urine is not sterile, the doctor may prescribe a different antibiotic. A urine culture taken 1 to 2 weeks later indicates whether or not the infection has been eradicated. Repeat infections are treated with long-term, low-dosage antibiotic therapy. (See *How to manage a urinary tract infection*, page 339.)

NEPHROTIC SYNDROME

A major risk of nephrotic syndrome: Progression to kidney failure.

What is this condition?

Nephrotic syndrome is a condition marked by excessive protein in the urine, other chemical abnormalities, and edema. Although nephrotic syndrome is not a disease itself, it is linked to defects of the capillaries in the kidney and indicates kidney damage. The chance of a cure is highly variable, depending on the underlying cause. In some forms, the syndrome may progress to kidney failure.

What causes it?

About 75% of nephrotic syndrome cases are caused by spontaneous inflammation and degeneration of the kidney. Other causes of nephrotic syndrome include diseases of the metabolism such as diabetes, autoimmune disorders such as lupus, and circulatory diseases such as congestive heart failure. It may also accompany sickle-cell anemia, renal vein thrombosis, and exposure to toxins such as mercury, gold, and bismuth.

What are its symptoms?

The main symptom of nephrotic syndrome is mild to severe edema of the ankles or lower back, or swelling around the eyes, especially in children. The edema may lead to sores, lung effusion, and swollen external genitalia. The person with nephrotic syndrome may also experience dizziness upon standing, lethargy, depression, and pallor. Major complications are malnutrition, infection, coagulation disorders, and blood clots in the veins.

How is it diagnosed?

If the doctor sees the edema, he or she will order urine tests for proteins and for debris such as waxy, fatty casts and oval fat bodies. The doctor will use blood tests that may show increased cholesterol, phospholipids, and triglycerides and decreased albumin levels. He or she will order a biopsy of kidney tissue.

How is it treated?

The doctor will work to correct the underlying cause of nephrotic syndrome. The person with nephrotic syndrome will be put on a diet to replace lost protein, with restricted sodium intake, diuretics for edema, and antibiotics for infection.

Some people respond to an 8-week course of corticosteroid therapy (such as Deltasone), followed by maintenance therapy. For others, the doctor may prescribe a combination course of Deltasone and Imuran or Cytoxan.

NEUROGENIC BLADDER

What do doctors call this condition?

Neurologic bladder dysfunction, neuropathic bladder

What is this condition?

Neurogenic bladder refers to all types of bladder problems caused by disruption of normal nerve impulses to the bladder. The complications that follow neurogenic bladder include lack of bladder control, failure to completely empty, urinary infection, stone formation, and kidney failure. A neurogenic bladder can be spastic or flaccid.

What causes it?

At one time, experts thought neurogenic bladder was caused by spinal cord injury. Now it appears to be linked to such conditions as acute infectious diseases, dementia, heavy metal toxicity, certain types of cancer, and many additional disorders. (See *What causes a neurogenic bladder?* page 342)

What are its symptoms?

Neurogenic bladder produces a wide range of effects, depending on the underlying cause and its effect on the structural integrity of the

What causes a neurogenic bladder?

If you've been diagnosed with neurogenic bladder, it may be useful to know what other conditions contribute to it. You may have heard that this disorder is caused mainly by spinal cord injury, but it's also linked to various underlying conditions that can affect bladder control.

Brain diseases
- Amyotrophic lateral sclerosis (Lou Gehrig's disease)
- Brain tumors
- Stroke
- Encephalopathy
- Multiple sclerosis (MS)
- Parkinson's disease

Peripheral nervous system diseases
- Diabetes
- Guillain-Barré syndrome

Spinal cord diseases
- Myelomeningocele
- Spina bifida
- Cord trauma or tumors
- Spinal stenosis

Other diseases
- Alcoholism
- Atherosclerosis and other vascular diseases
- Shingles
- Underactive thyroid, porphyria, and other metabolic disturbances
- Lupus and other connective tissue diseases

bladder. Usually, the person with this disorder has some degree of incontinence.

If the person has a spinal cord lesion, a spastic neurogenic bladder may produce involuntary or frequent scanty urination without a feeling of bladder fullness and, possibly, spontaneous spasms of the arms and legs, hypertension, and headaches. Flaccid neurogenic bladder may be linked to overflow incontinence, diminished anal sphincter tone, and a greatly distended bladder that the doctor can feel. The person may feel no bladder fullness because the senses are impaired.

How is it diagnosed?

The doctor will ask about the person's health history to determine if he or she has a condition or disorder that can cause neurogenic bladder. The doctor will also ask if the person has experienced incontinence or disruption in urination patterns.

Tests to evaluate the person's bladder function may include cystography (a picture of the voiding process) to check bladder neck function, urine backup, and continence; and studies of how urine is stored in the bladder and how well the bladder empties.

How is it treated?

The doctor will work to maintain the integrity of the upper urinary tract, control infection, and prevent urinary incontinence through evacuation of the bladder, drug therapy, surgery or, less commonly, neural blocks and electrical stimulation.

The person may be taught to empty his or her bladder by applying manual pressure over the lower abdomen. He or she may be taught how to insert and remove a catheter. Generally, a man can perform this procedure more easily, but a woman can learn self-catheterization with the help of a mirror. Intermittent self-catheterization, in conjunction with a bladder-retraining program, is especially useful for people with flaccid neurogenic bladder. (See *How to avoid bladder infection from a catheter*.)

If conservative treatment fails, the doctor may use surgery to correct structural problems by modifying the bladder neck, widening the urethra, removing part of the sphincter muscle, or building a new route for urine. Implantation of an artificial urinary sphincter may be necessary if permanent incontinence follows surgery for neurogenic bladder.

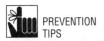

How to avoid bladder infection from a catheter

The catheter you wear increases your risk of developing a bladder infection. However, you can prevent or at least control infection by taking the following precautions.

Report warning signs
Notify the doctor immediately if you have any of the warning signs listed below:
- fever above 100° F (37.7° C)
- cloudy urine
- discharge around the catheter
- pain in the bladder area.

Don't give infection a chance
You may not always be able to prevent a bladder infection, but you can reduce your chances of getting one by following these guidelines:
- Drink at least eight 8-ounce glasses (2 quarts) of fluid a day. Include cranberry juice, which keeps urine acidic.
- Take the medicine prescribed by your doctor.
- Wash the catheter area with soap and water twice a day to keep it from becoming irritated or infected. Also wash your rectal area whenever you have a bowel movement. Dry your skin gently but thoroughly.
- If you're a woman, always wipe from front to back after bowel movements. Do the same when washing and drying the genital area. This prevents contamination of the catheter and urinary tract with bacteria from the rectum.
- Once a day, wash the drainage tubing and bag with soap and water. Rinse with a solution made from about one part white vinegar to seven parts water.
- Empty your leg drainage bag every 3 or 4 hours. Empty your bedside drainage bag at least every 8 hours.

- Always keep the drainage bag below bladder level.
- Never pull on the catheter. Disconnect it from the drainage tubing only to clean the bag.
- Notify the doctor immediately if you have urine leakage around the catheter, abdominal pain and fullness, scanty urine flow, or blood or particles in your urine.
- Never try to remove the catheter yourself unless the doctor or nurse has given you instructions.
- Keep your follow-up appointments with the doctor.

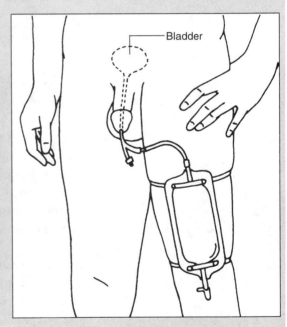

Bladder

POLYCYSTIC KIDNEY DISEASE

Getting proper treatment for polycystic kidney disease is crucial; without treatment, this condition can be rapidly fatal.

What is this condition?

Polycystic kidney disease is an inherited disorder marked by fluid-filled cysts that eventually replace healthy kidney tissue, causing severe enlargement and stopping kidney function. There appear to be two distinct forms. The infantile form causes stillbirth or early infant death. A few infants with this disease survive for 2 years. The adult form begins subtly but usually becomes obvious between ages 30 and 50 — rarely, in the person's 70s. The affected person's deterioration is more gradual but without treatment he or she will develop kidney failure.

The prognosis in adults is extremely variable. Progression may be slow, even after symptoms of kidney failure appear. However, polycystic kidney disease is usually fatal within 4 years, unless the person receives treatment with dialysis, kidney transplantation, or both.

What causes it?

While both types of polycystic kidney disease are genetically transmitted, the differences in age groups and inheritance patterns suggest that they are two unrelated disorders. Both types affect males and females equally.

What are its symptoms?

The doctor can identify a newborn with infantile polycystic disease by some facial characteristics such as skin folds around the eyes, a pointed nose, a small chin, and floppy, low-set ears. At birth, the infant has huge masses on both flanks that are symmetrical and tense. Signs of breathing distress and heart failure progress to kidney failure and death.

An adult with the disease may reach his or her 30s and 40s with only some vague symptoms, such as high blood pressure, excessive urination, and urinary tract infection. Later, the person develops definite symptoms related to the enlarging kidney mass, such as back pain, widening girth, and swollen or tender abdomen. Generally, about 10 years after symptoms appear, progressive compression of kidney structures by the enlarging mass causes death from kidney failure and uremic poisoning.

How is it diagnosed?

The doctor asks about the person's family history and symptoms and then does a physical exam to check for large, irregular masses on both the person's flanks. The doctor can feel the enlarged kidneys in a person with an advanced case. If the person has the above symptoms, the doctor may check for the following laboratory results:

- Scan with intravenous dye shows enlarged, misshapen kidneys and indentations caused by cysts.
- Ultrasound and a computed tomography scan (commonly called a CAT scan) show kidney enlargement and cysts; the CAT scan also shows multiple areas of cystic damage.
- Urinalysis and creatinine clearance tests evaluate the person's kidney function and indicate abnormalities.

How is it treated?

Polycystic kidney disease can't be cured. The doctor will work to preserve the functioning tissue in the kidney and prevent infections. If the person has high blood pressure, controlling it will help slow the loss of kidney function. Progressive kidney failure requires treatment similar to that for other types of severe kidney disease, including dialysis or, rarely, a kidney transplant.

If adult polycystic kidney disease is discovered in the early, asymptomatic stage, the person will have a urine culture and tests every 6 months to detect infection. When a urine culture detects infection, the doctor will prescribe prompt and vigorous antibiotic treatment (even when the person has no symptoms).

As kidney function worsens, some people may be candidates for dialysis, transplantation, or both. Cystic abscess or bleeding may require surgery to drain the kidney.

What can a person with polycystic kidney disease do?

Since polycystic kidney disease is usually relentlessly progressive, you may want to learn about the treatment for this disease, including dialysis. If you are a young adult or the parents of an infant with polycystic kidney disease, consider obtaining genetic counseling.

RENAL HYPERTENSION

What do doctors call this condition?
Renovascular hypertension

What is this condition?
Renal hypertension is an abnormal increase in a person's blood pressure due to narrowing of the kidney's major arteries or their branches or from narrowing of the kidney's internal arteries. It can be partial or complete, and the resulting blood pressure elevation can be benign or malignant. Approximately 5% to 10% of people diagnosed with high blood pressure have renal hypertension, and it is most common in those under age 30 or over age 50.

What causes it?
Narrowed arteries (especially in older men) and diseases of the renal artery wall layers are the primary causes in 95% of people with renal hypertension. Other causes include inflamed or defective arteries, a blood clot, injury, tumor, and aneurysm (swelling of a weakened blood vessel wall).

Blockage of the renal artery stimulates the affected kidney to release an enzyme, which starts a series of reactions involving the lungs, liver, veins, and arteries, eventually causing high blood pressure.

What are its symptoms?
The person with renal hypertension usually has symptoms common to other illnesses that cause high blood pressure such as headache, palpitations, fast heartbeat, anxiety, light-headedness, sensitivity to temperature extremes, and mental sluggishness. The worst complications include congestive heart failure, heart attack, stroke, and, occasionally, kidney failure.

How is it diagnosed?
The doctor will ask about the person's and the family's health histories and will also order several diagnostic scans to find abnormalities of blood flow through the kidneys and to check their size and shape. Blood samples from both the right and left renal veins are taken to measure the levels of the enzyme that triggers high blood pressure. A

If the kidney can't get enough blood, it releases an enzyme that sets off a complicated series of events leading to high blood pressure.

high level helps to determine whether one or both kidneys are involved and whether to use surgery.

How is it treated?

The doctor's first choice will be surgery to restore adequate circulation in the kidney and to control severe hypertension or severely reduced kidney function. The person may have a renal artery bypass,
arterioplasty, partial kidney removal, or, as a last resort, complete kidney removal.

Some people may be candidates for renal artery dilation with a
balloon catheter. The catheter is inserted and inflated to widen the
inside diameter of the vein, without the risks and longer recovery
time of surgery. If the doctor decides to treat the symptoms, the person may be given antihypertensives, diuretics, and a low-salt diet.

RENAL INFARCTION

What is this condition?

Renal infarction is the formation of a coagulated, damaged-tissue
area in one or both kidneys, caused by blockage of the kidney's blood
vessels. The location and size of the damaged area depend on the site
of blockage. Most often, infarction affects the renal cortex, but it can
extend into the medulla. (See *Sites where infarction strikes the kidney*,
page 348.) The person's recovery depends on how much of the kidney is damaged.

What causes it?

In most people with renal infarction, the blockage starts with a blood
clot that originates in the heart and lodges in a kidney artery. The clot
slows blood flow to part of the kidney tissue, which dies. The severity
of blood flow reduction determines whether or not the kidney damage will be short-term or chronic, as arterial narrowing progresses.

Besides heart disease, some people have a renal infarction linked to
artery diseases with or without blood clot formation, a clot from a
flank injury, and sickle-cell anemia.

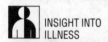

INSIGHT INTO
ILLNESS

Sites where infarction strikes the kidney

Renal infarction may damage tissues in the cortex, where urine is filtered from blood, or tissues in the medulla, where urine collects.

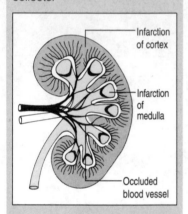

Infarction of cortex

Infarction of medulla

Occluded blood vessel

What are its symptoms?

Although some persons with kidney blockage may not have obvious symptoms, most have severe upper abdominal pain or gnawing flank pain and tenderness. The person may feel tenderness along the spine, and have fever, poor appetite, nausea, and vomiting. When a blocked artery causes renal infarction, the affected kidney is small and the doctor can't feel it with his or her hands.

High blood pressure, a common complication that may occur several days after infarction, is caused by the reduced blood flow, which stimulates the heart to work harder.

How is it diagnosed?

If the person has heart disease or some other diseases and typical symptoms, the doctor will suspect renal infarction. To be sure, the doctor will use several lab tests, including urinalysis, blood studies, angiography, and radioisotope scans.

How is it treated?

If the person has an infection in the blocked area or significant high blood pressure, the doctor may recommend surgery. The doctor may treat persistent high blood pressure with drugs and a low-sodium diet. More difficult cases may require drugs to break up blood clots or a catheter to remove an embolism.

RENAL VEIN CLOT

What do doctors call this condition?

Renal vein thrombosis

What is this condition?

A renal vein clot is a clot in the vein that carries blood from the kidney. It may cause kidney congestion, engorgement and, possibly, tissue death. The clot may affect one or both kidneys and may occur in an acute or a chronic form. A sudden clot that causes extensive damage may set off rapidly fatal kidney failure. Chronic clotting usually harms kidney function, causing tissue damage. If the clot affects both kidneys, the prognosis is poor.

If a person has less severe clotting that affects only one kidney or if the disorder is progressive and allows the body to develop new routes of circulation, he or she may recover with partial kidney function.

What causes it?

A renal vein clot commonly occurs because of a tumor that obstructs the renal vein. Other causes include clots from an abdominal injury or blood vessels of the legs, congestive heart failure, and inflammation of the arteries.

What are its symptoms?

The person with a renal vein clot will have either a sudden clot and pain or a slow-developing clot with other indicators. A sudden clot causes severe back pain and a tender abdomen. The person may also have fever, paleness, protein and blood in the urine, and swelling in the arms and legs. The doctor can feel the enlarged kidneys.

A slowly developing clot causes signs of kidney damage. Swelling of the extremities is possible, but the person usually does not feel pain. Other test results show protein and albumin in the person's urine.

How is it diagnosed?

The doctor can use intravenous pyelography to see the renal vein clot. In acute renal vein blockage, the kidneys appear enlarged and their excretory function diminishes. When intravenous dye is used, damaged kidney tissue appears on X-ray as a "smudge." In chronic blockage, the dye may show ureteral indentations caused by extra venous channels. The doctor may use renal arteriography and tissue biopsy to confirm the diagnosis. Other tests may include urinalysis, blood studies, and a venogram.

How is it treated?

If the person has a gradually developing clot in only one kidney, the chance of recovery is good. The doctor may prescribe drugs to break up the clots over a long period of treatment. Surgery must be performed within 24 hours of a clot formation to be effective. But, even quick surgery has limited success, since clots often travel into the small veins. Extensive bleeding in the kidney may require removal of tissue.

A sudden renal vein clot that causes extensive damage may cause rapidly fatal kidney failure.

URINARY REFLUX

What is this condition?

In urinary reflux, urine flows from the bladder back into the ureters and eventually into the kidneys. Because the bladder empties poorly, the person can get a urinary tract infection, possibly leading to kidney damage. Urinary reflux is most common during infancy in boys and during early childhood (ages 3 to 7) in girls. Urinary reflux from a birth defect is most prevalent in girls. If one child is diagnosed with inherited urinary reflux, there's a one-in-four chance that a brother or sister will eventually show reflux.

If one child is found to have urinary reflux, there's a one-in-four chance that a brother or sister has the problem — perhaps even an older sibling who shows no symptoms.

What causes it?

In people with urinary reflux, failure of a valve where the ureter enters the bladder allows urine to flow back into the ureter when the bladder contracts during voiding. The valve failure may be caused by disease or inherited flaws in the ureters or bladder, including short or absent parts of the ureter or a too-large ureteral opening.

What are its symptoms?

Urinary reflux gives most people the same symptoms as a urinary tract infection: frequency, urgency, burning urination, bloody or foul-smelling urine, and, in infants, dark, concentrated urine. If the person's upper urinary tract is involved, there's usually a high fever, chills, flank pain, vomiting, and general discomfort. In children, fever, nonspecific abdominal pain, and diarrhea may be the only apparent effects.

How is it diagnosed?

Symptoms of urinary tract infection are the first clues. In infants, bloody or strong-smelling urine may be the first indication. The doctor may be able to feel a hard, thickened bladder if the posterior urethral valves are causing an obstruction in male infants.

Using a dye and a scope, the doctor can see whether the ureter backs up colored water. Other lab studies may include urinalysis, blood tests, and X-rays with contrast dyes.

How is it treated?

The doctor will work to prevent tissue damage and kidney failure with antibiotic therapy and, when necessary, surgery. The surgery can create a normal valve effect at the junction by reimplanting the ureter into the bladder wall at a more oblique angle.

The drug therapy is usually effective for reflux that is linked to infection, neurogenic bladder, and, in children, to a short ureter (which becomes normal with age). Reflux related to infection usually abates after the infection is cured. However, 80% of girls with urinary reflux will have another urinary tract infection within a year.

Repeated reflux-related infection requires long-term preventive antibiotic therapy and careful follow-up (including diagnostic tests such as cystoscopy and intravenous pyelography every 4 to 6 months) to track the degree of reflux.

What can a person with urinary reflux do?

If you are diagnosed with urinary reflux, the nurse will teach you how to completely empty your bladder. Also, since your natural urge to urinate may be impaired, you should go to the bathroom every 2 to 3 hours whether or not you feel the urge.

WATER IN THE KIDNEY

What do doctors call this condition?

Hydronephrosis

What is this condition?

Water in the kidney is an abnormal widening of parts of one or both kidneys, caused by blocked urine flow. Although partial blockage and water in the kidney may not produce symptoms initially, the pressure that builds up behind the blockage eventually causes symptoms.

What causes it?

Almost any type of blockage in the urinary tract can cause water to build up in the kidney. The most common causes are benign prostrate changes, closing of the urethra, and kidney stones. Some people have a closed ureter or bladder outlet, congenital abnormalities, abdominal tumors, blood clots, or a damaged bladder. If the obstruction is in the urethra or bladder, it usually affects both kidneys. If it's below the bladder, the bladder expands to act as a buffer zone and delays symptoms. If the person's urine flow stops entirely, the kidney stops functioning.

What are its symptoms?

Symptoms depend on the obstruction's location in the kidney. Some people will have no symptoms or only mild pain and slightly decreased urinary flow. The pain may be on one side or both. Another person may have severe, colicky kidney pain or dull flank pain that radiates to the groin plus chemical changes in the urine. Other symptoms include nausea, vomiting, abdominal fullness, painful urination, dribbling, or hesitancy.

How is it diagnosed?

Because the person's symptoms may resemble other kidney disorders, the doctor will use tests with intravenous dye, ultrasound scans, and kidney function studies to confirm water in the kidney.

How is it treated?

The doctor first works to keep the kidney functioning and prevent infection. He or she may use surgery to remove the obstruction. If kidney function has already been affected, the doctor may put the person on a diet low in protein, sodium, and potassium. This diet is designed to stop the progression of kidney failure before surgery.

What can a person with water in the kidney do?

If you are diagnosed with the disorder, your most important task will be to keep it from progressing to irreversible kidney disease. If you are an older man, and especially if someone in your family has had benign prostrate trouble, have routine medical checkups.

Almost any blockage of the urinary tract can cause water to build up in the kidney. If no urine can flow, the kidney eventually stops functioning.

GYNECOLOGIC
DISORDERS

ABNORMAL ABSENCE OF MENSTRUATION

What do doctors call this condition?

Amenorrhea

What is this condition?

In the primary form of this disorder, a woman's first menstrual period (menarche) doesn't occur until age 18. In the secondary form, a woman doesn't menstruate for at least 3 months after menarche begins.

What causes it?

Absence of menstruation is normal before puberty, after menopause, or during pregnancy and lactation. It indicates a problem at any other time. It usually results from a failure to ovulate because of hormonal problems.

Abnormal absence of menstruation may also result from lack of a uterus, a damaged endometrium (surface lining of the uterus), or from ovarian, adrenal, or pituitary gland tumors. It's common in women with problems such as depression and poor appetite. Absence of menstruation may also result from malnutrition, intense exercise, and prolonged use of oral contraceptives.

How is it diagnosed?

A history of failure to menstruate in a woman over age 18 confirms primary absence of menstruation. Secondary absence of menstruation is indicated by a change is noted in the woman's established menstrual pattern (for example, absence of menstruation for 3 months). A thorough physical and pelvic exam rules out pregnancy, as well as anatomic abnormalities that may cause false absence of menstruation (called *cryptomenorrhea*), in which other symptoms of menstruation occur without external bleeding.

The doctor may order diagnostic tests, including administering pure progestins, such as Depo-Provera and progesterone, to evaluate uterine function. Blood and urine studies may reveal hormonal imbalances caused by lack of ovarian response to gonadotropins, failure of gonadotropin secretion, and abnormal thyroid levels. A complete medical workup, including appropriate X-rays, laparoscopy, and a biopsy, may disclose ovarian, adrenal, and pituitary tumors.

How is it treated?

The doctor will prescribe appropriate hormone replacement therapy to reestablish menstruation. If the disorder isn't related to hormone deficiency, treatment depends on the cause. For example, if it results from a tumor, surgery is usually required.

What can a woman with absence of menstruation do?

After treatment, keep an accurate record of your menstrual cycles to aid early detection if this condition recurs.

ABNORMAL PREMENOPAUSAL BLEEDING

What is this condition?

This condition refers to any vaginal bleeding that deviates from the normal menstrual cycle before menopause begins. These deviations include menstrual bleeding that's abnormally infrequent, abnormally frequent, excessive, deficient, or irregular (bleeding between periods). Occasionally, symptoms of menstruation occur without external bleeding (called *cryptomenorrhea*).

Premenopausal bleeding may merely be troublesome or can cause severe hemorrhage; the prognosis depends on the underlying cause. Abnormal bleeding patterns often respond to hormonal or other therapy.

Abnormal premenopausal bleeding may merely be troublesome — or it may lead to severe hemorrhage.

What causes it?

Causes of abnormal premenopausal bleeding vary:
- Abnormally frequent or infrequent bleeding usually results from failure to ovulate because of endocrine or other disorders.
- Excessive bleeding usually results from local lesions, such as uterine tumors, polyps in the endometrium (uterine lining), and endometrial hyperplasia. It may also result from inflammation of the uterus or fallopian tubes and failure to ovulate.
- Deficient bleeding results from local, endocrine, or other disorders or from blockage caused by partial obstruction by the hymen (a membrane at the vaginal opening) or cervical obstruction.

SELF-HELP

Advice for women with abnormal premenopausal bleeding

If you're diagnosed with this disorder, follow these guidelines.

Reduce bleeding

To minimize blood flow, avoid strenuous activity and lie down occasionally with your feet elevated.

Keep a log

- To help determine the cyclic pattern and amount of bleeding, record the dates of the bleeding and the number of tampons or pads you use per day.
- Immediately report abnormal bleeding to the doctor to help rule out major bleeding disorders, such as those that occur in abnormal pregnancy.

Follow up

To detect abnormal bleeding due to organic causes and to detect cancer early, have an annual Pap test and pelvic exam.

- Bleeding between periods is most commonly no more than a slight bleeding from the endometrium during ovulation. However, it may also result from local disorders, such as malignant uterine tumors, cervical erosions, polyps (which tend to bleed after intercourse), or inappropriate estrogen therapy. Complications of pregnancy can also cause premenopausal bleeding. Such bleeding may be mild or severe.
- Cryptomenorrhea may result from an abnormally closed hymen or cervical narrowing.

What are its symptoms?

Bleeding not associated with abnormal pregnancy is usually painless, but it may be severely painful. When bleeding is associated with abnormal pregnancy, other symptoms include nausea, breast tenderness, bloating, and fluid retention. Severe or prolonged bleeding causes anemia, especially in women with underlying disease (such as a blood disorder) and in women receiving anticoagulants.

How is it diagnosed?

The typical clinical picture confirms abnormal premenopausal bleeding. The doctor will take a health history. Special tests identify the underlying cause. These may include lab tests of blood hormone levels, endometrial sampling to rule out malignant tumors, a pelvic exam, and a Pap test. A complete blood count helps to eliminate anemia as a cause.

If testing rules out pelvic and hormonal causes of abnormal bleeding, further blood studies may help to determine clotting abnormalities.

How is it treated?

Treatment depends on the type of bleeding abnormality and its cause. Menstrual irregularity alone may not require therapy unless it interferes with the woman's attempt to achieve or avoid conception or leads to anemia. When it does require treatment, the drug Clomid induces ovulation. Electrocautery, chemical cautery, or cryosurgery can remove cervical polyps; dilation and curettage, uterine polyps. Organic disorders — such as cervical or uterine cancer — may require hysterectomy, radium or X-ray therapy, or both of these treatments, depending on the site and extent of the disease. Of course, anemia and infections require appropriate treatment. (See *Advice for women with abnormal premenopausal bleeding*.)

DYSFUNCTIONAL UTERINE BLEEDING

What is this condition?

Dysfunctional uterine bleeding refers to abnormal bleeding from the endometrium (surface lining of the uterus) that occurs without recognizable organic lesions. Prognosis varies with the cause. Dysfunctional uterine bleeding is the reason for almost 25% of all gynecologic surgeries.

What causes it?

Dysfunctional uterine bleeding usually results from an imbalance in hormonal-endometrial interactions, in which estrogen constantly stimulates the endometrium. Disorders that cause sustained high estrogen levels include polycystic ovary syndrome, obesity, immaturity of the hypothalamic-pituitary-ovarian mechanism (in sexually mature teenagers), and failure to ovulate (in women in their late 30s or early 40s).

What are its symptoms?

Dysfunctional uterine bleeding usually causes episodes of vaginal bleeding between periods; it may also cause heavy or prolonged periods (longer than 8 days) or shorten the menstrual cycle to less than 18 days. Such bleeding is unpredictable and can cause anemia. (See *How to tell when uterine bleeding is abnormal.*)

How is it diagnosed?

Dilatation and curettage (D&C) and biopsy results confirm the diagnosis. Blood tests help determine the need for blood or iron replacement.

Diagnostic studies must rule out other causes of excessive vaginal bleeding, including cancer, polyps, incomplete abortion, pregnancy, and infection.

How is it treated?

The primary treatment, high-dose estrogen-progestogen combination therapy (oral contraceptives), is designed to control endometrial growth and reestablish a normal menstrual cycle. These drugs are usually administered four times daily for 5 to 7 days, even though bleeding usually stops in 12 to 24 hours.

SELF-HELP

How to tell when uterine bleeding is abnormal

If you have episodes of uterine bleeding, you may wonder whether they're only a temporary upset in your menstrual cycle or an ongoing disorder requiring treatment.

When to get help

The timing, duration, and amount of bleeding determines whether the bleeding is abnormal. For example, you should seek medical attention if your bleeding episodes occur:
- between menstrual periods.
- as a consistently heavy or prolonged period (more than 8 days).
- as a consistently short menstrual cycle (fewer than 18 days).
- more than 1 year after your last menstrual period.
- after sexual intercourse.
- as consistent, bloody discharge.

STRAIGHT
TALK

What to expect with a D&C

Dilatation and curettage (or D&C) is a surgical procedure designed to control abnormal uterine bleeding and to determine its cause.

Before the procedure

Before you enter the hospital, you'll describe your health history and the doctor will give you a physical and a gynecologic exam. You'll have a Pap test and blood and urine tests to make sure you're ready for surgery.

You may be asked to shower with an antibacterial soap the night before the procedure; you also may be given an enema to clean your bowel — a precaution against infection. You'll probably be told not to eat or drink anything after midnight.

In the hospital, you'll be given a mild tranquilizer before surgery, and an intravenous line will be started to give you fluids or medicine you may need during the procedure.

During the procedure

If you get a general anesthetic to make you sleep through the procedure, you'll wake up in the recovery room in about an hour, and a nurse will check your progress. If you get a local anesthetic, you'll be awake during the procedure. Here's what to expect:

• The surgical team will help you lie on your back on the operating table. You'll put your legs in stirrups.

• The doctor will examine you internally. As he or she does, polyps (growths that can cause bleeding) may be removed and tissue samples taken from your cervix and uterus. (The tissue will be studied to find the reason for your bleeding.) Then the doctor will do the D&C using surgical instruments to stretch (dilate) your cervix and gently scrape the surface lining of the uterus (the endometrium).

If you feel temporary cramping, nausea, or light-headedness, breathe deeply and try to relax. It's unlikely you'll feel discomfort. However, if you do, tell the doctor, who will give you medicine.

After the procedure

When your anesthetic wears off, you'll feel mild to severe cramping, similar to a menstrual period. You may also have some lower back pain for 1 or 2 days. Here are some tips for your recovery:

• Ask your doctor or nurse to recommend a pain medicine.

• Use a sanitary napkin, *not* a tampon, for mild spotting or staining that may last a few days or more.

• Resume your normal activities, but ask your doctor about vigorous exercise.

• Don't have sexual intercourse until healing is complete — about 2 weeks.

• Report any of the following to your doctor: vaginal bleeding that resembles a menstrual period; fever; sharp, constant pelvic pain; increased pulse rate; or foul-smelling vaginal drainage. Also call the doctor if you just don't feel right.

• Be sure to make and keep your appointment for a checkup.

In women over age 35, endometrial biopsy is necessary before the start of estrogen therapy, to rule out endometrial cancer. Progestogen therapy is a necessary alternative in some women, such as those susceptible to the side effects of estrogen (thrombophlebitis, for example).

If drug therapy is ineffective, a D&C serves as a supplementary treatment that removes a large portion of the bleeding endometrium.

Also, a D&C can help determine the original cause of hormonal imbalance and can aid in planning further therapy.

Regardless of the primary treatment, the woman may need iron replacement or transfusions of packed cells or whole blood because of anemia caused by recurrent bleeding. (See *What to expect with a D&C.*)

What can a woman with dysfunctional uterine bleeding do?

If you have dysfunctional bleeding, follow these guidelines:

- Be sure to follow the prescribed hormonal therapy.
- Get regular checkups to determine if your treatment is effective.

ENDOMETRIOSIS

What is this condition?

In this condition, endometrial tissue occurs outside of its customary location: the lining of the uterine cavity. Called *ectopic* tissue, it's generally confined to the pelvic area, but it can appear anywhere in the body. This ectopic endometrial tissue responds to normal stimulation in the same way that the endometrium does. During menstruation, the ectopic tissue bleeds, which causes inflammation of the surrounding tissues. This inflammation causes fibrosis, leading to adhesions that produce pain and infertility.

Active endometriosis usually occurs between ages 30 and 40, especially in women who postpone childbearing; it's uncommon before age 20. Severe symptoms of endometriosis may develop rapidly or may develop over many years. This disorder usually becomes progressively severe during the menstrual years; after menopause, it tends to subside.

What causes it?

Although there are several theories to explain this disorder, its precise cause remains unknown.

What are its symptoms?

The classic symptom of endometriosis is painful menstruation, which may produce constant pain in the lower abdomen and in the

STRAIGHT
TALK

Questions women ask about endometriosis and pregnancy

Will endometriosis prevent me from getting pregnant?

That depends on how severe it is and where the implants and adhesions are located. If severe endometriosis affects your ovaries or fallopian tubes, it might make conception difficult or impossible. For instance, extensive blood-filled cysts around an ovary may prevent the egg from being released. Or adhesions in the fallopian tubes, pelvic peritoneum, or cul-de-sac may block the egg's path from the ovary to the uterus.

How can treatment help me get pregnant?

Medication can shrink the endometrial implants or suppress their growth. Laparoscopy can remove implants that interfere with conception. If you want to get pregnant, the doctor can prescribe drugs that won't affect your ability to ovulate. If you need surgery, the doctor will leave your uterus intact and preserve at least part of one ovary and fallopian tube.

Will I be able to get pregnant after laparoscopy?

With mild endometriosis, the pregnancy rate after surgery is about 70%; with moderate endometriosis, it's about 50%; and with severe endometriosis, it's about 30%. You can usually resume sexual intercourse a few days after a laparoscopy, when the bleeding stops. You can try to become pregnant as soon as the doctor gives the OK — usually when healing is complete and there's a better chance for a viable pregnancy. Until then, use a reliable means of contraception.

vagina, posterior pelvis, and back. This pain usually begins from 5 to 7 days before a period reaches its peak and lasts for 2 to 3 days.

Other clinical features depend on the location of the ectopic tissue:

- *ovaries* and *oviducts:* infertility and heavy menstrual flow
- *ovaries* or *cul-de-sac:* deep-thrust dyspareunia (painful intercourse)
- *bladder:* suprapubic pain, dysuria, and hematuria
- *rectovaginal septum* and *colon:* painful defecation, rectal bleeding with a menstrual period, and pain in the coccyx or sacrum (base of the spine)
- *small bowel* and *appendix:* nausea and vomiting, which worsen before menses, and abdominal cramps
- *cervix, vagina,* and *perineum:* bleeding from endometrial deposits in these areas during a menstrual period.

How is it diagnosed?

The doctor will perform a pelvic exam to detect endometriosis. He or she may be able to feel multiple tender nodules on the uterosacral ligaments or between the rectum and vagina or detect ovarian enlargement. Laparoscopy must confirm the diagnosis and determine the stage of the disease before treatment begins.

Comparing endometrial surgical procedures

Endometrial surgery involves laparoscopy, in which an illuminated tube is inserted through the abdominal wall to visualize the abdominal cavity. The surgeon can use this procedure along with laser surgery, cryosurgery, or electrocautery to remove endometrial implants (abnormal tissue fragments) and adhesions. These approaches don't require cutting with a knife. Therefore, healthy tissue is spared, bleeding is minimized, infection risk and swelling are reduced, and pain is minimized when nerve endings are quickly sealed by heat or cold.

Laser surgery

Laser energy can destroy deep-seated, widespread implants and adhesions. The surgeon may use an *argon laser* beam directed through a fiber-optic wave guide. This beam penetrates 1 to 2 millimeters but causes minimal scarring.

For shallow implants or adhesions, the surgeon may use a *carbon dioxide laser*. Focused through the laparoscope, this beam has to travel only 0.1 to 1.2 millimeters into the target tissue as it raises the tissue's intracellular water temperature to the flash point. In turn, the tissue vaporizes, and the intense heat causes blood vessels to clot. Suctioning through the laparoscope removes the vapor.

Cryosurgery

To destroy tissue by freezing, the surgeon uses the laparoscope to introduce a probe into the target area and then instills a refrigerant (such as liquid nitrogen or Freon) through an insulated tube to the probe's uninsulated tip. This causes clotting within the capillaries and localized tissue destruction when a frozen tissue ball forms around the probe's tip.

Electrocautery

The surgeon uses laparoscopy to apply a small, wire loop heated by a steady, direct electrical current to implants. This destroys a small amount of tissue on contact. The intense heat causes blood clotting.

How is it treated?

Treatment varies according to the stage of the disease and the woman's age and desire to have children. (See *Questions women ask about endometriosis and pregnancy*.) Conservative therapy for young women who want to have children includes androgens, such as Danocrine, which produce a temporary remission. Progestins and oral contraceptives also relieve symptoms. Gonadotropin-releasing hormone agonists, which work by inducing false menopause, are commonly used to provide a remission of disease. When ovarian masses are present, surgery must be performed to rule out cancer. Conservative surgery is possible, but the treatment of choice for women who don't want to bear children or for extensive disease is total removal of the uterus, fallopian tubes, and ovaries. (See *Comparing endometrial surgical procedures*.)

FIBROIDS

What do doctors call this condition?
Uterine leiomyomas, myomas

What is this condition?
The most common benign tumors in women, fibroids are smooth-muscle tumors that arise in the uterus. They usually occur in multiples in the uterine body, although they may appear on the cervix or on the round or broad ligament. (The term *fibroids* is somewhat misleading because these tumors consist of muscle cells, not fibrous tissue.)

Uterine fibroids occur in 20% to 25% of women of reproductive age and affect three times as many blacks as whites. The tumors become malignant in only 0.1% of women.

What causes them?
The cause of fibroids is unknown, but use of steroid hormones, including estrogen and progesterone, and several growth factors, including epidermal growth factor, have been implicated as a possible cause of fibroid growth. Fibroids typically arise after the first menstrual period and regress after menopause, suggesting that estrogen may promote fibroid growth.

What are the symptoms?
Fibroids may be located within the uterine wall or may protrude into the endometrial cavity of the uterus. Most fibroids produce no symptoms. The most common symptom is abnormal bleeding, which typically occurs as heavy menstrual bleeding. Uterine fibroids probably do not cause pain directly unless they bulge into the peritoneal cavity and become twisted. Pelvic pressure and impingement on nearby organs are common indications for treatment. Various reproductive disorders, including infertility, recurrent spontaneous abortion, and preterm labor, have been attributed to fibroids.

How are they diagnosed?
Clinical findings and the woman's history suggest uterine fibroids. Blood studies showing anemia from abnormal bleeding support the diagnosis. Bimanual exam may reveal an enlarged, firm, nontender, and irregularly contoured uterus. Ultrasound allows accurate assess-

ment of the dimensions, number, and location of tumors. Other diagnostic procedures include hysterosalpingography, dilation and curettage (D&C), endometrial biopsy, and laparoscopy.

How are they treated?

Treatment depends on the severity of symptoms, the size and location of the tumors and the woman's age, pregnancy status, desire to have children, and general health.

Treatment options include nonsurgical as well as surgical procedures. Nonsurgical methods include administration of gonadotropin-releasing hormone analogues, which profoundly depress blood estrogen levels and cause a 50% reduction in uterine volume.

Surgical options include abdominal, laparoscopic, or hysteroscopic myomectomy — for women who want to preserve their fertility — and hysterectomy, the definitive treatment for symptomatic women who have completed childbearing. (See *Advice for a woman with fibroids.*)

INFERTILITY

What is this condition?

Infertility refers to the inability to conceive a child after regular intercourse without contraception for at least 1 year. It affects approximately 10% to 15% of all couples in North America. About 40% to 50% of infertility is attributed to the female partner.

After extensive evaluation and treatment, about half of these infertile couples achieve pregnancy. In about 10% of the half who don't, doctors can't find a specific cause for infertility; in this group, the prognosis is poor if pregnancy isn't achieved after 3 years.

What causes it?

The causes of female infertility may be functional (lacking a physical or structural origin), anatomic, or psychological. (See *Sex-specific causes of infertility,* page 365.) Psychological problems probably account for relatively few cases of infertility. Occasionally, a woman who's under stress may stop ovulating; marital discord may also affect the frequency of sexual intercourse. However, psychological problems usually are a result, rather than a cause, of infertility.

SELF-HELP

Advice for a woman with fibroids

If you've been diagnosed with uterine fibroids, follow this advice.

Be alert for symptoms
Report any abnormal bleeding or pelvic pain to the doctor immediately.

Surgical considerations
- If you're scheduled for a multiple myomectomy (surgical removal of fibroids), understand that you may still be able to get pregnant.
- If you need a myomectomy but are pregnant and close to delivery, be aware that if the uterine cavity is entered during surgery, the baby may have to be delivered by cesarean section.
- Be aware that you won't experience premature menopause if your ovaries have been left intact.

What are its symptoms?

Inability to achieve pregnancy after having regular intercourse without contraception for at least 1 year suggests infertility.

How is it diagnosed?

The woman undergoes a complete physical exam and health history, which includes specific questions about her reproductive and sexual function, past diseases, mental state, previous surgery, types of contraception used in the past, and family history. For instance, if her history reveals irregular, painless menstrual periods, this may indicate that she's not ovulating. A history of pelvic inflammatory disease may suggest a blocked fallopian tube.

The doctor will order the following tests to assess ovulation:

- *Basal body temperature graph* shows a sustained rise in body temperature after ovulation until just before the menstrual period starts, showing the approximate time of ovulation.
- *Endometrial biopsy* (removal of tissue from the surface lining of the uterus), done on or about day 5 after the basal body temperature rises, provides evidence that ovulation has occurred.
- *Progesterone blood levels,* measured when they should be highest, can show inadequate progesterone production.

To assess the structure of the fallopian tubes, ovaries, and uterus, the doctor may perform the following procedures:

- *Hysterosalpingography* (an X-ray study of the uterus and fallopian tubes in which a radiopaque dye is injected through the cervix) may reveal a blocked fallopian tube or abnormalities of the uterine cavity.
- *Endoscopy* (visual inspection using an illuminated tube) confirms the results of hysterosalpingography and allows the doctor to examine the endometrial cavity and explore the front surface of the uterus, fallopian tubes, and ovaries. The doctor also may make a small incision in the abdominal wall (laparoscopy) to visualize the abdominal and pelvic areas.

The doctor may also order male-female interaction studies, including the following:

- *Postcoital tests* (Sim's and Huhner's tests) examine the cervical mucus for motile sperm cells after intercourse that has occurred at the middle of the woman's reproductive cycle (as close to ovulation as possible).
- *Immunologic or antibody testing* detects sperm-killing antibodies in the woman's blood. Further research is being conducted in this area.

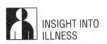

INSIGHT INTO
ILLNESS

Sex-specific causes of infertility

Many conditions can cause infertility in women or men; most are related to sex-specific anatomic and physiologic features.

Causes of female infertility

Female infertility usually stems from an ovulation problem, a blocked fallopian tube, an abnormal uterine condition, or abnormalities caused by one or more of the following:

- hormonal imbalances that prevent the ovary from releasing an egg regularly or at all or from producing enough hormone (progesterone) to support growth and maintain the uterine lining needed for a fertilized egg's implantation
- infection or inflammation (past, chronic, or current) that damages the ovaries and fallopian tubes, such as pelvic inflammatory disease, sexually transmitted diseases, appendicitis, childhood disease, or surgical trauma
- structural defects — for example, a uterus that's scarred by infection, abnormally shaped or positioned since birth, deformed by fibroids, exposed to diethylstilbestrol (also called DES), or injured by conization (removal of a cone of tissue for treatment or diagnosis)
- mucosal defects caused by infection, inadequate hormone levels, or antibodies to sperm, all of which prevent sperm from entering the uterus and traveling to the fallopian tubes
- endometriosis in which the endometrial tissue — normally confined to the uterus's inner lining — is

deposited outside the uterus on the ovaries or fallopian tubes, causing inflammation and scarring
- endocrine imbalances, such as elevated prolactin levels or pituitary, thyroid, or adrenal gland dysfunction.

Causes of male infertility

While some causes of male infertility remain unknown, others include:

- structural abnormalities, such as varicoceles (enlarged, varicose veins in the scrotum), which can affect sperm count and motility (ability to travel)
- infection, possibly from a sexually transmitted disease
- hormonal imbalances that reduce sperm production or decrease the sperm's motility in the female reproductive tract
- injury to the penis or testicles or congenital abnormalities that diminish the sperm count
- some prescription drugs known to affect sperm quality and, possibly, substances suspected of affecting sperm quality (such as alcohol, marijuana, cocaine, and tobacco)
- frequency of sexual intercourse — either too often or too seldom, which may decrease sperm count and motility
- heat (caused by wearing tight underwear or jeans, sitting in a hot tub or hot bath water, driving long distances, or fever-producing illnesses), which adversely affects sperm count and motility
- environmental agents, such as radiation and other industrial and environmental toxins
- psychological and emotional stress.

How is it treated?

Treatment depends on the underlying problem. If an overactive or underactive adrenal or thyroid gland is the cause of infertility, hormone therapy is necessary. For a progesterone deficiency, the woman receives progesterone replacement. A woman who's not ovulating is given the drug Clomid, human menopausal gonadotropins, or hu-

How in vitro fertilization works

For selected women, in vitro fertilization and embryo transfer can bypass the barriers to fertilization.

In this procedure, after the ovaries receive hormonal stimulation, the doctor may insert an illuminated tube through a small incision in the abdominal wall to visualize and withdraw fluid (containing eggs) from the ovarian follicles. (Or, to avoid this procedure and general anesthesia, the doctor may use ultrasound, first to visualize the ovarian follicles and then to guide a needle through the back of the vagina to retrieve fluid and eggs from the ovarian follicles.) The doctor then deposits the eggs in a test tube or a lab dish containing a culture medium.

Next, the doctor or a technician adds the sperm from the woman's husband (or a donor) to the dish. One to 2 days after insemination, the doctor transfers the now-fertilized egg or embryo to the woman's uterus, where it may implant and establish a pregnancy.

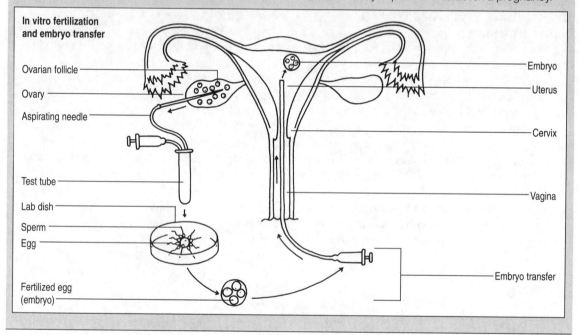

In vitro fertilization and embryo transfer

Ovarian follicle
Ovary
Aspirating needle
Test tube
Lab dish
Sperm
Egg
Fertilized egg (embryo)
Embryo
Uterus
Cervix
Vagina
Embryo transfer

man chorionic gonadotropin; typically, she ovulates several days after such treatment.

Surgery may correct certain anatomic causes of infertility, such as a blocked fallopian tube. It may also be done to remove tumors located within or near the hypothalamus or pituitary gland (structures in the brain). To treat endometriosis (abnormal tissue growth on the surface lining of the uterus), the woman receives drug therapy (Danocrine or Depo-Provera or noncyclic oral contraceptives), has surgery to remove the abnormal tissue, or undergoes a combination of both.

Other treatment options for infertility include use of a surrogate, frozen embryos, or in vitro fertilization. However, these options can be controversial and involve emotional and financial cost. (See *How in vitro fertilization works.*)

---

*I*NFLAMMATION OF THE VULVA AND VAGINA

What do doctors call this condition?
Vulvovaginitis

What is this condition?
Because vulva and vagina are located close together, inflammation of one structure usually causes inflammation of the other. Such inflammation may occur at any age and affects most women at some time. Prognosis is good with treatment.

What causes it?
Common causes of vaginal inflammation (vaginitis), with or without consequent vulval inflammation, include:
- infection with *Trichomonas vaginalis,* a protozoan, which is usually transmitted through sexual intercourse
- infection with *Candida albicans,* a fungus. Incidence rises during the secretory phase of the menstrual cycle. Such infection occurs twice as often in pregnant women as in nonpregnant women; it also commonly affects users of oral contraceptives, diabetics, and women receiving systemic therapy with broad-spectrum antibiotics.
- bacterial infection caused by *Gardnerella vaginalis* or *Neisseria gonorrhoeae* (gonorrhea)
- viral infection with venereal warts or herpesvirus type II, usually transmitted by sexual intercourse
- vaginal mucosa atrophy in menopausal women caused by decreasing levels of estrogen, which encourages bacterial invasion.

   Common causes of vulval inflammation include:
- parasitic infection with *Phthirus pubis* (crab louse)
- trauma (skin breakdown may lead to secondary infection)
- poor personal hygiene
- chemical irritations, or allergic reactions to douches, detergents, hygiene sprays, clothing, or toilet paper

- vulval atrophy in menopausal women caused by decreasing estrogen levels
- retention of a foreign body such as a tampon or diaphragm.

What are its symptoms?

In trichomonal vaginal inflammation, vaginal discharge is thin, bubbly, green-tinged, and malodorous. This infection causes marked irritation and itching and urinary symptoms, such as burning and frequency. *Candida* produces a thick, white, cottage cheese–like discharge and red, swollen mucous membranes, with white flecks adhering to the vaginal wall, and is often accompanied by intense itching. Gonorrhea may produce no symptoms at all or heavy pus discharge and difficult urination.

Acute vulval inflammation causes a mild-to-severe inflammatory reaction, including swelling, redness, burning, and itching. Severe pain on urination and painful intercourse may require immediate treatment. Herpes infection may cause painful ulcers or blisters during the active phase. Chronic vulval inflammation generally causes relatively mild inflammation, possibly associated with severe swelling that may involve the entire groin area.

How is it diagnosed?

Diagnosis of vaginal inflammation requires identification of the infectious organism during microscopic exam of vaginal discharge on a wet slide preparation (a drop of vaginal discharge placed in normal saline solution).

Diagnosis of vulvitis or suspected venereal disease may require a complete blood count, urinalysis, cytology screening, biopsy of chronic lesions to rule out malignant disease, and culture of discharge from acute lesions.

How is it treated?

Common therapeutic measures include the following:
- Flagyl, given orally, for the woman with trichomonal vaginal inflammation and all her sexual partners
- topical Micatin 2% or Mycelex 1% for candidal infection
- Flagyl for *Gardnerella*
- systemic antibiotic therapy for the woman with gonorrhea and for all her sexual partners as well
- Vibramycin or E-Mycin for chlamydial infection.

Cold compresses or cool sitz baths may provide relief from itching caused by acute vulval inflammation; severe inflammation may require warm compresses. Other therapy includes avoiding harsh, drying soaps, wearing loose clothing to promote air circulation, and applying topical corticosteroids to reduce inflammation. Chronic vulval inflammation may respond to topical hydrocortisone or antipruritics and good hygiene (especially in elderly or incontinent women). Topical estrogen ointments may be used to treat atrophic inflammation of the vulva and vagina. No cure currently exists for herpesvirus infections; however, oral and topical Zovirax may decrease the duration and symptoms of active lesions.

What can a woman with inflammation of the vulva and vagina do?

- Be sure to take medication for the length of time prescribed, even if your symptoms subside.
- After inserting a vaginal ointment or suppository, remain lying down for at least 30 minutes to promote absorption (insertion at bedtime is ideal). Wear a pad to prevent staining your underwear.
- Practice good hygiene. If you've had several episodes of inflammation of the vulva and vagina, wear all-cotton underpants. Avoid wearing tight-fitting pants and panty hose, which encourage the growth of the infecting organisms. (See *Tips for relieving vulvovaginal irritation.*)

MENOPAUSE

What is this condition?

Menopause is the cessation of menstruation. Between ages 45 and 55, as a woman's cyclic hormone production and function decline, menstruation ends naturally. However, it may end earlier because of illness or surgical removal of the uterus or both ovaries.

What causes it?

Menopause results from a complex syndrome of changes within the body, called the *climacteric*, which is caused by declining function of the ovaries.

SELF-HELP

Tips for relieving vulvovaginal irritation

If you have vulvovaginal irritation, following these tips can soothe the irritation and help you avoid recurrent infection:
- Shower daily, washing between showers with soap and water if discharge or odor seems excessive. Rinse soap away thoroughly.
- Avoid tub baths, especially with soap bubbles or oils.
- Change underwear daily.
- Avoid using feminine hygiene deodorant sprays, douches, perfumes, creams, or chemicals around the perineum.
- Use unscented, white toilet tissue and sanitary napkins.
- Wear white cotton underwear.
- Don't wear nylon panty hose without a cotton crotch or tight panties made of synthetic fabrics that inhibit ventilation.
- Change a wet bathing suit promptly instead of wearing it until it dries.
- Avoid contamination by wiping the perineal area from front to back each time you use the bathroom.
- Take antibiotics cautiously because some can cause a yeast infection.
- Consider using alternative birth control methods if oral contraceptives cause recurrent yeast infection.

Menopause results from a complex syndrome of changes within the body, called the climacteric, which is caused by declining ovarian function.

Classification

Three types of menopause — based on the cause — have been defined:

▪ *Physiologic menopause,* the normal loss of ovarian function caused by aging, starts in most women between ages 40 and 50 and results in infrequent ovulation, decreased menstrual function and, eventually, cessation of menstruation (typically between ages 45 and 55).

▪ *Pathologic (premature) menopause,* the gradual or abrupt cessation of menstruation before age 40, occurs with no known cause in about 5% of women in North America. However, certain diseases, especially severe infections and reproductive tract tumors, may cause this condition by seriously impairing ovarian function. Contributing factors include malnutrition, debilitation, extreme emotional stress, excessive radiation exposure, and surgical procedures that impair blood supply to the ovaries.

▪ *Artificial menopause* may follow radiation therapy or certain surgical procedures such as ovary removal.

What are its symptoms?

Many menopausal women have no symptoms, but some have severe symptoms. Loss of ovarian function and declining estrogen levels cause the following menstrual irregularities:

▪ decreased amount and duration of menstrual flow

▪ episodes of absent and abnormally frequent menstruation (possibly with excessive bleeding) or spotting.

These irregularities may last a few months or several years before menstruation stops permanently.

Menopause may cause changes in many body systems:

▪ *Reproductive system:* shrinkage of external genitalia and loss of subcutaneous fat, sometimes leading to shrinkage of the labia; shrinkage of the vaginal mucosa and flattening of the vaginal folds, possibly causing bleeding after intercourse or douching; vaginal itching and discharge; excessive vaginal dryness and painful intercourse because of decreased vaginal lubrication; shrinkage of the ovaries and their ducts; and progressive pelvic relaxation as estrogen loss causes the supporting structures to lose their tone

▪ *Urinary system:* bladder inflammation (from the effects of decreased estrogen), causing painful urination, urinary frequency and urgency, and incontinence

▪ *Breasts:* reduced size

Estrogen therapy: Mixed blessing?

To combat the symptoms of decreasing estrogen levels, some women receive estrogen replacement therapy during menopause. However, this therapy is controversial.

Those in favor of estrogen therapy claim that it successfully controls the physical and emotional symptoms of menopause. Opponents argue that it causes undesirable side effects, such as vaginal bleeding, breast tenderness, nausea, vomiting, abdominal bloating, and uterine cramps. At the heart of the controversy, however, is the increased risk of endometrial cancer in women who take supplemental estrogen.

Recent evidence

According to recent studies, these are the facts concerning estrogen use:

- Estrogen therapy has proven to be an effective treatment for two complaints associated with menopause — hot flashes and vaginal tissue shrinkage.

It also prevents osteoporosis by reducing bone resorption, and it decreases bone loss.

- The increased risk of cancer is directly linked to how long a woman takes estrogen. Taking it for more than 5 years increases the cancer risk by as much as 15 times in the general population; its use for less than 1 year only doubles the risk.
- Adding a progestin to estrogen therapy on a cyclic basis appears to reduce the risk of endometrial cancer.
- To minimize the risk of cancer, estrogen should be prescribed in the lowest possible dosage.
- Women who experience menopause prematurely or as a result of surgery may need estrogen replacement therapy to prevent osteoporosis.
- Smoking increases the risk of blood-clotting diseases in women who take estrogen.
- Women with family histories of gynecologic cancer should not take estrogen.

- *Skin, hair and nails:* poor skin elasticity and resilience (from lack of estrogen) loss of pubic and armpit hair and, occasionally, slight baldness
- *Nervous system:* hot flashes and night sweats (in about 60% of women), vertigo, fainting, rapid pulse, shortness of breath, ringing in the ears, emotional disturbances (irritability, nervousness, crying spells, fits of anger), and worsening of preexisting depression, anxiety, and compulsive, manic, or schizoid behavior.

Menopause may also induce hardening of the arteries; a decrease in the estrogen level contributes to osteoporosis (loss of bone mass). In pathologic and artificial menopause, menstruation often stops abruptly and may cause severe blood vessel disease and emotional disturbances.

How is it diagnosed?

The woman's history and typical symptoms suggest menopause. A Pap test may show the influence of estrogen deficiency on vaginal mucosa. A highly sensitive test method called *radioimmunoassay* shows characteristic hormone levels in the blood and urine. Hor-

SELF-HELP

Advice for women going through menopause

- If you're experiencing menopause, be aware that your bodily changes are normal and that you can still enjoy an active sex life.
- Continue to use contraception until the doctor confirms that your menstrual periods have stopped permanently.
- Immediately call your doctor if vaginal bleeding or spotting occurs after your menstrual periods have stopped.
- If you're receiving estrogen replacements, be sure to have regular medical checkups.
- If you feel very depressed or upset about menopause, seek psychological counseling.

mone measurement may also show an increase in the follicle-stimulating hormone of up to 15 times its normal level and an increase in luteinizing hormone production of up to 5 times its normal level.

To rule out organic disease in a woman with abnormal menstrual bleeding, the doctor performs a pelvic exam. Then, the doctor may remove tissue from the surface lining of the uterus and perform a uterine procedure called *dilatation and curettage* (or D&C).

How is it treated?

Estrogen is the treatment of choice to relieve hot flashes and symptoms caused by shrinkage of the vaginal tissue. Estrogen also improves mood, helps prevent osteoporosis, and may help prevent cardiovascular disease. Because of the controversy over the effect of estrogen replacement therapy on breast cancer, women should have screening mammograms before starting this therapy. (See *Estrogen therapy: Mixed blessing?* page 371.)

Estrogen replacement therapy may be administered in cycles or continuously. The doctor usually prescribes the lowest dosage that effectively treats symptoms and prevents osteoporosis. A woman with severe hot flashes may get a higher dosage for a limited period, followed by a gradual reduction of the standard dose.

In women who haven't had a hysterectomy (surgical uterus removal), adding a progestin (such as Depo-Provera) during the last 12 days of estrogen administration lowers the incidence of endometrial cancer and cell abnormalities.

Preferably, the woman takes estrogen in tablet form. However, skin patches reduce gastrointestinal side effects such as nausea, and topical estrogen relieves symptoms of vaginal tissue shrinkage. All women taking estrogen must have regular checkups to detect endometrial abnormalities early.

Some women shouldn't take estrogen — those with unexplained vaginal bleeding, liver disease, recent thrombosis, breast cancer, or endometrial cancer. To reduce the incidence of hot flashes, these women may receive Depo-Provera, Megace, or Catapres. Psychotherapy and drug therapy may relieve psychological disturbances. (See *Advice for women going through menopause.*)

OVARIAN CYSTS

What is this condition?

Ovarian cysts are usually noncancerous sacs that contain fluid or semisolid material. Although these cysts are usually small and produce no symptoms, they require thorough investigation to be sure they're not cancerous. Common types of ovarian cysts include follicular cysts, lutein cysts, and those associated with polycystic ovarian disease.

Ovarian cysts can develop any time between puberty and menopause, including during pregnancy. Some lutein cysts occur infrequently during early pregnancy. The prognosis for noncancerous ovarian cysts is excellent.

What causes them?

Follicular cysts are typically small and arise from follicles that have malfunctioned during the menstrual cycle. When such cysts persist into menopause, they secrete excessive amounts of estrogen in response to the hypersecretion of follicle-stimulating hormone and luteinizing hormone that normally occurs during menopause.

Granulosa-lutein cysts, which occur within the corpus luteum, are functional, nonneoplastic enlargements of the ovaries, caused by excessive accumulation of blood during the bleeding phase of the menstrual cycle. *Theca-lutein cysts* are commonly bilateral and filled with clear, straw-colored fluid; they're often associated with other types of ovarian tumors or hormone therapy.

Polycystic ovarian disease is part of the Stein-Leventhal syndrome and stems from endocrine abnormalities.

What are the symptoms?

Small ovarian cysts (such as follicular cysts) usually don't produce symptoms unless twisting or rupture causes abdominal tenderness, distention, and rigidity. Large or multiple cysts may induce mild pelvic discomfort, low back pain, painful intercourse, or abnormal uterine bleeding secondary to a disturbed ovulatory pattern. Ovarian cysts that become twisted cause acute abdominal pain similar to that of appendicitis.

Granulosa-lutein cysts that appear early in pregnancy may grow as large as 2 to 2½ inches (5 to 6 centimeters) in diameter and produce discomfort on one side of the pelvis and, if rupture occurs, massive one-sided bleeding within the abdomen. In nonpregnant women, these cysts may cause delayed menstruation, followed by prolonged or irregular bleeding. Polycystic ovarian disease may also produce secondary absence of menstruation, diminished menstrual flow, or infertility.

How are they diagnosed?

Generally, the doctor diagnoses ovarian cysts based on the woman's signs and symptoms. A physical exam and lab tests may also help detect certain types of cysts.

Visualization of the ovary through ultrasound, laparoscopy, or surgery (often for another condition) confirms ovarian cysts.

How are they treated?

Follicular cysts generally don't require treatment because they tend to disappear spontaneously within 60 days. However, if they interfere with daily activities, Clomid taken orally for 5 days or progesterone given intramuscularly (also for 5 days) reestablishes the ovarian hormonal cycle and induces ovulation. Oral contraceptives may also accelerate involution of functional cysts (including both types of lutein cysts and follicular cysts).

Treatment for granulosa-lutein cysts that occur during pregnancy is symptomatic because these cysts diminish during the third trimester and rarely require surgery. Theca-lutein cysts disappear spontaneously after elimination of hydatidiform mole or choriocarcinoma, or discontinuation of human chorionic gonadotropin or Clomid therapy.

Treatment of polycystic ovarian disease may include the administration of such drugs as Clomid to induce ovulation, Depo-Provera for 10 days of every month for the woman who doesn't want to become pregnant, or low-dose oral contraceptives for the woman who needs reliable contraception. Surgery may be necessary to remove a persistent or suspicious ovarian cyst.

What can a woman who's had ovarian cyst surgery do?

You'll be advised to increase your activities at home gradually — preferably over 4 to 6 weeks. Abstain from intercourse and use tampons and douches during this period.

PAINFUL MENSTRUATION

What do doctors call this condition?

Dysmenorrhea

What is this condition?

Painful menstruation is the most common gynecologic complaint and a leading cause of absenteeism from school (it affects 10% of high school girls each month) and work (it causes an estimated 140 million lost work hours a year). It can occur as a primary disorder or secondary to an underlying disease.

What causes it?

Although primary painful menstruation is unrelated to any identifiable cause, possible contributing factors include hormonal imbalances and psychological factors. The pain probably results from increased prostaglandin secretion that intensifies normal uterine contractions.

Painful menstruation may also stem from an underlying gynecologic disorder, such as endometriosis, cervical narrowing, uterine fibroids, uterine malposition, pelvic inflammatory disease, or pelvic tumors.

What are its symptoms?

Painful menstruation produces irregular, sharp, cramping pain in the lower abdomen, which usually radiates to the back, thighs, groin, and vulva. Such pain — sometimes compared with labor pains — typically starts with or immediately before menstrual flow and peaks within 24 hours. Painful menstruation may also occur with other signs of premenstrual syndrome (urinary frequency, nausea, vomiting, diarrhea, headache, chills, abdominal bloating, painful breasts, depression, and irritability).

How is it diagnosed?

A pelvic exam and a detailed history may suggest the cause of painful menstruation.

Primary painful menstruation is diagnosed when secondary causes are ruled out. Appropriate tests (such as laparoscopy, dilation and curettage, and X-rays) are used to diagnose underlying disorders in secondary painful menstruation.

SELF-HELP

Relieving menstrual cramps through exercise

Exercising several times a day can help relieve menstrual cramps. Do each exercise once and gradually work up to 10 repetitions. If you feel severe pain during any exercise, stop right away. If the pain continues, call your doctor.

Remember — to get the full benefit of these exercises, perform each one slowly. Try working them into your daily routine. For instance, exercise first thing in the morning, before dinner, or whenever you feel discomfort.

Use the instructions below as a guide.

Bicycling exercise
Swing your legs up to raise your hips and lower back off the floor. Support your hips with your hands, as shown. Your soles should be facing the ceiling. Now bend your knees and alternately move your legs in a pedaling motion. Return to the starting position.

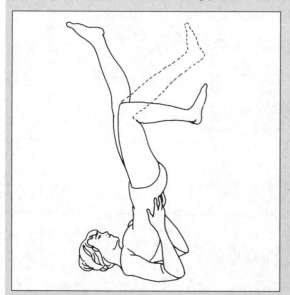

Modified sit-ups
Lie on your back with both knees bent. Curl up slowly, reaching forward with your arms. Try to raise your head and shoulders about 6 inches (25 centimeters) off the floor. Hold for about 3 seconds. Now, slowly curl back down.

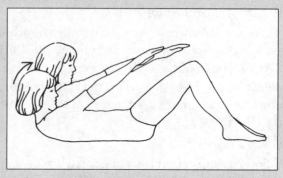

Elbow-to-knee stretches
Stand and clasp your hands behind your head. First, lift your left knee to your right elbow, or as close as you can. Then lower your leg. Next, lift your right knee to your left elbow, or as close as you can, and then lower your leg.

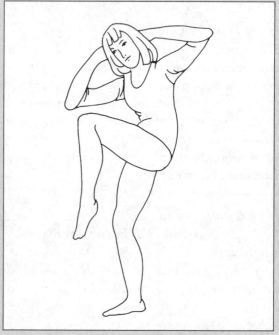

Relieving menstrual cramps through exercise *(continued)*

Trunk bends

Stand with your legs about 12 inches (30 centimeters) apart, keeping your knees slightly bent. Put your hands on your hips. First, bend forward as far as you can. Then return to the starting position.

Now, bend to the right as far as you can. Return to the starting position. Next, bend backward as far as possible. Return to the starting position. Finally, bend to the left as far as possible, and return to the starting position.

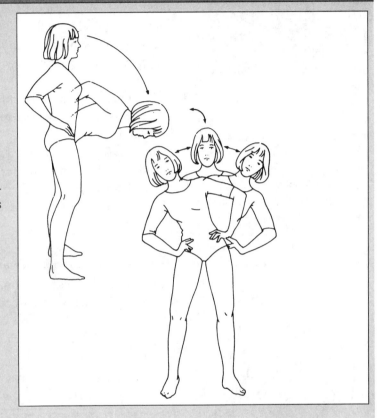

How is it treated?

Initial treatment aims to relieve pain. Pain relief measures may include the following:

▪ *pain relievers,* such as aspirin, for mild-to-moderate pain (most effective when taken 24 to 48 hours before the onset of menstruation). Aspirin is especially effective for treating painful menstruation because it also inhibits prostaglandin synthesis.

▪ *narcotics* if pain is severe (infrequently used).

▪ *prostaglandin inhibitors* (such as Ponstel and Advil) to relieve pain by decreasing the severity of uterine contractions.

▪ *heat* applied locally to the lower abdomen (may relieve discomfort in mature women but is not recommended in young adolescents because appendicitis may mimic painful menstruation).

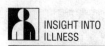

Where pelvic inflammatory disease strikes

Pelvic inflammatory disease can spread throughout the reproductive system and damage the endometrium, uterus, fallopian tubes, and ovaries. In severe cases, it may involve the peritoneum (the membrane covering the abdominal wall).

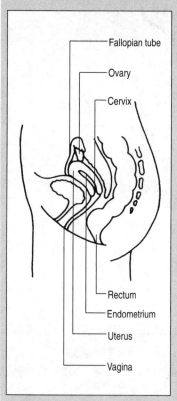

Fallopian tube

Ovary

Cervix

Rectum

Endometrium

Uterus

Vagina

For *primary painful menstruation,* administration of sex hormones is an effective alternative to treatment with antiprostaglandins or analgesics. Such therapy usually consists of oral contraceptives to relieve pain by suppressing ovulation. (However, women who are attempting pregnancy should rely on antiprostaglandin therapy instead of oral contraceptives to relieve symptoms of primary painful menstruation.)

Because persistent, severe menstrual pain may have a psychological cause, psychological evaluation and appropriate counseling may be helpful.

In *secondary painful menstruation,* treatment is designed to identify and correct the underlying cause. This may include surgical treatment of underlying disorders, such as endometriosis or fibroids. However, surgical treatment is recommended only after conservative therapy fails.

What can a woman with painful menstruation do?

To help deal with this condition, you'll want to keep a detailed record of your menstrual symptoms and seek further medical care if these symptoms persist. Also, you can learn exercises that help relieve cramps. (See *Relieving menstrual cramps through exercise,* pages 376 and 377.)

PELVIC INFLAMMATORY DISEASE

What is this condition?

Pelvic inflammatory disease is any acute, subacute, recurrent, or chronic infection of the oviducts and ovaries, with adjacent tissue involvement. It includes inflammation of the cervix, uterus, fallopian tubes, and ovaries, which can extend to the connective tissue lying between the broad ligaments. (See *Where pelvic inflammatory disease strikes.*)

Early diagnosis and treatment prevents damage to the reproductive system. Untreated, the disease may cause infertility and lead to potentially fatal blood infection, blood clots in the lungs, and shock.

What causes it?

Pelvic inflammatory disease can result from infection with bacteria, which invade the uterus when the defensive barrier formed by the cervical mucus is compromised. The breach may be caused by various procedures, such as insertion of an intrauterine device, biopsy instrument, or catheter. Other predisposing factors include abortion, pelvic surgery, and infection during or after pregnancy. (See *Who's at risk for pelvic inflammatory disease?*)

Bacteria may also enter the uterine cavity through the bloodstream or from drainage from a chronically infected fallopian tube, a pelvic abscess, a ruptured appendix, diverticulitis of the large intestine, or other infected areas.

The bacterium *Neisseria gonorrhoeae* most commonly causes pelvic inflammatory disease because it's most able to cross the cervical mucus barrier. Other common bacteria found in cervical mucus are staphylococci, streptococci, diphtheroids, chlamydiae, and coliforms, including *Escherichia coli* and *Pseudomonas*. Uterine infection can result from one or more of these bacteria, or it may follow overgrowth of normally nonpathogenic bacteria in an altered endometrial environment, as occurs in childbirth.

What are its symptoms?

Symptoms of pelvic inflammatory disease vary with the affected area but generally include excessive pus discharge from the vagina, sometimes accompanied by low-grade fever and malaise (particularly if gonorrhea is the cause). The woman experiences lower abdominal pain, and movement of the cervix or palpation of the fallopian tubes or ovaries may be extremely painful.

How is it diagnosed?

Diagnostic tests generally include:
- *Gram staining* of secretions from the endocervix or cul-de-sac to identify the bacterial agent; culture and sensitivity testing aids selection of the appropriate antibiotic. (Urethral and rectal secretions may also be cultured.)
- *ultrasound* to identify a tubal or uterine mass (simple X-rays seldom identify pelvic masses)
- *culdocentesis* (aspiration) to obtain peritoneal fluid or pus for culture and sensitivity testing.

Who's at risk for pelvic inflammatory disease?

Pelvic inflammatory disease is reported in over 1 million women annually in the United States. However, reporting this disease isn't mandatory, so the estimated incidence may run as high as 3 million cases annually.

Who gets it?
Pelvic inflammatory disease most commonly occurs between ages 15 and 24, especially among women who can't afford care and those with a poor understanding of sexually transmitted diseases. Adolescents are the group hardest hit by this disease.

What are the risk factors?
The risk of pelvic inflammatory disease increases with multiple sex partners, a history of cervical inflammation from gonorrheal or chlamydial infection, a history of the condition, and use of an intrauterine device, which may introduce infection. Another risk factor is failure to use a condom, spermicide, or diaphragm, which are barriers to infection, during sexual activity.

SELF-HELP

Advice for a woman with pelvic inflammatory disease

To avoid getting reinfected, comply with your prescribed treatment regimen. Here are some other important precautions.

Contain the damage
- Tell your sexual partners to get examined and, if necessary, treated for infection.
- Consult with your doctor about sexual activity because pelvic inflammatory disease may cause painful intercourse.

Encourage healing
To prevent infection after gynecologic procedures such as dilatation and curettage, avoid douching and intercourse for at least 7 days. Immediately report any fever, increased vaginal discharge, or pain.

In addition, the woman's history is significant. Pelvic inflammatory disease is typically associated with recent sexual intercourse, intrauterine device insertion, childbirth, or abortion.

How is it treated?

To prevent progression of pelvic inflammatory disease, antibiotic drug therapy begins immediately after culture specimens are obtained. Infection may become chronic if treated inadequately.

The guidelines of the Centers for Disease Control and Prevention for at-home treatment include a single dose of Mefoxin given along with Benemid, or a single dose of Rocephin. Each of these regimens is given with Vibramycin for 14 days.

The official guidelines for hospital treatment include Vibramycin alone or a combination of Cleocin and Garamycin.

Development of a pelvic abscess necessitates adequate drainage. A ruptured abscess is life-threatening. If this complication develops, the woman may need a total removal of her uterus, fallopian tubes, and ovaries. (See *Advice for a woman with pelvic inflammatory disease*.)

POSTMENOPAUSAL BLEEDING

What is this condition?

Postmenopausal bleeding is defined as bleeding from the reproductive tract that occurs 1 year or more after menstrual periods stop. Sites of bleeding include the vulva, vagina, cervix, and endometrium. Prognosis varies with the cause.

What causes it?

Postmenopausal bleeding may result from:
- *estrogen therapy* — when excessive amounts are given or when small amounts are given in the presence of a hypersensitive endometrium.
- *internal estrogen production* — especially when levels are high, as in persons with estrogen-producing ovarian tumors; however, in some persons, even slight fluctuation in estrogen levels may cause bleeding.
- *atrophic endometrium* — due to low estrogen levels.

- *atrophic vaginitis* — usually triggered by trauma during intercourse when estrogen is lacking.
- *aging* — which weakens blood vessels, produces degenerative tissue changes, and decreases resistance to infections.
- *cervical or endometrial cancer* — more common after age 60.
- *adenomatous hyperplasia* or *atypical adenomatous hyperplasia* — usually considered a premalignant lesion.

What are its symptoms?

Vaginal bleeding, the predominant symptom, ranges from spotting to outright hemorrhage; its duration also varies. Other symptoms depend on the cause. Excessive estrogen stimulation, for example, may also produce copious cervical mucus; estrogen deficiency may cause the vaginal mucosa to shrink.

How is it diagnosed?

The doctor will perform a physical exam (including a pelvic exam), obtain a detailed history, and order standard lab tests (such as complete blood count) and a cytologic exam of tissue specimens from the cervix and the endocervical canal. An endometrial biopsy or dilation and curettage reveals evidence of disease in the endometrium.

Diagnosis must rule out any underlying disease. For instance, evidence of elevated levels of endogenous estrogen may suggest an ovarian tumor. Before testing for estrogen levels, the woman must stop all sources of estrogen intake — including face and body creams that contain estrogen — to rule out excessive estrogen as a cause.

How is it treated?

Emergency treatment to control massive bleeding is rarely necessary, except in advanced cancer. Treatment may include dilation and curettage to relieve bleeding. Other therapy varies according to the underlying cause. Estrogen creams and suppositories are usually effective in correcting estrogen deficiency because they're rapidly absorbed. Hysterectomy is indicated for repeated episodes of postmenopausal bleeding from the endometrial cavity. Such bleeding may indicate endometrial cancer.

SELF-HELP

Identifying the many symptoms of PMS

Premenstrual syndrome (PMS) can cause diverse symptoms, affecting virtually any body system and triggering mental and emotional problems. The list below can help you pinpoint the pattern of symptoms that most closely matches your own experience with PMS.

Cardiovascular symptoms
Irregular heartbeat and palpitations

Nervous system symptoms
Clumsiness, dizziness, headache, seizures, slurred speech, and tingling or numbness in the hands

Digestive tract symptoms
Abdominal bloating or cramps, hemorrhoidal flare-ups, and nausea

Muscle and joint symptoms
Backache, joint swelling or pain, muscle aches, and stiff neck

Skin symptoms
Acne; oral, skin, or genital herpes; hives; and rash

Psychological symptoms
Absentmindedness, accident-proneness, anger, anxiety, confusion, crying, depression, fatigue, indecisiveness, insomnia, irritability, lethargy, low self-esteem, mood swings, panic, paranoia, sex-drive changes, suicidal thoughts, violence, and withdrawal

Other symptoms
Alcohol intolerance; asthma; breast tenderness and swelling; dry eyes; swelling; food cravings (salt, sweets); infections; lactation problems; noise, smell, and touch sensitivities; and urinary problems

PREMENSTRUAL SYNDROME (PMS)

What is this condition?

Premenstrual syndrome (PMS) refers to a complex of various symptoms that appear 7 to 14 days before a menstrual period starts and usually subside with its onset. The effects of PMS range from minimal discomfort to severe, disruptive symptoms. These may include nervousness, irritability, depression, and multiple physical complaints. Researchers believe that 70% to 90% of women experience PMS at some time during their childbearing years, usually between ages 25 and 45.

What causes it?

Many theories have been offered to explain the cause of PMS, including vitamin deficiencies and a progesterone deficiency during a certain phase of the menstrual cycle. But so far, no one knows for sure.

This suggests that PMS represents a variety of symptoms triggered by normal hormonal changes.

What are its symptoms?

The symptoms of PMS vary widely among women and may include any combination of the following:

- *behavioral* — mild-to-severe personality changes, nervousness, hostility, irritability, agitation, sleep disturbances, fatigue, sluggishness, and depression
- *physical* — breast tenderness or swelling, a bloated or tender abdomen, joint pain, headache, swelling, diarrhea or constipation, worsening of skin problems (such as acne or rashes), respiratory problems (such as asthma), or seizures. (See *Identifying the many symptoms of PMS.*)

How is it diagnosed?

The woman's history shows typical symptoms related to the menstrual cycle. Before diagnosing PMS, the doctor or nurse may ask her to record her menstrual symptoms and body temperature on a calendar for 2 to 3 months. Evaluating estrogen and progesterone levels helps to rule out hormonal imbalance. A psychological evaluation may be done to rule out or detect an underlying psychiatric disorder.

How is it treated?

The woman is taught about PMS and reassured that it's a real physical problem. Because treatment focuses mainly on relieving symptoms, each woman must learn to cope with her own set of symptoms.

Treatment may include diuretics to reduce excess fluid buildup, antidepressants, vitamins such as B complex, progestins, prostaglandin inhibitors, and nonsteroidal anti-inflammatory drugs. For treatment to be effective, a woman may have to eat a diet low in simple sugars, caffeine, and salt.

What can a woman with PMS do?

- Get a good night's sleep. If you're tired during the day, set aside time for regular breaks.
- Engage in regular exercise, such as walking, bicycling, or swimming. Try to work out three to five times a week, 20 to 30 minutes per session.

- Eat a well-balanced diet, and don't skip meals. Drink 6 to 8 glasses of fluid daily. Avoid caffeine-containing foods and beverages, and limit or avoid alcohol.
- Use stress-reduction techniques. If you have emotional problems you can't resolve on you own, seek a qualified counselor.
- See your doctor to rule out other possible causes of your symptoms.
- Ask your doctor or nurse for the names of local self-help groups for women with PMS.

PREGNANCY-RELATED DISORDERS

ABNORMAL VOMITING DURING PREGNANCY

What is this condition?

Unlike the nausea and vomiting a woman may normally have between the 6th and 12th weeks of pregnancy, this condition involves severe, constant nausea and vomiting that persist after the first trimester. If untreated, it produces substantial weight loss, starvation, dehydration, and other problems.

This condition occurs in about 1 in 200 pregnancies. The prognosis is good with appropriate treatment.

What causes it?

Although its cause is unknown, abnormal vomiting during pregnancy often affects women with conditions that produce high levels of a hormone called *human chorionic gonadotropin.* These conditions include cysts in the uterus or multiple pregnancy. Other possible causes include pancreatitis, bile duct disease, drug toxicity, inflammatory bowel disease, and vitamin deficiencies (especially of vitamin B_6).

What are its symptoms?

The cardinal symptoms of this disorder are constant nausea and vomiting. The vomit initially contains undigested food, mucus, and small amounts of bile; later, only bile and mucus; and finally, blood and material that resembles coffee grounds. Persistent vomiting causes substantial weight loss and eventual emaciation.

How is it diagnosed?

Diagnosis depends on a history of uncontrolled nausea and vomiting that persists beyond the first trimester, evidence of substantial weight loss, and other characteristic symptoms. Lab tests may also provide important evidence. Diagnosis must rule out other conditions with similar clinical effects.

How is it treated?

The woman with this condition may require hospitalization to correct electrolyte imbalances and prevent starvation. Intravenous feedings maintain nutrition until her condition improves. She progresses slowly to a clear liquid diet, then a full liquid diet and, finally, small, frequent meals of high-protein solid foods. Snacks help stabilize blood sugar levels, and vitamin B supplements help correct vitamin deficiency.

When vomiting stops and electrolyte balance has been restored, the pregnancy usually continues uneventfully, and most women feel better as they begin to regain normal weight. However, some continue to vomit throughout the pregnancy, requiring further treatment. If appropriate, some women may benefit from consultations with a clinical nurse specialist, a psychologist, or a psychiatrist.

What can a pregnant woman with abnormal vomiting do?

Eat dry foods if you have a poor appetite, and decrease your liquid intake during meals. To boost your appetite, try to have company and conversation at mealtimes. Stay upright for 45 minutes after eating to decrease the risk of vomiting.

Adolescent Pregnancy

What is this condition?

In the United States, an estimated 1 million adolescents become pregnant each year. Because up to 70% of them don't receive adequate prenatal care, and some are drug-dependent as well, they are apt to develop special problems, such as anemia and pregnancy-induced high blood pressure, and their pregnancies are more likely to result in death of the fetus or infant. Surviving infants are more likely to be premature or weigh very little at birth; be at high risk for birth injuries, childhood illness, and retardation or other neurologic defects; and to die soon after birth. (See *How maternal drug use affects infants,* page 388.) As a rule, the younger the mother, the greater the health risk for both mother and infant. Adolescents account for one-third of all abortions performed in the United States.

What causes it?

Adolescent pregnancy occurs at all socioeconomic levels. Contributing factors include ignorance about sexuality and contraception, precocious sexual activity, rebellion against parental influence, and a

In the United States, an estimated 1 million adolescents become pregnant each year. Most don't receive adequate prenatal care, and some are drug-dependent. Infant mortality is high.

How maternal drug use affects infants

An infant born to a drug-dependent mother is at risk for certain medical problems during the first 8 months of life — from mild to severe drug withdrawal symptoms to a host of complications affecting virtually every part of the body. The onset and severity of these problems depend on the type, amount, and duration of the mother's drug use. However, *any* drug the mother takes, including over-the-counter products, alcohol, and illicit drugs, may cross the placenta and enter the fetal circulation, where its concentration is 50% to 100% higher than in the mother. The table lists some common drug side effects.

BODY AREA	SIDE EFFECTS
Digestive tract	Diarrhea, vomiting, colic, feeding problems, susceptibility to inguinal hernia
Lungs	Croup, pneumonia, asthma, severe viral infection of the lower respiratory tract
Nervous system	Involuntary, rhythmic eye movements; squinting; abnormal head size; susceptibility to viral inflammation of the brain and spinal cord
Skin	Yeast infections, susceptibility to bacterial infection, allergic dermatitis, dry or moist greasy scales and yellowish skin crusts, bruising, skin hemorrhages
Other	Failure to thrive, middle ear infection, sudden infant death syndrome

desire to escape an unhappy family situation and to fulfill emotional needs unmet by the family.

What are its symptoms?

The pregnant adolescent experiences the same symptoms as an adult: absence of menstruation, nausea, vomiting, breast tenderness, and fatigue. However, she is much more likely to develop complications, such as poor weight gain, premature labor, pregnancy-induced hypertension, premature placental detachment, and toxemia of pregnancy (preeclampsia). Her infant is more likely to be of low birth weight.

How is it diagnosed?

A pregnancy test showing human chorionic gonadotropin in the blood or urine and a pelvic exam confirm pregnancy. Ultrasound and other tests can detect fetal heart sounds and assess the fetus's gestational age.

How is it treated?

The pregnant adolescent requires the same prenatal care as an adult. However, she also needs psychological support and close observation for signs of complications. (See *Helping a pregnant teenager.*)

BLOOD INCOMPATIBILITY BETWEEN MOTHER AND FETUS

What do doctors call this condition?

Erythroblastosis fetalis

What is this condition?

When the fetus's blood is incompatible with the mother's, the mother produces antibodies against the fetus's red blood cells. Intrauterine transfusions with human $Rh_o(D)$ immune human globulin can save 40% of fetuses with this disorder. However, in severe, untreated blood incompatibility, the prognosis is poor, especially if kernicterus (infiltration of parts of the brain and spinal cord with bilirubin) develops. About 70% of these infants die, usually within the first week of life; survivors inevitably develop severe nervous system damage.

What causes it?

Blood incompatibility between mother and fetus usually results from Rh isoimmunization — a condition that develops in approximately 7% of all pregnancies in the United States. Until treatment with human $Rh_o(D)$ immune human globulin became available, this condition was an important cause of kernicterus and neonatal death.

During her first pregnancy, a woman with Rh-negative blood factors becomes sensitized (during delivery or abortion) by exposure to Rh-positive fetal blood factors inherited from the father. In the next pregnancy that produces an Rh-positive fetus, increasing amounts of maternal anti-Rh-positive antibodies cross the placental barrier, attach to Rh-positive cells in the fetal blood, and destroy them.

To compensate for this, the fetus steps up the production of new red blood cells, which are attacked in their turn. Escalating red cell destruction releases large amounts of unconjugated bilirubin (a red cell component), which the fetal liver cannot properly process and excrete.

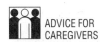

ADVICE FOR CAREGIVERS

Helping a pregnant teenager

To have a healthy baby, a pregnant teenager needs lots of help and support.

Help her maintain good health
Advise her to eat three well-balanced meals a day and to get plenty of rest. Between-meal snacks should be nutritious: fruits and raw vegetables, for instance, rather than cookies, cake, and chips.

Build her self-esteem
Help her to identify her own strengths and support systems for coping with pregnancy, birth, and parenting.

Prepare her for birth
Encourage her to attend prenatal classes. Educational films, hospital tours, and role-playing exercises will make her more informed and comfortable.

Help her get a new start
After giving birth, a teenager needs help to set realistic goals. If she'll give the infant up for adoption, she should clearly understand her legal rights. If she'll raise the infant, she needs to learn parenting skills, plan for child care and returning to school or a job, and work out her relationship with the father.

ABO incompatibility, another form of blood incompatibility between mother and fetus, is less severe. (See *Understanding ABO incompatibility*).

What are its symptoms?

An infant with this incompatibility disorder has liver problems. Jaundice (resulting from the fetal liver's failure to process bilirubin from the destroyed red cells) doesn't usually appear at birth but may occur 30 minutes to 24 hours later. A mildly affected infant is pale and has a mildly to moderately enlarged liver and spleen. Severely affected infants who survive birth usually have pallor, swelling, small reddish skin spots, an enlarged liver and spleen, grunting respirations, abnormal breath sounds, poor muscle tone, nervous system unresponsiveness, possible heart murmurs, a bile-stained umbilical cord, and yellow or meconium-stained amniotic fluid.

How is it diagnosed?

Diagnostic evaluation considers both prenatal and neonatal findings. Important factors to consider are:

- maternal history (for blood incompatibility–related stillbirths, abortions, previously affected children, or previous anti-Rh blood levels)
- blood typing and screening
- father's blood test results
- history of blood transfusion.

Other diagnostic tests that provide important information include amniotic fluid analysis and X-ray studies.

How is it treated?

Treatment depends on the degree of maternal sensitization and the effects of hemolytic disease on the fetus or newborn.

- Intrauterine-intraperitoneal blood transfusion is performed when amniotic fluid analysis suggests that the fetus is severely affected and that delivery is inappropriate because the fetus will be premature. A transabdominal puncture under fluoroscopy into the fetal peritoneal cavity allows infusion of group O, Rh-negative blood. This may be repeated every 2 weeks until the fetus is mature enough for delivery.
- Planned delivery is usually done 2 to 4 weeks before term date, depending on maternal history, serologic tests, and amniocentesis results; labor may be induced from the 34th to 38th week of gestation. During labor, the fetus should be monitored electronically; capillary

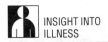

INSIGHT INTO
ILLNESS

Understanding ABO incompatibility

ABO incompatibility — a form of blood incompatibility between mother and fetus — occurs in about 25% of all pregnancies, most commonly among blacks.

In about 1% of cases, this disorder leads to destruction of red blood cells and jaundice in the newborn. ABO incompatibility is more common but less severe than Rh isoimmunization, another form of blood incompatibility.

Each blood group (A, B, AB, and O) has specific antigens on red blood cells and specific antibodies in the blood. The mother forms antibodies against fetal cells when the fetus has a different blood group. Infants with group A blood who are born to group O mothers account for about half of all cases of ABO incompatibility. ABO incompatibility is more likely to develop in firstborn infants.

Signs of ABO incompatibility in the newborn include jaundice (yellowish skin discoloration caused by too much bilirubin in the blood), which usually appears within 24 to 48 hours; mild anemia; and mild enlargement of the liver and spleen.

Diagnosis is based on the newborn's signs, the presence of different blood groups in the mother and newborn, a weak to moderate positive Coombs' test, and elevated serum bilirubin levels.

The newborn's umbilical cord hemoglobin and indirect bilirubin levels may indicate the need for an exchange transfusion. In this procedure, the newborn's blood is replaced with donor blood of the same group and Rh type as the mother's. Fortunately, because newborns with ABO incompatibility respond so well to fluorescent light therapy, few need exchange transfusions.

Blood group	Antigens on red blood cells	Antibodies in serum	Most common incompatible groups
A	A	Anti-B	Mother A, infant B or AB
B	B	Anti-A	Mother B, infant A or AB
AB	A and B	No antibodies	Mother AB
O	No antigens	Anti-A and B	Mother O, infant A or B

blood scalp sampling determines acid-base balance. Any indication of fetal distress calls for an immediate cesarean delivery.

■ The newborn's serum bilirubin levels are brought down by phenobarbital administered during the last 5 to 6 weeks of pregnancy; or by an albumin infusion, which helps bind bilirubin; or by phototherapy with ultraviolet light.

■ Administration of human $Rh_o(D)$ immune globulin can provide passive immunization, which prevents maternal Rh isoimmunization in Rh-negative women. However, it's ineffective if sensitization has already resulted from a previous pregnancy, abortion, or transfusion.

CARDIOVASCULAR DISEASE IN PREGNANCY

Cardiovascular disease ranks fourth (after infection, toxemia, and hemorrhage) among the leading causes of maternal death.

What is this condition?

Cardiovascular disease ranks fourth (after infection, toxemia, and hemorrhage) among the leading causes of maternal death. The physiologic stress of pregnancy and delivery is often more than a compromised heart can tolerate and often leads to death of the mother and child.

Approximately 1% to 2% of pregnant women have heart disease, but the incidence is rising because current medical treatment allows more women with rheumatic heart disease or congenital defects to reach childbearing age. With careful management, the prognosis for pregnant women with cardiovascular disease is good. Decompensation (the heart's failure to maintain adequate circulation) is the leading cause of maternal death. Infant mortality increases with decompensation, because uterine congestion, insufficient oxygenation, and the elevated carbon dioxide content of the blood not only endanger the fetus, but also frequently cause premature labor and delivery.

What causes it?

More than 80% of pregnant women who develop cardiovascular complications have a history of rheumatic heart disease. In the rest, these complications stem from congenital defects (10% to 15%) or coronary artery disease (2%).

The diseased heart is sometimes unable to meet the normal increased demands of pregnancy, which include a 25% increase in cardiac output (the amount of blood pumped by the heart per minute), a 40% to 50% increase in plasma volume, increased oxygen requirements, retention of salt and water, weight gain, and alterations in hemodynamics during delivery. This physiologic stress often leads to decompensation. The degree of decompensation depends on the woman's age, the duration of heart disease, and the functional capacity of her heart at the outset of pregnancy.

What are its symptoms?

The woman with cardiovascular disease during pregnancy will have distended neck veins, diastolic murmurs, moist crackles heard at the base of the lungs, an enlarged heart, and irregular heartbeats. Other typical symptoms may include bluish skin discoloration, pericardial friction rub, and pulse irregularities.

Decompensation may develop suddenly or gradually. As it progresses, the woman may experience swelling, increasing shortness of breath on exertion, palpitations, a smothering sensation, and coughing up blood.

How is it diagnosed?

Exam findings, including unusual heart sounds, irregular heartbeats, and an enlarged heart, suggest cardiovascular disease. To determine the extent and cause of the disease, an electrocardiogram, echocardiogram, or phonocardiogram may be performed. X-rays show heart enlargement and congestion in the lungs. Cardiac catheterization should be postponed until after delivery, unless surgery is necessary.

How is it treated?

The goal of therapy is to prevent complications and minimize the strain on the mother's heart, primarily through rest. This may require periodic hospitalization for women with moderate heart dysfunction or with symptoms of decompensation, toxemia, or infection. Older women or those with previous episodes of decompensation may require hospitalization and bed rest throughout the pregnancy.

Drug therapy, when necessary, will use the safest possible drugs in the lowest possible dosages to minimize harm to the fetus. Diuretics and drugs that increase blood pressure, blood volume, or cardiac output should be used with extreme caution. If an anticoagulant is needed, heparin is the drug of choice. Digoxin (also known as Lanoxin) and common antiarrhythmics, such as Cardioquin and Procan SR, are often required. The preventive use of antibiotics is reserved for women who are susceptible to endocarditis.

A therapeutic abortion may be considered for women with severe heart dysfunction, especially if decompensation occurs during the first trimester. Women hospitalized with heart failure usually follow a regimen of digoxin, oxygen, rest, sedation, diuretics, and restricted intake of sodium and fluids. If these measures fail to improve symptoms, heart surgery may be necessary. During labor, the woman may require oxygen and an analgesic for relief of pain and apprehension without adversely affecting the fetus or herself. Depending on which procedure would be less stressful for the woman's heart, delivery may be vaginal or by cesarean section.

Bed rest and medications already instituted should continue for at least 1 week after delivery because of a high incidence of decompensation, cardiovascular collapse, and maternal death during the early puerperal period.

Breast-feeding is undesirable for women with severe cardiovascular disease because it increases fluid and metabolic demands on the heart.

What can a pregnant woman with cardiovascular disease do?

Get plenty of rest and control your weight to decrease the strain on your heart. To prevent vascular congestion, limit your fluid and sodium intake. Take supplementary folic acid and iron to prevent anemia.

DIABETIC COMPLICATIONS DURING PREGNANCY

What is this condition?

Pregnancy places special demands on carbohydrate metabolism and increases the body's insulin requirement, even in a healthy mother. Thus, she may become prediabetic, or, if she's diabetic, runs the risk of aggravating her preexisting condition.

The prognosis of the mother and fetus is good if the mother's blood glucose (sugar) level is well controlled and ketosis and other complications are prevented. Infant morbidity and mortality depend on recognizing and successfully controlling low blood sugar, which may develop within hours after delivery.

What causes it?

In diabetes, glucose is inadequately used by the body, either because insulin is not synthesized by the pancreas (as in insulin-dependent diabetes) or because body tissues resist the hormonal action of endogenous insulin (as in non-insulin-dependent diabetes). During pregnancy, the fetus relies on the mother's glucose as a primary fuel source, but pregnancy triggers protective mechanisms that have anti-insulin effects: increased hormone production (placental lactogen, estrogen, and progesterone), which counteracts the effects of insulin; degradation of insulin by the placenta; and prolonged elevation of stress hormones (cortisol, epinephrine, and glucagon), which raises blood sugar levels.

Pregnancy places special demands on carbohydrate metabolism and increases the body's insulin requirement, even in a healthy mother. Thus, she may become prediabetic, or risk aggravating her preexisting disease.

In a normal pregnancy, an increase in anti-insulin factors is met by increased insulin production to maintain normal blood sugar levels. However, prediabetic or diabetic women can't produce enough insulin to overcome the insulin antagonist mechanisms of pregnancy, or their tissues are insulin-resistant. As insulin requirements rise toward term, a prediabetic woman may develop gestational diabetes, requiring dietary management and, possibly, administration of insulin to achieve glucose control; an insulin-dependent woman may need to increase her insulin dosage.

What are the symptoms?

Indications for diagnostic screening for maternal diabetes during pregnancy include obesity, excessive weight gain, excessive hunger or thirst, excessive urination, recurrent monilial infections, glucose in the urine, previous delivery of a large infant, excessive amniotic fluid, maternal high blood pressure, and a family history of diabetes.

Uncontrolled diabetes in a pregnant woman can cause stillbirth, fetal anomalies, premature delivery, and birth of an infant who is large or small for gestational age. Such infants are predisposed to severe episodes of low blood sugar shortly after birth and may also develop calcium deficiency, high levels of bilirubin in the blood, and respiratory distress syndrome.

How is it diagnosed?

The prevalence of gestational diabetes makes careful screening for high blood sugar appropriate in all pregnancies in each trimester. Abnormal blood sugar levels measured in a fasting person or after she has eaten, signs and symptoms, and the person's history suggest diabetes in women not previously diabetic.

A 3-hour glucose tolerance test confirms diabetes when two or more values are above normal.

Procedures to assess fetal status include stress and nonstress tests, ultrasound to determine fetal age and growth, and measurement of urine hormone levels.

How is it treated?

Treatment of both newly diagnosed and established diabetes is designed to maintain the woman's blood sugar levels within acceptable limits through dietary management and insulin administration. Most pregnant women with overt diabetes require hospitalization at the beginning of pregnancy to assess physical status, to check for

Managing diabetes during pregnancy

If you have diabetes and are pregnant, your therapy will include:
- making bimonthly visits to the obstetrician and the internist during the first 6 months of pregnancy (possibly weekly visits during the third trimester)
- maintaining blood sugar levels at or below 100 milligrams during the third trimester
- frequently monitoring your urine for glucose or ketones (ketosis presents a grave threat to your baby's nervous system)
- limiting weight gain to 3 to 3½ pounds (1.5 kilograms) per month during the last 6 months of pregnancy
- ensuring a daily protein intake of 2 grams per kilogram of body weight (or at least 80 grams per day during the second half of pregnancy); a daily intake of 30 to 40 calories per kilogram of body weight; a daily carbohydrate intake of 200 grams; and enough fat to provide 36% of total calories
- taking insulin if diet alone fails to control your blood sugar levels.

Insulin requirements may change from one trimester to the next and immediately after delivery. You shouldn't receive oral antidiabetic drugs because they may cause low blood sugar and congenital anomalies in your baby.

SELF-HELP

Advice for the pregnant woman with diabetes

Strict compliance with the prescribed treatment plan should ensure a favorable outcome. You can also take the following steps:

- Make sure your doctor monitors you often throughout your pregnancy.
- Adjust your insulin dosage as needed and as directed by your doctor.
- Talk to your doctor about the outlook for future pregnancies.

heart and kidney disease, and to regulate diabetes. (See *Managing diabetes during pregnancy,* page 395.)

Generally, the optimal time for delivery is between 37 and 39 weeks' gestation. An insulin-dependent diabetic woman requires hospitalization before delivery because bed rest promotes optimal circulation to the fetus and improves uterine muscle tone. In addition, hospitalization permits frequent monitoring of blood sugar levels and prompt intervention if complications develop.

Depending on fetal status and maternal history, the obstetrician may induce labor or perform a cesarean delivery. During labor and delivery, the woman with diabetes will receive a continuous intravenous infusion of dextrose with regular insulin in water. Maternal and fetal status must be monitored closely throughout labor. The woman may benefit from half her prepregnancy dosage of insulin before a cesarean delivery. Her insulin requirement will fall markedly after delivery. (See *Advice for the pregnant woman with diabetes.*)

ECTOPIC PREGNANCY

What is this condition?
Ectopic pregnancy is an abnormal pregnancy in which the fertilized egg is implanted outside, rather than within, the uterine cavity. The most common site is the fallopian tube — one of a pair of long, slender tubes extending from the uterus to the region of the ovary. (See *Where ectopic pregnancies occur.*)

With prompt diagnosis, appropriate surgery, and control of bleeding, the prognosis is good. Rarely, in an abdominal ectopic pregnancy, the fetus may even survive to term. Usually, the woman can achieve a normal subsequent pregnancy.

What causes it?
Ectopic pregnancy occurs when some conditions prevent or slow the passage of the fertilized egg through the fallopian tube and into the uterine cavity. Such conditions include:

- endosalpingitis, an inflammatory reaction that narrows the fallopian tube
- diverticulosis, the formation of blind pouches (diverticulae) that cause fallopian tube abnormalities

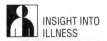

INSIGHT INTO
ILLNESS

Where ectopic pregnancies occur

In about 90% of women with an ectopic pregnancy, the fertilized egg is implanted in the fallopian tube — either in the fimbria (fringelike projections), ampulla (a dilated portion that takes a twisted path over the ovary), or isthmus (the portion extending from the upper outer angle of the uterus). Other possible sites of implantation include the interstitium of the uterus, the tubo-ovarian ligament, the ovary, the abdominal viscera, and the internal cervical os.

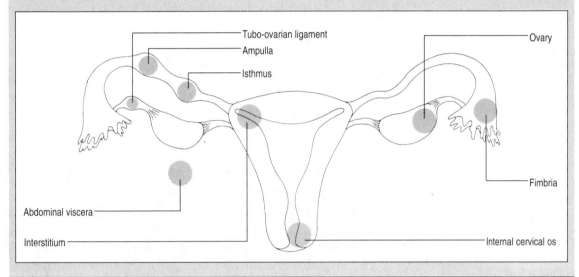

- tumors that press against the fallopian tube
- previous surgery, such as tubal ligation, or adhesions from previous abdominal or pelvic surgery.

Using an IUD for birth control may increase the risk of ectopic pregnancy by affecting the cells that line the uterus.

What are its symptoms?

Ectopic pregnancy sometimes causes symptoms of normal pregnancy but may cause no symptoms other than mild abdominal pain (especially if the pregnancy is in the abdomen). With fallopian tube pregnancy, the woman typically has abnormal menstrual periods (or no periods), followed by slight vaginal bleeding and pelvic pain on the side of the pregnancy. If the tube ruptures, she may have life-threatening complications, such as heavy bleeding, shock, and peritonitis (inflammation of the abdominal wall lining).

Ectopic pregnancy also may cause sharp pain the lower abdomen, possibly radiating to the shoulders and neck. This pain is commonly triggered by activities that increase abdominal pressure, such as a bowel movement. During a pelvic exam, the woman may feel extreme pain if her cervix is moved or if the examiner touches the structures adjoining the uterus. The uterus feels tender and abnormally soft.

How is it diagnosed?

The doctor may suspect ectopic pregnancy from the woman's history, symptoms, and pelvic exam results, and will confirm the diagnosis with a variety of serum tests, ultrasound scans, vaginal fluid analysis (culdocentesis), laparoscopy, and possibly exploratory laparotomy.

The doctor must also rule out certain conditions, such as uterine abortion, appendicitis, fallopian tube inflammation, and twisting of the ovary.

How is it treated?

If culdocentesis reveals blood in the abdominal wall lining, the doctor surgically removes the affected fallopian tube. If the woman wishes to have children, she can undergo microsurgery to repair the fallopian tube; the ovary is saved, if possible. However, if the ectopic pregnancy is in an ovary, the ovary must be removed. If the pregnancy is in an abnormal site within the uterus, a hysterectomy (removal of the uterus) may have to be performed. In an abdominal pregnancy, the fetus is surgically removed (except in rare cases, when the fetus survives to term or calcifies undetected in the abdominal cavity).

Supportive treatment includes transfusions of whole blood or packed red cells to replace excessive blood loss, intravenous antibiotics to treat infection, iron supplements, and a high-protein diet.

HYDATIDIFORM MOLE

What is this condition?

Hydatidiform mole is an uncommon chorionic tumor of the placenta. Its early signs — absence of menstrual periods and an enlarged uterus — mimic those of normal pregnancy; however, it eventually causes vaginal bleeding. Hydatidiform mole occurs in 1 in 1,500 to

2,000 pregnancies, most commonly in women over age 45. Incidence is highest in Asian women.

With prompt diagnosis and appropriate treatment, the prognosis is excellent. However, approximately 10% of women with this disorder develop chorionic cancer. Recurrence is possible in about 2% of cases.

What causes it?

The cause of hydatidiform mole is unknown, but death of the embryo and loss of fetal circulation seem to precede it. Despite the embryo's death, maternal circulation continues to nourish the trophoblast (tissue surrounding the embryo), but loss of fetal circulation causes abnormal fluid buildup within the villi. This converts some or all of the chorionic villi into a mass of clear vesicles, resembling a bunch of grapes.

What are its symptoms?

The early stages of this type of pregnancy typically seem normal, except that the uterus grows more rapidly than usual. The first obvious signs of trouble — absence of fetal heart tones, vaginal bleeding (ranging from spotting to hemorrhage), and lower abdominal cramps — mimic those of a miscarriage. The blood may contain hydatid vesicles; excessive vomiting is likely, and signs and symptoms of preeclampsia are possible. Other possible complications of hydatidiform mole include anemia, infection, miscarriage, uterine rupture, and choriocarcinoma.

How is it diagnosed?

Persistent bleeding and an abnormally enlarged uterus suggest hydatidiform mole. Diagnosis is based on the passage of hydatid vesicles, which allows microscopic confirmation. Without identification of hydatid vesicles, it's difficult to differentiate hydatidiform mole from other complications of pregnancy, particularly an impending miscarriage. Confirmation of hydatidiform mole requires a dilatation and curettage (called a *D & C*).

The diagnosis may also be supported by ultrasound studies, a pregnancy test, arteriography, chest X-ray (to rule out types of cancer), and other lab tests.

Types of hysterectomy

Surgeons perform three types of hysterectomy. The removed portion, shaded in the illustrations below, varies in each one. In each, though, the surgeon leaves the external genitals and vagina intact, enabling a woman to resume sexual relations.

Subtotal hysterectomy
This surgery removes all but the farthest portion of the uterus.

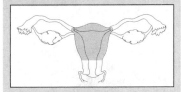

Total hysterectomy
The entire uterus and cervix are removed, and the woman will no longer menstruate.

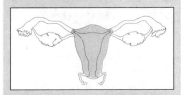

Total hysterectomy with salpingo-oophorectomy
All reproductive organs are removed, and the woman will no longer menstruate.

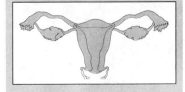

SELF-HELP

Advice for women following hydatidiform mole

After you've had surgery for this disorder, do the following.

Prevent further problems
- Promptly report any new symptoms — for example, a cough or coughing up of blood, suspected pregnancy, nausea, vomiting, or vaginal bleeding.
- Get regular follow-up checkups to help detect possible cancerous changes early.

Promote healing
Be sure to use contraceptives to prevent pregnancy for at least 1 year after your hormone levels return to normal and your regular ovulation and menstrual cycles are reestablished.

How is it treated?

Hydatidiform mole requires uterine evacuation by D & C, abdominal hysterectomy, or instrument or suction curettage, depending on the size of the uterus. (See *Types of hysterectomy*, page 399.) Intravenous Pitocin may be used to promote uterine contractions. Because this drug may act as an antidiuretic, the woman must be observed for respiratory complications.

Postoperative treatment varies, depending on the amount of blood lost and complications. If no complications develop, hospitalization is usually brief and normal activities can be resumed quickly.

Because of the possibility of choriocarcinoma developing after hydatidiform mole, scrupulous follow-up care is essential. Such care includes monitoring human chorionic gonadotropin levels until they return to normal and taking chest X-rays to check for cancer spread to the lungs. Another pregnancy should be postponed until at least 1 year after hormone levels return to normal. (See *Advice for women following hydatidiform mole.*)

MISCARRIAGE

What do doctors call this condition?

Spontaneous abortion

What is this condition?

A miscarriage refers to the spontaneous expulsion of the fetus from the uterus before the fetus can survive on its own. Up to 15% of all pregnancies and approximately 30% of first pregnancies end in miscarriage. At least 75% of miscarriages occur during the first trimester.

What causes it?

Miscarriage may result from fetal, placental, or maternal factors. *Fetal factors*, which usually cause miscarriage at 9 to 12 weeks' gestation, include defective development of the embryo due to abnormal chromosome division (most common cause of fetal death), faulty implantation of the fertilized ovum (egg), and failure of the endometrium to accept the fertilized ovum.

Placental factors usually cause miscarriage around the 14th week, when the placenta takes over the hormone production necessary to maintain the pregnancy. These factors include premature separation of the normally implanted placenta and abnormal placental implantation.

Maternal factors, which usually cause miscarriage between the 11th and 19th weeks, include a long list:

- maternal infection, severe malnutrition, drug ingestion, abnormalities of the reproductive organs (especially an incompetent cervix, in which the cervix dilates painlessly and bloodlessly in the second trimester)
- endocrine problems, such as a thyroid disorder
- trauma, including surgery involving the pelvic organs
- certain immune disorders or blood group incompatibility.

What are its symptoms?

Signs of an impending miscarriage may include a pink discharge for several days or a scant brown discharge for several weeks before the onset of cramps and increased vaginal bleeding. For a few hours, the cramps intensify and occur more frequently; then the cervix dilates to expel uterine contents. If expulsion is complete, cramps and bleeding subside. However, if any contents remain, cramps and bleeding continue.

How is it diagnosed?

Diagnosis of miscarriage is based on clinical evidence of expulsion of uterine contents, a pelvic exam, and lab studies. Decreased levels of human chorionic gonadotropin, a hormone that is present in the blood or urine during pregnancy, suggest miscarriage. A pelvic exam determines the size of the uterus and whether this size is consistent with the length of the pregnancy. Microscopic exam reveals evidence of products of conception. Lab tests reflect decreased hematocrit and hemoglobin levels due to blood loss.

How is it treated?

Uterine contents must be carefully examined before a treatment plan can be formulated. A miscarriage can't be prevented, except when the cause is an incompetent cervix. If bleeding is severe, the woman must be hospitalized and receive a blood transfusion. Initially, intravenous Pitocin stimulates uterine contractions. If any remnants remain in the uterus, dilatation and curettage (called a *D & C*) or dilatation and evacuation (called a *D & E*) should be performed.

STRAIGHT TALK

Questions women ask about pregnancy after miscarriage

I just had a miscarriage. What are my chances of having another one?

If this was your first miscarriage, your chances of having another one are no greater than any other woman's. If you've had two or more miscarriages or a late miscarriage (after 13 weeks of pregnancy), you may be more likely to have another one. Discuss your concerns with your doctor before becoming pregnant again.

Should I have any tests before getting pregnant again?

Unfortunately, no test can predict whether you'll have another miscarriage. However, if your doctor can test the tissues expelled in this miscarriage, he or she may be able to determine why you miscarried.

How soon can I try to get pregnant again?

Most experts advise waiting between 3 and 6 months because your body needs time to heal and get back to normal. Consider practicing birth control for a time. Your first and second menstrual periods may be a little late. If you don't have a period for 8 weeks, schedule a check-up with your doctor.

Advice for women following a miscarriage

Here are some points to help you recover from this traumatic event.

Communicating
- You and your partner should express your feelings about the miscarriage.
- See your doctor in 2 to 4 weeks for a follow-up exam.
- If this isn't your first miscarriage, you and your partner should get physical exams and possibly genetic counseling.

Watching for symptoms
- Vaginal bleeding or spotting will occur. Report any bleeding lasting longer than 10 days or excessive, bright-red blood. Also watch for signs of infection, such as fever above 100° F (37.8° C) and vaginal discharges.
- Avoid using tampons for 1 to 2 weeks.

Resuming daily activities
Step up daily activities, but avoid increasing vaginal bleeding or fatigue.

Resuming your sex life
Avoid sex for 1 to 2 weeks; then use a contraceptive. Wait two or three normal menstrual cycles after a miscarriage before trying to conceive.

A woman who's had several miscarriages because of an incompetent cervix may have it surgically reinforced 14 to 16 weeks after the last menstrual period. A few weeks before the estimated delivery date, the sutures are removed and the woman awaits the onset of labor. An alternative procedure, especially for a woman who wants to have more children, is to leave the sutures in place and to deliver the infant by cesarean section. (See *Questions women ask about pregnancy after miscarriage,* page 401, and *Advice for women following a miscarriage.*)

PLACENTAL SEPARATION

What do doctors call this condition?
Abruptio placentae

What is this condition?
In this condition, the placenta separates from the uterine wall prematurely, usually after the 20th week of gestation, producing hemorrhage. This separation, a common cause of bleeding during the second half of pregnancy, occurs most often in women over age 35 who've had multiple pregnancies.

The prognosis for the fetus depends on gestational age and amount of blood lost; the mother's prognosis is good if hemorrhage can be controlled. A firm diagnosis in the presence of heavy maternal bleeding generally requires termination of pregnancy.

What causes it?
The cause of placental separation is unknown. Predisposing factors include trauma (such as a direct blow to the uterus or bleeding due to needle puncture of the placenta during amniocentesis), chronic or pregnancy-induced high blood pressure, having more than five children, short umbilical cord, dietary deficiency, smoking, advanced maternal age, and pressure on the vena cava from an enlarged uterus.

In placental separation, blood vessels at the placental bed rupture spontaneously because of a lack of resiliency or abnormal changes in uterine vasculature. High blood pressure complicates the situation, as does an enlarged uterus, which can't contract enough to seal off the torn vessels. Consequently, bleeding continues unchecked, possibly shearing off the placenta partially or completely.

What are its symptoms?

Placental separation produces a wide range of symptoms, depending on the extent of placental separation and the amount of blood that the mother loses.

Mild placental separation (marginal separation) develops gradually and produces mild to moderate bleeding, vague lower abdominal discomfort, mild to moderate abdominal tenderness, and uterine irritability. Fetal heart tones remain strong and regular.

Moderate placental separation (about 50% placental separation) may develop gradually or abruptly and produces continuous abdominal pain, moderate dark red vaginal bleeding, a tender uterus that remains firm between contractions, barely audible or irregular and slowed fetal heart tones and, possibly, signs of shock. Labor usually starts within 2 hours and often proceeds rapidly.

Severe placental separation (70% placental separation) develops abruptly and causes agonizing, unremitting uterine pain (described as tearing or knifelike); a boardlike, tender uterus; moderate vaginal bleeding; rapidly progressive shock; and absence of fetal heart tones. (See *Degrees of placental separation.*)

In addition to hemorrhage and shock, other complications may include kidney failure and disseminated intravascular coagulation. Death of the mother and fetus may result.

How is it diagnosed?

Diagnostic measures for placental separation include observation of signs and symptoms, a pelvic exam, and ultrasound. Decreased hemoglobin and platelet counts support the diagnosis.

How is it treated?

Treatment of placental separation is designed to assess, control, and restore the amount of blood lost; to deliver a viable infant; and to prevent blood clotting disorders. Immediate measures include starting an intravenous infusion of appropriate fluids to offset fluid losses, monitoring fluid status, various blood studies, electronic fetal monitoring, and monitoring of maternal vital signs and vaginal bleeding.

After these measures, prompt delivery by cesarean section is necessary if the fetus is in distress. If the fetus is not in distress, monitoring continues; delivery is usually performed at the first sign of fetal distress.

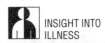

INSIGHT INTO ILLNESS

Degrees of placental separation

Mild separation

Here, bleeding develops between the placenta and uterine wall.

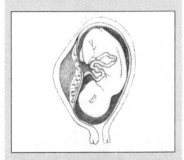

Moderate separation

Here, hemorrhage occurs through the vagina.

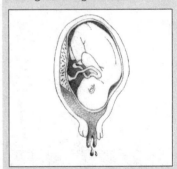

Severe separation

Here, hemorrhage also occurs.

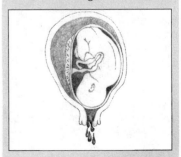

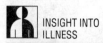

INSIGHT INTO
ILLNESS

Three types of placenta previa

In *low marginal implantation,* a small placental edge can be felt through the internal os (which opens into the cervical canal).

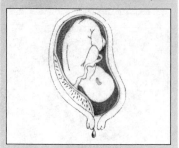

In *partial placenta previa,* the placenta partially caps the internal os.

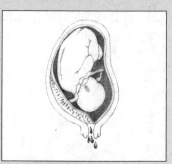

In *total placenta previa,* the internal os is covered entirely.

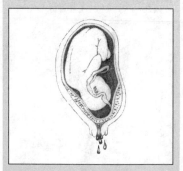

PLACENTA PREVIA

What is this condition?

In placenta previa, the placenta is implanted in the lower uterine segment, where it encroaches on the internal cervical os. This disorder, one of the most common causes of bleeding during the second half of pregnancy, occurs in approximately 1 in 200 pregnancies, more commonly in women who've had several children already.

Generally, termination of pregnancy is necessary when placenta previa is accompanied by heavy maternal bleeding. The mother's prognosis is good if hemorrhage can be controlled; the fetus's prognosis depends on gestational age and the amount of blood lost.

What causes it?

Although the specific cause of placenta previa is unknown, factors that may affect the site of the placenta's attachment to the uterine wall include early or late fertilization, receptivity and adequacy of the uterine lining, multiple pregnancy, previous uterine surgery, and advanced maternal age.

The placenta may cover all (total, complete, or central), part (partial or incomplete), or a fraction (marginal or low-lying) of the internal cervical opening. The degree of placenta previa depends largely on the extent of cervical dilation at the time of examination, because the dilating cervix gradually uncovers the placenta. (See *Three types of placenta previa.*)

What are its symptoms?

Placenta previa usually produces painless bleeding in the third trimester (often the first complaint). Although the fetus's head does not descend properly, the fetus remains active and has good heart tones. Complications of placenta previa include shock and maternal or fetal death.

How is it diagnosed?

Diagnostic measures include ultrasound scanning to determine the placenta's position and a pelvic exam performed immediately before delivery to confirm the diagnosis.

Supportive findings include:
- minimal descent of the fetal presenting part
- decreased hemoglobin levels due to blood loss

- various ultrasound studies to locate the placenta (X-ray studies, which are riskier, may be done only when ultrasound is unavailable).

How is it treated?

Treatment of placenta previa is designed to assess, control, and restore the amount of blood lost; to deliver a viable infant; and to prevent blood clotting disorders. Immediate measures include starting an intravenous infusion of appropriate fluids, performing various blood studies, initiating electronic fetal monitoring, monitoring maternal vital signs, and assessing the amount of vaginal bleeding.

After these measures, if the fetus is premature, it must be observed carefully to allow more time to mature. If clinical evaluation confirms complete placenta previa, the woman is usually hospitalized because of the increased risk of bleeding. As soon as the fetus is sufficiently mature, or if severe bleeding occurs, immediate delivery by cesarean section may be necessary. Vaginal delivery is considered only when the bleeding is minimal and the placenta previa is marginal, or when labor is rapid.

PREGNANCY-INDUCED HIGH BLOOD PRESSURE

What do doctors call this condition?

Toxemia of pregnancy, preeclampsia, eclampsia

What is this condition?

Pregnancy-induced high blood pressure, a potentially life-threatening disorder, usually develops late in the second or third trimester. *Preeclampsia,* the nonconvulsive form of the disorder, develops in about 7% of pregnancies. It may be mild or severe and is more common in low socioeconomic groups. *Eclampsia,* the convulsive form, affects about 5% of women with preeclampsia; of these, about 15% die from toxemia itself or its complications. The fetal mortality rate is high because of the increased incidence of premature delivery.

What causes it?

The cause of pregnancy-induced high blood pressure is unknown, but it appears to be related to inadequate prenatal care (especially poor nutrition), first pregnancies, multiple pregnancies, and preexisting diabetes or high blood pressure. Age is also a factor: Adolescents and women having their first child over age 35 are at higher risk for preeclampsia.

What are its symptoms?

Mild preeclampsia generally produces high blood pressure, excessive proteins in the urine, generalized swelling, and weight gain of more than 3 pounds (1.36 kilograms) per week during the second trimester or more than 1 pound (0.45 kilogram) per week during the third trimester.

Severe preeclampsia is marked by more pronounced high blood pressure and even higher levels of protein in the urine, eventually leading to decreased urine output. Hemolysis, elevated liver enzymes, and a low platelet count (the HELLP syndrome) are often present in severe preeclampsia. Other symptoms that may indicate worsening preeclampsia include blurred vision, stomach pain or heartburn, irritability, emotional tension, and a severe frontal headache.

In eclampsia, all the symptoms of preeclampsia are magnified and are associated with seizures and, possibly, coma, premature labor, stillbirth, kidney failure, and liver damage.

How is it diagnosed?

The following findings suggest mild preeclampsia:
- high blood pressure (140 systolic, or an increase of 30 or more points above the woman's normal systolic pressure, measured on two occasions 6 hours apart; 90 diastolic, or an increase of 15 or more points above the woman's normal diastolic pressure, measured on two occasions 6 hours apart)
- urine protein levels higher than 500 milligrams per 24 hours.

These findings suggest severe preeclampsia:
- higher blood pressure readings (160/110 or higher on two occasions 6 hours apart) while the woman is on bed rest
- urine protein levels of 5 grams or more per 24 hours
- urine output less than or equal to 400 milliliters per 24 hours
- possibly hyperactive deep tendon reflexes.

The presence of seizures along with typical symptoms of severe preeclampsia strongly suggests eclampsia.

SELF-HELP

Making the most of bed rest

Your doctor has prescribed bed rest to help control your blood pressure. Bed rest may prevent your heart from beating faster. If your heart rate slows down, less blood will be pumped into your arteries. This may keep your blood pressure stable.

As long as your high blood pressure remains mild, you can manage it at home. But if you don't get better in 3 or 4 days, the doctor will probably admit you to the hospital. That way, you'll be sure to get the proper rest and care.

Most important: Stay in bed

Bed rest means lying quietly in a darkened room with as little stimulation as possible. You should lie on your left side to help increase the blood flow to your baby. Leave your bed only to go to the bathroom.

Get help

Ask your family and friends to help by preparing meals, doing the laundry, shopping, and cleaning. If no help is available, ask the doctor or nurse to help you arrange for a home health care aide or volunteer.

If you have young children, ask a family member or friend to babysit or, better yet, to keep them for several days. This can be an exciting experience for children if they view it as a "vacation."

Do what you can

Staying in bed doesn't mean you can't do anything. You can still plan meals, balance your checkbook, pay bills, read, or watch television. Any activity is fine, as long as you lie in bed and the activity doesn't cause excitement or stress.

The bottom line

Staying in bed is hard when you're used to being active and when you have a house and family that need attention. But it's worth it. Following your doctor's orders will help you deliver a healthy baby and will keep you healthy, too.

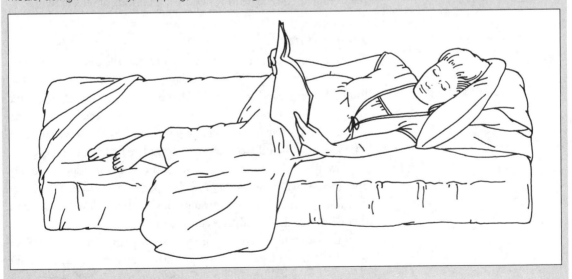

STRAIGHT TALK

Questions pregnant women ask about treating high blood pressure

I've always been active, but now my doctor says I can't exercise. Why not?

Most pregnant women with high blood pressure are advised to restrict activities; some are even ordered to stay in bed. That's because exercise increases your heart rate, causing it to pump more and more blood into your arteries and circulatory system. This increased force causes your blood pressure to rise even higher.

Why do I have to cut back on salty foods?

Large amounts of salt absorbed into your blood can cause your kidneys to retain water. When this happens, the blood exerts more force against the artery walls and your blood pressure increases. Besides re-

ducing your salt intake, try to eat a well-balanced diet that's high in protein (including meat, fish, poultry, eggs, milk, cheese, and nuts).

I've been resting at home, but now my doctor says I have to go to the hospital. Why?

Obviously, your doctor has decided that conservative treatment isn't working and that your condition is progressing to a more serious stage. This can affect your health and your baby's life.

By admitting you to the hospital, the doctor can monitor your baby's health and your blood pressure, diet, and activity much more closely. You can also receive medication to help you relax, lower your blood pressure, and reduce the likelihood of seizures.

During the crisis, real-time ultrasound and stress and nonstress tests evaluate the fetus's well-being. Electronic monitoring reveals stable or increased fetal heart tones during periods of fetal activity.

How is it treated?

Treatment of preeclampsia is designed to halt the disorder's progress, to prevent the early effects of eclampsia — seizures, residual high blood pressure, and kidney shutdown — and to ensure the fetus's survival. Some doctors induce labor promptly, especially if the woman is near term, whereas others follow a more conservative approach. Therapy may include sedatives and complete bed rest to relieve anxiety, lower blood pressure, and evaluate the woman's response to therapy. (See *Making the most of bed rest,* page 407.) If the kidneys are working normally, a high-protein, low-sodium, low-carbohydrate diet with increased fluids is recommended.

If the woman's blood pressure persistently rises above 160/100 despite bed rest and sedatives, or if central nervous system irritability increases, magnesium sulfate may be given to produce general sedation, promote urine excretion, reduce blood pressure, and prevent seizures. If the woman's condition doesn't improve, or if the fetus's life is endangered, cesarean section or induction of labor may be required to terminate the pregnancy.

Emergency treatment of eclamptic seizures consists of immediate intravenous administration of Valium followed by magnesium sulfate, oxygen administration, and electronic fetal monitoring. After the woman's condition stabilizes, a cesarean section may be performed. (See *Questions pregnant women ask about treating high blood pressure.*)

PREMATURE LABOR

What is this condition?

Premature labor is the onset of rhythmic uterine contractions that produce cervical changes (dilation and effacement) after fetal viability but before fetal maturity. It usually occurs between the 26th and 37th week of gestation. Approximately 5% to 10% of pregnancies end in premature labor, which is responsible for about 75% of newborn deaths and many birth defects.

What causes it?

Possible causes of premature labor may include "breaking water," or premature rupture of the membranes (occurs in 30% to 50% of cases), preeclampsia, chronic hypertensive vascular disease, excessive amniotic fluid, multiple pregnancy, placenta previa, placental separation, incompetent cervix, abdominal surgery, trauma, structural anomalies of the uterus, infections (such as German measles or toxoplasmosis), congenital adrenal hyperplasia, and death of the fetus.

Other important predisposing factors include:

- *Fetal stimulation:* Genetically imprinted information tells the fetus that nutrition is inadequate and that a change in environment is required for its well-being; this provokes labor.
- *Progesterone deficiency:* Decreased placental production of progesterone — thought to be the hormone that maintains pregnancy — triggers labor.
- *Oxytocin sensitivity:* Labor begins because the myometrium becomes hypersensitive to oxytocin, the hormone that normally induces uterine contractions.

Approximately 5% to 10% of pregnancies end prematurely. Premature labor accounts for about 75% of newborn deaths and many birth defects.

- *Myometrial oxygen deficiency:* The fetus becomes increasingly proficient in obtaining oxygen, depriving the myometrium of the oxygen and energy it needs to function normally, thus making the myometrium irritable.
- *Maternal genetics:* A genetic defect in the mother shortens gestation and precipitates premature labor.

What are its symptoms?

Like labor at term, premature labor produces rhythmic uterine contractions, cervical dilation and effacement, possible rupture of the membranes, expulsion of the cervical mucus plug, and a bloody discharge.

How is it diagnosed?

Premature labor is confirmed by the combined results of a prenatal history, a physical exam, signs and symptoms, and ultrasound (if available) showing the position of the fetus in relation to the mother's pelvis. A vaginal exam confirms progressive cervical effacement and dilation.

How is it treated?

Treatment is designed to suppress premature labor when tests show immature fetal lung development, cervical dilation of less than 1.5 inches (4 centimeters), and the absence of any factors that would prevent continuation of the pregnancy. Measures consist of bed rest and, when necessary, drug therapy.

Beta-adrenergic stimulants, such as Bricanyl, Vasodilan, or Yutopar, inhibit uterine contractions. Side effects include rapid heart rate (mother and fetus) and high blood pressure (mother). Magnesium sulfate relaxes the uterine muscle and may produce side effects in the mother, such as drowsiness, slurred speech, flushing, decreased reflexes, gastrointestinal symptoms, and a slow respiratory rate. Side effects in the fetus or newborn may include central nervous system depression, decreased respiratory rate, and decreased sucking reflex.

Maternal factors that jeopardize the fetus and make premature delivery the preferred choice include intrauterine infection, placental separation, placental insufficiency, and severe preeclampsia. Among the fetal problems that become more dangerous as pregnancy nears term are severe isoimmunization and congenital anomalies.

Treatment and delivery require intensive team effort, focusing on:
- continuously assessing the infant's health through fetal monitoring
- avoiding amniotomy (surgical rupture of fetal membranes), if possible, to prevent cord prolapse or damage to the infant's tender skull
- maintaining adequate hydration through I.V. fluids
- avoiding sedatives and narcotics that might harm the infant. Morphine or Demerol may be required to minimize pain; these drugs have little effect on uterine contractions but depress central nervous system function and may cause fetal respiratory depression. They should be administered in the smallest dose possible and only when extremely necessary.

Preventing premature labor requires good prenatal care, adequate nutrition, and proper rest. A procedure that reinforces an incompetent cervix may be done at 14 to 18 weeks' gestation to help prevent premature labor in women with a history of this disorder.

*P*REMATURE RUPTURE OF THE MEMBRANES

What is this condition?

Premature rupture of the membranes ("breaking water") is a spontaneous break or tear in the amniochorial sac before onset of regular contractions, resulting in progressive cervical dilation. This condition occurs in nearly 10% of all pregnancies over 20 weeks' gestation. Labor usually starts within 24 hours after the membranes rupture, and more than 80% of these infants are mature.

The latent period (between membrane rupture and onset of labor) is generally brief when the membranes rupture near term; when the infant is premature, this period is prolonged, which increases the risk of death from maternal infection and fetal infection.

What causes it?

Although the cause of this condition is unknown, malpresentation and a contracted pelvis commonly accompany the rupture. Predisposing factors may include:
- poor nutrition and hygiene and lack of proper prenatal care
- incompetent cervix (perhaps as a result of abortions)

Premature rupture of the membranes occurs in nearly 10% of all pregnancies over 20 weeks' gestation. Labor usually starts within 24 hours, and more than 80% of these infants are mature.

- increased intrauterine tension due to excessive amniotic fluid or multiple pregnancies
- defects in the amniochorial membranes' tensile strength
- uterine infection.

What are its symptoms?

Typically, premature rupture of the membranes causes blood-tinged amniotic fluid to leak or gush from the vagina. Maternal fever, fetal rapid heart rate, and a foul-smelling vaginal discharge indicate infection.

How is it diagnosed?

Characteristic passage of amniotic fluid confirms this condition. A physical exam shows amniotic fluid in the vagina. Examination of this fluid helps determine appropriate management. The physical exam also determines the presence of multiple pregnancies, and helps determine fetal presentation and size.

How is it treated?

Treatment of this condition depends on fetal age and the risk of infection. In a term pregnancy, if spontaneous labor and vaginal delivery don't occur within a relatively short time (usually within 24 hours after the membranes rupture), the doctor usually tries to induce labor; if induction fails, cesarean delivery is usually necessary. Cesarean hysterectomy is recommended for women with a severe uterine infection.

Management of a preterm pregnancy of less than 34 weeks is controversial. However, with advances in technology, a conservative approach has now proved effective. In a preterm pregnancy of 28 to 34 weeks, treatment includes hospitalization and observation of the mother and fetus for signs of infection while awaiting fetal maturation. If tests confirm infection, labor must be induced, followed by intravenous administration of antibiotics. The newborn may also require antibiotics.

What can a woman with premature rupture of the membranes do?

If you think your membranes have ruptured, call your doctor right away. Don't use a douche or have sexual intercourse.

11

SEXUAL DISORDERS

AROUSAL AND ORGASMIC DISORDERS

What are these conditions?

Arousal and orgasmic disorders are disorders of female sexual function. A woman with *arousal disorder* can't experience sexual pleasure because she can't reach or maintain the physical responses of sexual excitement — vaginal lubrication, blood vessel congestion in the genital area, and swelling of external genitalia. In *orgasmic disorder*, the woman becomes sexually excited but can't reach orgasm or has a delayed orgasm. These problems are considered disorders only if they persist or recur.

The prognosis is good when these disorders are temporary or mild and result from misinformation or stress. However, when they're caused by intense anxiety, relationship problems, psychological disturbances, or drug or alcohol abuse in either partner, the prognosis is less certain.

What causes them?

Any of the following factors, alone or in combination, may cause arousal or orgasmic disorder:

- drugs (central nervous system depressants, alcohol, street drugs and, rarely, oral contraceptives)
- disease (illness of the body as a whole, endocrine or nervous system diseases, or diseases that impair muscle tone or muscle contraction)
- gynecologic factors (chronic vaginal or pelvic infection or pain, congenital abnormalities, and genital cancers)
- psychological factors (performance anxiety, guilt, depression, or subconscious conflicts about sexuality)
- relationship problems (poor communication, hostility toward the partner, fear of abandonment, or boredom with sex)
- stress and fatigue.

What are their symptoms?

The woman with an arousal disorder has slight sexual desire and responds poorly to stimulation. Typically, she lacks vaginal lubrication and signs of congested blood vessels in the genital area.

In an orgasmic disorder, the main symptom is an inability to achieve an orgasm, either totally or under certain circumstances. Many women experience orgasm through masturbation or other means but not through intercourse alone. Others achieve orgasm with some partners but not with others.

How are they diagnosed?

To rule out physical causes of arousal or orgasmic disorders, the doctor performs a thorough physical exam, orders lab tests, and takes a medical history. When physical causes are absent, a complete psychosexual history is the most important tool. (See *What the therapist will ask about arousal or orgasmic disorder.*)

How are they treated?

An arousal disorder is hard to treat, especially if the woman has never experienced sexual pleasure. Therapy aims to help her relax and become aware of her feelings about sex, as well as to eliminate guilt and fear of rejection. Specific measures usually include *sensate focus exercises,* which emphasize touching and awareness of sensual feelings all over the body — not just in the genital area — and minimize the importance of intercourse and orgasm.

In orgasmic disorder, the goal is to help the woman overcome her inhibition of the orgasmic reflex. Treatment may include experiential therapy, psychoanalysis, or behavior modification. The therapist may teach the woman self-stimulation and distraction techniques, such as focusing attention on fantasies, breathing patterns, or muscle contractions to relieve anxiety. Gradually, the therapist involves the woman's sexual partner in the treatment sessions; some therapists treat the couple as a unit from the outset.

What can a woman with arousal or orgasmic disorder do?

Consult a doctor, nurse, psychologist, social worker, or counselor trained in sex therapy. The therapist should be certified by the American Association of Sex Educators, Counselors, and Therapists or by the Society for Sex Therapy and Research. If not, ask about the therapist's credentials.

CHANCROID

What do doctors call this condition?

Soft chancre

What is this condition?

Chancroid is a sexually transmitted disease marked by painful genital ulcers and swollen, possibly ulcerated, lymph nodes in the groin area.

What the therapist will ask about arousal or orgasmic disorder

To find the cause of either of these disorders, the therapist takes the woman's psychosexual history. Typically, the therapist will ask about the following subjects.

Sex education
- The woman's level of sex education and previous sexual response patterns
- Her contraceptive practices and reproductive goals

Attitude about sex
- The woman's feelings during childhood and adolescence about sex in general and, specifically, about masturbation, incest, rape, sexual fantasies, and homosexual or heterosexual practices
- Her level of family stress or fatigue
- Her present relationship, including her partner's attitude toward sex

Psychological health
- The woman's self-esteem and body image
- Any history of psychotherapy

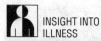

INSIGHT INTO
ILLNESS

What a chancroidal lesion looks like

Chancroid produces a soft, painful sore called a *chancre*, similar to that of syphilis. If the disease isn't treated, buboes — large, inflamed lymph glands — may form and the lymph glands at the top of the thigh may become inflamed.

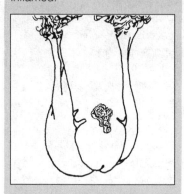

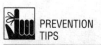

PREVENTION
TIPS

Avoiding chancroid

Protect yourself by following these three tips:
- Don't have sex with an infected person.
- Use condoms during sexual activity.
- Wash your genital area with soap and water after sex.

This infection occurs worldwide but is most common in tropical countries. It affects men more often than women.

Chancroidal ulcers may heal by themselves and usually respond well to treatment if there are no secondary infections. A high rate of HIV infection has been reported among people with chancroid.

What causes it?

Chancroid is caused by a bacterium and is transmitted through sexual contact. Poor hygiene may predispose men — especially those who are uncircumcised — to this disease.

What are its symptoms?

After a 3- to 5-day incubation period, a small pimple erupts at the site of entry, usually the groin or inner thigh; in men, it may appear on the penis; in women, on the vulva, vagina, or cervix. Occasionally, it may erupt on the tongue, lip, breast, or navel. The pimple rapidly breaks out into an ulcer, becoming painful, soft, and foul-smelling; it bleeds easily and produces pus. It's gray and shallow, with irregular edges, and measures up to 1 inch (2.5 centimeters) in diameter. (See *What a chancroidal lesion looks like.*)

Within 2 to 3 weeks, lymph nodes in the groin area become swollen, creating pus-filled, inflamed nodes that may rupture into large ulcers or buboes. Headache and malaise occur in 50% of people with chancroid. During the healing stage, phimosis (narrowed orifice of the foreskin) may develop.

How is it diagnosed?

Lab tests provide evidence of the disease but are not 100% reliable. A biopsy (removal and analysis of tissue) confirms the diagnosis but is reserved for resistant cases or cases in which cancer is suspected. Additional tests may be performed to rule out other sexually transmitted diseases that cause similar ulcers. Testing for HIV infection should be done at the time of diagnosis.

How is it treated?

The treatment of choice includes the following drugs: Zithromax, E-mycin, or Rocephin. The safety of Zithromax for pregnant or breast-feeding women has not been established. Aspiration of fluid-filled nodes helps prevent spreading the infection.

What can a person with chancroid do?

Don't apply lotions, creams, or oils on or near your genitalia or on other lesion sites. Avoid sexual contact until healing is complete (usually about 2 weeks after treatment begins). Wash your genitalia daily with soap and water. If you're an uncircumcised man, you should retract the foreskin for thorough cleaning. (See *Avoiding chancroid.*)

CHLAMYDIAL INFECTIONS

What are these conditions?

Chlamydial infections — including urethritis in men and urethritis and cervicitis in women — comprise a group of infections linked to one bacteria: *Chlamydia trachomatis.* These infections are the most common sexually transmitted diseases in the North America, affecting more than 4 million people each year.

Untreated chlamydial infections can lead to such complications as acute inflammation of the epididymis (in men) and of the fallopian tubes (in women), pelvic inflammatory disease and, eventually, sterility.

What causes them?

Transmission of *C. trachomatis* bacteria primarily follows vaginal or rectal intercourse or oral-genital contact with an infected person. Because symptoms commonly appear late in the course of the disease, transmission usually occurs unknowingly.

Children born of mothers who have chlamydial infections may contract associated conjunctivitis, ear infections, and pneumonia during passage through the birth canal.

What are their symptoms?

Both men and women with chlamydial infections may have no symptoms or may show signs of infection during the physical exam. Individual signs and symptoms vary with the specific type of chlamydial infection. (See *Symptoms of chlamydial infection.*)

How are they diagnosed?

Lab tests provide a definite diagnosis of chlamydial infection. A swab culture from the site of infection (urethra, cervix, or rectum) estab-

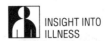
INSIGHT INTO ILLNESS

Symptoms of chlamydial infection

Chlamydial infection may cause inflammation of various parts of the body. Symptoms vary with the location of the infection.

Cervix
Cervical erosion, vaginal discharge containing mucus and pus, pelvic pain, pain during intercourse

Fallopian tubes or uterus
Pain and tenderness of the abdomen, cervix, uterus, and lymph nodes; chills; fever; breakthrough bleeding; bleeding after intercourse; vaginal discharge; pain when urinating

Urethra
Frequent, painful urination; redness, tenderness, discharge, and itching of the urinary opening of the penis

Epididymis
Painful swelling of the scrotum, discharge from the penis

Prostate
Lower back pain, frequent and painful urination, nighttime urination, painful ejaculation

Rectum and anus
Diarrhea, rectal spasms, anal itching, ulcers in the colon, rectal discharge containing blood, mucus, or pus

SELF-HELP

Advice for a person with a chlamydial infection

If you've been diagnosed with chlamydia, consider the following.

Comply with treatment

Make sure you understand the prescribed medication regimen. Complete the entire course of drug therapy even after your symptoms subside.

Keep clean

- To prevent reinfection during treatment, abstain from sexual intercourse until you and your partner are cured.
- Practice meticulous personal hygiene. To prevent contaminating your eyes, avoid touching any discharge, and wash and dry your hands thoroughly before touching your eyes.

Spread the word

Inform sexual contacts of your infection so they can receive appropriate treatment.

Follow up

- Return to the doctor for follow-up testing.
- Consider getting tested for HIV infection.

lishes a diagnosis of urethritis, cervicitis, salpingitis, endometritis, or proctitis.

How are they treated?

The recommended first-line treatment for adults and adolescents with a chlamydial infection is Vibramycin by mouth for 7 days or a single dose of Zithromax by mouth.

For pregnant women with a chlamydial infection, E-Mycin is the treatment of choice. (See *Advice for a person with a chlamydial infection.*)

GENITAL HERPES

What is this condition?

Genital herpes is a viral infection that causes acute inflammation of the genitalia. The first episode usually is self-limiting but may cause painful genital symptoms or even disease of the body as a whole. After the initial episode, the virus remains dormant in the body, causing recurrent outbreaks. These recurrences, which tend to be milder, may be triggered by stress, illness, and overexposure to sunlight.

What causes it?

The usual cause of genital herpes is infection with herpes simplex virus type 2. Typically, the disease spreads through sexual intercourse, oral-genital sexual activity, kissing, and hand-to-body contact. Pregnant women may pass the infection to their newborns during vaginal delivery.

What are its symptoms?

About 3 to 7 days after a person is infected with herpes simplex virus, fluid-filled blisters appear, usually on the cervix and possibly on the labia, skin around the rectum, external genitalia, or vagina of the woman and on the penis or foreskin of the man. Blisters may also appear on the mouth or anus. Usually painless at first, the blisters soon erupt into painful ulcers with yellow oozing centers. Often, the lymph glands located along the top of the thigh become tender.

During the initial infection, the person may also have fever, a general ill feeling, painful urination and, in women, a white vaginal discharge.

How is it diagnosed?

The doctor diagnoses genital herpes by examining the person and taking a history. Lab tests may show characteristic antibody and cell findings. The diagnosis is confirmed if the virus appears in fluid from blisters, or is implicated in tests that identify specific antigens.

How is it treated?

The drug Zovirax is effective against genital herpes. The doctor will prescribe oral Zovirax for people with first-time infections or frequent recurrences. Some people take it daily for prevention; used daily, it reduces the frequency of recurrences by at least 50%. People hospitalized with severe genital herpes and those with weak immune systems who have potentially life-threatening herpes infection may receive intravenous Zovirax. (See *Advice for a person with genital herpes.*)

GENITAL WARTS

What do doctors call this condition?

Venereal warts, condylomata acuminata

What is this condition?

Genital warts are projections from the skin surface called *papillomas,* marked by fibrous tissue overgrowth from the upper layers of the skin. They are uncommon before puberty and after menopause. Certain types of human papillomavirus infection have been associated with certain types of genital and cervical cancer.

What causes it?

Infection with one of the more than 60 known strains of human papillomavirus causes genital warts. The viruses are transmitted through sexual contact. Genital warts grow rapidly in the presence of heavy perspiration, poor hygiene, or pregnancy and often accompany other genital infections.

What are its symptoms?

After a 1- to 6-month incubation period (usually 2 months), genital warts develop on moist surfaces: in men, on the subpreputial sac,

SELF-HELP

Advice for a person with genital herpes

Here are some things you can do on your own:
- Get adequate rest and nutrition.
- Keep the ulcers dry.
- Avoid sexual intercourse during the active stage of the disease (while lesions are present), and use condoms during all sexual exposures. Encourage your sexual partners to be examined by a doctor.
- If you're female, get a Pap smear every 6 months.
- If you're pregnant, be aware that your newborn is at risk for infection during vaginal delivery. Talk to your doctor about cesarean delivery.
- Contact the Herpes Resource Center for support.

SELF-HELP

Advice for a person with genital warts

- Wash off the medication with soap and water 4 to 6 hours after applying it.
- Abstain from sexual intercourse or use a condom until healing is complete.
- Encourage sexual partners to be examined for human papillomavirus, HIV, and other sexually transmitted diseases.
- If you're female, get an annual Pap smear.

within the urethral meatus and, less commonly, on the penile shaft; in women, on the vulva and on vaginal and cervical walls. In both sexes, papillomas spread to the perineum and the perianal area.

These painless warts start as tiny red or pink swellings that grow, sometimes to 4 inches (10 centimeters). Typically, numerous swellings give them a cauliflower-like appearance.

How is it diagnosed?

Microscopic examination of scrapings from wart cells helps to distinguish genital warts. Applying 5% acetic acid (white vinegar) to the warts turns them white.

How is it treated?

Initial treatment must clear up any associated genital infections. Warts often disappear by themselves. Topical drug therapy with Podoben removes small warts. (Podoben should not be given to pregnant women.) Warts larger than 1 inch (2.5 centimeters) are generally removed by cauterizing or cryosurgery. There's no permanent cure for human papillomavirus. Relapses are common. (See *Advice for a person with genital warts.*)

GONORRHEA

What is this condition?

A common venereal disease that affects both sexes, gonorrhea is an infection of the genitourinary tract (especially the urethra and cervix) and, occasionally, the rectum, pharynx, and eyes. Untreated gonorrhea can spread through the blood to the joints, tendons, membranes of the spinal cord and brain, and the interior membrane lining of the heart; in women, it can also lead to chronic pelvic inflammatory disease and sterility.

After adequate treatment, the prognosis for both men and women is excellent, although reinfection is common. Gonorrhea is especially prevalent among young people (between ages 19 and 25) and people with multiple sexual partners.

What causes it?

Transmission of *Neisseria gonorrhoeae,* the organism that causes gonorrhea, almost always follows sexual contact with an infected person. Children born of infected mothers can contract neonatal gonococcal conjunctivitis as they pass through the birth canal. Children and adults with gonorrhea can get this type of conjunctivitis by touching their eyes with contaminated hands.

What are its symptoms?

Although many infected men may have no symptoms, after 3 to 6 days, some develop symptoms of urethritis, including painful urination and a pus-filled urethral discharge, with redness and swelling at the infection site. Most infected women remain symptom-free, but some develop inflammation and a greenish yellow discharge from the cervix — the most common gonorrheal symptoms in women. Other signs and symptoms vary according to the infection site. (See *Symptoms of gonorrhea.*)

Signs of neonatal conjunctivitis include swollen eyelids, conjunctival infection in both eyes, and a heavy pus-filled discharge 2 to 3 days after birth. Adult conjunctivitis, most common in men, causes conjunctival redness and swelling in one eye. Untreated gonococcal conjunctivitis can progress to blindness.

How is it diagnosed?

A culture from the infected body part usually establishes the diagnosis by isolating the organism. A lab test called a *Gram stain* supports the diagnosis and may be sufficient to confirm gonorrhea in men. A culture of scrapings from the eye confirms gonococcal conjunctivitis.

How is it treated?

For adults and adolescents, the recommended treatment for uncomplicated gonorrhea caused by *N. gonorrhoeae* is Rocephin by intramuscular injection. Treatment of concurrent chlamydial infection may require Vibramycin taken orally. A single dose of Rocephin followed by E-Mycin for 7 days is recommended for pregnant women and those allergic to penicillin. Other drugs may be used to treat complications.

Drug therapy should be continued for 24 to 48 hours after improvement begins; usually a full week of antibiotics is required, although the doctor may switch to different medications to finish treatment.

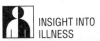 INSIGHT INTO ILLNESS

Symptoms of gonorrhea

The effects of gonorrhea depend on which body sites become infected.

Urethra
Painful urination, urinary frequency and incontinence, pus-filled discharge, itching, red and swollen urinary opening

Vulva
Occasional itching, burning, and pain due to discharge from an adjacent infected area

Vagina
Most common site in children over age 1; engorgement, redness, swelling, and profuse pus-filled discharge

Pelvis
Severe pelvic and lower abdominal pain, muscular rigidity, tenderness, and abdominal distention; as the infection spreads, nausea, vomiting, and fever possible

Liver
Pain in the upper right area of the stomach

Additional possible sites
Sore throat, inflamed tonsils, and, at the rectum, burning, itching and bloody discharge containing mucus and pus

SELF-HELP

Advice for a person with gonorrhea

Be aware that until cultures are negative, you're still infectious and can transmit gonorrhea.

In the meantime
• Inform sexual contacts of your infection so they can seek treatment, even if cultures are negative. Avoid sexual intercourse until treatment is complete.
• To prevent another episode of gonorrhea, avoid sex with anyone suspected of being infected, use condoms during intercourse, wash your genitalia with soap and water before and after intercourse, and avoid sharing washcloths or douche equipment.

Routine instillation of 1% silver nitrate or Ilotycin drops into the eyes of newborns has greatly reduced the incidence of gonococcal neonatal conjunctivitis. (See *Advice for a person with gonorrhea*.)

HYPOGONADISM

What is this condition?
Hypogonadism results from decreased androgen production in men, which may impair sperm production and cause infertility, and inhibit the development of normal secondary sex characteristics. The symptoms of androgen deficiency depend on the person's age at onset.

What causes it?
Primary (hypergonadotropic) hypogonadism results from damage to testicular structures, specifically the Leydig cells, which secrete testosterone, and the seminiferous tubules, which produce sperm. The pituitary gland responds to this damage by secreting more gonadotropins to try to maintain sperm production. Primary hypogonadism occurs in persons with Klinefelter's syndrome, Reifenstein's syndrome, Turner's syndrome, and Sertoli-cell–only syndrome.

Secondary (hypogonadotropic) hypogonadism results from impairment of a complex hormonal regulatory mechanism between the pituitary gland and hypothalamus that reduces gonadotropin secretion. Secondary hypogonadism occurs in persons with hypopituitarism, isolated follicle-stimulating hormone deficiency, isolated luteinizing hormone deficiency, Kallmann's syndrome, and Prader-Willi syndrome.

Depending on the person's age at onset, hypogonadism may cause eunuchism (complete gonadal failure) or eunuchoidism (partial failure).

What are its symptoms?
Symptoms vary with the specific cause of hypogonadism. In a child, some characteristic findings include delayed closure of the epiphyses (ends of long bones) and immature bone age; delayed puberty; infantile penis and small, soft testicles; below-average muscle development and strength; fine, sparse facial hair; scant or absent underarm, pubic, and body hair; and a high-pitched, effeminate voice. In an adult,

hypogonadism diminishes the sex drive and potency and causes regression of secondary sex characteristics.

How is it diagnosed?

An accurate diagnosis requires a detailed history, a physical exam, and hormonal studies. Chromosomal analysis may determine the specific cause. Testicular biopsy and semen analysis determine sperm production, identify impaired sperm formation, and assess low levels of testosterone.

How is it treated?

Treatment depends on the underlying cause and may consist of hormone replacement, especially with testosterone, methyltestosterone, or human chorionic gonadotropin for primary hypogonadism and with human chorionic gonadotropin alone for secondary hypogonadism. Fertility cannot be restored after permanent testicular damage. However, eunuchism resulting from pituitary-hypothalamic dysfunction can be corrected when administration of gonadotropins stimulates normal testicular function. (See *Advice for the parents of a boy with hypogonadism.*)

 SELF-HELP

Advice for the parents of a boy with hypogonadism

If your child has been diagnosed with this condition, here's how you can help.

Seek counseling
- Seek a counseling environment where you will feel comfortable expressing your feelings and concerns about your son's delayed development.
- Make every possible effort to promote your child's self-confidence.

Quiz the doctor
Make sure you and your child fully understand hormonal replacement therapy, including expected side effects, such as acne and water retention. Ask your doctor to clarify anything you don't understand.

IMPOTENCE

What is this condition?

Impotence refers to a man's inability to reach or maintain erection of the penis sufficient to complete intercourse. It's called *primary impotence* if he has never achieved a sufficient erection or *secondary impotence* if he has successfully completed intercourse in the past despite present inability. Secondary impotence is more common and less serious than primary impotence.

In response to stress, a man may have situational impotence, a temporary condition. About half of adult men probably experience temporary periods of impotence, which aren't considered dysfunctional.

Impotence affects all age-groups but becomes more common with advancing age. The prognosis depends on the severity and duration of impotence and on the underlying cause.

What a therapist will ask about impotence

To help pinpoint the cause of impotence, a therapist may ask a man these questions:

- Do you have an erection periodically? At night? In the early morning?
- Can you have an erection through sexual activities other than intercourse?
- When did the impotence start? What was your life like at that time?
- Did the problem occur suddenly or gradually?
- Are you taking any drugs?

What causes it?

Emotional and mental factors account for at least half of all cases of impotence; physical factors account for the rest. In some men, all of these factors coexist, so it's hard to isolate the main cause.

Emotional and mental causes fall into two main categories. *Personal sexual anxieties* generally involve guilt, fear, depression, or feelings of inadequacy resulting from previous traumatic sexual experience, rejection by parents or peers, exaggerated religious orthodoxy, incest, or homosexual experiences. *Interpersonal sexual anxieties* reflect a disturbed sexual relationship and may stem from differences in sexual preferences between partners, lack of communication, ignorance of sexual function, or nonsexual personal conflicts.

Physical causes of impotence include chronic diseases, such as heart and lung disease, diabetes, MS, or kidney failure; spinal cord injury; complications of surgery; drug or alcohol use; and genital or central nervous system defects.

What are its symptoms?

The man with partial impotence can't achieve a full erection. The man with intermittent impotence sometimes is potent with the same partner. The man with selective impotence is potent only with certain women.

Some men become impotent suddenly; others, gradually. If the underlying cause isn't physical, the man may still be able to achieve an erection through masturbation.

When impotence stems from emotional or mental factors, the man may experience anxiety, sweating, and palpitations, or he may lose interest in sex. He may also suffer extreme depression (this may cause the impotence or result from it).

How is it diagnosed?

Typically, the health care professional takes a detailed sexual history to help distinguish between physical and nonphysical factors that may be causing impotence. (See *What a therapist will ask about impotence.*) The health care provider also must rule out other disorders, such as diabetes and problems involving the blood vessels, nervous system, or urinary and genital structures.

How is it treated?

Sex therapy, which should include both partners, may cure impotence stemming from emotional or mental factors. This type of therapy usually includes exercises that restrict the couple's sexual activity while encouraging foreplay. It also includes improving verbal communication skills, eliminating unreasonable guilt, and reevaluating attitudes toward sex and sexual roles.

When impotence results from physical factors, treatment aims to reverse the underlying cause, if possible. If it can't be reversed, psychological counseling may help the couple deal realistically with their situation and explore alternatives for sexual expression. Some men who are physically impotent may benefit from penile implants.

MALE INFERTILITY

What is this condition?
Male infertility — inability of a man to reproduce — is suspected whenever a couple fails to achieve pregnancy after about 1 year of regular unprotected intercourse. Male infertility accounts, in whole or in part, for 40% to 50% of infertility problems in North America.

What causes it?
Numerous factors, including anatomic and hormonal abnormalities, can cause male infertility.

What are its symptoms?
The obvious sign of male infertility is failure to impregnate a fertile woman. An infertile man may also have shrunken testicles, or an empty or swollen scrotum; inflamed seminal vesicles (pouches that secrete seminal fluid, which keeps sperm cells viable after ejaculation); abnormal masses on the spermatic cord and vas deferens (a tube that forms part of the spermatic cord); abnormal growths on the penis; hypospadias (a congenital defect in which the urinary opening is on the underside, rather than the tip, of the penis); or prostate enlargement.

How is it diagnosed?
The doctor obtains a detailed history, which may reveal abnormal sexual development, delayed puberty, infertility in previous relationships, and a medical history of prolonged fever, mumps, impaired

In one form or other, male infertility accounts for 40% to 50% of infertility problems in North America.

PREVENTION
TIPS

Guarding against male infertility

Here are some steps a male can take to prevent infertility:
- Have regular physical exams.
- Protect your testicles during athletic activity.
- Get early treatment for sexually transmitted diseases.
- Have surgery to correct anatomic defects that could affect your fertility.

nutritional status, previous surgery, or injury to the genitalia. After a thorough history and physical exam, the most conclusive test for male infertility is semen analysis.

The doctor also may order other lab tests, such as studies of the organs that control hormone secretion and sperm formation, and measurement of testosterone levels in the blood. He or she may also perform a biopsy (removal and analysis of testicular tissue) and may order X-rays of the reproductive system.

How is it treated?

If male infertility stems from an anatomic problem or infection, it's treated by correcting the underlying problem. For instance, enlarged varicose veins in the scrotum must be surgically repaired or removed.

If infertility results from sexual dysfunction, treatment includes education, counseling or therapy (on sexual techniques, frequency of intercourse, and reproductive physiology), and proper nutrition with vitamin supplements. Men with decreased levels of follicle-stimulating hormone (which stimulates sperm formation) may respond to vitamin B therapy; those with decreased levels of luteinizing hormone (also active in sperm formation) may respond to therapy with chorionic gonadotropin (a hormonal substance that stimulates testicular function). Men with normal or elevated levels of luteinizing hormone require low doses of testosterone. Those with decreased testosterone levels, reduced semen motility, and a low sperm count may respond to chorionic gonadotropin.

Men with a low sperm count who have a normal history and physical exam, normal hormone study results, and no signs of disease need emotional support and counseling, adequate nutrition, vitamin supplements, and hormone therapy with chorionic gonadotropin and testosterone.

What can an infertile man do?

If you have a low sperm count, avoid activities that may impair normal sperm development by raising scrotal temperature, such as wearing tight underwear and athletic supporters, taking hot tub baths, or habitually riding a bicycle. Be aware that a cool scrotal temperature is essential for adequate sperm development. (See *Guarding against male infertility*.)

If possible, consider participating in support groups where you can share your feelings and concerns with other couples with the same problem.

PAINFUL INTERCOURSE

What do doctors call this condition?
Dyspareunia

What is this condition?
Genital pain associated with intercourse may be mild, or it may be severe enough to affect enjoyment of intercourse. Painful intercourse is commonly associated with physical problems; less commonly, with psychological disorders. The prognosis is good if the underlying cause can be treated successfully.

What causes it?
Painful intercourse may result from either physical or psychological causes. (See *When sex hurts: The possible reasons.*)

What are its symptoms?
Painful intercourse produces discomfort, ranging from mild aches to severe pain before, during, or after intercourse. It also may be associated with vaginal itching or burning.

How is it diagnosed?
A physical exam and lab tests help determine the underlying cause. Diagnosis also depends on a detailed sexual history to elicit physical and temporal factors contributing to the pain.

How is it treated?
Treatment of physical causes may include creams and water-soluble gels for inadequate lubrication, appropriate medications for infections, excision of scars on the hymen, and gentle stretching of painful vaginal scars. The woman may be advised to change her position during intercourse to reduce pain on deep penetration.

Treatment of psychologically based painful intercourse varies with the particular person. Sensate focus exercises deemphasize intercourse itself and teach appropriate foreplay techniques. Teaching contraception methods can reduce the fear of pregnancy; teaching about sexual activity during pregnancy can relieve fear of harming the fetus.

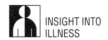 INSIGHT INTO ILLNESS

When sex hurts: The possible reasons

Persistent pain during sex may result from physical or psychological factors.

Physical causes
- Intact hymen
- Deformities or lesions of the introitus or vagina
- Tipping backward of the uterus
- Genital, rectal, or pelvic scar tissue
- Acute or chronic infections of the genitourinary tract
- Disorders of organs surrounding the genitourinary tract
- Abnormal growth and function of the tissue on the surface lining of the uterus
- Cancer
- Lack of vaginal lubrication
- Allergic reactions to contraceptives

Psychological causes
- Fear of pain or injury during sex
- Recollection of a previous painful experience
- Guilt about sex
- Fear of pregnancy or of injury to the fetus during pregnancy
- Anxiety caused by a new sexual partner or technique
- Fatigue

PREMATURE EJACULATION

What is this condition?

Premature ejaculation refers to a man's inability to control his ejaculatory reflex during sexual intercourse, resulting in persistently early ejaculation. This common sexual disorder affects men in all age-groups.

What causes it?

Premature ejaculation may result from anxiety and is often linked to previous sexual experiences. Other psychological factors may include ambivalence toward or unconscious hatred of women, a negative sexual relationship in which the man unconsciously denies his partner sexual fulfillment, and guilty feelings about sex.

Premature ejaculation can also occur in emotionally healthy men with stable, positive relationships. Rarely, it may be linked to an underlying neurologic disorder, such as multiple sclerosis, or to an inflammatory process such as prostatitis.

What are its symptoms?

The man with this disorder may be unable to prolong foreplay, or he may be able to prolong foreplay but ejaculates as soon as penetration occurs. Some men may exhibit signs of severe inadequacy or self-doubt in addition to general anxiety and guilt. With other men, the complaint lies solely with the sexual partner, who may believe that the male is indifferent to her sexual needs.

How is it diagnosed?

The physical exam and lab test results are usually normal because most men with this complaint are quite healthy. However, a detailed sexual history can be valuable in making a diagnosis. A history of adequate ejaculatory control without evidence of psychological problems suggests an organic cause.

How is it treated?

Masters and Johnson have developed a highly successful, intensive program that combines insight therapy, behavioral techniques, and experiential sessions involving both sexual partners. The program, designed to help the man focus on the sensations of an impending orgasm, continues for 2 weeks or longer and typically includes:

- *mutual physical exam,* which increases the couple's awareness of anatomy and physiology while reducing shameful feelings about sexual parts of the body
- *sensate focus exercises,* which allow each partner to caress the other's body, without intercourse, and to focus on the pleasurable sensations of touch
- *Semans squeeze technique,* which helps the man gain control of ejaculatory tension by having the woman squeeze his penis every few minutes during a touching exercise that is designed to delay ejaculation.

Another method, called the *stop-and-start technique,* involves intercourse with pelvic thrusting by the woman, who is in the superior position. She continues thrusting until orgasmic sensations start, then stops and restarts to help her partner control ejaculation. Eventually, the couple is allowed to achieve orgasm.

What can a man with premature ejaculation do?

- Be aware that this is a common disorder that does not reflect on your masculinity.
- Be aware that the condition is reversible.

A variety of behavioral and experiential techniques has been developed to successfully treat premature ejaculation.

Syphilis

What is this condition?

A chronic sexually transmitted disease, syphilis begins in the mucous membranes and quickly becomes systemic, spreading to nearby lymph nodes and the bloodstream. This disease, when untreated, is characterized by progressive stages: primary, secondary, latent, and late (formerly called tertiary).

About 34,000 cases of primary and secondary syphilis are reported each year in the United States. Incidence is highest among urban populations, especially in people between ages 15 and 39, drug users, and those infected with HIV. Untreated syphilis leads to crippling or death, but the prognosis is excellent with early treatment.

What causes it?

Infection by the organism *Treponema pallidum* causes syphilis. The disease spreads primarily through sexual contact during the primary, secondary, and early latent stages of infection. An infected mother can pass the disease to her fetus.

What are its symptoms?

Primary syphilis develops after an incubation period of about 3 weeks. Initially, one or more chancres (small, fluid-filled lesions) erupt on the genitalia; others may erupt on the anus, fingers, lips, tongue, nipples, tonsils, or eyelids. Usually painless, these chancres start as pimples and then erode; they have hardened, raised edges and clear bases. Chancres typically disappear after 3 to 6 weeks, even when untreated. They're usually associated with lymph node disease on one or both sides of the body. In women, chancres may be overlooked because they often develop internally, on the cervix or vaginal wall.

Secondary syphilis is marked by development of symmetrical lesions on mucous membranes and skin and general lymphadenopathy, which may develop within a few days or up to 8 weeks after the first chancres appear. The rash of secondary syphilis varies in appearance. Lesions are of uniform size, well defined, and generalized. Macules often erupt between rolls of fat on the trunk and on the arms, palms, soles, face, and scalp. In warm, moist areas (perineum, scrotum, vulva, between rolls of fat), the lesions enlarge and erode, producing highly contagious pink or grayish white lesions.

Mild constitutional symptoms, which appear during the secondary stage, may include headache, malaise, lack of appetite, weight loss, nausea, vomiting, sore throat, and possibly a mild fever. Hair loss may occur, with or without treatment, and is usually temporary. Nails become brittle and pitted.

Latent syphilis lacks clinical symptoms but is detected in a serologic test for syphilis. Because infectious lesions may reappear when the infection is less than 4 years old, early latent syphilis is considered contagious. About two-thirds of people are symptom-free in the latent stage and remain so until death. The rest develop characteristic late-stage symptoms.

Late syphilis is the final destructive but noninfectious stage of the disease. It has three subtypes, any or all of which may affect the person: late benign syphilis, cardiovascular syphilis, and neurosyphilis. Late benign syphilis produces lesions 1 to 10 years after infection. They may appear on the skin, bones, mucous membranes, upper respiratory tract, liver, or stomach. In severe cases, late benign syphilis results in destruction of bones or organs, which eventually causes death. (See *When syphilis attacks the heart and nervous system.*)

How is it diagnosed?

Microscopic identification of *T. pallidum* from a lesion confirms the diagnosis. Other tests may identify this organism in tissue, eye fluid, cerebrospinal fluid, tracheobronchial secretions, and discharges from lesions.

Additional procedures may include the Venereal Disease Research Laboratory (VDRL) slide test, the rapid plasma reagin test, and cerebrospinal fluid analysis.

How is it treated?

The treatment of choice is penicillin by intramuscular injection. Persons who are allergic to penicillin may be treated with Achromycin or Vibramycin by mouth for 15 days for early syphilis or for 30 days for late infections. Pregnant women should not be given Achromycin.

What can a person with syphilis do?

- Be sure to complete the entire course of drug therapy, even after symptoms subside.
- Arrange for testing after 3, 6, 12, and 24 months to detect possible relapse. If you've been treated for latent or late syphilis, have blood tests every 6 month for 2 years.
- Inform sexual partners of your infection so they can receive treatment.
- Get tested for HIV.

TESTICULAR TWISTING

What do doctors call this condition?

Testicular torsion

What is this condition?

This condition involves an abnormal twisting of the spermatic cord caused by rotation of a testicle or the mesorchium (a fold in the area

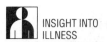
INSIGHT INTO
ILLNESS

When syphilis attacks the heart and nervous system

Heart

When this disorder affects the heart, it's called *cardiovascular syphilis.* This type of syphilis develops about 10 years after the initial infection in approximately 10% of people with untreated late syphilis. It may lead to inflammation of the aorta, the large artery that carries blood from the heart to the rest of the body. Some people have no symptoms; others have an aneurysm or backflow of blood from the aorta into the heart.

Nervous system

Symptoms of *neurosyphilis,* which develop in about 8% of people with untreated late syphilis, appear from 5 to 35 years after infection. They include inflammation of the brain and spinal cord membranes and widespread central nervous system damage, which may include personality changes, arm and leg weakness, and even paralysis.

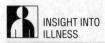

Twisted testicle

In one form of testicular twisting, the spermatic cord rotates above the testicle, causing strangulation. Eventually, this may lead to local destruction of tissue.

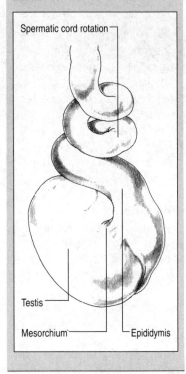

Spermatic cord rotation

Testis

Mesorchium   Epididymis

between the testicle and epididymis), which causes strangulation and, if untreated, eventual infarction (tissue death) in the testicle. This twisting almost always occurs only on one side.

Testicular twisting is most common between ages 12 and 18, but it may occur at any age. The prognosis is good with early detection and prompt treatment.

What causes it?

Normally, the tunica vaginalis (internal pouch) envelops the testicle and attaches to the epididymis and spermatic cord. Testicular twisting may result from an abnormality of the tunica, in which the testicle is abnormally positioned, or from a narrowing of supporting tissues. In newborns, loose attachment of the tunica vaginalis to the scrotal lining may cause spermatic cord rotation above the testicle. A sudden forceful contraction of the cremaster muscle may precipitate this condition. (See *Twisted testicle*.)

What are its symptoms?

Twisting produces excruciating pain in the affected testicle.

How is it diagnosed?

A physical exam reveals tense, tender swelling in the scrotum or inguinal canal and hyperemia of the overlying skin. Ultrasound helps distinguish testicular twisting from strangulated hernia, undescended testicles, or epididymitis.

How is it treated?

Treatment consists of immediate surgical repair by orchiopexy (fixation of a viable testicle to the scrotum) or orchiectomy (excision of a nonviable testicle).

TRICHOMONIASIS

What is this condition?

An infection of the lower genitourinary tract, trichomoniasis affects about 15% of sexually active women and 10% of sexually active men. It occurs worldwide. In women, the condition may be acute or chronic. Recurrence is minimized when sexual partners are treated as well.

What causes it?

The infecting organism, *Trichomonas vaginalis,* causes the disease in women by infecting the vagina, the urethra, and, possibly, the endocervix, Bartholin's glands, Skene's glands, or the bladder. In men, it infects the lower urethra and, possibly, the prostate gland, seminal vesicles, or epididymis.

Use of oral contraceptives, pregnancy, bacterial overgrowth, cervical or vaginal lesions, or frequent douching may predispose a woman to trichomoniasis.

Trichomoniasis is usually transmitted by sexual intercourse; less often, by contaminated douche equipment or moist washcloths.

What are its symptoms?

Approximately 70% of women — including those with chronic infections — and most men with trichomoniasis have no symptoms. In women, acute infection may produce various signs, such as a gray or greenish yellow, possibly frothy vaginal discharge with an unpleasant odor. Other effects include severe itching, redness, swelling, tenderness, painful intercourse, painful urination, urinary frequency and, occasionally, postcoital spotting, excessive menstrual bleeding, or painful menstruation.

Such symptoms may persist for a week to several months and may be more pronounced just after menstruation or during pregnancy. If trichomoniasis is untreated, symptoms may subside but the infection persists.

In men, trichomoniasis may produce mild to severe transient urethritis, possibly with painful urination and urinary frequency.

How is it diagnosed?

Direct microscopic examination of vaginal or seminal discharge and examination of clear urine specimens may reveal the infecting organism. A physical exam of the vagina and cervix may reveal signs of illness.

How is it treated?

The treatment of choice for trichomoniasis is oral Flagyl to both sexual partners. Oral Flagyl may not be safe during the first trimester of pregnancy. Sitz baths may be used to help relieve symptoms.

Tips on dealing with trichomoniasis

To help speed your recovery from this infection — and to prevent reinfection — follow these suggestions:

- Don't douche before being examined for trichomoniasis.
- Abstain from sexual intercourse until you're cured. Encourage your sexual partner to get treatment.
- Avoid using tampons until the infection is gone.
- Don't drink alcoholic beverages while taking Flagyl. Combining alcohol with this drug may provoke a serious reaction that includes confusion, headache, cramps, vomiting, and seizures. Also, be aware that Flagyl turns your urine dark brown.
- Avoid over-the-counter douches and vaginal sprays because chronic use can alter the vaginal pH.
- Scrub the bathtub with a disinfecting cleanser before and after sitz baths.
- To reduce the risk of bacterial growth in the genitourinary tract, wear loose-fitting, cotton underwear that allows ventilation; bacteria flourish in a warm, dark, moist environment.

After treatment, both sexual partners must have a follow-up exam to check for residual signs of infection. (See *Tips on dealing with trichomoniasis.*)

UNDESCENDED TESTICLES

What do doctors call this condition?
Cryptorchidism

What is this condition?
In this congenital disorder, one or both of a newborn's testicles fail to descend into the scrotum. Although this condition may occur on both sides, it more commonly affects the right testis.

Because the testicles normally descend into the scrotum during the eighth month of gestation, undescended testicles most commonly affects premature newborns. In about 80% of affected infants, the testicles descend spontaneously during the first year; in the rest, the testicles may or may not descend later.

If the bilateral condition persists untreated into adolescence, it may result in sterility, make the testicles more vulnerable to injury, and significantly increase the risk of testicular cancer.

What causes it?
The reason the testicles fail to descend into the scrotum is still unexplained. Some evidence seems to implicate hormonal factors.

What are its symptoms?
In the young boy with one-sided undescended testicles, the testicle on the affected side can't be felt in the scrotum during examination, and the scrotum may appear underdeveloped. On the unaffected side, the scrotum occasionally appears enlarged because of compensatory overgrowth. After puberty, uncorrected bilateral undescended testicles prevents sperm formation and results in infertility.

How is it diagnosed?
A physical exam confirms undescended testicles after lab tests determine the infant's sex. A test to measure the hormone gonadotropin in

the blood confirms the presence of testicles by assessing the appropriate level of circulating hormone.

How is it treated?

If the testicles don't descend spontaneously by age 1, surgery is generally required. A procedure called *orchiopexy* secures the testicles in the scrotum and is commonly performed before the boy reaches age 4 (optimum age is 1 to 2 years). Orchiopexy prevents sterility and excessive injury from abnormal positioning. It also prevents harmful psychological effects.

VAGINAL SPASMS

What do doctors call this condition?

Vaginismus

What is this condition?

Vaginal spasms are involuntary spastic constrictions of the lower vaginal muscles, usually caused by fear of vaginal penetration. It may coexist with painful intercourse and, if severe, may prevent successful intercourse. The condition affects women of all ages and backgrounds. The prognosis is excellent for a motivated woman who doesn't have untreatable physical abnormalities.

What causes it?

Vaginal spasms may be physical or psychological in origin. They may occur spontaneously as a protective reflex to pain, or they may result from organic causes, such as hymen abnormalities, genital herpes, obstetric injury, and atrophic vaginitis.

Psychological causes may include:
- childhood and adolescent exposure to rigid, punitive, and guilt-ridden attitudes toward sex
- fears resulting from painful or traumatic sexual experiences, such as incest or rape
- early traumatic experience with pelvic exams
- fear of pregnancy, venereal disease, or cancer.

What are its symptoms?

The woman with this disorder typically experiences muscle spasms with pain when any object—such as a tampon, diaphragm, or speculum—is inserted into her vagina. She may express a lack of interest in sex or have a normal level of sexual desire.

How is it diagnosed?

Diagnosis requires a sexual history and pelvic exam to rule out physical disorders. The sexual history includes early childhood experiences and family attitudes toward sex, previous and current sexual responses, contraceptive practices and reproductive goals, the woman's feelings about her sexual partner, and specific details about the pain she feels on insertion of any object into the vagina.

A carefully performed pelvic exam confirms the diagnosis by showing involuntary constriction of the muscles surrounding the outer portion of the vagina.

How is it treated?

Treatment is designed to eliminate abnormal muscle constriction and underlying psychological problems. In Masters and Johnson therapy, the woman inserts a graduated series of dilators into her vagina while tensing and relaxing her pelvic muscles. She controls the time the dilator is left in place and dilator movement. Together with her sexual partner, she begins sensate focus and counseling therapy to increase sexual responsiveness, improve communication skills, and resolve any underlying conflicts.

12

HORMONE AND GLAND DISORDERS

ACROMEGALY AND GIGANTISM

What do doctors call these conditions?
Hyperpituitarism

What are these conditions?
Acromegaly and gigantism are chronic, progressive diseases marked by hormonal dysfunction and startling skeletal overgrowth. Acromegaly causes bones to thicken and grow transversely. Gigantism causes proportional overgrowth of all body tissues. These disorders usually reduce life expectancy unless treated in a timely fashion.

The earliest signs of acromegaly are swelling and enlargement of the arms, legs, and face. This rare disorder occurs in men and women equally, usually between ages 30 and 50.

Gigantism causes remarkable height increases of as much as 6 inches (15 centimeters) a year. Infants and children may grow to three times the normal height for their age; adults may ultimately reach a height of more than 6 feet 8 inches (2 meters).

What causes them?
Typically, oversecretion of human growth hormone produces changes throughout the body, resulting in acromegaly or, when oversecretion occurs before puberty, gigantism. Tumors of the anterior pituitary gland may cause this oversecretion, but the causes of the tumors themselves remain unclear. Occasionally, levels of human growth hormone are elevated in more than one family member, suggesting the possibility of a genetic cause.

What are their symptoms?
Acromegaly develops slowly and typically produces profuse sweating, oily skin, hypermetabolism, and excessive hair growth. Severe headache, central nervous system impairment, loss of sharp vision, and blindness may also result.

Oversecretion of human growth hormone produces cartilaginous and connective tissue overgrowth, resulting in a characteristic hulking appearance, with an enlarged ridge over the eye and thickened ears and nose. The jaw may project so much that chewing becomes difficult.

Enlargement of the larynx and paranasal sinuses and thickening of the tongue cause the voice to sound deep and hollow. Fingertips display an arrowhead appearance on X-rays, and the fingers are thickened. Irritability, hostility, and various psychological disturbances may occur.

Prolonged effects of human growth hormone oversecretion include bowlegs, barrel chest, arthritis, osteoporosis, kyphosis, high blood pressure, and hardening of the arteries. Both gigantism and acromegaly may also cause symptoms similar to those of diabetes.

Gigantism develops abruptly, producing some of the same skeletal abnormalities seen in acromegaly. As the disease progresses, the pituitary tumor enlarges and invades normal tissue, thereby causing the organ involved to stop functioning.

How are they diagnosed?

The doctor will observe a person with acromegaly or gigantism for characteristic features. He or she will order blood tests to measure levels of human growth hormone, which are usually elevated. However, results of this test may be misleading.

A lab test called the *glucose suppression test* may be ordered to obtain more reliable information. Glucose normally suppresses the secretion of growth hormone. If an infusion of glucose does not suppress the hormone level, it may indicate acromegaly or gigantism.

In addition, skull X-rays, computed tomography scan (commonly called a CAT scan), arteriography, and magnetic resonance imaging (commonly called MRI) determine the presence and extent of the pituitary lesion. Bone X-rays showing a thickening of the cranium and of the long bones, as well as osteoarthritis in the spine, support this diagnosis.

How are they treated?

Treatment aims to limit human growth hormone secretion by pituitary radiation therapy or by surgery to remove the underlying tumor. In acromegaly, surgery is mandatory when a tumor causes blindness or other severe neurologic disturbances. Postoperative therapy often requires replacement of thyroid hormones, cortisone, and gonadal hormones. Additional treatment may include administration of Parlodel and Sandostatin, which inhibit human growth hormone synthesis. (See *Advice for the person with acromegaly or gigantism.*)

 SELF-HELP

Advice for the person with acromegaly or gigantism

Here are some points to consider if you have one or the other of these conditions.

Daily activities
- If you have late-stage acromegaly and a weak hand clasp, ask family members or others to help with such tasks as cutting food.
- Keep your skin dry — but avoid using an oily lotion because your skin is already oily.

Following the treatment
- If the doctor has prescribed continuing hormone replacement therapy, make sure you understand which hormones you are to take and why, as well as the correct dosages and administration times. And don't suddenly stop taking the hormones.
- Be aware that the disease can cause inexplicable mood changes, which can be modified with treatment.
- Wear a medical identification bracelet at all times, and bring your hormone replacement schedule with you whenever you return to the hospital.

ADDISON'S DISEASE

What do doctors call this condition?
Adrenal hypofunction, adrenal insufficiency

What is this condition?
In this disorder, the adrenal glands don't secrete enough steroid hormones. A relatively uncommon disorder, Addison's disease can occur at any age and in both sexes. With early diagnosis and adequate replacement of the steroid hormones, the prognosis for Addison's disease is good.

Adrenal crisis (also known as *addisonian crisis*), a critical shortage of steroid hormones, generally follows acute stress, sepsis, injury, surgery, or failure of people with chronic adrenal insufficiency to take steroids. Because it's a medical emergency, adrenal crisis requires immediate, vigorous treatment.

What causes it?
Addison's disease occurs when more than 90% of both adrenal glands are destroyed. In primary Addison's disease, such destruction usually results from an autoimmune process in which circulating antibodies react specifically against the adrenal tissue. Other possible causes include tuberculosis, adrenal gland surgery, hemorrhage, and certain cancers or infections. Rarely, a person inherits a predisposition for developing Addison's disease and other endocrine disorders.

Secondary Addison's disease results from a disorder outside the gland (such as a pituitary tumor).

What are its symptoms?
Addison's disease typically causes weakness, fatigue, weight loss, and gastrointestinal disturbances, such as nausea, vomiting, loss of appetite, and chronic diarrhea. Also, it usually causes a conspicuous bronze skin discoloration — almost like a deep suntan — most noticeable in the creases of the hands, but also on the hand joints, elbows, and knees. It may darken scars and increase pigmentation of the mucous membranes.

The disorder may affect the heart and blood vessels, causing low blood pressure and a weak, irregular pulse. Other possible symptoms include a reduced tolerance for stress (even when minor), poor coor-

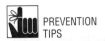

PREVENTION
TIPS

How to avoid adrenal crisis

Even if you follow your treatment plan for Addison's disease carefully, unexpected situations can create stress and worsen your condition. Because your adrenal glands can't respond to increased demands, you'll need to prepare for stressful situations and know what to do to prevent adrenal crisis.

Take precautions

• Always wear or carry medical identification with your name, the name of your disorder, and the phone numbers of your doctor and a responsible person.

• Always carry a clearly labeled emergency kit, especially when you travel. Double-check to make sure the kit contains a syringe and needle, 100 milligrams of hydrocortisone, and instructions for use.

• Don't exercise strenuously in hot, humid weather. If you start to sweat heavily, drink more fluids, and add salt to your food.

• Follow your doctor's directions for increasing your daily doses of prescribed steroids during stressful times—emotional crisis, overexertion, infection, illness, or injury.

• Balance active periods with rest.

Eat right

• Eat regularly. Don't skip meals or go for a long time without food.

• Be sure to maintain a high-carbohydrate, high-protein diet with up to 8 grams of sodium (salt) daily. If you sweat a lot, you can use even more salt.

Recognize warning signs

Notify your doctor immediately (or go directly to the nearest hospital emergency room) if you develop any of the following warning signs of adrenal crisis:

• apathy or restlessness, anxiety, confusion, dizziness, or headache

• unusually pale or cool, clammy skin

• fever

• rapid breathing and heart rate

• unusual fatigue or weakness

• loss of appetite, stomach cramps, diarrhea, nausea, and vomiting

• dehydration or reduced urine output.

If you can't reach your doctor or get to a hospital at once, give yourself an injection of 100 milligrams of hydrocortisone under the skin. Then get medical help.

Plan ahead

Instruct a family member or a friend to give you an injection of 100 milligrams of hydrocortisone under the skin if he or she finds you unconscious or unable to take your medicine by mouth. This person should then get you medical help immediately.

dination, and a craving for salty food. In women, Addison's disease may retard the growth of underarm and pubic hair, reduce the libido, and, in severe cases, cause menstruation to stop.

Secondary Addison's disease produces symptoms similar to those of the primary type but doesn't cause hyperpigmentation.

Adrenal crisis produces profound weakness, fatigue, nausea, vomiting, low blood pressure, dehydration and, occasionally, high fever followed by hypothermia. If untreated, this condition can progress to vascular collapse, kidney failure, coma, and death.

How is it diagnosed?

Lab tests are key to diagnosing Addison's disease. The doctor will require blood samples to measure plasma cortisol levels to confirm adrenal insufficiency. If secondary Addison's disease is suspected, he or she may order a special test called the *metyrapone test*. For primary or secondary Addison's disease, the doctor will probably order a cor-ticotropin stimulation test.

How is it treated?

Lifelong hormone replacement therapy with steroid drugs is the pri-mary treatment for people with Addison's disease. The person usually receives the drugs cortisone or hydrocortisone. He or she may also require treatment with drugs to prevent dangerous dehydration and low blood pressure. Such drugs may include desoxycorticosterone or fludrocortisone.

Adrenal crisis constitutes a medical emergency and requires im-mediate medical intervention. Interventions include large doses of hydrocortisone. With proper treatment, adrenal crisis usually sub-sides quickly. (See *How to avoid adrenal crisis,* page 441, and *Taking steroids safely.*)

CUSHING'S SYNDROME

What is this condition?

Cushing's syndrome is a cluster of abnormalities caused when the adrenal glands secrete excessive steroid hormones. Its unmistakable signs include rapidly developing fatty tissue in the face, neck, and trunk and purple streaks on the skin.

Cushing's syndrome is most common in women. The prognosis depends on the underlying cause of the problem.

What causes it?

In most cases, Cushing's syndrome results from an overproduction of a hormone called *corticotropin*. This hormone stimulates the adrenal gland to produce the hormone cortisol and, to a lesser extent, the hormones called *androgens* and *aldosterone*.

Too much corticotropin may stem from excessive production of the hormone (a phenomenon called *Cushing's disease*), a tumor in another organ that produces corticotropin, or the consumption of large amounts of prescribed steroids.

In other people, the disorder results from a tumor in the adrenal gland that secretes cortisol and that's usually benign. In infants, the usual cause of Cushing's syndrome is cancer of the adrenal gland.

What are its symptoms?

Like most hormonal disorders, Cushing's syndrome induces changes throughout the body. Signs and symptoms may include the following:
- *endocrine and metabolic systems:* diabetes with decreased sugar tolerance, fasting high blood sugar, and glucose in the urine
- *musculoskeletal system:* muscle weakness, pathologic fractures; skeletal growth retardation in children
- *skin:* purplish streaks; bruises; fat pads above the clavicles, over the upper back ("buffalo hump"), on the face ("moon face"), and throughout the trunk, with slender arms and legs; poor wound healing; and acne and abnormal hairiness in women. (See *How Cushing's syndrome affects the body.*)
- *digestive system:* peptic ulcer and decreased stomach mucus
- *nervous system:* irritability and moodiness, ranging from euphoric behavior to depression or psychosis; insomnia
- *heart and blood vessels:* high blood pressure, an enlarged heart, bleeding
- *immune system:* increased susceptibility to infection, decreased resistance to stress
- *kidneys and bladder:* sodium and fluid retention; increased potassium excretion; inhibited antidiuretic hormone secretion; kidney stones
- *reproductive system:* increased androgen production, with clitoral enlargement, mild virilism, and absent or decreased menstruation in females; sexual dysfunction.

How is it diagnosed?

Lab tests measuring levels of hormones in the blood are crucial to diagnosing Cushing's syndrome. If results indicate the need for further tests, your doctor may order another lab test, called the *dexamethasone suppression test*, to confirm the diagnosis.

Another dexamethasone suppression test may be administered to determine if Cushing's syndrome results from a pituitary problem (Cushing's disease). Ultrasound, a computed tomography scan (com-

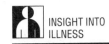

INSIGHT INTO ILLNESS

How Cushing's syndrome affects the body

The increased cortisol levels in Cushing's syndrome affect the entire body. Besides the effects illustrated here, a person with Cushing's syndrome may also have thin skin, high blood pressure, and osteoporosis.

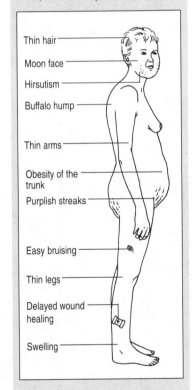

Thin hair
Moon face
Hirsutism
Buffalo hump
Thin arms
Obesity of the trunk
Purplish streaks
Easy bruising
Thin legs
Delayed wound healing
Swelling

monly called a CAT scan), or angiography can help to localize tumors in the adrenal gland. A CAT scan or magnetic resonance imaging (also called MRI) of the head may help identify pituitary tumors.

How is it treated?

Treatment to restore hormone balance and reverse Cushing's syndrome may include radiation, drug therapy, or surgery. For example, people with poorly controlled diabetes, osteoporosis, and severe pathologic fractures may require radiation or surgical removal of the pituitary gland. If the person fails to respond, his or her adrenal glands may be removed.

The drugs Cytadren and Nizoral may reduce cortisol levels and are beneficial in relieving symptoms of Cushing's syndrome. Cytadren alone, or in combination with Metopirone, may also be useful in treating adrenal cancer that has spread.

Cortisol therapy is essential during and after surgery to help the person tolerate the physiologic stress imposed by removal of the pituitary or adrenal glands. If normal cortisol production resumes, steroid therapy may be gradually tapered and eventually discontinued. However, removal of both adrenal glands or of the entire pituitary gland requires lifelong steroid replacement therapy to correct hormonal deficiencies.

What can a person with Cushing's syndrome do?

Following surgical removal of the adrenal or pituitary glands, the doctor will prescribe replacement steroids. Follow necessary precautions for undergoing this type of drug therapy:

- Be aware that you'll need lifelong drug therapy.
- Take prescribed steroids with antacids or meals to minimize stomach upset. (Usually, it helps to take two-thirds of the dose in the morning and the remainder in the early afternoon.)
- Carry a medical identification card.
- Immediately report stressful situations, such as infections, which call for an increase in the steroid dosage. (See *How to detect and prevent infection.*)
- Watch closely for signs of an inadequate steroid dosage (fatigue, weakness, dizziness) and steroid overdose (severe swelling, weight gain). Never abruptly discontinue taking steroids — this may cause a fatal adrenal crisis.

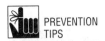

How to detect and prevent infection

If you have Cushing's syndrome, you're an easy target for infection. That's one reason why you should be alert for the warning signs of infection and take steps to prevent infection.

Warning signs

Infection can worsen quickly. Call your doctor at once if any of these warning signs occur:

- fever
- cough that produces foul-smelling or colored (green, yellow, brown, pink, or red) sputum
- unusual fatigue or weakness
- increasing breathing difficulty
- cuts or scrapes that are red or swollen, feel tender, or begin draining
- confusion, decreased alertness, or memory loss.

Preventive steps

To help prevent infection, follow these steps:

- Eat well-balanced, nutritious meals. Don't skip meals or eat extra ones.

- Drink at least six glasses of water a day unless your doctor directs otherwise.
- Get 7 to 8 hours of sleep at night, and rest frequently during the day.
- Take your medicine *exactly* as your doctor directs.
- If possible, avoid anyone who has a cold or the flu, and stay away from crowds. If you can't avoid someone who's sick, wear a disposable surgical mask when you're around the person. You can usually buy disposable masks at drugstores.
- Check with your doctor about getting a flu shot.
- Avoid exposure to inhaled pollutants — for example, cigarette smoke, harmful industrial fumes, and car exhaust.
- Carefully wash your hands before meals. Also wash them after touching tissues soiled with mucus and before and after using the bathroom, handling money, or petting an animal.
- Avoid cuts and other accidental injuries. If you do cut or scrape yourself, wash the area with soap and water, and cover it with a dry, sterile bandage. If the wound doesn't heal within a few days, call your doctor.

DIABETES INSIPIDUS

What do doctors call this condition?

Pituitary diabetes insipidus

What is this condition?

A disorder of water metabolism, diabetes insipidus results from a deficiency of a hormone called *vasopressin* or *antidiuretic hormone*. It's characterized by excessive consumption of fluids and profuse urination. The disorder has no relationship to the much better-known form of diabetes called *diabetes mellitus*.

Diabetes insipidus may start in childhood or early adulthood and is more common in men than in women. If the person with diabetes

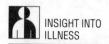

Two forms of diabetes insipidus

Diabetes insipidus may result from various disorders or from the use of certain drugs. Some forms of the disorder, such as nephrogenic diabetes insipidus, are inherited. Sometimes, the cause is never discovered. Some known causes of diabetes insipidus appear below.

Causes of neurogenic diabetes insipidus
- Autoimmune disorders and diseases such as leukemia
- Alcohol and drugs such as Dilantin
- Head injury such as a basilar skull fracture
- Infections, such as encephalitis or meningitis
- Surgery involving the pituitary gland
- A cancerous tumor that has spread to the brain
- Blood vessel abnormalities, such as an aneurysm or blood clot formation

Causes of nephrogenic diabetes insipidus
- Chronic kidney disorders, such as polycystic disease, advanced kidney failure, or blockage in one of the tubes that carry urine from the kidney to the bladder
- Such drugs as Fungizone, Declomycin, and Lithane
- Electrolyte imbalances, such as a decreased blood potassium level or an increased blood calcium level
- Blood disorders such as sickle cell syndrome
- Infections such as a serious kidney infection
- Kwashiorkor (a malnutrition disease)

insipidus doesn't have complications, the prognosis is good, and he or she can usually lead a normal life.

What causes it?

Diabetes insipidus usually results from damage to the pituitary gland. This damage may result from a brain tumor, neurosurgery, a skull fracture, or head injury. Another form of the disorder, called *nephrogenic diabetes insipidus*, originates with kidney problems. (See *Two forms of diabetes insipidus*.)

What are its symptoms?

Typically, the person abruptly begins to urinate profuse amounts: usually 4 to 16 quarts per day of diluted urine, but sometimes as much as 30 quarts per day. As a result, the person is extremely thirsty and drinks large quantities of water to compensate for the body's fluid losses. This disorder may also result in nighttime urination and, in severe cases, extreme fatigue from inadequate rest due to frequent voiding and excessive thirst.

Other characteristic features of diabetes insipidus include symptoms of dehydration (poor tissue turgor, dry mucous membranes, constipation, muscle weakness, dizziness, and low blood pressure).

How is it diagnosed?

To diagnose diabetes insipidus, the doctor will order a urinalysis to evaluate the physical characteristics of the person's urine. In diabetes insipidus, the urine contains a high percentage of water.

Another test, called a *water deprivation test*, provides further information about the person's condition. In this test, baseline vital signs and weight are taken, and urine and blood analyses are done. Then the person is deprived of fluids. Hourly measurements then record the total volume of urine output, body weight, and the physical characteristics of his or her urine. Throughout the test, blood pressure and pulse rate are carefully monitored. Also during the course of the test, the person receives an injection of vasopressin; the response to this injection helps to determine if diabetes insipidus results from a problem with the person's pituitary gland or a problem with his or her kidney.

How is it treated?

Until the cause is identified and eliminated, administration of various forms of vasopressin or of a vasopressin stimulant can control fluid balance and prevent dehydration:

- *Pitressin* is a liquid preparation that's administered under the skin or in the muscle several times a day because it's effective for only 2 to 6 hours. This form of the drug is used in acute disease and as a diagnostic agent.
- *DDAVP* can be given as a nasal spray or by an intravenous injection or injection under the skin. This drug is effective for 8 to 20 hours, depending on the dosage. (See *Coping with diabetes insipidus.*)

 SELF-HELP

Coping with diabetes insipidus

While undergoing treatment for the disorder, follow this advice.

Watch fluids carefully
- Make sure you know how much fluid you consume and how much urine you void. If necessary, ask your doctor and nurse to clarify their instructions.
- To prevent retaining too much fluid, use the nasal spray form of DDAVP only *after* you start urinating frequently.

Watch your weight
Report any weight gain to your doctor. An increase in weight may mean that your medication dosage is too high.

Be prepared
Wear a medical identification bracelet and carry your medication with you at all times.

DIABETES MELLITUS

What is this condition?

Diabetes mellitus is a chronic disease in which the body produces little or no insulin or resists the insulin that it does produce. Insulin transports glucose into the cells for use as energy and storage as glycogen. It also stimulates protein synthesis and free fatty acid storage in the fat deposits. When a person lacks sufficient insulin, body tissues have less access to essential nutrients for fuel and storage.

The incidence of diabetes mellitus is equal in men and women and rises with age. The disease increases the risk of heart attack, stroke, kidney failure, and peripheral blood vessel disease. What's more, it's a major cause of blindness in adults.

Classifying diabetes

There are two main forms of diabetes mellitus: *Type I* or *insulin-dependent,* and the more prevalent *Type II* or *non-insulin-dependent.* Type I usually occurs before age 30, although it may strike at any age. The person with this type is usually thin and needs insulin injections and dietary modifications to control his or her blood sugar level. Type II usually occurs in obese adults over age 40. It's most often treated with diet and exercise (possibly in combination with drugs that lower the blood sugar level), although treatment sometimes includes insulin therapy.

What causes it?

The cause of diabetes mellitus remains unknown, but genetic factors may play a part in development of the disease. In Type I diabetes, cells in the pancreas that produce insulin are damaged, possibly because of an immune system problem. Consequently, these cells are able to produce very little or no insulin.

In Type II diabetes, the cells in the pancreas are still able to produce insulin, but not enough to meet the body's needs. People with this type of diabetes are usually obese.

Other forms of diabetes, called secondary diabetes, may be caused by pregnancy, physical or emotional stress, or the use of certain medications.

What are its symptoms?

All types of diabetes produce similar symptoms. The most common symptom is fatigue, caused by energy deficiency and abnormal processing of fats, carbohydrates, and proteins. Insulin deficiency causes high blood sugar. High blood sugar, in turn, causes increased and frequent urination, dehydration, excessive thirst, dry mucous membranes, and dry skin. Some people with diabetes may experience weight loss, as fat and muscles are burned up to provide energy and excessive amounts of glucose are excreted in the urine.

Symptoms of Type I diabetes may develop rapidly within weeks or months. Symptoms of Type II diabetes usually develop more gradually and may not appear until many years after the onset of the disease.

If not properly managed, diabetes may also lead to dangerous metabolic crises, such as *ketoacidosis* and *hyperosmolar nonketotic syndrome*. These crises result from excessive amounts of glucose in the blood and may lead to fluid loss and shock.

Long-term effects of diabetes may include retinal changes, kidney problems, atherosclerosis (plaque buildup in the arteries), and nervous system problems, such as pain or numbness in hands and feet or paralysis of the stomach resulting in nausea. Other nervous system effects include impotence, nighttime diarrhea, and dizziness when rising to an upright position (due to low blood pressure).

High levels of sugar in the blood encourage bacterial growth and reduce resistance to infection, possibly leading to skin and urinary tract infections and vaginal inflammation.

How is it diagnosed?

When making a diagnosis of diabetes mellitus, the doctor observes the person for symptoms of uncontrolled diabetes. He or she will order blood tests to measure sugar levels. A blood sugar level equal to or above 200 milligrams per deciliter suggests diabetes mellitus. Another test for diabetes mellitus, called the *fasting plasma glucose test*, requires fasting for 12 or 14 hours before blood is drawn.

An eye examination may show retinal abnormalities. Other diagnostic and monitoring tests include urinalysis and additional blood tests.

How is it treated?

The goal of treatment is to normalize the person's blood sugar level. In Type I, this is achieved with insulin injections, diet, and exercise. The person may receive insulin in a single-dose, mixed-dose, split-mixed dose, or multiple-dose regimen. For a multiple-dose regimen, an insulin pump may be used. Insulin may be rapid-acting (regular), intermediate-acting (NPH), long-acting (ultralente), or a combination of rapid-acting and intermediate-acting (Mixtard); it may be standard or purified, and it may be derived from beef, pork, or human sources. Today, purified human insulin is commonly used.

A person with either Type I or Type II diabetes must follow a strict diet to meet nutritional needs, control blood sugar levels, and reach and maintain appropriate weight. The person must follow the diet consistently and eat meals at regular times.

For an obese person with Type II diabetes, dietary measures aim to promote weight reduction. In many cases, diet alone may be sufficient to control Type II diabetes. Alternatively, a person with Type II

What's new in diabetes treatments

If you have diabetes mellitus, you'll be glad to know that new investigative treatments are being developed to improve monitoring and control of blood sugar levels.

Glycemic index

This form of diet therapy links blood sugar fluctuations with specific foods. It also identifies low-fat, starchy foods that people with diabetes can eat to increase their carbohydrate intake without triggering high blood sugar. The person must comply with therapy by measuring his or her blood sugar level after every meal and snack.

Implantable probes and pumps

These devices, designed to monitor blood sugar levels and automatically deliver the correct insulin dose, permit more precise blood sugar control. However, possible clogging of these devices and unreliable insulin secretion are drawbacks.

Sandimmune therapy

A promising treatment for Type I diabetes, Sandimmune therapy aims to prevent islet beta-cell destruction. This drug may prevent circulating islet-cell antibodies in the blood from attacking islet cells. However, the drug can also be harmful to the kidneys and liver.

Pancreatic islet-cell grafts

A graft (transplant) of islet cells, the cells in the pancreas that produce insulin, may help control blood sugar metabolism and prevent or resolve diabetic complications involving the small blood vessels. However, successful grafting requires pure, undamaged islet cells, which are hard to obtain.

Pancreas transplant

Because of the high risk of rejection, people receiving a pancreas transplant must take drugs that suppress the immune system. Unfortunately, these drugs eventually can cause more problems, including infection and damage to the liver and kidneys. Consequently, most people selected for a pancreas transplant are already receiving immunosuppressants for a previous transplant. They also face a greater health risk from diabetic complications than from long-term immunosuppression.

diabetes may take oral antidiabetic drugs to stimulate the body's insulin production, increase the cells' sensitivity to insulin, and stop the formation of carbohydrates from noncarbohydrate sources in the liver.

Some people with diabetes may be candidates for pancreas transplantation to help them produce insulin. But this procedure is experimental and requires long-term use of drugs that suppress the immune system. (See *What's new in diabetes treatments*.)

Treating complications

A diabetic with kidney failure may receive dialysis or a kidney transplant. A person with retinal abnormalities may undergo a procedure called *photocoagulation*, in which a laser or xenon arc light is used to cause condensation of protein material in the eye. Blood vessel disease may require vascular surgery.

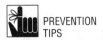
PREVENTION
TIPS

Avoiding diabetic complications

There's no way around it. Controlling your diabetes means checking your blood sugar levels daily and making the following good health habits a way of life.

Keep your heart healthy

Because diabetes raises your risk of heart disease, take care of your heart by following these American Heart Association guidelines:
- Maintain a normal weight.
- Exercise regularly, following your doctor's recommendations.
- Help control your blood pressure and cholesterol levels by eating a low-fat, high-fiber diet, as your doctor prescribes.

Have your eyes checked

Have your eyes examined by an ophthalmologist at least once a year. He may detect any diabetes-related damage (which can cause blindness) before symptoms appear.

Care for your teeth

Schedule regular dental checkups and follow good home care to minimize the dental problems that may result from diabetes, such as gum disease and abscesses. If you have any bleeding, pain, or soreness in your gums or teeth, report this to the dentist immediately. Brush your teeth after every meal and floss daily. If you wear dentures, clean them thoroughly every day, and make sure they fit properly.

Provide skin care

Breaks in your skin can increase your risk of infection. So check your skin daily for cuts and irritated areas, and see your doctor if necessary. Bathe daily with warm water and a mild soap, and apply a lanolin-based lotion afterward to prevent dryness. Pat your skin thoroughly dry, taking extra care between your toes and in any other areas where skin surfaces touch. Always wear cotton underwear to allow moisture to evaporate and help prevent skin breakdown.

Prevent foot problems

Diabetes can reduce blood flow to your feet and dull their ability to feel heat, cold, or pain. To help prevent foot problems, wear comfortable shoes and avoid walking barefoot. Follow your doctor's or nurse's instructions to prevent foot problems.

Check your urine

Because symptoms of kidney disease usually don't appear until the problem is advanced, your doctor will check your urine routinely for protein, which can signal kidney disease. Don't delay telling him if you have symptoms of a urinary tract infection: burning, painful or difficult urination, or blood or pus in the urine.

Have regular checkups

See your doctor regularly so he or she can detect early signs of complications and start treatment promptly.

What can a person with diabetes mellitus do?

- Be sure to comply with your prescribed treatment program. (See *Avoiding diabetic complications*.)
- Make sure you understand — and follow — your doctor's instructions on managing minor illnesses, such as a cold, flu, or upset stomach. (For instance, you may need to increase your insulin dosage.)

- For more information on this disease, contact the Juvenile Diabetes Foundation or the American Diabetes Association.

DWARFISM

What do doctors call this condition?

Hypopituitarism, panhypopituitarism

What is this condition?

Dwarfism is characterized by dysfunction of the endocrine system, sexual immaturity and, in children, slowed growth. It results from deficiency of the hormones secreted by the front (anterior) portion of the pituitary, a cherry-sized gland in the base of the brain.

Partial dwarfism and complete dwarfism occur in both adults and children. In children, these disorders may cause late puberty. The prognosis may be good if the child receives adequate hormone replacement therapy and the underlying cause is corrected.

What causes it?

The most common cause of *primary dwarfism* is a tumor. Other causes include congenital defects (an absent or undeveloped pituitary gland); localized destruction of pituitary tissue (usually from heavy bleeding after childbirth); or partial or total pituitary removal by surgery, radiation therapy, or chemical agents. Rarely, dwarfism results from tuberculosis or other granulomatous diseases. Sometimes, primary dwarfism has no identifiable cause.

Secondary dwarfism stems from insufficient production of releasing hormones by the hypothalamus, a crucial brain structure that regulates many body functions. This hormone deficiency may have no known cause, or it may result from infection, trauma, or a tumor.

What are its symptoms?

Symptoms of dwarfism develop slowly and vary with the severity of the disorder and the number of deficient hormones. In adults, dwarfism may cause:

- absence of menstruation
- impotence

- infertility
- decreased sex drive
- diabetes insipidus (a metabolic disorder marked by profuse urination and excessive thirst)
- an underactive thyroid (causing tiredness, sluggishness, sensitivity to cold, and menstrual disturbances)
- low blood sugar
- appetite loss
- nausea
- stomach pain
- dizziness when rising to an upright position.

In children, dwarfism causes slowed growth or late puberty. Dwarfism usually isn't apparent at birth, but signs start to appear during the first few months; by age 6 months, growth retardation is obvious. Although these children generally enjoy good health, they may be chubby because of fat deposits in the lower trunk, their secondary teeth may come in late, and they may have low blood sugar. They continue to grow at less than half the normal rate — sometimes until their 20s or 30s — to an average height of 4 feet (1.2 meters), but their proportions are normal.

When dwarfism strikes before puberty, it prevents development of secondary sex characteristics (including facial and body hair). In men, it causes undersized testicles, penis, and prostate gland; absent or minimal sex drive; and inability to initiate and maintain an erection. In women, it usually causes immature breast development, sparse or absent pubic and underarm hair, and absence of menstruation.

Neurologic symptoms associated with dwarfism may include headache, vision problems and, possibly, blindness. Acute dwarfism resulting from surgery or infection is often accompanied by fever, low blood pressure, vomiting, and low blood sugar. (See *A dangerous form of dwarfism.*)

How is it diagnosed?

The doctor evaluates the person to confirm hormonal deficiency due to impairment or destruction of the pituitary gland. He or she must rule out diseases of the hypothalamus, adrenal glands, ovaries or testicles, and thyroid. Some people may undergo special tests to help pinpoint the source of low levels of the hormone cortisol. These tests require careful medical supervision because they may trigger a dangerous condition called *adrenal crisis.*

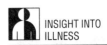
INSIGHT INTO ILLNESS

A dangerous form of dwarfism

Partial or total failure of all six vital hormones secreted by the anterior pituitary gland may cause a form of dwarfism known as *panhypopituitarism.*

This condition may cause a host of mental and physical abnormalities, including psychosis, sluggishness, low blood pressure, a slow pulse, anemia, and appetite loss. Unfortunately, symptoms don't become apparent until 75% of the pituitary gland is destroyed. Unless it's diagnosed and treated promptly, panhypopituitarism is fatal.

The doctor may also order lab tests to measure growth hormone levels in the person's blood after administering regular insulin or Larodopa. In most people, these substances trigger increased secretion of growth hormone. Persistently low growth-hormone levels confirm growth hormone deficiency.

Computed tomography scan (commonly called a CAT scan), magnetic resonance imaging (commonly called MRI), or an X-ray study of the brain's blood vessels can reveal whether a tumor is the cause of dwarfism.

How is it treated?

The most effective treatment for dwarfism is replacement of hormones secreted by the adrenal glands, ovaries or testicles, and thyroid. Hormone replacement therapy includes cortisol, thyroxine, and androgen or cyclic estrogen. To boost fertility, a person of reproductive age may receive follicle-stimulating hormone and human chorionic gonadotropin.

Protropin therapy

The drug Protropin, the main treatment for dwarfism, stimulates growth increases of up to 4 to 6 inches (10 to 15 centimeters) during the first year of treatment. After that, the child's growth rate tapers off. Protropin has limited value after puberty. Occasionally, a child becomes unresponsive to Protropin, even in larger doses. In these children, small doses of androgen may again stimulate growth, but extreme caution is needed to prevent premature closure of the heads of long bones. Children with dwarfism may also need replacement of adrenal and thyroid hormones and, as they approach puberty, sex hormones. (See *Helping a child with dwarfism.*)

GRAVES' DISEASE

What do doctors call this condition?

Hyperthyroidism, Basedow's disease, thyrotoxicosis

What is this condition?

Graves' disease is a metabolic imbalance resulting from overproduction of thyroid hormones. This disorder causes increased production of the hormone thyroxine, enlarges the thyroid gland (goiter), and causes numerous changes in body systems. Graves' disease occurs most often between ages 30 and 40, especially in people with a family history of thyroid abnormalities; only 5% of people with the disorder are younger than age 15.

With treatment, most people can lead normal lives. However, thyroid storm — an acute exacerbation of Graves' disease — is a medical emergency that may lead to life-threatening heart, liver, or kidney failure. (See *What happens in thyroid storm.*)

What causes it?

Graves' disease may result from both genetic and immunologic influences. For example, certain twins have a higher risk for Graves' disease, suggesting a genetic link. This disease occasionally coexists with abnormal iodine metabolism and other endocrine disorders, such as diabetes, thyroiditis, and hyperparathyroidism.

In latent Graves' disease, excessive dietary intake of iodine and, possibly, stress can precipitate clinical hyperthyroidism. Unless the disorder is properly treated, stress — including surgery, infection, toxemia of pregnancy, and diabetic ketoacidosis — can precipitate thyroid storm.

What are its symptoms?

Classic symptoms include goiter (an enlarged thyroid), nervousness, heat intolerance, weight loss despite increased appetite, sweating, diarrhea, tremor, and palpitations.

Abnormally protruding eyeballs are a classic sign but don't occur in all cases. (See *How Graves' disease affects the body,* page 456.)

How is it diagnosed?

Diagnosing Graves' disease is usually uncomplicated. If your doctor suspects that you have it, he or she will carefully review your history, perform a physical exam, and order routine hormone tests. These tests confirm Graves' disease by showing increased levels of the thyroid hormones thyroxine and triiodothyronine and other characteristic features of the illness. Ultrasound test may confirm eye problems caused by Graves' disease.

How is it treated?

Antithyroid drugs, radioactive iodine, and surgery are primary treatments for Graves' disease. Which one is used depends on the size of

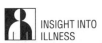
INSIGHT INTO ILLNESS

What happens in thyroid storm

Thyroid storm is a complication of Graves' disease. Signs and symptoms include extreme irritability, high blood pressure, rapid heart rate, vomiting, fever up to 106° F (41.1° C), delirium, and coma. Left untreated, it's invariably fatal.

Thyroid storm begins suddenly and may be caused by a stressful event, such as injury, surgery, or infection. Other less common predisposing factors include:
- insulin-induced low blood sugar or diabetic ketoacidosis
- stroke
- heart attack
- blood clot in the lungs
- sudden cessation of antithyroid drug therapy
- initiation of radioactive iodine therapy
- preeclampsia
- excessive intake of synthetic thyroid hormone after partial thyroidectomy (removal of part of the thyroid gland).

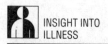

INSIGHT INTO
ILLNESS

How Graves' disease affects the body

Graves' disease can have a profound effect on many different parts of the body, as follows.

Nervous system
Difficulty concentrating, excitability or nervousness, fine tremor, shaky handwriting, clumsiness, emotional instability, and mood swings

Eyes
Abnormal protrusion of the eyeballs; occasional inflammation of conjunctivas, corneas, or eye muscles; double vision; and increased tearing

Skin
Smooth, warm, flushed skin (the person sleeps with minimal covers and little clothing); raised patches of skin that are itchy and sometimes painful; and occasional nodules

Hair and nails
Fine, soft hair; premature graying and increased hair loss in both sexes; nails that break easily or become separated from the nailbed

Heart and blood vessels
Rapid heart rate; full, bounding pulse; enlarged heart; heart rhythm irregularities (especially in elderly people); and, occasionally, a heart murmur

Lungs
Shortness of breath on exertion and at rest

Digestive system
Nausea and vomiting; increased defecation; soft stools or, with severe disease, diarrhea; liver enlargement; and possible loss of appetite

Muscles and bones
Weakness, fatigue, muscle wasting, possible paralysis, and occasional swelling

Reproductive system
In women — infrequent or absent menstrual periods, decreased fertility, and a higher incidence of miscarriage; in men — abnormal breast enlargement; in both sexes — diminished sex drive

the goiter, the causes, the person's age and whether he or she plans to have children, and how long surgery will be delayed (if the person is a candidate).

Drug therapy

Antithyroid drug therapy is used for children, young adults, pregnant women, and people who refuse surgery or radioactive iodine treatment. These drugs include propylthiouracil (PTU) and Tapazole, which block thyroid hormone synthesis. Although symptoms subside within 4 to 8 weeks after such therapy begins, the person must continue the medication for 6 months to 2 years. Many people must take the drug Inderal at the same time to prevent a rapid heart rate and other side effects of treatment.

Pregnant women should receive the lowest possible dosage of antithyroid medication to minimize the risk of thyroid hormone insufficiency in the fetus. Because Graves' disease sometimes worsens after childbirth, continuous control of the mother's thyroid function is essential. The mother receiving low-dose antithyroid treatment may breast-feed as long as the infant's thyroid function is checked periodically.

Radioactive iodine treatment in the form of a single oral dose of iodine 131 is another major therapy for Graves' disease and is the preferred treatment for people who don't plan to have children. During treatment, the thyroid gland picks up the radioactive element as it does regular iodine. The radioactivity destroys some of the cells that normally concentrate iodine and produce thyroxine, thus decreasing thyroid hormone production and normalizing thyroid size and function. In most people, hypermetabolic symptoms diminish from 6 to 8 weeks after such treatment; others may require a second dose.

Surgery

Thyroidectomy — surgery to remove part of the thyroid gland — reduces its ability to produce hormone. Surgery is the preferred treatment for people with a large goiter who chronically relapse after drug therapy and for people who refuse or aren't candidates for iodine 131 treatment. (See *Questions people ask about thyroidectomy*.)

After surgery or treatment with radioactive iodine, regular lifelong medical supervision is necessary because many people develop thyroid insufficiency, sometimes years after treatment.

Other treatments

Therapy for eye problems caused by Graves' disease includes local applications of topical medications but may require high doses of corticosteroids. A person with severe eyeball bulging that causes pressure on the optic nerve may require external beam radiation therapy or surgical decompression to lessen pressure,

Treatment of thyroid storm includes administration of an antithyroid drug, intravenous Inderal, a steroid, and an iodide drug. Supportive measures include administration of nutrients, vitamins, fluids, and sedatives. (See *Advice for the person with Graves' disease*, page 458.)

STRAIGHT
TALK

Questions people ask about thyroidectomy

I know the thyroid gland is located near my voice box. Will removing my thyroid change my voice?
It shouldn't. After surgery, you may notice some slight hoarseness for a few days. However, there's a small chance that surgery may injure the recurrent laryngeal nerve, which could cause a permanent change in your voice.

Are there other risks?
Very few. But you should learn how to recognize them so they can be corrected promptly. After surgery, the main risks are bleeding, infection, and breathing difficulty. There's also a slight chance that surgery may injure the nearby parathyroid glands, which help to control your body's calcium supply.

After my thyroid is removed, will I have to keep taking medication?
That depends. If your surgeon removes all or most of your thyroid, you may need to take thyroid hormone medication to replace what your body can no longer make. On the other hand, if you have enough healthy thyroid gland remaining, you won't need this medication.

SELF-HELP

Advice for the person with Graves' disease

Monitor yourself closely

- If you're pregnant, watch closely during the first 3 months for signs of miscarriage (spotting, occasional mild cramps). Report such signs immediately.
- Get plenty of bed rest, and keep your room cool, quiet, and dark. If you have difficulty breathing, you'll be most comfortable sitting upright.
- Remember that extreme nervousness may produce bizarre behavior. Be aware that such behavior will probably subside with treatment.
- To promote weight gain, eat a balanced diet, with six meals a day. If you have swelling, eat a low-salt diet.
- Watch for signs of thyroid storm (an increased pulse, hyperactivity, fever, vomiting, and high blood pressure).
- If you have protruding eyeballs or other eye problems, wear sunglasses or eyepatches to protect your eyes from light. Moisten your eyes often with isotonic eyedrops. If you have severe eyelid retraction, avoid sudden movements that might cause the lid to slip behind the eyeball. Report signs of decreased visual clarity.

Getting the most out of treatment

- If iodide is part of your treatment, mix it with milk, juice, or water to prevent stomach upset, and drink it through a straw to prevent tooth discoloration.
- After thyroid removal, be sure to have regular medical checkups because hypothyroidism may develop 2 to 4 weeks after surgery. Report symptoms of hypothyroidism: fatigue, forgetfulness, sensitivity to cold, unexplained weight gain, and constipation.
- After radioactive iodine therapy, don't spit or cough freely because your saliva will remain radioactive for 24 hours. Your serum thyroxine levels must be measured repeatedly.
- If you're taking propylthiouracil (PTU) or Tapazole, have a complete blood count periodically to detect abnormalities. Take these medications with meals to minimize stomach upset, and avoid over-the-counter cough preparations because many contain iodine.
- If you're taking Inderal, watch for symptoms of low blood pressure, such as dizziness and decreased urine output. To prevent dizziness, rise slowly to a standing position.

*H*YPERPARATHYROIDISM

What is this condition?

In hyperparathyroidism, one or more of the four parathyroid glands (pea-sized organs located behind the thyroid) are overactive, causing excessive secretion of parathyroid hormone. This results in bone loss and leads to excessive calcium and a shortage of phosphates in the blood. Consequently, the kidneys and gastrointestinal system absorb more calcium.

What causes it?

Hyperparathyroidism may be classified as primary or secondary. In *primary hyperparathyroidism*, one or more of the parathyroid glands become enlarged. The most common cause is an adenoma, a type of benign tumor. Other causes include genetic disorders or multiple endocrine neoplasia (a rare disorder that causes the endocrine glands to become overactive). Primary hyperparathyroidism usually occurs between ages 30 and 50 but can also occur in children and the elderly. It affects women two to three times more often than men.

Secondary hyperparathyroidism is marked by excessive production of parathyroid hormone. This type of hyperparathyroidism results from a condition outside the parathyroid glands that decreases the level of calcium in the body. Such conditions include rickets, vitamin D deficiency, chronic kidney failure, or osteomalacia (softening of the bones).

What are its symptoms?

Symptoms of primary hyperparathyroidism may include:
- *kidney:* excessive urination (one of the most common effects)
- *bones and joints:* chronic lower back pain and easy fracturing due to bone degeneration; bone tenderness; pain associated with calcium buildup in joints, erosion of joint surfaces, and cartilage fractures
- *digestive tract:* severe epigastric pain radiating to the back caused by pancreatitis; abdominal pain, appetite loss, and nausea caused by peptic ulcers
- *muscles:* marked muscle weakness and wasting, particularly in the legs
- *nervous system:* psychomotor and personality disturbances, depression, overt psychosis, stupor and, possibly, coma
- *other:* skin destruction, cataracts, anemia, and calcification under the skin.

In secondary hyperparathyroidism, decreased levels of calcium in the blood may produce the same features of calcium imbalance, with skeletal deformities of the long bones (rickets, for example), as well as symptoms of the underlying disease.

How is it diagnosed?

A diagnosis of primary disease is confirmed by lab tests revealing high levels of parathyroid hormone and calcium in the blood. X-rays typically show diffuse demineralization of bones, bone cysts, outer cortical bone absorption, and subperiosteal erosion of the phalanges and distal clavicles. Microscopic examination of the bone typically shows increased bone turnover. Lab tests show elevated urine and blood calcium, chloride, and alkaline phosphatase levels and decreased blood phosphorus levels.

In secondary disease, lab findings show normal or slightly decreased serum calcium levels and variable serum phosphorus levels, especially when hyperparathyroidism is due to rickets, osteomalacia, or kidney disease. The person's history may reveal a family history of kidney disease, seizure disorders, or drug ingestion. Other lab studies and physical exam findings identify the cause of secondary hyperparathyroidism.

How is it treated?

Treatment varies, depending on the cause of the disease. Treatment for primary hyperparathyroidism may include surgery to remove the adenoma or, depending on the extent of hyperplasia, all but half of one parathyroid gland (necessary to maintain normal parathyroid hormone levels). Such surgery may relieve bone pain within 3 days. However, kidney damage may be irreversible.

If surgery isn't feasible or necessary, the following treatments can decrease calcium levels:

- forcing fluids
- limiting dietary intake of calcium
- promoting sodium and calcium excretion through forced diuresis using normal saline solution, Lasix, or Edecrin
- administering sodium, potassium phosphate, calcitonin, Mithracin, or biphosphonates.

Treatment of secondary hyperparathyroidism must correct the underlying cause. It consists of vitamin D therapy or, in the person with kidney disease, administration of an oral calcium preparation for hyperphosphatemia. In the person with kidney failure, dialysis is necessary to lower calcium levels and may have to continue for life. In the person with chronic secondary hyperparathyroidism, the enlarged glands may not revert to normal size and function even after calcium levels have been controlled.

What can a person with hyperparathyroidism do?

Be sure to receive periodic medical follow-up through lab tests. If your condition wasn't corrected surgically, make sure you avoid calcium-containing antacids and thiazide diuretics (such as Diuril).

HYPOPARATHYROIDISM

What is this condition?

Hypoparathyroidism is a deficiency of parathyroid hormone caused by disease, injury, or congenital malfunction of the parathyroid glands (pea-sized organs located behind the thyroid). Since these glands primarily regulate calcium balance, hypoparathyroidism causes calcium depletion, producing neuromuscular symptoms ranging from numbness and tingling in the arms and legs to tetany. The side effects are usually correctable with replacement therapy. However, some complications of long-term calcium deficiency, such as cataracts and calcifications within brain tissue, are irreversible.

What causes it?

Hypoparathyroidism may occur suddenly or exist as a chronic condition. There are three classifications of hypoparathyroidism:

- *Idiopathic hypoparathyroidism* may result from a genetic disorder or being born without any parathyroid glands.
- *Acquired hypoparathyroidism* often results from accidental removal of or injury to one or more parathyroid glands during surgery or, rarely, from massive thyroid radiation. Other possible causes include poor iron metabolism, lesions in various body systems, tuberculosis, cancer, or trauma.
- *Reversible hypoparathyroidism* may result from impaired hormone synthesis due to insufficient magnesium, from suppression of normal gland function due to excessive calcium, or from subnormal parathyroid function.

What are its symptoms?

Although mild hypoparathyroidism may cause no symptoms, it usually produces a calcium deficiency and high levels of phosphate in the blood, which affect the central nervous system as well as other body systems. Chronic hypoparathyroidism typically causes neuromuscular irritability, increased deep tendon reflexes, Chvostek's sign (hyperirritability of the facial nerve that causes severe pain when it's tapped), difficulty swallowing, organic brain syndrome, psychosis, mental deficiency in children, and tetany (tingling, muscle tension, and spasms) that may be severe.

SELF-HELP

Coping with hypoparathyroidism

To help you recover from this condition, follow this advice.

Diet
Maintain a high-calcium, low-phosphorus diet. Ask your doctor which foods are permitted.

Drug therapy
If you're on drug therapy, make sure to have your blood calcium levels checked at least three times a year. Watch for signs of high blood calcium, such as confusion, appetite loss, stomach pain, and muscle pain and weakness. Keep medications away from light and heat.

Skin care
If you have scaly skin, apply cream to soften it. Keep your nails trimmed to prevent them from splitting.

Other symptoms include abdominal pain; dry, lusterless hair; spontaneous hair loss; brittle fingernails that develop ridges or fall out; dry, scaly skin; cataracts; and weakened tooth enamel, which causes teeth to stain, crack, and decay easily. Depletion of blood calcium may result in irregular heartbeats and, eventually, congestive heart failure.

How is it diagnosed?
A diagnosis of hypoparathyroidism is confirmed when lab test results show reduced levels of parathyroid hormone, calcium, and phosphorus in the blood and electrocardiograph results show changes consistent with calcium depletion.

The doctor may also perform a test using a blood pressure cuff on the upper arm to help elicit possible signs of hypoparathyroidism.

How is it treated?
Treatment includes vitamin D (necessary for calcium absorption) and calcium supplements. Such therapy is usually lifelong, except for the reversible form of the disease. If the person can't tolerate the pure form of vitamin D, alternatives include Hytakerol or Rocaltrol. (See *Coping with hypoparathyroidism.*)

Acute, life-threatening tetany requires immediate intravenous administration of 10% calcium gluconate to raise serum calcium levels. The person who's awake and able to cooperate can help raise serum calcium levels by breathing into a paper bag and then inhaling his or her own carbon dioxide; this produces hypoventilation and mild respiratory acidosis. Sedatives and antiseizure drugs may control spasms until calcium levels rise. Chronic tetany requires maintenance therapy with oral calcium and vitamin D supplements.

Hypothyroidism in Adults

What is this condition?
In this disorder, thyroid hormone levels in the blood are too low because of a problem in the pituitary gland, thyroid gland, or hypothalamus (a crucial brain structure that governs many body functions). Hypothyroidism is most common in women. In the United States, the incidence is rising significantly in people ages 40 to 50.

STRAIGHT
TALK

Questions people ask about thyroid hormone replacement

Why should I tell my other doctors and my pharmacist that I have hypothyroidism?
Because hypothyroidism slows your metabolism, prolonging the effects of any medications you take. This increases your risk of having a serious drug reaction. To prevent this, your doctor (or dentist) may have to reduce the dosage of your other medications.

Thyroid hormone may also change the effectiveness of certain medications you take. Again, your doctor may need to adjust the dosage of these medications.

Why do I feel nervous and restless now after taking my medication, when I was tired and slow-moving before?
You may be taking too much thyroid hormone. Tell your doctor about these symptoms. Also tell him or her if your hands become shaky, if you have trouble sleeping, or if you experience palpitations, unexplained weight loss, rash, or a change in appetite or bowel habits. These symptoms could also mean that your dosage needs to be adjusted.

Be patient. It will take time for your doctor to find the right medication dosage for you.

Will taking thyroid hormone medication affect my other health problems?
Possibly. If you have heart disease, taking thyroid hormone may put added stress on your heart. Thyroid hormone treatment also may interfere with successful therapy for diabetes or Addison's disease. Tell you doctor if you have either of these. Ask him or her what special precautions, if any, you should take. Your doctor will closely monitor your condition, so you don't have to worry.

How long will I need to take thyroid hormone medication?
For your body to function properly and for you to feel well, you'll need to take it for the rest of your life.

What causes it?

Hypothyroidism in adults is caused by inadequate production of thyroid hormone. Usually, this stems from thyroid gland dysfunction resulting from surgery (thyroidectomy), radiation therapy (particularly with radioactive iodine), inflammation, or chronic autoimmune thyroiditis (also called *Hashimoto's disease)*. Hypothyroidism may also occur if the pituitary gland fails to produce thyroid-stimulating hormone or if the hypothalamus fails to produce thyrotropin-releasing hormone.

Other causes include congenital errors of thyroid hormone synthesis, iodine deficiency (usually dietary), or use of antithyroid medications such as propylthiouracil (PTU).

What are its symptoms?

Early symptoms of hypothyroidism are typically vague and include fatigue, forgetfulness, sensitivity to cold, unexplained weight gain, and constipation. Eventually, the person may experience mentally in-

SELF-HELP

Coping with hypothyroidism

To help you progress with therapy, follow this advice.

Eat sensibly
- Eat a high-fiber, low-calorie diet.
- Exercise regularly to prevent constipation and promote weight loss.

Take your medication
- Continue your course of thyroid medication even if your symptoms subside.
- After thyroid replacement therapy begins, watch for symptoms of an overactive thyroid, such as restlessness, sweating, and excessive weight loss.

Watch for warning signs
- Call your doctor right away if you have signs of infection such as a fever.
- Also call your doctor if you have symptoms of aggravated cardiovascular disease, such as chest pain and a fast pulse.

Spread the word
Make sure any doctor who prescribes drugs for you knows you have hypothyroidism.

stability; dry, flaky, inelastic skin; puffy face, hands, and feet; hoarseness; swelling around the eyes; drooping eyelids; dry, sparse hair; and thick, brittle nails.

Other common symptoms include appetite loss, a swollen abdomen, abnormally heavy or long menstrual periods, decreased sex drive, infertility, impaired coordination, tremors, and involuntary rhythmic movements of the eyes.

Myxedema coma

In people with hypothyroidism, infection, exposure to cold, and use of sedatives may trigger myxedema coma. This life-threatening emergency compromises many body systems. Myxedema coma usually develops gradually, but it may arise suddenly if stress aggravates severe or prolonged hypothyroidism. Without prompt treatment, myxedema coma can lead to shock and death.

Symptoms of myxedema coma include stupor, abnormally slow and shallow breathing, low levels of sodium and sugar in the blood, low blood pressure, and a reduced body temperature.

How is it diagnosed?

Radioimmunoassay, a highly sensitive lab test, confirms hypothyroidism by showing low levels of the thyroid hormones triiodothyronine and thyroxine. Other lab findings that support this diagnosis include an increased level of thyroid-stimulating hormone when hypothyroidism is due to thyroid insufficiency; a decreased thyroid-stimulating hormone level when hypothyroidism is due to hypothalamic or pituitary insufficiency; and elevated blood cholesterol and triglyceride levels.

How is it treated?

The person with hypothyroidism receives gradual thyroid hormone replacement with Levoxine and, occasionally, Cytomel.

A person with myxedema coma receives treatment to support vital functions while restoring normal thyroid function. To support blood pressure and increase the pulse rate, Levoxine and hydrocortisone are given intravenously. To restore normal breathing, the person receives supplemental oxygen and respiratory support. Other supportive measures include fluid replacement and antibiotics for infection. (See *Questions people ask about thyroid hormone replacement*, page 463, and *Coping with hypothyroidism*.)

HYPOTHYROIDISM IN CHILDREN

What do doctors call this condition?
Congenital hypothyroidism, infantile cretinism

What is this condition?
Hypothyroidism in children is a deficiency of thyroid hormone secretion during fetal development or early infancy. Untreated hypothyroidism is characterized in infants by respiratory difficulties, persistent jaundice, and hoarse crying; in older children, by stunted growth (dwarfism), bone and muscle dystrophy, and mental deficiency.

Early diagnosis and treatment offer the best prognosis; infants treated before age 3 months usually grow and develop normally. However, hypothyroid children who remain untreated beyond age 3 months and children with acquired hypothyroidism who remain untreated beyond age 2 years suffer irreversible mental retardation; their skeletal abnormalities are reversible with treatment. Hypothyroidism occurs three times more often in girls than in boys.

What causes it?
In infants, hypothyroidism usually results from defective embryonic development that causes congenital absence or underdevelopment of the thyroid gland. The next most common cause can be traced to an inherited enzymatic defect in the synthesis of the thyroid hormone thyroxine. Less frequently, antithyroid drugs taken during pregnancy produce hypothyroidism in infants. In children older than age 2, hypothyroidism usually results from chronic autoimmune thyroiditis.

What are its symptoms?
At birth, the weight and length of an infant with hypothyroidism appear normal, but characteristic signs of hypothyroidism develop by age 3 to 6 months. Breast-fed infants don't show most symptoms until they're weaned because breast milk contains small amounts of thyroid hormone.

Symptoms in infants
Typically, an infant with hypothyroidism sleeps excessively, cries rarely (except for occasional hoarse crying), and is generally inactive.

Because of this, the parents may describe the child as a "good baby — no trouble at all." However, such behavior actually results from a decreased metabolism and progressive mental impairment.

The infant with hypothyroidism also has abnormal deep-tendon reflexes; hypotonic abdominal muscles; a protruding abdomen; slow, awkward movements; feeding difficulties; constipation; and jaundice.

A large, protruding tongue obstructs respiration, making breathing loud and noisy and forcing the child to breathe through an open mouth. The child may have shortness of breath on exertion, anemia, abnormal facial features, and a dull expression, resulting from mental retardation. The skin is cold and mottled because of poor circulation, and the hair is dry, brittle, and dull. Teeth erupt late and tend to decay early; body temperature is below normal; and pulse rate is slow.

Symptoms in children

In the child who gets hypothyroidism after age 2 years, appropriate treatment will likely prevent mental retardation. However, growth retardation becomes apparent in short stature, obesity, and a head that appears abnormally large because the arms and legs are stunted. An older child may show delayed or accelerated sexual development.

How is it diagnosed?

Lab tests help determine levels of thyroid hormones. A high serum level of thyroid-stimulating hormone, associated with low levels of thyroxine and triiodothyronine, points to hypothyroidism. Since early diagnosis and treatment can minimize the effects of hypothyroidism, many states require measurement of thyroid hormone levels at birth.

Electrocardiography shows slow heart rate and electrocardiographic changes in untreated infants. Thyroid scan and radioactive iodine uptake tests show decreased uptake levels and confirm the absence of thyroid tissue in hypothyroid children. Hip, knee, and thigh X-rays reveal delayed skeletal development that is markedly inappropriate for the child's age.

How is it treated?

Early detection is mandatory to prevent irreversible mental retardation and permit normal physical development.

Treatment in infants under age 1 year consists of replacement therapy with oral Levoxine, starting with moderate doses. Dosage gradually increases to levels sufficient for lifelong maintenance. (However, a rapid increase in dosage may precipitate thyrotoxicity.)

Infants with untreated hypothyroidism suffer respiratory problems, persistent jaundice, and hoarse crying. Older children have stunted growth, bone and muscle dystrophy, and mental deficiency.

Doses are proportionately higher in children than in adults because children metabolize thyroid hormone more quickly. Older children also receive Levoxine.

What can the parents of a child with hypothyroidism do?

- Be aware that your child will require lifelong treatment with thyroid supplements. Stay alert for signs of overdose: rapid pulse, irritability, insomnia, fever, sweating, and weight loss. To prevent further mental impairment, be sure to comply with your child's treatment program.
- Focus on your child's strengths, not weaknesses. Provide stimulating activities to help the child reach maximum potential.

INFLAMMATION OF THE THYROID

What do doctors call this condition?
Thyroiditis

What is this condition?
When bacteria or viruses invade the body, they may attack the thyroid and cause it to become inflamed. Thyroid gland inflammation occurs in several forms: as a long-term autoimmune inflammation, as a self-limiting subacute granulomatous inflammation, or as several miscellaneous disorders (acute suppurative, chronic infective, and chronic noninfective inflammations). A postpartum form strikes women within 1 year after delivery. Inflammation of the thyroid is more common in women than in men.

What causes it?
Autoimmune inflammation of the thyroid results from the immune system's response to thyroid antigens that occur naturally in the blood. *Subacute granulomatous inflammation of the thyroid* usually follows mumps, influenza, coxsackievirus, or adenovirus infection.

Miscellaneous forms may result from a variety of causes. *Acute suppurative thyroiditis* may be caused by bacterial invasion of the gland. *Chronic infective thyroiditis* may be caused by tuberculosis, syphilis, actinomycosis, or other infectious agents. *Chronic noninfective thyroiditis* may be caused by sarcoidosis or amyloidosis.

What are its symptoms?

The autoimmune form usually does not produce symptoms. It commonly occurs in women, with peak incidence in middle age. It's the most prevalent cause of spontaneous hypothyroidism.

In subacute granulomatous inflammation, moderate thyroid enlargement may follow an upper respiratory tract infection or a sore throat. The thyroid may be painful and tender, and the person may have difficulty swallowing.

Clinical effects of miscellaneous inflammation are characteristic of pus-forming infection: fever, pain, tenderness, and reddened skin over the gland.

How is it diagnosed?

Lab tests are the key to accurate diagnosis. Test results vary according to the type of thyroid inflammation.

How is it treated?

Appropriate treatment varies with the type of thyroid inflammation. Drug therapy includes Levoxine for accompanying hypothyroidism, pain relievers and anti-inflammatory drugs for mild, subacute granulomatous inflammation, Inderal for transient hyperthyroidism, and steroids for severe episodes of acute inflammation. Suppurative inflammation requires antibiotic therapy.

What can a person with inflammation of the thyroid do?

■ Watch for and report symptoms of hypothyroidism (sluggishness, restlessness, sensitivity to cold, forgetfulness, dry skin).

■ Be aware that you'll need lifelong thyroid hormone therapy if hypothyroidism occurs. If you're taking this medication, watch for signs of overdose, such as nervousness and palpitations.

PHEOCHROMOCYTOMA

What is this condition?

A pheochromocytoma is a tumor of the adrenal medulla, the central core of the adrenal gland that secretes two hormones: epinephrine and norepinephrine. These hormones are called *catecholamines.* This tumor causes the adrenal medulla to produce an excess amount of catecholamines, resulting in high blood pressure, increased metabolism, and increased blood sugar.

The disorder affects all races and both sexes, occurring primarily between ages 30 and 40. It's potentially fatal, but the prognosis is generally good with treatment. However, pheochromocytoma-induced kidney damage is irreversible.

What causes it?

A pheochromocytoma may result from an inherited genetic trait. According to some estimates, about 0.5% of newly diagnosed people with high blood pressure have pheochromocytoma. Although this tumor is usually benign, it may be malignant in as many as 10% of these people.

What are its symptoms?

The most important sign of pheochromocytoma is persistent or recurrent high blood pressure. Common symptoms include palpitations, fast pulse, headache, sweating, pallor, warmth or flushing, numbness and tingling, tremor, nervousness, feelings of impending doom, abdominal pain, rapid breathing, nausea, and vomiting.

Other common effects of this disorder are postural hypotension (abnormally low blood pressure when a person stands up) and a paradoxical response to drugs used to treat high blood pressure (the drugs cause blood pressure to rise instead of decrease). The person may also develop high blood sugar and hypermetabolism. People with hypermetabolism may show marked weight loss, although some people with pheochromocytoma are obese.

Symptoms may occur as seldom as once every 2 months or as often as 25 times a day. They may occur spontaneously or may follow certain precipitating events, such as changes in posture, exercise, laughing, smoking, induction of anesthesia, urination, a change in environmental or body temperature, or pregnancy. A person who has

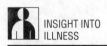

Pheochromocytoma in pregnancy

Often, pheochromocytoma is diagnosed during pregnancy, when uterine pressure on the tumor induces more frequent attacks; such attacks can prove fatal for both mother and fetus as a result of stroke, acute pulmonary edema, irregular heartbeats, or a lack of oxygen supply to tissues.

The risk of miscarriage is high in such women, but most fetal deaths occur during labor or immediately after birth.

periodic attacks may have no symptoms during a latent phase. (See *Pheochromocytoma in pregnancy*.)

How is it diagnosed?

The doctor makes a diagnosis based on the patient's health history, a physical exam, and lab tests. He or she will suspect pheochromocytoma if a person has a history of acute episodes of high blood pressure, headache, sweating, and palpitations, especially if the person also has high blood sugar, sugar in the urine, or hypermetabolism.

In rare cases, the doctor may be able to feel the tumor during inspection. Diagnosis is confirmed by a test of urine collected over a 24-hour period showing elevated levels of catecholamines.

Angiography (X-ray studies of blood vessels using contrast dye) demonstrates an adrenal medullary tumor (but the procedure may precipitate a hypertensive crisis). Various kidney function studies, adrenal venography, or computed tomography scan (commonly called a CAT scan) help to localize the tumor.

How is it treated?

Surgical removal of the tumor is the treatment of choice. To decrease blood pressure, drugs such as alpha-adrenergic blockers or Demser are given 1 to 2 weeks before surgery. A beta-adrenergic blocker such as Inderal may also be used. After surgery, intravenous fluids, plasma volume expanders, vasopressors and, possibly, transfusions may be required to treat low blood pressure. Persistent high blood pressure can occur immediately after surgery.

If surgery isn't feasible, alpha- and beta-adrenergic blockers — such as Dibenzyline and Inderal, respectively — are beneficial in controlling catecholamine effects and preventing attacks.

Management of an acute attack or hypertensive crisis requires intravenous Regitine or Nitropress to normalize blood pressure.

What can a person with pheochromocytoma do?

■ Report headaches, palpitations, nervousness, or other symptoms of an acute attack.
■ If the doctor suspects your disease was inherited, other members of your family should be evaluated for it.

SIMPLE GOITER

What do doctors call this condition?
Nontoxic goiter

What is this condition?
Simple goiter is an enlargement of the thyroid gland — the butterfly-shaped gland in the front of the neck — that's not caused by inflammation or abnormal growth of new tissue. Simple goiter is more common in women than men, especially during adolescence, pregnancy, and menopause, when the body's demand for thyroid hormone increases. With appropriate treatment, the prognosis is good.

What causes it?
Simple goiter occurs when the thyroid gland can't secrete enough thyroid hormone to meet the body's needs. To compensate, the thyroid gland enlarges. Such compensation usually overcomes mild to moderate hormonal deficiency. Goiter probably results from impaired hormone synthesis within the thyroid and depletion of the gland's iodine level, which makes it more sensitive to thyroid-stimulating hormone.

Classifying goiter
Simple goiter is commonly classified as endemic or sporadic. *Endemic goiter* usually results from too little iodine in the diet, as occurs from iodine-depleted soil or malnutrition. Using iodized salt prevents this deficiency.

Sporadic goiter is caused by eating large amounts of foods or taking drugs that decrease production of the thyroid hormone thyroxine. Such foods include rutabagas, cabbage, soybeans, peanuts, peaches, peas, strawberries, spinach, and radishes. Goiter-causing drugs include propylthiouracil (PTU), iodides, Butazolidin, Pabanol, cobalt, and Lithane. In a pregnant woman, such substances may cross the placenta and affect the fetus.

What are its symptoms?
In simple goiter, the thyroid may be mildly enlarged, or it may be huge and misshapen. Simple goiter doesn't affect metabolism, so the symptoms arise solely from the enlarged gland. The person's neck

Endemic goiter usually results from too little iodine in the diet; using iodized salt prevents this deficiency. Sporadic goiter typically is caused by eating large amounts of foods, or taking drugs that decrease thyroxine production.

Advice for the person with simple goiter

If you have simple goiter, follow the guidelines below.

Maintain a consistent drug schedule

To maintain constant thyroid hormone levels, take your prescribed thyroid hormone medication at the same time each day. Immediately report symptoms of excess thyroid hormones, such as an increased pulse, palpitations, diarrhea, sweating, tremors, agitation, and shortness of breath.

Have some salt

If you have an endemic goiter, use iodized salt to supply the daily 150 to 300 micrograms of iodine needed to prevent goiter.

may be swollen; if the gland compresses the windpipe and esophagus, difficulty breathing and swallowing may occur. A large goiter may impede blood flow through the veins, causing them to swell. Blocked veins may cause dizziness or fainting when the person raises his or her arms above the head.

How is it diagnosed?

The doctor reviews the medical history and performs a physical exam to rule out disorders with similar symptoms, such as Graves' disease, Hashimoto's disease, and thyroid cancer. A detailed history also may reveal goiter-causing foods or medications or geographic factors.

Lab test results that suggest goiter include:
- a normal-to-high level of thyroid-stimulating hormone
- low-normal or normal thyroxine levels
- normal or increased uptake of radioactive iodine

How is it treated?

The goal of treatment is to reduce an enlarged thyroid. The treatment of choice is thyroid hormone replacement with Levoid, a preparation that inhibits secretion of thyroid-stimulating hormone and allows the gland to rest. Small doses of iodide commonly relieve goiter caused by iodine deficiency. A person with sporadic goiter must avoid goiter-causing drugs and foods.

For a large goiter that doesn't respond to treatment, the surgeon may have to remove part of the thyroid. (See *Advice for the person with simple goiter.*)

EYE DISORDERS

AGE-RELATED MACULAR DEGENERATION

Among the elderly, macular degeneration is one of the leading causes of blindness.

What is this condition?

Macular degeneration — atrophy or degeneration of the macular disk, located near the center of the retina — accounts for about 12% of all cases of blindness in North America and for about 17% of new cases. Among the elderly, macular degeneration is one of the leading causes of blindness.

Two types of age-related macular degeneration occur. The dry form is characterized by atrophic pigment epithelial changes and is most often associated with slow, progressive, and mild vision loss. The wet form causes rapidly progressive and severe vision loss.

What causes it?

Age-related macular degeneration results from hardening and obstruction of the retina's arteries, probably reflecting normal degenerative changes. No predisposing conditions have been identified. However, it may be hereditary.

What are its symptoms?

The person notices a change in central vision, such as a blank spot in the center of the page when reading.

How is it diagnosed?

An eye examination may reveal dramatic macular changes. In an angiogram of the eye, sequential photographs may show leaking vessels as a special dye flows into the tissues from the network of blood vessels behind the retina. An Amsler's grid test reveals visual field loss.

How is it treated?

Laser photocoagulation can reduce the incidence of severe vision loss in some people.

What can a person with age-related macular degeneration do?

Be aware that special devices, such as low-vision optical aids, are available to improve your quality of life if you still have adequate peripheral vision.

BLEPHARITIS

What is this condition?

A common eye inflammation, especially in children, blepharitis produces a red-rimmed appearance on the margins of the eyelids. It often involves both eyes and can affect both upper and lower eyelids.

The two forms of the disorder are *seborrheic (nonulcerative) blepharitis*, characterized by greasy scales, and *staphylococcal (ulcerative) blepharitis*, in which dry scales with tiny ulcerated areas appear along the lid margins. Both types may coexist.

Blepharitis tends to recur and become chronic. It can be controlled if treatment begins before other eye structures are involved.

What causes it?

Seborrheic blepharitis generally results from seborrhea of the scalp, eyebrows, and ears; staphylococcal blepharitis, from *Staphylococcus aureus* infection. Blepharitis may also result from infestations of body lice (pediculosis) on the brows and lashes, which irritates the lid margins.

What are its symptoms?

Typically, the person complains of itching, burning, a foreign-body sensation, and sticky, crusted eyelids on waking. This constant irritation leads to unconscious rubbing of the eyes (causing reddened rims) or continual blinking. Other signs include greasy scales in seborrheic blepharitis; flaky scales on lashes, loss of lashes, and ulcerated areas on lid margins in staphylococcal blepharitis; and nits (louse eggs) on lashes if the person has pediculosis.

How is it diagnosed?

Diagnosis depends on the person's history and symptoms. In staphylococcal blepharitis, culture of the ulcerated lid margin shows *S. aureus*. In pediculosis, lash examination reveals nits.

How is it treated?

Early treatment is essential to prevent recurrence or complications. Treatment depends on the type of blepharitis:

- *seborrheic blepharitis:* daily shampooing (using a mild shampoo on a damp applicator stick or a washcloth) to remove scales from the lid

SELF-HELP

Tips for managing blepharitis

You can control this common eyelid inflammation or prevent it from getting worse. Just follow these directions:

- Remove scales from your lid margins daily, using an applicator stick or a clean washcloth.
- Apply warm compresses. To do this, fill a clean bowl with warm water. Then immerse a clean cloth in the water and wring it out. Place the warm cloth against your closed eyelid, taking care not to burn your skin. Hold the compress in place until it cools. Continue this procedure for 15 minutes.

margins and frequent shampooing of the scalp and eyebrows (see *Tips for managing blepharitis*)

- *staphylococcal blepharitis:* sulfonamide eye ointment or an appropriate antibiotic
- *blepharitis resulting from pediculosis:* removal of nits (with forceps) or application of ophthalmic Eserine Sulfate or another ointment as an insecticide (this may cause pupil constriction and, possibly, headache, conjunctival irritation, and blurred vision from the film of ointment on the cornea).

BULGING EYES

What do doctors call this condition?

Besides bulging eyes, doctors call this condition exophthalmos or proptosis.

What is this condition?

In a person with this condition, one or both of the eyeballs protrude or appear to bulge forward. The prognosis depends on the underlying cause.

What causes it?

Bulging eyes commonly result from Graves' disease, a thyroid disorder that causes the eyeballs to be displaced forward and the lids to retract. When only one eye is affected, another possible cause is traumatic injury, such as fracture of the ethmoid bone, which allows air from the adjacent sinus cavity to enter the orbital tissue, displacing soft tissue and the eyeball. Bulging eyes may also stem from hemorrhage, varicosities, blood clots, and swelling, all of which similarly displace one or both eyeballs.

Other causes include infection, cancer, cysts, and paralysis of certain eye muscles.

What are its symptoms?

The obvious sign is a bulging eyeball, commonly accompanied by double vision. The person may blink infrequently. Other symptoms depend on the cause.

How is it diagnosed?

This disorder is usually obvious on physical examination; a special device that shows the degree of eyeball projection and misalignment between the eyes can confirm the diagnosis.

How is it treated?

Treatment hinges on the cause of the condition. For instance, if the condition stems from Graves' disease, treatment may include anti-thyroid drug therapy or partial or total removal of the thyroid gland, initial high doses of steroids, and protective eye lubricants.

Surgery may be done to correct lid retraction or preserve vision.

CATARACT

What is this condition?

A cataract is a clouding of the lens of the eye, which is normally transparent. This clouding makes vision fuzzy. (See *How a cataract blurs vision.*) A common cause of vision loss, cataracts usually affect both eyes — except for traumatic cataracts, which usually occur in just one eye.

A disorder of aging, cataracts are most common in people over age 70. The prognosis is generally good; surgery improves vision in 95% of people with the disorder.

What causes it?

Cataracts have various causes:

- *Senile cataracts* develop in the elderly, probably from chemical changes in the lens of the eye.
- *Congenital cataracts* occur in newborns as genetic defects or may result from German measles contracted by the mother during the first trimester of pregnancy.
- *Traumatic cataracts* develop after a foreign body injures the lens with enough force to allow eye fluids to enter the lens capsule.
- *Complicated cataracts* result from other eye disorders (such as inflammation of the uveal tract in the eye, glaucoma, or a detached retina) or from a systemic disease such as diabetes, underactive parathyroid glands, or a skin inflammation called atopic dermatitis.

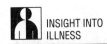

INSIGHT INTO ILLNESS

How a cataract blurs vision

In the normal eye, light shining on the cornea passes through the pupil and the clear lens and is focused upside down on the retina. The retina converts light into electrical impulses, and the optic nerve collects and sends these impulses to the brain, which interprets the image the right way up.

In an eye with a cataract, light shining through the cornea is blocked by a cloudy lens. As a result, a blurred image is cast onto the retina, and a hazy image travels to the brain.

Understanding lens replacement options

If you're scheduled for cataract surgery, be aware that removing the clouded lens won't restore your vision on its own. You'll need a device to replace the missing lens. Most often, the doctor uses a lens implant to correct vision. Occasionally, a contact lens may be an option.

Without a lens implant, your vision will be blurred after surgery. You must wait 4 to 8 weeks after surgery until the doctor can prescribe contact lenses or reading glasses or both.

Lens implant

With this lens, you'll probably have clear distance vision immediately, but you'll need reading glasses for near vision. The lens implant, which corrects vision to 20/20 in some people, provides normal depth perception and peripheral vision with no distortion.

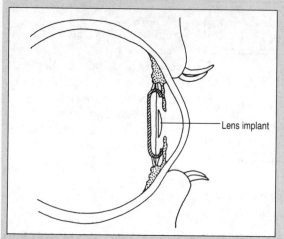

Lens implant

Contact lens

A contact lens provides normal depth perception and peripheral vision. But not everyone can wear a

lens comfortably. Moreover, learning to insert and remove the lens requires patience, perseverance, and a steady hand.

You'll also need to clean and care for the lens. Even an extended-wear lens, which you can wear continually for up to 7 days, must be checked, cleaned, and reinserted by the doctor at regular intervals. Expect minimal distortion.

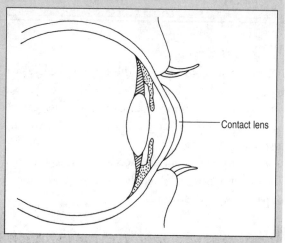

Contact lens

These cataracts can also result from exposure to ionizing radiation or infrared rays.

- *Toxic cataracts* result from toxicity from certain drugs (such as Orasone, ergot alkaloids, and phenothiazines) or certain chemicals (such as dinitrophenol and naphthalene).

What are its symptoms?

Typically, a cataract causes painless, gradual blurring of vision and vision loss. As it progresses, the normally black pupil turns milky white. Other symptoms include blinding glare from headlights when driving at night, poor reading vision, and an unpleasant glare and poor vision in bright sunlight. If the central part of the lens is cloudy, vision is better in dim light than in bright light.

How is it diagnosed?

Shining a penlight into the eye reveals the white area of an advanced cataract behind the pupil. To confirm the diagnosis, the doctor performs ophthalmoscopic and slit-lamp exams.

How is it treated?

To restore sight, the cataract must be removed. Usually, this is done in one of the following same-day surgical procedures:

- *Extracapsular cataract extraction* removes the front lens capsule, leaving the rear lens capsule intact. Then an intraocular lens is implanted where the person's own lens used to be. This procedure can be done in people of all ages.
- *Phacoemulsification* fragments the cloudy lens with ultrasonic vibrations; lens debris is removed by suction.
- *Discission and aspiration* can still be used for children with soft cataracts but the procedure is obsolete.

A person with an intraocular lens implant has clear distance vision once the eye patch is removed but needs corrective reading glasses or contact lenses for reading. Glasses or lenses are fitted 4 to 8 weeks after surgery. (See *Understanding lens replacement options*.)

After surgery, the person must care for the eye properly. (See *Avoiding complications after cataract surgery*.)

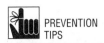 PREVENTION TIPS

Avoiding complications after cataract surgery

To prevent accidental eye injury, you'll have a patch and shield on your eye for up to 24 hours after surgery, until you see the doctor the next day. Then for several weeks, you'll wear an eye shield (a plastic or metal shield with perforations) or glasses during the day and an eye shield at night.

To speed healing

- Sleep on your unaffected side.
- Avoid activities that increase pressure within your eye, such as straining when defecating.
- Don't get soap or unsterile water in your eyes.
- Follow the activity restrictions specified by your doctor.
- Call your doctor immediately if you experience sharp eye pain.

CHALAZION

What is this condition?

A chalazion is an enlarged gland in the upper or lower eyelid. This common eye disorder usually develops over several weeks. A chalazion may become large enough to press on the eyeball, causing astigmatism.

A chalazion is generally benign and chronic, and can occur at any age. In some people, it's apt to recur. A large chalazion seldom subsides spontaneously.

Tips for treating a chalazion

To speed the healing process, do the following:
- Clean your eyelids with water and mild baby shampoo applied with a cotton applicator.
- Apply warm compresses to your eyelid, as instructed by your doctor. Take special care to avoid burning your skin. Always use a clean cloth and discard used compresses. Start applying warm compresses at the first sign of lid irritation.

What causes it?

A meibomian (sebaceous) gland in the eyelid becomes inflamed; eventually the gland's duct becomes plugged, causing the characteristic swelling of a chalazion.

What are its symptoms?

A chalazion occurs as a painless, hard lump that usually points toward the conjunctival side of the eyelid.

How is it diagnosed?

The doctor will examine the eye and palpate the eyelid to disclose a small bump or nodule. Frequently recurring chalazions, especially in an adult, require a biopsy to rule out meibomian cancer.

How is it treated?

Initially, the doctor will apply warm compresses to open the duct of the gland. Sometimes he'll instill sulfonamide eyedrops. (See *Tips for treating a chalazion.*)

If such therapy fails, or if the chalazion presses on the eyeball or causes a severe cosmetic problem, steroid injection or incision and curettage under local anesthesia may be necessary.

CORNEAL ABRASION

What is this condition?

Corneal abrasion is a scratch on the surface lining of the cornea — the transparent, convex, front portion of the eye. The most common eye injury, corneal abrasion has a good prognosis if properly treated.

What causes it?

Corneal abrasion usually occurs when a foreign body, such as a bit of dust or dirt, lodges under the eyelid. Even if the particle is washed out by tears, it may still injure the cornea. For instance, a tiny piece of metal that gets in the eye of a worker who neglects to wear protective eyewear quickly forms a rust ring on the cornea and abrades it. Corneal abrasions are also common in people who fall asleep wearing hard contact lenses.

A corneal scratch from a fingernail, a piece of paper, or another organic substance may cause a persistent wound. The lining doesn't always heal properly, and recurrent corneal erosion may develop, with delayed effects that are more severe than the original injury.

What are the symptoms?

Typically, corneal abrasion causes redness, pain, increased tearing, and a sensation of something in the eye, even after the offending particle falls out. A corneal abrasion may also affect vision. Because the cornea is richly endowed with nerve endings, symptoms are more severe than the size of the injury would suggest.

How is it diagnosed?

Diagnosis is based on typical symptoms and a history of eye injury or prolonged wearing of contact lenses. The doctor will examine the eye with a penlight to reveal a foreign body on the cornea; to check for a foreign body embedded under the lid, he or she will gently turn the eyelid inside out. To confirm the diagnosis, the doctor may stain the cornea with fluorescein, a dye that makes the injured area look green when examined with a penlight.

How is it treated?

To remove a deeply embedded foreign body, the doctor uses a spadelike device after applying a topical anesthetic. To remove a rust ring on the cornea, the doctor uses an ophthalmic burr, an abrasive device. When only partial removal is possible, healing of the epithelium lifts the ring to the surface and allows complete removal the next day.

After the foreign body is removed, antibiotic eyedrops must be instilled in the affected eye every 3 to 4 hours. Applying a pressure patch prevents further corneal irritation when the person blinks, except where abrasion is caused by contact lenses. (See *Coping with a corneal abrasion.*)

 SELF-HELP

Coping with a corneal abrasion

A scratched cornea usually heals in 24 to 48 hours. By following these suggestions, you can help it heal without complications.

Using an eye patch
If the doctor has instructed you to wear an eye patch, be sure to leave the patch in place for 12 to 24 hours. Be aware that the patch alters your depth perception, so you'll need to use caution in everyday activities, such as climbing stairs and stepping off a curb.

Applying medication
Learn how to instill prescribed antibiotic eyedrops properly, since an untreated corneal infection can lead to ulceration and permanent vision loss.

CORNEAL ULCER

What is this condition?

A major cause of blindness worldwide, corneal ulcers produce scarring or perforation of the cornea. They occur in the central or marginal areas of the cornea, but marginal ulcers are the most common form. A person may have one or several ulcers, of varied size and shape. Prompt treatment (within hours of onset) can prevent visual impairment.

What causes it?

A corneal ulcer generally results from infections by protozoa, bacteria, viruses, or fungi. Other causes include trauma, exposure, vitamin A deficiency, toxins, and allergens.

What are its symptoms?

Typically, a corneal ulcer causes pain (aggravated by blinking) and sensitivity to light, followed by increased tearing. Eventually, a central corneal ulcer blurs vision markedly. Bacterial ulcers may produce a pus-filled discharge.

How is it diagnosed?

A history of trauma or use of contact lenses and a penlight exam that reveals an irregular corneal surface suggest a corneal ulcer. Fluorescein dye, instilled in the conjunctival sac, stains the outline of the ulcer and confirms the diagnosis. Cultures of corneal scraping may identify the causative bacterium or fungus.

How is it treated?

Treatment aims to relieve pain and eliminate the underlying cause of the ulcer, as follows:

- *Pseudomonas aeruginosa:* the antibiotics Aerosporin and Garamycin, given topically and by subconjunctival injection, or Geocillin and Tobrex given intravenously. Since this type of corneal ulcer spreads so rapidly, it can cause corneal perforation and loss of vision within 48 hours. Immediate treatment and isolation of hospitalized patients are required. Eye coverings are never used when treating bacterial corneal ulcers.
- *herpes simplex type 1 virus:* hourly topical application of Herplex or Vira-A Ophthalmic. Corneal ulcers resulting from a viral infection often recur.
- *varicella-zoster virus:* a topical sulfonamide ointment applied 3 to 4 times daily to prevent secondary infection. These lesions are typically painful, so the person also receives pain relievers.
- *fungi:* instillation of Natacyn eyedrops for *Fusarium, Cephalosporium,* and *Candida*

■ *vitamin A deficiency:* correction of dietary deficiency or malabsorption of vitamin A

■ *neurotropic ulcers or exposure keratitis:* frequent instillation of artificial tears or lubricating ointments and use of a plastic bubble eye shield.

Prompt treatment is essential for all forms of corneal ulcer to prevent complications and permanent vision problems or blindness.

CROSS-EYE

What do doctors call this condition?
Strabismus or squint

What is this condition?
Cross-eye is a misalignment of the eye caused by the absence of normal, parallel, or coordinated eye movement. In children, it may be *concomitant,* in which the degree of deviation doesn't vary with the direction of gaze; *inconcomitant,* in which the degree of deviation varies with the direction of gaze; *congenital* (present at birth or during the first 6 months); or *acquired* (present during the first 2½ years.)

Cross-eye can also be latent (phoria) — apparent only when the child is tired or sick — or manifest (tropia). In tropias, the eyes deviate in one of four ways: esotropia (eyes deviate inward), exotropia (eyes deviate outward), hypertropia (eyes deviate upward), and hypotropia (eyes deviate downward).

The prognosis for correction varies with the timing of treatment and the onset of the disorder. Muscle imbalances may be corrected by glasses, patching, or surgery, depending on the cause. However, residual defects in vision and extraocular muscle alignment may persist even after treatment.

Cross-eye affects about 2% of the population. Its incidence is higher in people with central nervous system disorders, such as cerebral palsy, mental retardation, and Down syndrome.

What causes it?
Cross-eye is frequently inherited, but its cause is unknown. Controversy exists over whether or not amblyopia (lazy eye) causes or results from cross-eye. Strabismic amblyopia is characterized by loss of central vision

When to have surgery?

The timing of surgery for cross-eye varies. For instance, a 6-month-old infant with equal visual acuity and a large inward deviation of one eye will have surgery to correct cross-eye. But a child with unequal visual acuity and acquired cross-eye will have the affected eye patched until visual acuity is equal and then undergo surgery.

in one eye that typically leads to esotropia. It may result from far-sightedness or unequal refractive power. Esotropia may result from muscle imbalance and may be congenital or acquired. In accommodative esotropia, the child's attempt to compensate for farsightedness affects the convergent reflex, and the eyes cross.

Misalignment of the eyes suppresses vision in one of the eyes, causing amblyopia if it develops early in life.

What are its symptoms?

Misalignment of the eyes can be detected by an external eye exam when deviation is obvious or by ophthalmoscopic observation of the corneal light reflex in the center of the pupils. Cross-eye also causes double vision and other visual disturbances, which is often the reason the person seeks medical help.

How is it diagnosed?

Parents of children with cross-eye typically seek medical advice. Older people with cross-eye commonly seek treatment to correct double vision or improve their appearance. A detailed history is essential not only for the diagnosis but for treatment. Eye tests also help diagnose cross-eye.

How is it treated?

Initial treatment depends on the type of cross-eye. In strabismic amblyopia, therapy includes patching the normal eye and prescribing corrective glasses to keep the abnormal eye straight and to counteract farsightedness.

Surgery is often necessary for cosmetic and psychological reasons to correct cross-eye due to basic esotropia, or residual accommodative esotropia after correction with glasses. The timing of surgery varies from person to person. (See *When to have surgery?*)

Surgical correction consists of moving or shortening the muscle. A new procedure uses an adjustable suture. Eye exercises and corrective glasses may still be necessary; surgery may have to be repeated.

DROOPING EYELID

What do doctors call this condition?

Ptosis

What is this condition?

A drooping eyelid may be present at birth or develop later in life. It can affect one or both eyes and be constant or intermittent. A severely drooping eyelid usually responds well to treatment, and a slightly drooping eyelid may require no treatment at all.

What causes it?

If present at birth, a drooping eyelid is genetically transmitted or results from a failure of the levator muscles of the eyelids to develop. This condition usually affects one eyelid.

An acquired drooping eyelid may result from any of the following:
- age (involutional drooping eyelid, the most common form)
- mechanical factors that make the eyelid heavy, such as swelling or an extra fatty fold
- myogenic factors, such as muscular dystrophy or myasthenia gravis
- neurogenic (paralytic) factors from injury, diabetes, or carotid aneurysm
- nutritional problems, such as thiamine (vitamin B_1) deficiency in chronic alcoholism.

What are its symptoms?

An infant with a congenital drooping eyelid has a smooth, flat upper eyelid, without the eyelid fold normally produced by the pull of the levator muscle.

A child with one drooping eyelid that covers the pupil may develop a lazy eye from disuse or lack of eye stimulation. A child with two drooping eyelids may elevate the brow in an attempt to compensate, wrinkling the forehead in an effort to raise the upper lid. To see, the child may tilt the head backward.

How is it diagnosed?

A physical exam shows the severity of drooping eyelid. Additional tests determine the underlying cause.

Taking precautions after eyelid surgery

If you've had surgery to treat a drooping eyelid, here's what you can do to aid the healing process:

- Immediately tell the doctor about any bleeding on the pressure patch.
- Take special precautions to prevent accidental injury to the surgical site until healing is complete (in about 6 weeks). If the suture line is damaged, the drooping eyelid may recur.

How is it treated?

A slightly drooping eyelid that doesn't cause deformity or vision loss requires no treatment. A severely drooping eyelid that interferes with vision or is cosmetically undesirable usually requires surgery to fix the weak levator muscles. (See *Taking precautions after eyelid surgery*.)

Surgery to correct congenital drooping eyelid is usually performed at age 3 or 4, but it may be done earlier if both eyelids droop. If surgery is undesirable, special glasses with an attached suspended crutch on the frames may elevate the eyelid.

The underlying cause of drooping eyelid also is treated.

EXTRAOCULAR MOTOR NERVE PALSIES

What are these conditions?

Extraocular motor nerve palsies are dysfunctions of the third, fourth, and sixth cranial nerves, which are involved with movement and focusing of the eyes.

What causes them?

The most common causes of extraocular motor nerve palsies are diabetic neuropathy and pressure from an aneurysm or a brain tumor. Other causes vary, depending on which cranial nerve is involved.

What are their symptoms?

The most characteristic symptom is double vision of recent onset. Typically, the person with third nerve palsy exhibits drooping eyelid, an eye that looks outward, dilated pupils, and an inability to adjust to light.

The person with fourth nerve palsy has double vision and cannot rotate the eye downward or upward; wryneck may develop from repeatedly tilting the head to the affected side to compensate for double vision.

Sixth nerve palsy causes one eye to turn; the eye cannot abduct beyond the midline. To compensate for double vision, the person turns the head to the unaffected side and develops wryneck.

How are they diagnosed?

The doctor will perform a complete neuro-ophthalmologic exam and obtain a thorough history. Differential diagnosis of third, fourth, or sixth nerve palsy depends on the specific motor defect. For all extraocular motor nerve palsies, skull X-rays and a computed tomography scan (called a CAT scan) rule out tumors. The person is also evaluated for an aneurysm or diabetes. If sixth nerve palsy results from infection, cultures identify the causative organism and determine the choice of an antibiotic.

How are they treated?

Treatment depends on the underlying cause. Neurosurgery is necessary if the cause is a brain tumor or an aneurysm. For infection, massive doses of antibiotics may be appropriate. After treatment of the primary condition, the person may need to perform exercises that stretch the neck muscles.

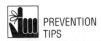

PREVENTION TIPS

Glaucoma screening

For early detection and prevention of glaucoma, everyone over age 35 — especially people with a family history of glaucoma — should have an annual eye exam with tonometry to measure intraocular pressure.

GLAUCOMA

What is this condition?

In glaucoma, the eye is affected by abnormally high internal (intraocular) pressure. Glaucoma can damage the optic nerve, which conducts visual impulses to the brain for sight perception. If untreated, it can lead to gradual vision loss and, ultimately, blindness.

Glaucoma occurs in several forms: chronic open-angle, acute closed-angle, congenital (an inherited disorder), and secondary (resulting from other causes).

Glaucoma affects about 2% of the North American population over age 40 and accounts for 12% of all new cases of blindness. Its incidence is highest among blacks. With early treatment, the prognosis is good.

What causes it?

Chronic open-angle glaucoma results from too much aqueous humor (a fluid in the front of the eye). This form of glaucoma often runs in families and accounts for about 90% of all cases.

Questions people ask about trabeculectomy

Now that I've had surgery for glaucoma, can I stop using my eyedrops?
Not unless your doctor says so. In fact, you may need to continue using them indefinitely because surgery only relieves the buildup of pressure within your eye. If you've been putting drops in the opposite eye, continue to do so. That's because glaucoma often affects both eyes.

Will I see better after surgery?
Unfortunately, you won't. Your optic nerve was permanently damaged. The surgery aims to prevent further vision loss.

Why does the doctor want to keep testing my vision?
Visual field tests keep track of glaucoma, a disease that robs your vision like a "thief in the night." In other words, you may not be aware of any further vision loss until after it happens. However, visual field tests detect even tiny losses. Your doctor will use these tests to determine if and when to adjust your glaucoma medication to prevent further vision loss.

Acute closed-angle (narrow-angle) glaucoma can result from blocked drainage of aqueous humor due to narrow angles between the front part of the iris and the rear surface of the cornea; shallow anterior chambers (the spaces behind the cornea and in front of the iris); thickening of the iris that causes angle closure when the pupils are dilated; or a bulging iris that causes the angle to close. Unless treated promptly, this form of glaucoma leads to blindness in 3 to 5 days.

Secondary glaucoma can result from inflammation of the membrane covering the eye, trauma, or drugs (such as steroids.) Growth of new blood vessels in the angle can result from a blocked vein or diabetes.

What are the symptoms?

Chronic open-angle glaucoma usually affects both eyes; it develops and progresses gradually. Symptoms arise late in the disease and include mild aching in the eyes, loss of peripheral vision, seeing halos around lights, and reduced visual acuity (especially at night) that eyeglasses don't correct.

Acute closed-angle glaucoma typically begins suddenly; in fact, it's an emergency. Symptoms may include inflammation and pain in one eye, pressure over the eye, moderate pupil dilation that doesn't react to light, a cloudy cornea, blurring, reduced visual acuity, abnormal sensitivity to light, and seeing halos around lights. This form of glaucoma may be mistaken for stomach upset because increased intraocular pressure may cause nausea and vomiting.

How is it diagnosed?

Loss of peripheral vision and changes in the optic disk (a blind spot in the surface of the retina) confirm glaucoma. The doctor may also order the following diagnostic tests:

- *Tonometry* measures intraocular pressure by determining the eyeball's resistance to indentation by an applied force from a handheld device. Normal pressure ranges from 8 to 21 millimeters of mercury. However, people who fall in this normal range can develop symptoms of glaucoma, and people with abnormally high pressure may have no symptoms. (See *Glaucoma screening,* page 487.)
- *Slit-lamp exam* allows the doctor to examine the frontal structures of the eye, including the cornea, iris, and lens.
- *Gonioscopy* involves use of a special instrument that determines the angle of the eye's anterior chamber to distinguish between chronic open-angle and acute closed-angle glaucoma. In chronic open-angle

glaucoma, the angle is normal. However, in older people, partial angle closure may also occur, so two forms of glaucoma may coexist.

- *Ophthalmoscopy* allows the doctor to look at the deepest part of the eye, where cupping and shrinkage of the optic disk are visible in chronic open-angle glaucoma. These changes appear later in chronic closed-angle glaucoma if the disease is not brought under control. In acute closed-angle glaucoma, the optic disk looks pale.
- *Perimetry or visual field tests* reveal peripheral vision loss, pinpointing the extent of chronic open-angle deterioration.

How is it treated?

In chronic open-angle glaucoma, treatment initially aims to reduce aqueous humor production. The doctor may prescribe the following drugs:

- beta blockers, such as Timoptic or Betoptic
- epinephrine to lower intraocular pressure
- diuretics, such as Diamox.

Drug treatment also includes eyedrops that constrict the pupil, such as Pilocar, to help drain aqueous humor.

People who don't respond to drugs may be candidates for argon laser trabeculoplasty or a surgical filtering procedure called trabeculectomy. In trabeculoplasty, an argon laser beam is focused on a certain part of the eye, producing a thermal burn that improves aqueous humor drainage. In trabeculectomy, some eye tissue and part of the iris are removed to allow aqueous humor to drain under the conjunctiva. (See *Questions people ask about trabeculectomy.*)

Acute closed-angle glaucoma is an emergency that must be treated immediately. If drugs don't lower the intraocular pressure enough, the doctor uses a laser to cut into the iris or removes a peripheral part of the iris to preserve vision. To prevent an acute episode of glaucoma in the normal eye, preventive iris surgery is performed a few days later on this eye. Before surgery, the person receives drugs to help lower intraocular pressure.

What can a person with glaucoma do?

Closely follow the prescribed drug regimen to prevent optic disk changes, vision loss, and increased intraocular pressure. (See *Questions people ask about glaucoma.*)

STRAIGHT TALK

Questions people ask about glaucoma

What is intraocular pressure?

It's the force exerted by the fluids within your eyeball, called aqueous humor and vitreous humor. *Aqueous humor* is the clear fluid in the front of your eye that is constantly being produced and reabsorbed. *Vitreous humor* is a jellylike substance in the back of your eye. Its volume stays constant.

What causes increased intraocular pressure?

Intraocular pressure rises when the aqueous humor doesn't drain normally or when too much aqueous humor is being produced. It can rise suddenly if the opening between the iris and the lens narrows, causing a buildup of aqueous humor. Or it can rise slowly if some other part of the eye's drainage system malfunctions.

Will I go blind?

If your intraocular pressure isn't lowered and permanently brought under control, you will go blind. Persistently high intraocular pressure impairs blood supply to the optic nerve, eventually causing blindness. The doctor will choose a treatment to try to lower your intraocular pressure and save your vision.

INFLAMMATION OF THE CORNEA

What do doctors call this condition?

Keratitis

What is this condition?

Inflammation of the cornea (the transparent covering of the eye) may be acute or chronic and superficial or deep. Superficial inflammation is fairly common and may develop at any age. The prognosis is good with treatment. Without treatment, recurrent inflammation of the cornea may lead to blindness.

What causes it?

Inflammation of the cornea usually results from infection by herpes simplex virus type 1 (known as *dendritic* inflammation of the cornea). It may also result from exposure caused by the person's inability to close the eyelids, or from congenital syphilis (known as *interstitial* inflammation of the cornea). Less commonly, it stems from bacterial or fungal infections.

What are its symptoms?

Usually occurring in one eye, inflammation of the cornea produces cloudy areas in the corneal tissue, mild irritation, tearing, and sensitivity to light. An infection in the center of the cornea may produce blurred vision. When inflammation results from exposure, it usually affects the lower portion of the cornea.

How is it diagnosed?

The doctor will perform a slit-lamp exam to confirm inflammation of the cornea. To determine if the inflammation results from herpes virus infection, the doctor will stain the eye with a fluorescein-impregnated strip, which produces one or more small, dendritic (branchlike) lesions. Touching the cornea with cotton reveals reduced corneal sensation.

Vision testing may show slightly decreased acuity. The person's history may reveal a recent infection of the upper respiratory tract accompanied by cold sores. (See *Anticipating flare-ups.*)

How is it treated?

Acute inflammation caused by the herpes virus is treated with Herplex eyedrops and ointment or Vira-A Ophthalmic ointment; recurrent herpetic inflammations are treated with Viroptic solution. A broad-spectrum antibiotic may prevent secondary bacterial infection. Chronic dendritic inflammation may respond more quickly to Vira-A. Long-term topical therapy may be necessary. (Corticosteroid therapy should not be used in dendritic inflammation or any other viral or fungal disease of the cornea.) Treatment of fungal inflammation consists of Natacyn.

Inflammation due to exposure requires application of moisturizing ointment to the exposed cornea and a plastic bubble eye shield or eye patch. Treatment of severe corneal scarring may include a cornea transplant.

OPTIC ATROPHY

What is this condition?

Optic atrophy is degeneration of the optic nerve; it can develop spontaneously (primary form) or follow inflammation or swelling of the nerve head (secondary form). This condition may subside without treatment, but the nerve degeneration is irreversible.

What causes it?

Optic atrophy usually results from central nervous system disorders, such as:
- pressure on the optic nerve from an aneurysm or an intraorbital or intracranial tumor
- optic neuritis, which may occur in multiple sclerosis or other degenerative neurologic disorders.

What are its symptoms?

Optic atrophy causes painless loss of visual acuity or visual field defects, or both. Loss of vision may be abrupt or gradual, depending on the cause.

How is it diagnosed?

Slit-lamp examination and ophthalmoscopy confirm the diagnosis. Visual field testing reveals an abnormal blind spot (scotoma) and, possibly, a major visual field deficit.

How is it treated?

Optic atrophy is irreversible, so treatment generally consists of correcting the underlying cause to prevent further vision loss. Steroids may be given to decrease inflammation and swelling if a space-occupying lesion is the cause. In multiple sclerosis, optic neuritis often subsides spontaneously.

PINKEYE

What do doctors call this condition?

Conjunctivitis

What is this condition?

Pinkeye is an inflammation of the conjunctiva — the delicate membrane that lines the eyelids and covers the exposed surface of the eyeball. This disorder is usually harmless, but it can become chronic. In the Western hemisphere, it's probably the most common eye disorder.

What causes it?

Pinkeye usually results from infection, allergy, or chemical reactions. (See *Questions people ask about pinkeye*.)

Allergic and chemical causes include pollen, grass, topical medications, air pollutants, smoke, and occupational irritants (acids and alkalies). Seasonal or warm-weather pinkeye is caused by an allergy to an unidentified substance. This form of pinkeye, which affects both eyes, usually begins before puberty and lasts about 10 years. Sometimes, it's associated with other allergy symptoms commonly related to grass or pollen sensitivity.

STRAIGHT
TALK

Questions people ask about pinkeye

Why do I get pinkeye so often?
Pinkeye commonly results from a bacterial or viral infection. Without realizing it, you may be contaminating your eyes with infected fingers, towels, washcloths, contact lenses, or eye makeup. To prevent recurrent infections, avoid touching or rubbing either the infected or the uninfected eye with your fingers. And don't share washcloths and towels with family members. Also, make a habit of washing your hands frequently.

If someone else in my family gets pinkeye, can they use my medicine?
No, they shouldn't share your medicine. The doctor prescribed your medicine especially for your condition. Just because another family member has similar symptoms doesn't mean he has the same type of pinkeye — or should use the same medicine as you.

Can I use the same eyedrops or ointment if I get pinkeye again?
No. When your pinkeye has improved, throw your medicine away. Leftover medicine may lose its effectiveness with time. Moreover, it can become contaminated with harmful germs. Besides, your new symptoms may stem from another type of pinkeye and require different medicine. See a doctor about your new symptoms — don't try to diagnose and treat yourself.

Ever since I began wearing soft contact lenses, I've had a series of pinkeye infections. Do you think my lenses are causing these infections?
Your lenses probably aren't, but your cleaning methods or solution may be. Make sure you precisely follow the manufacturer's directions for the lens cleaning solution.

Also, check the product's expiration date to make sure that your solution isn't too old. An old solution may be ineffective or contaminated.

And *never* moisten your lenses with anything but a sterile solution. For instance, don't moisten them with saliva before putting them in your eyes.

What are its symptoms?

Pinkeye commonly causes redness of the conjunctiva, making the eyes look pink. Some people also have eye discharge, tearing, and pain; children may have a sore throat or fever. If the cornea is also inflamed, the eyes may be sensitive to light.

Pinkeye rarely affects vision. It usually starts in one eye and rapidly spreads to the other by contamination of towels, washcloths, or the person's hands.

Acute bacterial pinkeye usually lasts only 2 weeks. Typical symptoms are itching, burning, and a foreign body sensation in the eye. The eyelids show a crust of sticky discharge that contains mucus and pus.

Pinkeye caused by a virus leads to profuse tearing, a little discharge, and an enlarged lymph gland in front of the ear. Some viruses

SELF-HELP

Getting over pinkeye

Read the following guidelines to speed healing, protect family members, and prevent a recurrence of pinkeye.

Getting better

- Don't rub the infected eye because this can spread the infection to the other eye and to other people.
- Apply warm compresses and therapeutic ointment or drops, as your doctor prescribes. Wash your hands before using the medication, and use clean washcloths or towels frequently so you don't infect the other eye.
- Don't flush your eye with water or other fluids because this will spread the infection.
- When using eyedrops and ointments, be sure not to touch the tip of the bottle to your eye or lashes.

Protecting others

- Wash your hands regularly with soap and warm water. Some forms of pinkeye are highly contagious.
- Don't share washcloths, towels, or pillows because these items can spread the infection to others.

Avoiding another infection

- To prevent a recurrence, wear safety glasses if you work near chemical irritants.

take a chronic course and cause severe disabling disease, while others last just 2 to 3 weeks.

How is it diagnosed?

A physical exam usually reveals redness and swelling of blood vessels in the conjunctiva. The doctor may take a specimen of conjunctival scrapings to determine if pinkeye is bacterial, viral, or allergic.

How is it treated?

Treatment of pinkeye varies with the cause. In bacterial pink eye, the doctor prescribes a topical antibiotic or sulfonamide. Although viral pinkeye resists treatment, eyedrops may prevent a secondary infection. Herpes simplex infection generally responds to Herplex or Vira-A Ophthalmic ointment, but it may persist for 2 to 3 weeks. Allergic pinkeye is treated with eyedrops that constrict the blood vessels, cold compresses to relieve itching and, occasionally, oral antihistamines. (See *Getting over pinkeye.*)

RETINAL DETACHMENT

What is this condition?

Retinal detachment occurs when the layers of the retina become separated, creating a subretinal space that then fills with subretinal fluid. Retinal detachment usually involves only one eye, but it may involve the other eye later.

Surgical reattachment is often successful. However, the prognosis for good vision depends on the area of the retina that's affected.

What causes it?

Any breach of the retina allows the liquid vitreous humor of the eyeball to seep between the retinal layers, separating the retina from its blood supply. In adults, retinal detachment usually results from age-related degenerative changes, which cause a spontaneous retinal opening.

Predisposing factors include nearsightedness, cataract surgery, tumors, systemic diseases, and traumatic injury. The influence of trau-

Scleral buckling: Two-step treatment for retinal detachment

Treating retinal detachment is a two-step process. First, the surgeon repairs the retinal hole or tear; then he re-attaches the retina.

Repairing the retinal hole or tear

Using cryotherapy, photocoagulation, or diathermy, the surgeon creates a sterile inflammatory reaction that seals the retinal hole or tear and achieves retinal readherence.

Reattaching the retina

The surgeon then performs scleral buckling. This procedure applies external pressure to the separated retinal layers to reunite the retina with its blood supply.

First, the surgeon severs the superior rectus muscle. This allows him to place an explant (a silicone plate or sponge) over the site of readherence. He keeps the explant in place with a circling band. Pressure exerted on the explant indents or "buckles" the eyeball, gently pushing the choroid and retina closer together.

This reunites the retina with its blood supply and prevents vitreous humor from seeping between the detached retinal layers. (Seepage can lead to further detachment and possible blindness.)

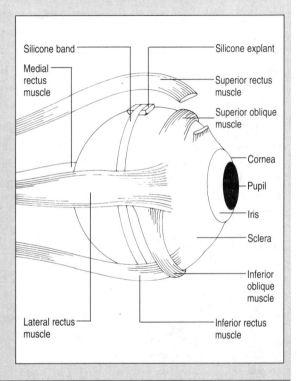

matic injury may explain why retinal detachment is twice as common in males. Retinal detachment is rare in children.

What are its symptoms?

Initially, the person may complain of floating spots and recurrent flashes of light. But as detachment progresses, gradual, painless vision loss occurs. This vision loss may be described as a veil, curtain, or cobweb effect that eliminates a portion of the visual field.

How is it diagnosed?

Ophthalmoscopy reveals the usually transparent retina as gray and opaque; in severe detachment, it reveals folds in the retina and ballooning out of the area.

Understanding laser surgery for retinal disorders

You may wonder if laser surgery is for real. This proven space-age technique can indeed repair retinal tears and detachments quickly — with minimal pain and complications.

How the laser works

A laser generates monochromatic light waves, then amplifies and focuses their energy levels by, among other things, deflecting them in a series of mirrors to obtain a finely focused, high-energy beam that is useful for microsurgical work.

How it's used

To mend retinal holes, tears, and detachments, eye surgeons use heat-generating thermal lasers to condense protein material and vaporize fluids. For example, the argon laser produces a short-wavelength, blue-green beam that's highly effective on blood and pigment. This makes it ideal for repairing the vascular retina or for containing an existing localized detachment with tiny laser burn scars, limiting its size and preventing further damage.

How is it treated?

Treatment depends on the location and severity of the detachment. It may include restricting eye movements and positioning the person's head so that the tear or hole lies below the rest of the eye. Retinal detachment usually requires scleral buckling to reattach the retina and, possibly, replacement of the vitreous humor with silicone, oil, air, or gas. (See *Scleral buckling: Two-step treatment for retinal detachment,* page 495.) A hole in the peripheral retina can be treated with cryothermy; in the posterior portion, with laser therapy. (See *Understanding laser surgery for retinal disorders.*)

What can a person with retinal detachment do?

- Learn the proper method for instilling eyedrops.
- Be sure to comply with prescribed therapy and follow-up care.
- Wear dark glasses to compensate for light sensitivity.

STYE

What do doctors call this condition?

Besides stye, doctors call this condition hordeolum.

What is this condition?

A stye is a localized red, swollen, and tender abscess of the eyelid glands. It can occur outside or inside the eye.

A stye can occur at any age. Generally, this infection responds well to treatment but tends to recur. An untreated stye can eventually lead to cellulitis of the eyelid.

What causes it?

A stye is caused by infection of the eyelid glands by *Staphylococcus* bacteria.

What are its symptoms?

Typically, a stye produces redness, swelling, and pain. An abscess frequently forms at the lid margin, with an eyelash pointing outward from its center. A pus-filled discharge is typically present.

How is it diagnosed?

Visual examination generally confirms the infection. Culture of pus from the abscess usually reveals a staphylococcal organism.

How is it treated?

Treatment consists of warm compresses applied for 10 to 15 minutes, 4 times a day, for up to 4 days to promote drainage of the abscess and to relieve pain and inflammation. (See *How to treat a stye.*)

Drug therapy includes a topical sulfonamide or antibiotic eyedrops or ointment and, occasionally, a systemic antibiotic. If conservative treatment fails, incision and drainage may be necessary.

UVEITIS

What is this condition?

Uveitis is an inflammation of one uveal tract of the eye. (The uveal tract consists of the iris, choroid, and related tissue structures.) The disorder occurs as *anterior uveitis,* which affects the iris (iritis) or both the iris and the ciliary body (iridocyclitis); as *posterior uveitis,* which affects the choroid (choroiditis) or both the choroid and the retina (chorioretinitis); or as *panuveitis,* which affects the entire uveal tract.

Untreated anterior uveitis progresses to posterior uveitis, causing scarring, cataracts, and glaucoma. With immediate treatment, anterior uveitis usually subsides after a few days to several weeks; however, recurrence is likely. Posterior uveitis generally causes some residual vision loss and markedly blurred vision.

What causes it?

In most cases, the cause of uveitis is unknown. But it can result from allergy, bacteria, viruses, fungi, chemicals, traumatic injury, surgery, or systemic diseases, such as rheumatoid arthritis, ankylosing spondylitis, and toxoplasmosis.

What are its symptoms?

Anterior uveitis produces moderate to severe pain in one eye; severe ciliary congestion; sensitivity to light; tearing; a small, nonreactive pupil; and blurred vision. Posterior uveitis begins insidiously, with

SELF-HELP

How to treat a stye

To promote healing, your doctor will instruct you to place warm compresses on your eye several times a day and to apply eyedrops. Here are some other suggestions that will ensure proper self-care.

Avoid reinfection
- Use a clean cloth for each application of warm compresses, and dispose of the cloth or launder it separately.
- Don't squeeze the stye; this spreads the infection and may cause a skin infection called cellulitis.

Apply medication properly
Closely follow your doctor's instructions when instilling eyedrops or ointment into the space between your lower eyelid and the conjunctiva.

Coping with uveitis

To safeguard your vision and prevent complications of uveitis, you'll need to follow your doctor's instructions closely. The following suggestions can help you to combat this eye inflammation.

Comply wth therapy
- Get plenty of rest during the acute disease phase.
- Closely follow the doctor's instructions for instilling eyedrops.
- Wear dark glasses to ease the discomfort of light sensitivity.
- Watch for and report side effects of systemic corticosteroids — for example, swelling and muscle weakness.

Follow up
Be sure to get follow-up care because uveitis is likely to recur. Seek treatment at the first signs of iritis — pain, excessive tearing, light sensitivity, and reduced visual acuity.

complaints of slightly decreased or blurred vision or floating spots. Pain and sensitivity to light may also occur.

How is it diagnosed?

In anterior and posterior uveitis, a slit-lamp exam shows a "flare and cell" pattern, which looks like light passing through smoke. It also shows an increased number of cells over the inflamed area. With a special lens, the doctor can also use slit-lamp and ophthalmoscopic exams to identify active inflammatory fundus lesions involving the retina or choroid.

In posterior uveitis, serologic tests can reveal if toxoplasmosis is the cause.

How is it treated?

Uveitis requires vigorous and prompt management, which includes treatment of any known underlying cause and application of eyedrops or ointment, such as 1% Atropisol or steroids. For severe uveitis, therapy includes oral steroids. However, long-term steroid therapy can cause increased intraocular pressure and increased risk of cataracts. (See *Coping with uveitis*.)

VASCULAR RETINOPATHIES

What are these conditions?

Vascular retinopathies are eye conditions that result from poor blood supply to the eyes. The five types of vascular retinopathy are central retinal vein occlusion, diabetic retinopathy, hypertensive retinopathy, sickle cell retinopathy, and central retinal artery occlusion.

What causes them?

When one of the arteries that supplies blood to the retina becomes blocked, blood flow diminishes. This damages the eye and causes vision problems.

Causes of *central retinal vein occlusion* include external compression of the retinal vein, injury, diabetes, blood clots, granulomatous diseases, infections, glaucoma, and atherosclerosis. This form of vascular retinopathy is most prevalent in elderly people.

Diabetic retinopathy results from juvenile or adult diabetes. Microcirculatory changes occur more rapidly when diabetes is poorly controlled. About 75% of people with juvenile diabetes develop retinopathy within 20 years of the disease's onset. In adults with diabetes, incidence increases with the duration of diabetes. This condition is a leading cause of acquired adult blindness.

Hypertensive retinopathy results from prolonged high blood pressure, producing retinal vasospasm and consequent damage and narrowing of retinal blood vessels.

Sickle cell retinopathy results from the impaired ability of sickled cells to pass through the tiny capillary blood vessels, producing obstructions. This results in microaneurysms, chorioretinal tissue death, and retinal detachment.

Central retinal artery occlusion may have an unknown cause or may result from embolism, atherosclerosis, infection, or conditions that slow the blood flow, such as temporal arteritis, a narrowed carotid artery, and heart failure. This rare type of retinopathy occurs in one eye and affects elderly people.

What are their symptoms?

Central retinal vein occlusion reduces vision, allowing perception of only hand movement and light. This condition is painless, except when it results in secondary neovascular glaucoma (uncontrolled proliferation of weak blood vessels). The prognosis is poor — 5% to 20% of people with this type of vascular retinopathy develop secondary glaucoma within 4 months.

Nonproliferative diabetic retinopathy produces changes in the lining of the retinal blood vessels that cause the vessels to leak plasma or fatty substances, which decrease or block blood flow within the retina. This disorder may also produce microaneurysms and small hemorrhages. Although some people with nonproliferative retinopathy lack symptoms, others have significant loss of central visual acuity (necessary for reading and driving) and diminished night vision.

Proliferative diabetic retinopathy causes fragile new blood vessels on the disk and elsewhere. These vessels can grow into the vitreous and then rupture, causing sudden vision loss. Scar tissue that may form along the new blood vessels can pull on the retina, causing macular distortion and even retinal detachment.

Symptoms of hypertensive retinopathy depend on the location of retinopathy. For example, mild visual disturbances, such as blurred vision, result from retinopathy located near the macula (a spot near

About 75% of people with juvenile diabetes develop retinopathy within 20 years of the disease's onset. This condition is a leading cause of acquired adult blindness.

the center of the retina concerned with visual acuity). Without treatment, 50% of people become blind within 5 years. With treatment, the prognosis varies with the severity of the disorder. Severe, prolonged disease eventually causes blindness; mild, prolonged disease causes visual defects.

Central retinal artery occlusion causes sudden, painless vision loss (partial or complete) in one eye. This condition typically causes permanent blindness. However, some people experience spontaneous resolution within hours and regain partial vision.

How are they diagnosed?

Appropriate diagnostic tests depend on the type of vascular retinopathy. Evaluation includes determination of visual acuity and ophthalmoscopic examination.

How are they treated?

Treatment approaches depend on the type of retinopathy. Therapy for central retinal vein occlusion may include aspirin, which acts as a mild anticoagulant. Laser photocoagulation can reduce the risk of glaucoma for some people.

Treatment of nonproliferative diabetic retinopathy is prophylactic. Careful control of blood sugar levels during the first 5 years of the disease may delay its onset or reduce its severity. For people with early symptoms of microaneurysms, therapy includes frequent eye exams (3 to 4 times a year) to monitor their condition. For children with diabetes, therapy includes an annual eye exam by an ophthalmologist.

The best treatment for proliferative diabetic retinopathy is laser photocoagulation, which cauterizes the leaking blood vessels. Despite treatment, neovascularization doesn't always regress and vitreous hemorrhage, with or without retinal detachment, may follow. If the blood isn't absorbed in 3 to 6 months, vitrectomy may restore partial vision.

Treatment of hypertensive retinopathy includes control of blood pressure with appropriate drugs, diet, and exercise.

No particular treatment has been shown to control central retinal artery occlusion. To lower intraocular pressure, therapy includes Diamox, eyeball massage and, possibly, anterior chamber paracentesis. Another treatment, inhalation of carbogen (95% oxygen and 5% carbon dioxide), improves retinal oxygenation.

14

EAR, NOSE, AND THROAT DISORDERS

ADENOID ENLARGEMENT

What is this condition?

Adenoid enlargement is excessive growth of the tissue of the nasopharynx, the upper part of the pharynx that connects with the nasal passages. This disorder also may be called *adenoid hypertrophy or hyperplasia.*

Normally, adenoidal tissue is small at birth ($\frac{3}{4}$ to $1\frac{1}{4}$ inches, or 2 to 3 centimeters), grows until the child reaches adolescence, and then begins to slowly shrink. In adenoid enlargement, however, this tissue continues to grow. Adenoid enlargement is a fairly common childhood condition.

What causes it?

The precise cause of adenoid enlargement is unknown, but factors that may contribute to it include heredity, repeated infection, chronic nasal congestion, persistent allergy, insufficient aeration, and inefficient nasal breathing. Inflammation resulting from repeated infection increases the risk of obstructed breathing.

What are its symptoms?

Typically, adenoid enlargement causes symptoms of obstructed breathing, including mouth breathing, snoring at night, and frequent, prolonged nasal congestion.

Persistent mouth breathing during the formative years produces distinctive changes in facial features — a slightly elongated face, open mouth, highly arched palate, shortened upper lip, and a vacant expression. Occasionally, the child is incapable of mouth breathing, snores loudly at night, and may eventually show effects of nocturnal respiratory insufficiency, such as nasal flaring. The child may develop a lung condition called *pulmonary hypertension* and a heart disease caused by pulmonary hypertension called *cor pulmonale.* Adenoid enlargement may also predispose the child to middle ear infection, which in turn can lead to fluctuating conductive hearing loss. Retained nasal secretions from adenoidal inflammation can lead to sinus infection.

How is it diagnosed?

The doctor can confirm this disorder using X-rays and by examining the nasal passages and the pharynx using an instrument called an *endoscope.*

Persistent mouth breathing in a child's formative years produces changes in facial features — a slightly elongated face, open mouth, highly arched palate, shortened upper lip, and a vacant expression.

How is it treated?

Surgical adenoid removal (adenoidectomy) is the treatment of choice for adenoid enlargement and is commonly recommended for a person with prolonged mouth breathing, nasal speech, facial features associated with adenoid enlargement, recurrent middle ear infection, constant nasopharyngitis, and nighttime respiratory distress. This procedure usually eliminates recurrent nasal infections and ear complications and reverses any secondary hearing loss. (See *Preparing for your child's adenoid surgery.*)

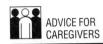

ADVICE FOR CAREGIVERS

Preparing for your child's adenoid surgery

If your child will have adenoids removed, he or she will probably need to be hospitalized for 2 nights. Ask the doctor or nurse if the hospital will let you stay with your child and participate in the child's care. Be aware that after surgery, your child may temporarily have a nasal voice.

HEARING LOSS

What is this condition?

In hearing loss, a mechanical or nerve-related condition impedes the transmission of sound waves. Hearing loss may be partial or total. Sometimes, it's inherited. In other cases, it's brought on by aging, disease, or exposure to loud noise.

Hearing loss takes one of three main forms.

- In *conductive loss,* some condition — for example, buildup of earwax in the ear canal — interferes with the function of external and middle ear structures. (See *How to remove earwax,* page 504.)
- In *sensorineural loss,* inner ear structures or the pathway leading from the inner ear is damaged.
- In *mixed hearing loss,* both conductive and sensorineural losses are present.

What causes it?

The cause of hearing loss varies.

Congenital hearing loss

This form of hearing loss may be inherited as a genetic disorder. In newborns, it may also result from injury, toxicity, or infection during delivery or the mother's pregnancy. Premature and low-birth-weight infants are most likely to have structural or functional hearing losses.

Predisposing factors for a congenital hearing loss include a family history of hearing loss or known hereditary disorders (for example, irregular bone development in the inner ear), the mother's exposure during pregnancy to German measles or syphilis or to drugs that

SELF-HELP

How to remove earwax

One potential cause of hearing loss is buildup of earwax, a natural substance created by oil glands in the ear canal. The amount and consistency of earwax vary in each person.

If your ears are draining, if you have pain, or if you've had ear surgery, the doctor may remove the wax from your ears.

Drops that dissolve wax

If the doctor tells you to clean or irrigate your own ears using an agent that dissolves earwax, such as Debrox or Cerumenex, put the drug in your ears twice a day for 3 to 4 days. The usual dose is 5 to 10 drops. Clean or irrigate your ear after using Debrox. If you're using Cerumenex, fill the ear canal and insert a cotton plug; then flush or clean the ear canal after 15 to 30 minutes.

When to get help

Don't use either of these drugs if your eardrum is perforated or your ear canal is red. Call the doctor if you have pain or if your hearing doesn't improve after cleaning.

For general cleaning, use a wet washcloth placed over your fingertip for your outer ear. Never insert anything into your ear canal to clean it.

damage hearing, prolonged lack of oxygen to the fetus during delivery, and congenital abnormalities of the ears, nose, or throat. (See *Preventing congenital hearing loss.*)

Sudden deafness

Sudden deafness is the abrupt loss of hearing in a person who had no previous hearing difficulty. This condition is considered a medical emergency because prompt treatment may restore full hearing. Its causes and predisposing factors include:

- acute infections, especially mumps, and other bacterial and viral infections (such as measles, German measles, the flu, shingles, and infectious mononucleosis)
- diabetes, an underactive thyroid, and high fat and cholesterol levels
- high blood pressure and hardening of the arteries
- head injury or brain tumors
- drugs that can damage hearing
- neurologic disorders, such as MS and neurosyphilis
- blood diseases, such as leukemia and abnormally increased blood clotting.

Noise-induced hearing loss

This form of hearing loss, which may be temporary or permanent, may occur in someone who's exposed to loud noise (85 to 90 decibels) for a prolonged period or to extremely loud noise (greater than 90 decibels) for a brief time. Noise-induced hearing loss is common in workers subjected to constant industrial noise and in military personnel, hunters, and rock musicians. (See *How to prevent hearing loss,* pages 506 and 507.)

Presbycusis

This progressive hearing loss comes with aging. It's caused by the loss of hair cells in the organ of Corti — the hearing sense organ in the innermost part of the ear.

What are its symptoms?

Although a congenital hearing loss may not be obvious at birth, a poor response to sound generally becomes apparent within 2 to 3 days. As the child grows older, hearing loss impairs speech development.

A person with a conductive hearing loss has decreased sensitivity to sound but no change in sound clarity. His or her hearing is normal if the volume is increased to compensate for the loss. Typically, the person has a quiet speaking voice and a normal ability to discriminate sounds, but may have trouble hearing when chewing.

A person with a sensorineural hearing loss has poor sound discrimination, poor hearing in noisy areas, and difficulty hearing high-frequency sounds. The person may complain that others mumble or shout and may have tinkling or ringing in the ears.

Sudden deafness may cause symptoms of conductive, sensorineural, or mixed hearing loss, depending on the cause. A person with noise-induced hearing loss has symptoms of sensorineural hearing loss. Initially, the person can't hear certain frequencies (around 4,000 hertz). With continued exposure, the person eventually loses hearing of all frequencies.

Presbycusis usually causes ringing in the ears and an inability to understand speech.

How is it diagnosed?

Usually, the person's medical, family, and occupational histories and a complete hearing exam provide ample evidence of hearing loss. These histories may also suggest possible causes or predisposing factors.

A doctor or an audiologist may perform various tests — Weber test, Rinne test, and specialized hearing tests — to determine if the person has conductive, sensorineural, or mixed hearing loss.

How is it treated?

To treat congenital hearing loss, the doctor first tries to determine the underlying cause. If the hearing loss doesn't improve with surgery, the person is taught to communicate through sign language, lip reading, or other effective means.

To treat sudden deafness, the doctor must promptly identify and treat the underlying cause.

To treat noise-induced hearing loss, the doctor tells the person to rest overnight. This usually restores normal hearing in people who've been exposed to noise levels above 90 decibels for several hours — but not in those who've been exposed to such noise repeatedly. As hearing deteriorates, the person must undergo speech and hearing rehabilitation. Hearing aids rarely help a person with noise-induced hearing loss.

A person with presbycusis usually needs a hearing aid.

What can the family of a person with hearing loss do?

- If the person is older, speak slowly and distinctly in a low tone. Avoid shouting.

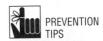

PREVENTION TIPS

Preventing congenital hearing loss

Before pregnancy
To avoid the possibility of giving birth to a child with a hearing defect, the prospective mother should be immunized against German measles as soon as possible to reduce the risk of being exposed during pregnancy.

During pregnancy
Pregnant women should be taught about the dangers of exposure to drugs, chemicals, or infections that can cause hearing loss.

During labor and delivery
Women should be carefully monitored to make sure that the fetus isn't being deprived of oxygen.

SELF-HELP

How to prevent hearing loss

A chief cause of hearing loss is overexposure to loud noise. Unfortunately, we're constantly bombarded by noise — from things like motor vehicles, power tools, appliances, televisions, and radios. But we can take steps to protect our hearing.

How? By covering our ears or wearing hearing protectors when we expect to be exposed to loud noise and by avoiding loud music or other noisy situations as much as possible.

How much noise is too much?

First, consider how sound is measured. It's calculated two ways — by frequency (pitch) and intensity (loudness). *Frequency* is measured in sound vibrations per second, or hertz (Hz). For example, a boat whistle has a frequency of about 250 Hz, and a bird singing has a frequency of about 4,000 Hz.

Intensity is measured in decibels (dB). A conversational voice measures about 65 dB. A shout measures 90 dB or more. A jackhammer registers 100 to 120 dB. Loud rock music is 120 to 130 dB, and an explosion registers 140 dB or more.

Low-intensity sounds are harmless and often quite pleasant. Sounds at or above the 85 to 90 dB range — called the caution or action zone — are dangerous.

If the noise occurs 3 feet (1 meter) away and you have to raise your voice to be heard, the level is probably about 85 dB. Constant exposure to noise at this level can cause permanent hearing loss. So can short exposure to extremely loud noise (greater than 140 dB), a condition called *acoustic trauma.*

Hearing loss can occur if you're exposed to a large *dosage* of noise. Dosage equals intensity (amount of noise exposure) times duration (over a period of time). When noise is less intense and of shorter duration, the hair cells in the ear's organ of Corti aren't damaged as much, and hearing is less affected.

The Occupational Safety and Health Administration has set the following standards for safe noise levels:

AMOUNT OF NOISE	MAXIMUM EXPOSURE TIME
90 dB	8 hours
95 dB	4 hours
100 dB	2 hours
105 dB	1 hour
110 dB	½ hour
115 dB	¼ hour

Wearing hearing protectors

Earplugs and earmuffs help prevent hearing loss by decreasing the amount of sound entering the ear. Wear them when you'll be exposed to sounds above the caution zone — for example, when using loud appliances, power tools, lawn mowers, tractors, or jackhammers; when shooting a gun; and when you're around motorcycles, snowmobiles, speedboats, or other noisy vehicles.

Although ear protectors may seem inconvenient or uncomfortable at first, wearing them now will preserve your hearing in the future. Here are some tips for using hearing protectors.

Disposable plugs

These plugs are placed inside the ear canal to block out noise. They also help keep dirt from entering the ear. Almost invisible, they're available in several styles. Try different plugs to find the most comfortable kind. Look for pliability and a snug fit. Never break off the tips.

Wash your hands before shaping and inserting plugs. If they're inserted correctly, your voice should sound louder to you. If they contain wax, dirt, or grease, throw them away and use a new pair.

How to prevent hearing loss *(continued)*

Reusable plugs

Placed inside the ear canal, these plugs block out noise and help keep dirt from entering the ear. They're available in several styles. Some are joined by a string to prevent their loss. Make sure that the plugs fit snugly in the ear canal and that they're comfortable.

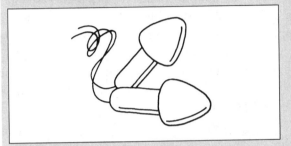

Before inserting the plugs, wash your hands and inspect the plugs for dirt. Wash them if necessary. If you use them all day at work, wash them every day; then rinse, dry, and store them in a plastic case or clean pill bottle. Replace them when they harden or discolor.

Headband plugs

These plugs are placed in your ears with the headband under your chin. The plugs should fit snugly yet comfortably.

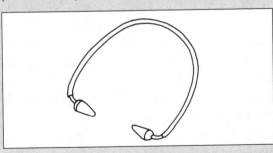

Wash the entire headband often. Don't twist or bend it — this will interfere with the fit of the earplugs. Store the headband safely.

Earmuffs

Earmuffs are placed over your ears with the band over your head. Cushioned muffs form a seal around the ear, completely blocking out noise. The cushions are foam- or liquid-filled. Don't loosen the earmuffs — this reduces their effectiveness. They may not fit correctly if you wear glasses.

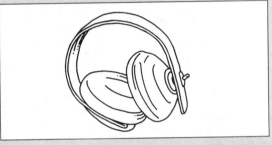

Remove the cushions for washing often. Inspect them periodically to see if they need replacing (they harden with use). Store the earmuffs in a safe place.

Other tips

Here are some hearing protection hints:
- When shopping for appliances, ask about decibel levels.
- Run appliances one at a time.
- Cover your ears when you're near noise, such as that from sirens or subways.
- Avoid loud music, and don't listen to music with earphones.
- Give your ears an occasional vacation. Turn off the TV and read a book.

- Provide emotional support and encouragement to the person who's learning how to use a hearing aid.
- If the person can read lips, stand directly in front of him or her when speaking and speak slowly and distinctly. Approach within the person's visual range, and get his or her attention by raising your arm or waving. Touching may startle the person.

INFECTIOUS MYRINGITIS

What is this condition?

Infectious myringitis is an inflammation of the eardrum. Acute infectious myringitis is characterized by inflammation, bleeding, and drainage of fluid into the tissue at the end of the external ear canal and the eardrum. This self-limiting disorder (which resolves spontaneously within 3 days to 2 weeks) often follows acute middle ear infection or upper respiratory tract infection. Epidemics of myringitis frequently occur among children.

Chronic granular myringitis, a rare inflammation of the eardrum, causes gradual hearing loss. Without specific treatment, this condition can lead to closing of the ear canal.

This self-limiting disorder goes away spontaneously within 3 days to 2 weeks. It often follows acute middle ear infection or upper respiratory tract infection. Epidemics of myringitis frequently occur among children.

What causes it?

Acute infectious myringitis usually follows viral infection, but may also result from infection with bacteria or any other organism that may cause acute middle ear infection. Rarely, myringitis may follow certain types of pneumonia. The cause of chronic granular myringitis is unknown.

What are its symptoms?

Acute infectious myringitis begins with severe ear pain, commonly accompanied by tenderness over the mastoid process, a bone located behind and below the ear. Small, reddened, inflamed blebs form in the canal, on the eardrum and, with bacterial invasion, in the middle ear. Spontaneous rupture of these blebs may cause bloody discharge. Fever and hearing loss are rare.

Chronic granular myringitis produces itching, a pus-filled discharge, and gradual hearing loss.

How is it diagnosed?

The doctor will diagnose the acute disorder based on the person's history and physical exam findings. Culture and sensitivity tests identify causative organisms.

How is it treated?

Hospitalization is usually not required for acute infectious myringitis. The doctor will try to relieve the person's pain with analgesics, such as aspirin or Tylenol, and application of heat to the external ear. Codeine may be given for severe pain. The doctor will prevent or treat secondary infection with systemic or topical antibiotics. Incision of blebs and evacuation of serum and blood may relieve pressure and help drain the discharge but do not speed recovery.

The doctor will treat chronic granular myringitis systemically with antibiotics or locally with anti-inflammatory–antibiotic eardrops, as well as with surgical excision and cautery if needed. If stenosis (narrowing) is present, surgical reconstruction is necessary. (See *Speeding your recovery from infectious myringitis*.)

INFLAMMATION OF THE MASTOID

What do doctors call this condition?
Mastoiditis

What is this condition?
This disorder occurs when the mastoid process, a bone located behind and below the ear, becomes infected. Although the prognosis is good with early treatment, possible complications include meningitis, facial paralysis, brain abscess, hearing loss, and a pus-producing infection of the labyrinth of the inner ear.

What causes it?
Inflammation of the mastoid is caused by infection with bacteria, such as pneumococci, *Haemophilus influenzae, Moraxella catarrhalis,* beta-hemolytic streptococci, staphylococci, and gram-negative organisms. Inflammation of the mastoid is usually a complication of chronic middle ear infection. Less often, it develops after acute middle ear infection.

What are its symptoms?
The main symptoms are a dull ache and tenderness in the area of the mastoid process, low-grade fever, and a thick, pus-filled discharge that gradually becomes more profuse, possibly leading to external ear infection. Redness and swelling behind the external ear may push the external ear out from the head. Pressure within the swollen mastoid

SELF-HELP

Speeding your recovery from infectious myringitis

To rid yourself of this painful infection, be sure to take all of your prescribed antibiotics. Make sure you understand your doctor's instructions for using antibiotic eardrops. If you're uncertain about how to put drops in your ear, call the doctor or nurse for clarification.

The best defense
To help prevent myringitis from recurring, seek prompt treatment for any symptoms of middle ear infection. The symptoms include sneezing, coughing, fever, and severe, deep, throbbing pain.

cavity may cause swelling and blockage of the external ear canal, leading to conductive hearing loss.

How is it diagnosed?

To confirm inflammation of the mastoid, the doctor takes X-rays of the mastoid area and examines the ear. During the exam, the external ear canal is cleaned. Persistent oozing into the canal indicates perforation of the eardrum.

How is it treated?

The doctor will treat an inflamed mastoid with intravenous antibiotics. If bone damage is minimal, the doctor may perform a procedure called a *myringotomy*, in which the eardrum is punctured to drain pus-filled fluid and provide a specimen of discharge for culture and sensitivity testing.

Surgical treatment may be necessary. Recurrent or persistent infection or signs of intracranial complications require simple mastoidectomy. This procedure involves removing the diseased bone and cleaning the affected area, after which a drain is inserted.

A chronically inflamed mastoid requires radical mastoidectomy (removal of the posterior wall of the ear canal, remnants of the eardrum, and two small bones in the ear, the malleus and the incus). Radical mastoidectomy (seldom needed because of antibiotic therapy) doesn't drastically affect the person's hearing because significant hearing loss has already occurred. With either operation, the person continues oral antibiotic therapy for several weeks after surgery and hospital discharge.

LABYRINTHITIS

What is this condition?

This rare disorder is an inflammation of the labyrinth of the inner ear. It frequently incapacitates the person by causing severe vertigo that lasts for 3 to 5 days. Symptoms gradually subside over a 3- to 6-week period.

What causes it?

Labyrinthitis is usually caused by viral infection. It may be a primary infection, the result of injury, or a complication of the flu, middle ear infection, or meningitis. In chronic middle ear infection, a cystlike formation called a *cholesteatoma* erodes the bone of the labyrinth, allowing bacteria to enter from the middle ear.

What are its symptoms?

Because the inner ear controls both hearing and balance, this infection typically produces severe vertigo (with any movement of the head) and hearing loss. Vertigo begins gradually but peaks within 48 hours, causing loss of balance and falling in the direction of the affected ear.

Other symptoms include spontaneous nystagmus, with jerking movements of the eyes toward the unaffected ear; nausea, vomiting, and giddiness; with cholesteatoma, signs of middle ear disease; and with severe bacterial infection, pus-filled drainage. To minimize giddiness and nystagmus, the person may assume a characteristic posture — lying on the side of the unaffected ear and looking in the direction of the affected ear.

How is it diagnosed?

The doctor may diagnose labyrinthitis based on a person's signs and symptoms and history of upper respiratory infection. The doctor will typically order culture and sensitivity testing to identify the infecting organism if pus-filled drainage is present. The person may also undergo audiometric testing.

How is it treated?

Treatment of labyrinthitis seeks to control symptoms and may include bed rest, with the head immobilized between pillows; the anti-vertigo drug Antivert; and massive doses of antibiotics to combat pus-producing labyrinthitis. The person may receive oral fluids to prevent dehydration from vomiting. For severe nausea and vomiting, intravenous fluids may be necessary.

If these measures fail, the doctor will surgically remove the cholesteatoma and drain the infected areas of the middle and inner ear.

Early and vigorous treatment of predisposing conditions, such as middle ear infection and any local or systemic infection, can prevent labyrinthitis.

SELF-HELP

Tips on coping with laryngitis

To help get over a bout of laryngitis, use medicated throat lozenges and be sure to complete the full course of prescribed antibiotics.

The best defense

To prevent a recurrence, use a vaporizer or humidifier during the winter to put more moisture into room air. During the summer, avoid air conditioning because it removes moisture from the air. If you're a smoker, stop smoking.

What can a person with labyrinthitis do?

Be aware that recovery may take as long as 6 weeks. During this time, limit activities that vertigo may make hazardous.

LARYNGITIS

What is this condition?

A common disorder, laryngitis is an acute or chronic inflammation of the larynx (voice box). Acute laryngitis may occur as an isolated infection or as part of a generalized upper respiratory tract infection.

What causes it?

Acute laryngitis usually is caused by infection (mainly viral) or excessive use of the voice. Thus, it's an occupational hazard for teachers, public speakers, singers, and others. It may also result from leisure activities (such as cheering at a sports event) or from inhaling smoke, fumes, or caustic chemicals.

Causes of chronic laryngitis include chronic upper respiratory tract disorders (sinus inflammation, bronchitis, nasal polyps, allergy), mouth breathing, smoking, constant exposure to dust or other irritants, and alcohol abuse.

What are its symptoms?

Acute laryngitis typically starts with hoarseness, which ranges from mild to complete loss of the voice. The person may also have pain (especially when swallowing or speaking), dry cough, fever, a swollen larynx, and an overall ill feeling.

In chronic laryngitis, persistent hoarseness is usually the only symptom.

How is it diagnosed?

To confirm laryngitis, the doctor examines the inside of the person's larynx by observing its reflection in a special mirror. This exam typically shows that the vocal cords are red, inflamed, and, occasionally, bleeding, with rounded rather than sharp edges. The doctor may also note a discharge and, in severe cases, take a culture of the discharge.

How is it treated?

Resting the voice is the primary treatment. For viral infection, the doctor prescribes analgesics and throat lozenges to relieve pain. (See *Tips on coping with laryngitis.*) To treat bacterial infection, the doctor prescribes an antibiotic. (See *Questions people ask about treating laryngitis.*)

A person with severe, acute laryngitis may need to be hospitalized. If swelling of the larynx causes a blocked airway, the doctor may perform a tracheotomy, cutting the trachea to gain access to the airway below the blockage.

In chronic laryngitis, the doctor prescribes treatment to correct the underlying cause.

MÉNIÈRE'S DISEASE

What is this condition?

Ménière's disease is a dysfunction of the labyrinth of the inner ear. It causes severe vertigo, hearing loss, and tinnitus (ringing in the ears). It usually affects adults between ages 30 and 60, men slightly more often than women. After multiple attacks over several years, this disorder leads to residual tinnitus and hearing loss.

What causes it?

Although its cause is unknown, this disease may result from overproduction or decreased absorption of endolymph, the fluid contained in the labyrinth of the ear. (See *What happens in Ménière's disease,* page 514.)

This condition may stem from autonomic nervous system dysfunction that temporarily constricts blood vessels supplying the inner ear. In some women, premenstrual water retention may trigger attacks of Ménière's disease.

What are its symptoms?

Ménière's disease produces three characteristic effects: severe vertigo, tinnitus, and hearing loss. Fullness or a blocked feeling in the ear is also quite common. Sudden, violent attacks last from 10 minutes to several hours. During an acute attack, other symptoms include severe

STRAIGHT TALK

Questions people ask about treating laryngitis

Will gargling help me get my voice back?

No. The larynx is below the epiglottis, which separates the throat from the windpipe. As a result, the gargling solution never reaches the larynx. But gargling may soothe your throat if it's sore.

Will cough medicine help my condition?

Only if you're coughing or clearing your throat frequently because of an allergy or a cold. If frequent coughing and throat clearing are irritating the inflamed larynx, a cough suppressant may help.

If I quit smoking, will this help my throat?

Definitely. Laryngitis is an inflammation of the larynx, and cigarette smoke irritates the inflamed larynx. The key to treatment is avoiding irritants like cigarettes that worsen inflammation.

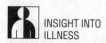

INSIGHT INTO
ILLNESS

What happens in Ménière's disease

Sound waves enter the ear canal and strike the eardrum, causing it to vibrate and creating pressure on the ossicles (three small bones in the middle ear). The ossicles, in turn, vibrate, transmitting sound waves to the inner ear.

The inner ear is small enough to fit inside a marble. It contains two structures: the cochlea and the semicircular canals. Together, these structures form the labyrinth, named for its complicated twists, bends, and turns. The snail-shaped cochlea converts sound waves into nerve impulses, which travel to the brain. The loop-shaped semicircular canals detect changes in balance and body orientation.

In Ménière's disease, fluid pressure within the labyrinth rises. This causes hearing loss, dizziness, and related symptoms.

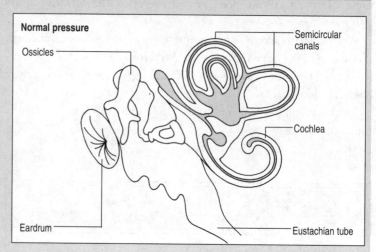

Normal pressure

Ossicles

Semicircular canals

Cochlea

Eardrum

Eustachian tube

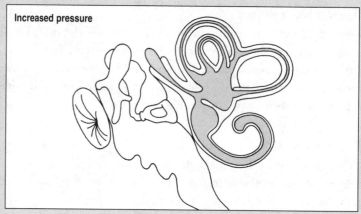

Increased pressure

---

nausea, vomiting, sweating, giddiness, and nystagmus (involuntary movement of the eyeball). Also, vertigo may cause loss of balance and falling to the affected side. To ease these symptoms, the person may assume a characteristic posture: lying on the unaffected ear and looking in the direction of the affected ear.

Initially, the person may not experience any symptoms between attacks, except for residual tinnitus that worsens during an attack. Such attacks may occur several times a year, or remissions may last as long as several years. Eventually, these attacks become less frequent as hearing loss progresses (usually in one ear); they may cease when hearing loss is total.

How is it diagnosed?

The presence of all three characteristic symptoms suggests Ménière's disease. The doctor also orders hearing tests and X-rays of the internal ear.

How is it treated?

The doctor will usually first prescribe drugs to treat Ménière's disease. Treatment with a drug called atropine may stop an attack in 20 to 30 minutes. Epinephrine or Benadryl may be necessary in a severe attack. Dramamine, Antivert, Benadryl, or Valium may be effective in a milder attack.

Long-term management includes use of a diuretic or vasodilator and restricted salt (sodium) intake (less than 2 grams per day). Preventive treatment with antihistamines or mild sedatives (phenobarbital, Valium) may also be helpful.

If Ménière's disease persists after 2 years of treatment, causes incapacitating vertigo, or resists medical management, surgery may be necessary. Destruction of the affected labyrinth permanently relieves symptoms but leads to irreversible hearing loss.

The doctor will order systemic streptomycin only when the disease affects both ears and no other treatment can be considered.

MIDDLE EAR INFECTION

What do doctors call this condition?

Otitis media

What is this condition?

Middle ear infection refers to infection of the tiny cavity in the temporal bone that contains three small bones (the malleus, incus, and stapes). Middle ear infection may be acute or chronic, suppurative (pus-producing) or secretory (secretion-producing).

Acute middle ear infection is common in children. Its incidence rises during the winter, when respiratory tract infections are com-

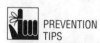

Guarding against middle ear infection

If you're susceptible to middle ear infections, following these suggestions may help you prevent them.

Practicing prevention

• Learn how to recognize the symptoms of upper respiratory infections, which often precede middle ear infection. Report these symptoms promptly so they can be treated early.

• To keep the eustachian tube open, perform Valsalva's maneuver several times daily: Inhale deeply, hold your breath, and strain hard for at least 10 seconds before exhaling.

• If you have allergies, get prompt treatment.

Preventing middle ear infection in infants

Don't feed your infant in a supine position or put him or her to bed with a bottle. Doing so allows bacteria and fungi from the nose and throat to flow backward, setting the stage for middle ear infection.

mon. With prompt treatment, the prognosis is excellent; however, prolonged fluid buildup in the middle ear causes *chronic middle ear infection,* with possible puncturing of the eardrum, which transmits sound vibrations to the inner ear.

Chronic suppurative middle ear infection may lead to scarring, adhesions, and severe ear damage. *Chronic secretory middle ear infection,* with its persistent inflammation and pressure, may cause conductive hearing loss.

What causes it?

Middle ear infection is caused by disruption of the eustachian tube, which joins the eardrum with the throat area behind the nose (nasopharynx).

Causes of suppurative infection

Suppurative middle ear infection usually is caused by bacterial infection, as bacteria from the nose flow backward through the eustachian tube and enter the middle ear. Other causes include changes in position and allergic reactions. Children are predisposed to suppurative infection because they have wider, shorter, and more horizontal eustachian tubes. (See *Guarding against middle ear infection.*)

Chronic suppurative middle ear infection may occur if acute episodes of middle ear infection aren't treated adequately or if the infection is caused by resistant strains of bacteria.

Causes of secretory infection

Secretory middle ear infection is caused by a blocked eustachian tube. This causes negative pressure to build up in the middle ear, allowing fluid from blood vessels to enter. (See *Where fluid collects in middle ear infection.*) Such fluid may result from a viral infection or an allergy. It may also follow a pressure injury, caused by inability to equalize pressures between the environment and the middle ear. In a person with an upper respiratory infection, this may happen during rapid descent in an airplane. It may also occur in a scuba diver who rapidly rises to the water surface.

Chronic secretory infection is caused by a mechanical obstruction (such as from overgrowth of adenoidal tissue or from tumors), swelling (such as in allergic rhinitis or chronic sinus infection), or inadequate treatment of acute suppurative infection.

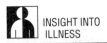

INSIGHT INTO
ILLNESS

Where fluid collects in middle ear infection

Normally, the eustachian tube equalizes pressure in the middle ear. But a blocked eustachian tube or backward flow of fluid can cause a vacuum in the middle ear space, hindering drainage of secretions and allowing them to collect. If the secretions remain sterile, the fluid may be thin and watery (in secretory middle ear infection); if infectious organisms enter the middle ear space, the fluid may contain pus (in acute suppurative middle ear infection).

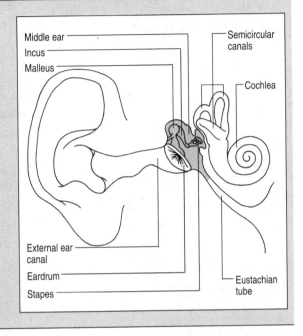

What are its symptoms?

Acute suppurative middle ear infection causes sneezing, coughing, mild to very high fever, hearing loss (usually mild), dizziness, nausea, vomiting, and severe, deep, throbbing pain. Some people also have a bulging eardrum; if the eardrum ruptures, they'll have swelling and drainage of pus in the ear canal. However, many people have no symptoms.

Acute secretory middle ear infection causes severe conductive hearing loss. The person may also have a sensation of fullness in the ear and popping, crackling, or clicking sounds when swallowing or moving the jaw. Fluid buildup may cause the person to hear an echo when speaking and to have a vague feeling of top-heaviness.

Eventually, chronic middle ear infection causes thickening and scarring of the eardrum, impairs the eardrum's movement, and leads to a cystlike mass in the middle ear. If the chronic infection is suppurative, a painless discharge of pus occurs.

Questions parents ask about middle ear infection

The doctor says my child has a temporary hearing loss. When will hearing return?

Your child's hearing should return to normal once the infection or eustachian tube blockage is relieved. Make sure your child takes the medication as the doctor directs. If your child's having surgery, remember to follow the doctor's directions afterward.

How many times must my child get an ear infection before the doctor will recommend tubes?

The doctor usually advises insertion of the tympanostomy tubes you're talking about after a child has been treated with antibiotics for 1 to 3 months without improved hearing. Or the doctor may recommend their use after a child has had frequent ear infections, even without a hearing loss.

Now that my child has tubes in the ears, how will I detect an infection?

If the tubes function normally, you'll see drainage from the outer ear canal. However, if the tubes are clogged, your child may respond as usual to infection. That is, he or she may tug at the ear, feel feverish, and act restless and irritable.

How is it diagnosed?

To diagnose middle ear infection, the doctor takes the person's history and examines the inside of the ear. Findings vary with the type of infection present. In some cases, the doctor may perform a test called *pneumatic otoscopy* to detect decreased eardrum movement — but this procedure can be painful. The pain pattern aids diagnosis. In acute suppurative infection, for example, pulling on the earlobe *doesn't* worsen the pain.

In chronic middle ear infection, the person has a history of recurrent or unresolved middle ear infection. An ear exam shows a thickened and possibly scarred eardrum with decreased mobility. Pneumatic otoscopy may show decreased or absent movement of the eardrum.

A history of recent air travel or scuba diving suggests a condition called *barotitis media* — middle ear infection caused by exposure to differing atmospheric pressures.

How is it treated?

Treatment of middle ear infection depends on which type of infection is present.

Treating acute suppurative infection

The doctor prescribes an antibiotic — typically, Totacillin or Amoxil. People who are allergic to penicillin derivatives may receive Ceclor or Bactrim.

Usually, an operation called *myringotomy* is done to treat severe, painful bulging of the eardrum. In this procedure, the doctor cuts into the eardrum and gently suctions fluid or pus from the middle ear to relieve pressure.

Broad-spectrum antibiotics can help prevent acute suppurative middle ear infection in people at high risk for the disorder. In those with recurring middle ear infection, the doctor will use antibiotics with discretion to prevent development of resistant strains of bacteria.

Treating acute secretory infection

The only required treatment may be inflating the eustachian tube by performing Valsalva's maneuver several times a day. To perform this maneuver, the person inhales deeply, holds his or her breath, and strains hard before exhaling.

Otherwise, decongestant therapy may help. The person should continue using decongestants for at least 2 weeks and may even need to use them indefinitely, with periodic evaluation. If decongestant therapy fails, the doctor performs myringotomy and removes middle ear fluid, then inserts a polyethylene tube into the eardrum to equalize pressure immediately. The tube falls out spontaneously after 9 to 12 months. (See *Questions parents ask about middle ear infection.*) At the same time, any underlying cause is treated. For instance, some people must eliminate allergens or have enlarged adenoids removed.

Treating chronic middle ear infection

The doctor prescribes antibiotics for acute flare-ups of middle ear infection. Depending on circumstances, other measures may include eliminating eustachian tube blockage, treating external ear infection, using a graft to surgically restore a perforated eardrum, or surgically reconstructing the hearing mechanism of the middle ear. Some people must undergo surgery to remove the mastoid process or to remove a cyst in the middle ear. (See *Caring for a child with middle ear infection.*)

ADVICE FOR CAREGIVERS

Caring for a child with middle ear infection

To help your child's recovery, follow this advice.
- Make sure your child completes the full course of prescribed antibiotic treatment.
- If the doctor prescribes decongestants, make sure you understand — and follow — the instructions for instilling them.
- Apply heat to your child's ear to relieve pain.
- If your child has acute secretory middle ear infection, watch for and immediately report pain and fever — signs of secondary infection.
- If your child has undergone surgery to reconstruct the hearing mechanism of the middle ear, don't let him or her get the ear wet when bathing. Warn your child against blowing his or her nose.

MOTION SICKNESS

What is this condition?

Motion sickness is a loss of equilibrium characterized by nausea and vomiting. This loss of equilibrium is caused by irregular or rhythmic movements or from the sensation of motion. Removing the stimulus restores normal equilibrium.

What causes it?

Motion sickness may result from excessive stimulation of the labyrinthine receptors of the inner ear by certain motions, such as those experienced in a car, boat, plane, or swing. It may also be caused by confusion in the brain from conflicting sensory input. For example, a visual stimulus may conflict with the message being sent to the brain by the labyrinthine receptors of the inner ear.

Predisposing factors include tension or fear, offensive odors, or sights and sounds associated with a previous attack. Motion sickness caused by cars, elevators, trains, and swings is most common in children; boats and airplanes mostly affect adults. People who suffer from one kind of motion sickness aren't necessarily susceptible to other types.

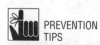

Minimizing motion sickness

Obviously, the best way to avoid motion sickness is to avoid traveling. Of course, that's not possible for most of us. But the following suggestions can help you reduce your risk of getting sick during a trip.

Drugs that help
- Take an antiemetic 30 to 60 minutes before traveling, or apply a Transderm-Scop patch at least 4 hours before traveling. (*Note:* If you have prostate enlargement or glaucoma, be sure to consult your doctor or pharmacist before taking antiemetics.)
- Avoid eating or drinking for at least 4 hours before a trip.
- Pick a seat where motion is least apparent — near the wing section in an aircraft, in the center of a boat, or in the front seat of an automobile.

Watch the horizon
- Keep your head still and your eyes closed or focused on a distant and stationary object, such as the horizon.
- If your child tends to get motion sickness, put him or her in an elevated car seat. This may prevent the child from getting sick by letting him or her see out the front window.

What are its symptoms?

Typically, motion sickness causes nausea, vomiting, headache, dizziness, fatigue, sweating and, occasionally, difficult breathing leading to a sensation of suffocation. These symptoms usually subside when the motion causing them stops, but they may persist for several hours or days.

How is it treated?

The best way to treat the disorder is to stop the motion that's causing it. If this isn't possible, the person will benefit from lying down, closing his or her eyes, and trying to sleep. Drugs that prevent or treat nausea or vomiting, such as Dramamine, Marezine, Antivert, and the Transderm-Scop patch, may prevent or relieve motion sickness. (See *Minimizing motion sickness.*)

NASAL PAPILLOMAS

What is this condition?

A papilloma is a benign overgrowth of tissue within the mucosa lining the inside of the nose.

Inverted papillomas grow into the tissue underlying the nose. They are sometimes associated with squamous cell cancer.

Exophytic papillomas, which also tend to occur singly, arise from epithelial tissue, commonly on the surface of the nasal septum (the wall between the nostrils).

Both types of papillomas are most prevalent in males. Recurrence is likely, even after the papilloma is surgically removed.

What causes it?

A papilloma may arise as a benign precursor of a tumor or as a response to tissue injury or viral infection. The exact cause is unknown.

What are its symptoms?

Both types of papilloma typically produce symptoms related to one-sided nasal obstruction — stuffiness, postnasal drip, headache, shortness of breath, difficulty breathing and, rarely, severe respiratory distress, nasal drainage, and infection. Nosebleeds are most likely to occur with exophytic papillomas.

How is it diagnosed?

An exam of the nasal mucosa may indicate the presence of papillomas. Lab exam of tissue removed in surgery confirms the diagnosis.

How is it treated?

The most effective treatment for papillomas is surgical removal, possibly with laser surgery. The surgeon must carefully inspect adjacent tissues and sinuses to rule out spread of papillomas. Aspirin or Tylenol and decongestants may relieve symptoms. (See *What you should know about treating nasal papillomas.*)

NASAL POLYPS

What is this condition?

Nasal polyps are benign and swollen growths that appear in the nose. Numerous polyps may occur in both sides of the nose. They may become large and numerous enough to cause nasal distention and enlargement of the bony framework, possibly blocking the airway. They are more common in adults than in children and tend to recur.

What causes it?

Nasal polyps usually result from the continuous pressure resulting from a chronic allergy that causes prolonged mucous membrane swelling in the nose and sinuses. Other predisposing factors include chronic sinus infection, chronic rhinitis, and recurrent nasal infections. (See *Preventing nasal polyps,* page 522.)

What are its symptoms?

Nasal blockage is the primary symptom of nasal polyps. The blockage causes loss of the sense of smell, a sensation of fullness in the face, nasal discharge, headache, and shortness of breath. Other symptoms usually mimic those of allergic rhinitis.

How is it diagnosed?

The doctor will use X-rays of the sinuses and nasal passages and will examine the nose with a nasal speculum to help diagnose nasal polyps.

 SELF-HELP

What you should know about treating nasal papillomas

Nasal papillomas can cause nosebleeds and may require surgery. The following tips can help you cope with nosebleeds, know what to expect after surgery, and avoid recurrences.

When nosebleed occurs

If you have a nosebleed, sit upright and spit blood into a container. Pinch the lower part of your nose closed for 15 minutes while you breathe through your mouth. Apply ice compresses to your nose. If the bleeding doesn't stop, notify the doctor.

If you have surgery

- After surgery, be aware that you won't be permitted to blow your nose. Nasal packing is usually removed 12 to 24 hours after surgery.
- Because papillomas tend to recur, seek medical attention at the first sign of nasal discomfort, discharge, or congestion that doesn't subside with conservative treatment.
- Make regular follow-up visits to the doctor to detect early signs of recurrence.

How is it treated?

The doctor will prescribe steroid drugs to be administered either by direct injection into the polyps or by local spray to temporarily shrink the polyps. The doctor may also treat the underlying cause, using antihistamines to control allergy and antibiotics if infection is present. Local application of an astringent shrinks swollen tissue.

Unfortunately, medical treatment alone is rarely effective in alleviating nasal polyps. Consequently, the doctor will surgically remove the polyps, usually using local anesthesia. Laser surgery is being used more frequently for polyp removal.

NOSEBLEED

What do doctors call this condition?

Epistaxis

What is this condition?

A nosebleed may be a primary disorder or may result from another condition. In children, bleeding generally originates in the anterior nasal septum and tends to be mild. In adults, it's most likely to originate in the posterior septum and can be severe. Nosebleeds are twice as common in children as in adults.

What causes it?

A nosebleed usually occurs after an injury, such as a blow to the nose, nose picking, or insertion of a foreign body into the nose. Less commonly, it occurs as a complication of nasal polyps or acute or chronic infections, such as sinusitis or rhinitis, which cause congestion and eventual bleeding of the capillary blood vessels. It may also result from inhalation of chemicals that irritate the nasal mucosa. (See *Questions people ask about nosebleeds.*)

Factors that predispose a person to nosebleeds include use of blood-thinning drugs (called *anticoagulants*), high blood pressure, chronic aspirin use, high altitudes and dry climates, sclerotic vessel disease, Hodgkin's disease, certain cancers, scurvy, vitamin K deficiency, rheumatic fever, blood disorders (hemophilia, purpura, leukemia, and anemias), and a bleeding disorder called *hemorrhagic telangiectasia.*

STRAIGHT
TALK

Questions people ask about nosebleeds

Why do I always seem to get nosebleeds in the spring?

An allergy may trigger springtime nosebleeds. This is especially true if a winter of forced-air heating leaves your nasal cavity dry and irritated and prone to bleeding.

To prevent nosebleeds, try to avoid known irritants. Also consider adding moisture to the air you breathe with a room or whole-house humidifier. Another home remedy may help too. Just dab a small amount of Vaseline inside your nose to help keep it moist. If you think you have an allergy, talk with your doctor before you begin taking any medications to control it.

My sister thinks I must have high blood pressure because I get nosebleeds. Is she right?

Not necessarily. Experts disagree on whether high blood pressure causes nosebleeds. In people who have high blood pressure, blood vessel degenera-

tion from hardening of the arteries is the primary cause of nosebleeds. People with high blood pressure usually have more serious nosebleeds because of increased pressure on the blood vessels. As a result, they often require medical treatment to stop the bleeding. Consult your doctor to identify the exact cause of your nosebleeds. Then follow your doctor's recommendations to keep the nosebleeds from recurring.

Sometimes I vomit when I have a nosebleed. Why does this happen?

Swallowing blood from a nosebleed can upset your stomach and cause vomiting. You can prevent this by sitting up rather than lying down during a nosebleed and by holding your head slightly forward. Also spit out — rather than swallow — any blood that comes into your mouth. Finally, avoid drinking fluids if you have any blood in your mouth, throat, or stomach. Doing so may cause vomiting.

What are its symptoms?

Blood oozing from the nostrils usually originates in the anterior nose and is bright red. Blood from the back of the throat originates in the posterior area and may be dark or bright red (and is often mistaken for hemoptysis, expectorated blood that is usually a sign of a respiratory disease). A nosebleed generally occurs only in one nostril, except when it's caused by a blood disorder or severe injury. In a severe nosebleed, blood may seep behind the nasal septum and may appear in the middle ear and in the corners of the eyes.

Associated symptoms depend on the severity of bleeding. Moderate blood loss may cause light-headedness, dizziness, and slight respiratory difficulty. Severe bleeding causes low blood pressure, rapid and bounding pulse, difficulty breathing, and pallor. Bleeding is considered severe if it lasts longer than 10 minutes after pressure is applied and may cause blood loss as great as 1 liter per hour in adults.

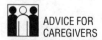

ADVICE FOR
CAREGIVERS

Teaching your child how to stop a nosebleed

Even a minor bump on a child's nose can start a nosebleed. To keep your child from panicking, teach him how to stop the bleeding. Here are some steps to follow.

Apply pressure

When your child's nose bleeds, show him how to pinch the lower half of his nose tightly shut between the thumb and fingers. Tell him to breathe through his mouth while holding his nose like this for about 10 minutes.

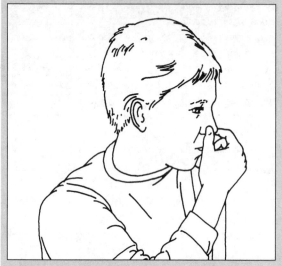

If your child's hand or fingers tire, advise switching hands by placing the thumb and fingers of the rested hand above the fingers of the tired hand. Tell him to start pinching with the rested hand as he lets go with the tired hand. Then he can slide his fingers down the nose until they're pinching the lower half of the nose as before.

Practice pinching each other's noses. This way you'll both learn how much pressure to apply. And you'll know how your fingers feel when they're in the right position.

Watch to be sure your child compresses the entire lower half of his nose — not just the tip.

Sit still, be calm — and other tips

Teach your child to sit down — quietly and calmly — whenever his nose starts to bleed. Show him how to tilt his head slightly forward so that he doesn't swallow or choke on blood.

Warn him not to tilt his head backward, not to lie down, and not to stuff a tissue in his nose.

Direct him to spit out any blood that gets in his mouth or throat. Tell him to spit into a container if possible. This will allow you or another supervising adult to estimate the blood loss.

Reassure your child that he can resume playing when the bleeding stops, but tell him to play quietly, not vigorously, to keep the bleeding from starting again.

Remind your child not to pick or blow his nose after a nosebleed because the bleeding may recur.

Get help

Instruct your child to get help from an adult if a nosebleed doesn't stop after 10 minutes or if bleeding starts again. Direct him to stay calm and to walk (not run) to find help. Tell him to hold his head straight or bent slightly downward and to keep applying pressure on his nose until he finds help.

How is it diagnosed?

Although simple observation confirms a nosebleed, inspection with a bright light and nasal speculum is necessary to locate the site of bleeding. The doctor may also order blood tests to evaluate blood count and clotting ability.

When making a diagnosis, the doctor must check for an underlying disorder that may cause nosebleed, especially disseminated intravascular coagulation (a condition marked by bleeding at multiple sites within the body) and rheumatic fever. Bruises or concomitant bleeding elsewhere probably indicates a blood disorder.

How is it treated?

For anterior bleeding, the doctor will recommend applying a cotton ball saturated with epinephrine to the bleeding site and applying external pressure to the nose. The doctor may then cauterize the bleeding site with electrocautery or silver nitrate stick. If these measures don't control the bleeding, petrolatum gauze nasal packing may be inserted.

For posterior bleeding, the doctor will insert gauze packing through the nose or postnasal packing through the mouth, depending on the bleeding site. (Gauze packing generally remains in place for 24 to 48 hours; postnasal packing, for 3 to 5 days.) An alternative method, the nasal balloon catheter, also controls bleeding effectively. The doctor may also prescribe antibiotics if packing must remain in place for longer than 24 hours.

If local measures fail to control bleeding, additional treatment may include supplemental vitamin K. A person with severe bleeding may require blood transfusions and surgery to close off a bleeding artery.

What can a person with nosebleeds do?

■ To control a nosebleed, sit upright. Then press the soft portion of the nostrils against the septum continuously for 5 to 10 minutes. Apply an ice collar or cold, wet compresses to the nose. If bleeding continues after 10 minutes of pressure, notify the doctor. Breathe through your mouth. Don't swallow blood, talk, or blow your nose. (See *Teaching your child how to stop a nosebleed.*)

■ Know that a nosebleed usually looks worse than it is. (See *Tips for avoiding nosebleeds.*)

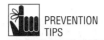 PREVENTION
TIPS

OTOSCLEROSIS

What is this condition?

The most common cause of conductive deafness, otosclerosis is the slow formation of spongy bone in the inner ear. It occurs more often in whites and is two times more common in females than in males. Onset usually occurs between ages 15 and 50. With surgery, the prognosis is good.

What causes it?

Otosclerosis appears to result from genetic factors. Many people report a family history of hearing loss. Pregnancy may trigger onset of this condition.

What are its symptoms?

This disorder causes progressive hearing loss in one ear, which may advance to deafness in both ears. Other symptoms include ringing in the ears and hearing conversation better in a noisy environment than in a quiet one.

How is it diagnosed?

Early diagnosis is based on a Rinne test that shows bone conduction lasting longer than air conduction (normally, the reverse is true). As otosclerosis progresses, bone conduction also deteriorates. Audiometric testing reveals hearing loss ranging from 60 decibels in early stages to total loss. The Weber test detects sound lateralizing to the more affected ear. Physical exam reveals a normal eardrum.

How is it treated?

The doctor will perform a stapedectomy (removal of the stapes, one of the small bones of the middle ear that contributes to the transmission of sound) and insert a prosthesis to restore partial or total hearing. This procedure is performed on one ear at a time, starting with the ear that has suffered greater damage. Alternative surgery includes stapedotomy (creation of a small hole in the stapes' footplate), through which a wire and piston are inserted.

After surgery, the person is hospitalized for 2 or 3 days and receives antibiotics to prevent infection. (See *How to speed your recovery after ear surgery*.)

If surgery isn't possible, a hearing aid (air conduction aid with molded ear insert receiver) enables the person to hear conversation in normal surroundings, although this therapy isn't as effective as stapedectomy.

SEPTAL PERFORATION AND DEVIATION

What is this condition?

Perforated septum is a hole in the nasal septum between the two air passages. Deviated septum is a shift of the nasal septum from the midline and is common in most adults. Deviated septum may be severe enough to block the passage of air through the nostrils. With surgical correction, the prognosis for either perforated or deviated septum is good.

What causes it?

Generally, perforated septum is caused by traumatic irritation, most commonly from excessive nose picking. Less often, repeated cauterization for nosebleed or from penetrating septal injury causes the condition. It may also be caused by infection called *perichondritis* that gradually erodes the perichondrial layer and cartilage, finally forming an ulcer that perforates the septum.

Other causes of septal perforation include syphilis, tuberculosis, untreated septal hematoma, chronic nasal infections, nasal cancer, granuloma, and chronic sinus infections, as well as inhaling irritating chemicals or snorting cocaine.

Deviated septum commonly develops during normal growth, as the septum shifts from one side to the other. Consequently, few adults have perfectly straight septa. Nasal trauma resulting from a fall, a blow to the nose, or surgery exaggerates the deviation. Congenital deviated septum is rare.

How to speed your recovery after ear surgery

If you plan to have an operation to treat otosclerosis, the following suggestions can speed your recovery and help you avoid complications:

- After surgery, avoid loud noises and sudden pressure changes (such as those that occur while diving or flying) until healing is complete (usually in 6 months).
- Don't blow your nose for at least 1 week after surgery to prevent contaminated air and bacteria from entering the eustachian tube.
- Take steps to protect your ears against the cold.
- Avoid activities that cause dizziness, such as straining, bending, and heavy lifting.
- If possible, avoid contact with anyone who has an upper respiratory infection.
- Make sure you understand — and follow — your doctor's instructions for changing the external ear dressing (eye or gauze pad) and caring for the incision.
- Complete the prescribed course of antibiotic therapy, and return for scheduled follow-up care.

Dealing with a perforated or deviated septum

Here are some tips for treating nosebleeds and other problems related to septal disorders.

Home care

• To treat a nosebleed, sit upright and spit any blood into a container. While breathing through your mouth, pinch the lower half of your nose tightly shut for 10 to 15 minutes, and apply ice packs. If bleeding persists, notify the doctor.

• If you have a septal perforation or a severe septal deviation, don't blow your nose. To relieve nasal congestion, use saline nose drops and install a room humidifier. Take decongestants, as instructed by the doctor.

If you have surgery

• After surgery, don't blow your nose; doing so may cause bruising and swelling, even after nasal packing is removed. Limit physical activity for 2 or 3 days. If you're a smoker, stop smoking for at least 2 days.

• Sneeze with your mouth open and avoid bending over at the waist. Stoop to pick up fallen objects.

What are its symptoms?

A small septal perforation rarely causes symptoms but may produce a whistle when the person inhales. A large perforation causes rhinitis, nosebleeds, nasal crusting, and watery discharge.

The person with a deviated septum may develop a crooked nose because the midline deflects to one side. The predominant symptom of severe deflection, however, is nasal obstruction. Other symptoms include a sensation of fullness in the face, shortness of breath, nasal discharge, recurring nosebleeds, infection, sinus infection, and headache.

How is it diagnosed?

Although clinical features suggest septal perforation or deviation, confirmation requires inspection of the nasal mucosa with bright light and a nasal speculum.

How is it treated?

The doctor will treat the symptoms of perforated septum by prescribing decongestants to reduce nasal congestion, local application of lanolin or Vaseline to prevent ulceration and crusting, and antibiotics to combat infection. The doctor may also recommend surgery to graft part of the perichondrial layer over the perforation. Also, a plastic or Silastic "button" prosthesis may be used to close the perforation.

Symptomatic treatment of deviated septum usually includes analgesics to relieve headache, decongestants to minimize secretions, and as necessary, vasoconstrictors, nasal packing, or cautery to control hemorrhage. (See *Dealing with a perforated or deviated septum*.) Manipulation of the nasal septum at birth can correct congenital deviated septum.

Surgical procedures that may be performed to correct the problem include:

• *reconstruction of the nasal septum by submucous resection* to reposition the nasal septal cartilage and relieve nasal obstruction

• *rhinoplasty* to correct nasal structure deformity by intranasal incisions

• *septoplasty* to relieve nasal obstruction and enhance cosmetic appearance.

SINUS INFECTION

What do doctors call this condition?
Sinusitis

What is this condition?
Sinus infection refers to infection of the paranasal sinuses — the four pairs of air pockets that drain into the nose. (See *Learning about your sinuses,* page 530.) Sinus infection may be acute, subacute, chronic, allergic, or hyperplastic. In this last, the number of sinus cells is abnormally increased.

What causes it?
Sinus infection usually is caused by viral or bacterial infection. Acute sinus infection is primarily caused by the common cold; it lingers in the subacute form in only about 10% of cases. Chronic sinus infection follows persistent bacterial infection.

Predisposing factors for sinus infection include any condition that interferes with sinus drainage and ventilation, such as:
- chronic nasal swelling
- a deviated septum
- thickened mucus
- nasal polyps
- allergic inflammation of the nasal mucous membranes (allergic rhinitis)
- a weakened state from chemotherapy, malnutrition, diabetes, a blood disease, chronic steroid use, or a depressed immune system.

Bacterial sinus invasion commonly is caused by the conditions listed above or after a viral infection. It may also result from swimming in polluted water.

Allergic sinus infection accompanies allergic rhinitis. Hyperplastic sinus infection is a combination of pus-producing acute sinus infection and allergic sinus infection or allergic rhinitis.

What are its symptoms?
Symptoms vary depending on the type of sinus infection.

Learning about your sinuses

Until your symptoms struck, you probably never thought about your sinuses. Now you may think of nothing else. Read over this information to understand what these structures do, where they're located, and why they're causing you so much trouble.

What do the sinuses do?

The sinuses are small, air-filled pockets in the facial bones that lend shape to the face without adding weight to the head. They also act as resonating chambers for the voice.

Where are the sinuses located?

The four pairs of sinuses — frontal, ethmoid, maxillary, and sphenoid — lie alongside the nose on both sides of your face.

Why do sinuses hurt?

Pain from sinus infection occurs when the mucus-producing membranes lining the sinuses become inflamed (from infection or blockage). Normally, mucus drains into the nose through tiny bone channels called *ostia*. In sinus infection, these openings become blocked, causing infection, facial pain, a stuffy nose, and other symptoms.

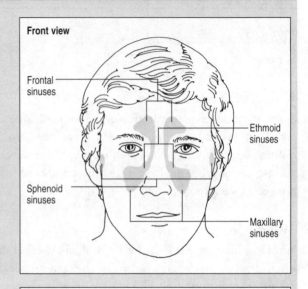

Front view

Frontal sinuses

Ethmoid sinuses

Sphenoid sinuses

Maxillary sinuses

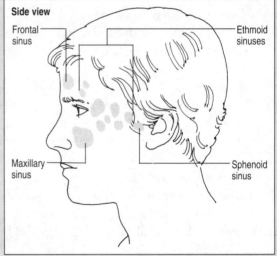

Side view

Frontal sinus

Ethmoid sinuses

Maxillary sinus

Sphenoid sinus

Acute sinus infection

The main symptom of this type of sinus infection is a stuffy nose, followed by gradually increasing pressure in the affected sinus. For 24 to 48 hours after symptoms first appear, the person may have a runny nose. Later, the nasal discharge contains pus. Other symptoms include an overall ill feeling, sore throat, headache, and slight fever (temperature of 99° to 99.5° F [37.2° to 37.5° C]). Pain location

SELF-HELP

Learning about sinus surgeries

You may have lots of concerns before you decide to undergo sinus surgery. The information below will help you to understand the types of sinus operations.

Maxillary sinus surgery

• The *antral window procedure* creates an intranasal opening in the sinus to allow secretions and pus to drain through the nose.
• The *Caldwell-Luc operation* removes diseased mucosa in the maxillary sinus through an incision inside the upper lip.

Ethmoid sinus surgery

• *Ethmoidectomy* removes all infected tissue through an external or intranasal incision into the ethmoid sinus. This connects the ethmoid air cells, improving drainage.
• *Endoscopic sinus surgery* removes diseased tissue and improves drainage by a tube called an endoscope, which is introduced through the nose into the ethmoid sinus. (This procedure may also reach the sphenoid and maxillary sinuses.)

Sphenoid sinus surgery

Sphenoethmoidectomy removes infected sphenoid sinus tissue through an external incision in the ethmoid sinus.

Frontal sinus surgery

• *Frontoethmoidectomy* removes infected frontal sinus tissue through an extended external ethmoidectomy.
• The *osteoplastic flap procedure* directly drains the frontal sinuses through an incision across the skull and behind the hairline.

Related surgeries

• *Submucous resection* repairs a deviated septum through an intranasal incision. This eliminates sinus drainage blockage.
• *Polypectomy* removes obstructive nasal polyps through an intranasal incision. Despite removal, nasal polyps commonly recur.

depends on the affected sinus, but may occur over the cheeks and upper teeth, over the eyes, over the eyebrows, or behind the eyes.

Subacute sinus infection

In this type of sinus infection, pus-filled nasal drainage lasts longer than 3 weeks after an acute infection subsides. Other symptoms include stuffy nose, vague facial discomfort, fatigue, and a nonproductive cough.

Chronic sinus infection

Symptoms of chronic sinus infection resemble those of acute sinus infection, except that the chronic form causes continuous mucus- and pus-filled discharge.

SELF-HELP

Advice for a person with sinus infection

Here are some pointers to help you recover from this condition.

Home care

- Get plenty of rest, and drink plenty of fluids to help your sinuses drain.
- To relieve pain and aid sinus drainage, apply warm compresses over the sinus area continuously, or four times daily for 2-hour intervals.
- Take prescribed pain relievers and antihistamines as needed.
- Finish the complete course of prescribed antibiotics, even if your symptoms disappear.
- Watch for and report complications, such as vomiting, chills, fever, swelling of the forehead or eyelids, blurred or double vision, or personality changes.

If you have surgery

If you're going to have sinus surgery, you'll have nasal packing for 12 to 24 hours afterward. You'll have to breathe through your mouth and you won't be able to blow your nose. Even after the packing is removed, blowing your nose may cause bleeding and swelling. Also, if you're a smoker, you must not smoke for at least 2 or 3 days after surgery.

Allergic sinus infection

The major symptoms of this type of infection are sneezing, a headache in the front of the head, watery nasal discharge, and a stuffy, burning, itchy nose.

Hyperplastic sinus infection

This type of infection causes a chronically stuffy nose and headache.

How is it diagnosed?

To diagnose sinus infection, the doctor examines the inside of the person's nose. The doctor may also take sinus X-rays, perform a sinus puncture (rare), or order ultrasound or a computed tomography scan (commonly called a CAT scan).

How is it treated?

The doctor may try a variety of treatments, depending on the type of sinus infection.

Acute sinus infection

Usually, the doctor prescribes local decongestants before trying oral decongestants and may also recommend inhaling steam. To combat pus-producing or persistent infection, the doctor will prescribe antibiotics, usually for 2 to 3 weeks, because sinus infection is deep seated. Applying heat to the sinus area may also help relieve pain and congestion.

Subacute sinus infection

In subacute sinus infection, antibiotics and decongestants may be helpful.

Allergic sinus infection

To treat allergic sinus infection, the doctor must also treat allergic rhinitis. Typically, the doctor prescribes antihistamines, orders skin testing to identify the cause of allergy, and may prescribe immunotherapy, which desensitizes the person to the offending allergens by administering them in increasingly large doses. Severe allergic symptoms may call for steroids and epinephrine.

Chronic and hyperplastic sinus infection

In both these types of infection, the doctor may prescribe antihistamines, antibiotics, and a steroid nasal spray to relieve pain and congestion. If irrigation fails to relieve symptoms, sinus surgery may be necessary. (See *Learning about sinus surgeries,* page 531, and *Advice for a person with sinus infection.*)

SORE THROAT

What do doctors call this condition?
Pharyngitis

What is this condition?
The most common throat disorder, sore throat is an acute or chronic inflammation of the pharynx, the passage between the mouth cavity and the esophagus. It's widespread among adults who live or work in dusty or very dry environments, use their voices excessively, habitually use tobacco or alcohol, or suffer from chronic sinus infection, persistent coughs, or allergies.

What causes it?
Sore throat is usually caused by a virus. The most common bacterial cause is group A beta-hemolytic streptococci. Other common causes include *Mycoplasma* and *Chlamydia*. (See *Questions people ask about a sore throat*.)

What are its symptoms?
The person has a sore throat and slight difficulty in swallowing. Swallowing saliva is usually more painful than swallowing food. Sore throat may also cause the sensation of a lump in the throat as well as a constant, aggravating urge to swallow. Other symptoms may include mild fever, headache, muscle and joint pain, and a runny nose. A sore throat usually subsides in 3 to 10 days.

How is it diagnosed?
Physical exam of the pharynx reveals generalized redness and inflammation. Bacterial sore throat usually produces a large amount of drainage.

A throat culture may be performed to identify bacterial organisms that may be the cause of the inflammation.

How is it treated?
Treatment of acute viral sore throat is usually symptomatic, and consists mainly of rest, warm saline gargles, throat lozenges containing a mild anesthetic, plenty of fluids, and analgesics as needed. If the per-

STRAIGHT TALK

Questions people ask about a sore throat

What's the difference between a sore throat and a strep throat?
"Sore throat" is a general term for a symptom you feel. A strep throat is a specific type of sore throat caused by infection with streptococcal bacteria. Strep throat requires antibiotic treatment. Other sore throats vary in their causes and treatments.

I've been told I'm a strep carrier. What does this mean?
Some people harbor streptococcal bacteria in their throats — even though they lack symptoms or have completed antibiotic treatment. You may remain a carrier for several months or longer after an acute strep infection. While you're a carrier, the harmful bacteria are greatly reduced in strength and number, so prolonged treatment isn't necessary and your risk of spreading the infection to others is small.

At the end of my workday, my throat hurts. Why?
Irritants in your workplace could be to blame. You may breathe chemical fumes that directly irritate your throat or cause postnasal drip, which in turn causes a sore throat. If the irritant is strong, others may be affected, too. Or you may be allergic to some substance at work.

Will a tonsillectomy prevent a sore throat?

If your child has frequent bouts of sore throat, you may wonder if having his or her tonsils removed will prevent a recurrence. The answer, simply, is no.

A tonsillectomy — surgical removal of the palatine tonsils — was commonly performed on children 25 years ago, but it's not routinely done today. A sore throat may still occur even if the tonsils are removed. Also, the tonsils, which are made of lymph tissue, actually help to protect the body from systemic infections.

Occasionally, a tonsillectomy is needed if the tonsils are chronically enlarged and interfere with breathing or swallowing. However, the procedure isn't advised for children under age 3.

son can't swallow fluids, he or she may have to go into the hospital for intravenous hydration.

The doctor will treat suspected bacterial sore throat with penicillin or another broad-spectrum antibiotic. The person will begin receiving antibiotic therapy while waiting for results of the throat culture. If the culture is positive (or if bacterial infection is suspected despite negative culture results), penicillin therapy will be continued for 10 days. Continued antibiotic therapy helps to prevent acute rheumatic fever.

Chronic sore throat requires the same supportive measures as acute sore throat but with greater emphasis on eliminating the underlying cause, such as an allergen. Preventive measures include providing room humidity and avoiding excessive air conditioner use. In addition, the person should be urged to stop smoking. (See *Will a tonsillectomy prevent a sore throat?* and *Coping with sore throat.*)

SWIMMER'S EAR

What do doctors call this condition?
External ear infection, otitis externa

What is this condition?
Swimmer's ear is an inflammation of the skin of the external ear canal and the folds of skin and cartilage known as the *auricle* or *pinna* (this is the part of the ear we see). It may be acute or chronic and is most common in the summer. With treatment, acute swimmer's ear usually subsides within 7 days. This disorder tends to recur.

What causes it?
Swimmer's ear usually is caused by bacteria, such as *Pseudomonas, Proteus vulgaris,* streptococci, and *Staphylococcus aureus.* Sometimes, swimmer's ear is caused by fungi, such as *Aspergillus niger* and *Candida albicans.* Fungal swimmer's ear is most common in the tropics.

Occasionally, chronic swimmer's ear is caused by dermatologic conditions, such as seborrhea or psoriasis.

Predisposing factors include:

- swimming in polluted water, after which earwax creates a culture medium for the waterborne organism (See *How to prevent swimmer's ear,* page 536.)
- cleaning the ear canal with a cotton swab, bobby pin, finger, or other foreign object, which irritates the ear canal and may introduce the infecting microorganism
- exposure to dust, hair care products, or other irritants, which causes the person to scratch the ear, excoriating the auricle and ear canal
- regular use of earphones, earplugs, or earmuffs, which trap moisture in the ear canal, creating a culture medium for infection
- chronic drainage from a perforated eardrum.

What are its symptoms?

A person with acute swimmer's ear will have moderate to severe pain that is exacerbated by manipulating the external ear, clenching the teeth, opening the mouth, or chewing. Other symptoms may include fever, foul-smelling discharge from the ear, regional cellulitis, and partial hearing loss.

Fungal swimmer's ear may not cause symptoms, although *A. niger* produces a black or gray, blotting paper–like growth in the ear canal. In chronic swimmer's ear, itching replaces pain, and may lead to scaling and skin thickening. Discharge from the ear may also be present.

How is it diagnosed?

Physical exam confirms swimmer's ear. In acute swimmer's ear, otoscopy reveals a swollen external ear canal (sometimes to the point of complete closure), periauricular lymphadenopathy (tender lymph nodes in front of or behind the external ear, or in the upper neck), and, occasionally, regional cellulitis.

In fungal swimmer's ear, removal of growth shows thick red epithelium. Microscopic exam or culture and sensitivity tests can identify the causative organism and determine antibiotic treatment. Pain on palpation of external ear structures distinguishes acute swimmer's ear from middle ear infection.

In chronic swimmer's ear, physical exam shows thick red epithelium in the ear canal. Severe chronic swimmer's ear may reflect underlying diabetes, underactive thyroid, or kidney infection.

SELF-HELP

Coping with sore throat

- Take pain relievers such as aspirin, and gargle with warm salt water, as prescribed by your doctor.
- Drink plenty of fluids.
- If you have an acute bacterial sore throat, be sure to complete the full course of antibiotic therapy.
- If you have a chronic sore throat, minimize sources of throat irritation in the environment, for example, by using a bedside humidifier.
- If you smoke, stop smoking. Ask your doctor or nurse for names of local self-help groups to stop smoking.

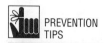

How to prevent swimmer's ear

If your child has repeated bouts of swimmer's ear, you'd like to prevent it before it gets started or stop it before it gets worse. Here are some hints that may help.

Avoiding the infection

- Cut back on the time you allow your child to stay in the water — especially if the infection keeps coming back. Typically, you should let your child swim for no longer than 1 hour.
- Allow between 1 and 2 hours for his ears to dry before letting him go back in the water.
- If he complains of water in his ear, show him how to shake or tap his head to release water trapped in the ear canal. Then show him how to blot the excess water with the corner of a towel.

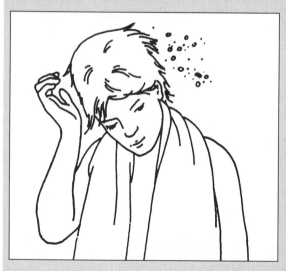

- Let your child take short baths or showers every day, but insist that he dry his ears afterward using a small dab of cotton rather than a cotton-tipped swab. (Swabs are too big for a child's ears. They can injure the ear canal and make an infection worse.)
- Try using a drying solution made of equal parts water, vinegar, and rubbing alcohol. Put a few drops in your child's ear after a shower, after swimming, and when he goes to bed. Let the solution stay in the ear for at least 5 minutes each time. Gently wiggle the ear to help the drops seep deeper into the ear canal. This will help to evaporate moisture remaining in the ear canal.
- If your child has symptoms of a middle ear infection, get prompt treatment to prevent perforation of the eardrum.

Nipping swimmer's ear in the bud

If your child's ear starts itching or causes pain despite these measures, follow these simple steps to keep it from getting worse:

- Call your child's doctor, who may prescribe medicine or may advise you to put a homemade drying solution in your child's ear.
- Keep him out of the water for at least 1 week — longer if pain, itching, and swelling don't clear up within that time.
- Dry his ears immediately after he showers or bathes and shampoos his hair. Then apply eardrops as directed by the doctor.

How is it treated?

To relieve the pain of acute swimmer's ear, treatment may include heat therapy to the region around the external ear (heat lamp, heating pad, or hot, damp compresses) and drug therapy with codeine and aspirin or Tylenol. After cleaning the ear and removing debris, the doctor may prescribe antibiotic eardrops (with or without hydrocortisone). If fever persists or regional cellulitis develops, a systemic antibiotic is necessary.

As with other forms of this disorder, fungal swimmer's ear requires careful cleaning of the ear. The doctor will prescribe a cream to treat swimmer's ear resulting from candidal organisms. Using slightly acidic eardrops creates an unfavorable environment in the ear canal for most fungi, as well as *Pseudomonas.* No specific treatment exists for swimmer's ear caused by *A. niger,* except repeated cleaning of the ear canal with baby oil.

In chronic swimmer's ear, primary treatment consists of cleaning the ear and removing debris. Supplemental therapy includes antibiotic eardrops or antibiotic ointment or cream (neomycin, bacitracin, or polymyxin B, possibly combined with hydrocortisone).

For mild chronic swimmer's ear, treatment may include antibiotic eardrops once or twice weekly and wearing specially fitted earplugs while showering, shampooing, or swimming.

THROAT ABSCESS

What is this condition?

A throat abscess is a localized accumulation of pus that may occur around the tonsils or in the back of the pharynx. With treatment, the prognosis for a person with throat abscess is good.

What causes it?

Abscess around the tonsils is a complication of acute tonsillitis, usually after streptococcal or staphylococcal infection. It occurs more often in adolescents and young adults than in children.

Acute abscess in the back of the pharynx is caused by infection in the lymph glands, which may follow an upper respiratory bacterial infection. Because these lymph glands, present at birth, start to become smaller after age 2, this condition most commonly affects infants and children under age 2.

Chronic abscesses in the back of the throat may result from tuberculosis of the cervical spine and may occur at any age.

What are its symptoms?

The person with an abscess around the tonsils will have severe throat pain, occasional ear pain on the same side as the abscess, and tenderness of the submandibular gland. Difficulty swallowing causes drooling. Tightening of the jaw muscles may occur as a result of swelling and spreading of the infection. Other symptoms include fever, chills, malaise, rancid breath, nausea, muffled speech, and dehydration.

The person with an abscess in the back of the pharynx will have pain, difficulty swallowing, and fever. When the abscess is located in the upper pharynx, the person may develop nasal obstruction. When the abscess is located in the lower pharynx, the person may develop difficult and noisy breathing. Children may experience drooling and muffled crying. A very large abscess may press on the larynx, causing swelling, or may erode into major vessels, causing sudden death from asphyxia or aspiration.

How is it diagnosed?

The doctor bases the diagnosis on the person's health history and on a throat exam. A person with an abscess around the tonsils commonly has a history of bacterial pharyngitis. A lab culture may reveal streptococcal or staphylococcal infection.

A person with an abscess in the back of the pharynx commonly has a history of nasopharyngitis or pharyngitis. The doctor will also take X-rays of the larynx and may order culture and sensitivity tests to isolate the causative organism and determine the appropriate antibiotic treatment.

How is it treated?

If an abscess around the tonsils is caught early, treatment consists of large doses of penicillin or another antibiotic. For late-stage abscess, primary treatment is usually incision and drainage under local anesthesia, followed by antibiotic therapy for 7 to 10 days. Tonsillectomy, scheduled no sooner than 1 month after healing, prevents recurrence but is recommended only after several episodes.

If a person has an acute abscess in the back of the pharynx, the doctor will make an incision to drain the abscess through the pharyngeal wall. In chronic conditions, drainage is performed through an external incision behind the adjacent neck muscles. Postoperative drug therapy includes antibiotics (usually penicillin) and analgesics.

What can a person with a throat abscess do?

After incision and drainage, the doctor may prescribe antibiotics, pain relievers, and fever-reducing medications. Be sure to complete the full course of prescribed antibiotic therapy. To promote healing, use warm salt water gargles or throat irrigations for 24 to 36 hours. Get adequate rest. (See *Gargling with warm salt water.*)

TONSILLITIS

What is this condition?

Tonsillitis is inflammation of the tonsils. It can be acute or chronic. The uncomplicated acute form usually lasts 4 to 6 days and commonly affects children between ages 5 and 10. The presence of proven chronic tonsillitis justifies surgical removal (tonsillectomy), the only effective treatment. Tonsils tend to grow during childhood and shrink after puberty.

What causes it?

Tonsillitis usually is caused by infection with bacteria known as *group A beta-hemolytic streptococci*. It may result from other bacteria or viruses or from oral anaerobes.

What are its symptoms?

Acute tonsillitis commonly begins with a mild to severe sore throat. A very young child, unable to complain about a sore throat, may stop eating. Tonsillitis may also produce difficulty swallowing, fever, swelling and tenderness of the lymph glands in the submandibular area, muscle and joint pain, chills, malaise, headache, and pain (frequently felt in the ears). Excess secretions may cause the child to complain of a constant urge to swallow; the back of the throat may feel constricted. Such discomfort usually subsides after 72 hours.

Chronic tonsillitis produces a recurrent sore throat and pus-filled drainage in the tonsillar crypts. Frequent attacks of acute tonsillitis may also occur. Complications include obstruction from swollen tonsils and an abscess around the tonsils.

 SELF-HELP

Gargling with warm salt water

After an incision to drain a throat abscess, you may be instructed to gargle with warm salt water. Proper gargling helps to relieve throat irritation, remove secretions, and promote healing. Here's how to do it:

- Run tap water until it's 100° to 120° F (37.8° to 48.9° C). Try to gargle with water that's as warm as you can stand it.
- Mix 1 cup of warm tap water with 1 to 2 teaspoons of salt. Stir until the salt is dissolved.
- Take a mouthful of this solution and tip your head back, allowing the fluid to flow gently against the walls of your throat.
- Agitate the solution at the back of your throat by forcing air through it. Do this for as long as you can.
- Spit out this mouthful of salt water and repeat this process three more times. (You don't have to use the whole cup of water.)

Easing the discomfort of tonsillitis

If your child has tonsillitis, his or her sore throat and poor appetite may be a challenge for you to cope with. Here are some ways you can ease your child's discomfort and ensure his or her well-being.

Home care
• Make sure your child drinks plenty of fluids, especially if he or she has a fever. Offer ice cream and flavored drinks and ices.
• Be sure your child completes the prescribed course of antibiotic therapy.

If your child has surgery
• If your child is going to have surgery, find out if the hospital will let a parent stay overnight.
• After surgery, provide plenty of nonirritating fluids. Instruct your child to take frequent deep breaths.
• Expect a white scab to form in the throat 5 to 10 days after the operation.
• Notify the doctor if your child has bleeding, ear discomfort, or a fever that lasts longer than 3 days.

How is it diagnosed?

Diagnostic confirmation requires a thorough throat exam. The doctor notes generalized inflammation of the pharyngeal wall, swollen tonsils, and the presence of drainage with pus. The person may also have a swollen, inflamed uvula (the small, fleshy mass hanging down in the back of the mouth).

Lab tests are also important in making a diagnosis. Cultures may determine the infecting organism and indicate appropriate antibiotic therapy.

How is it treated?

To treat acute tonsillitis, the doctor will prescribe rest, adequate fluid intake, aspirin or Tylenol and, if the person has a bacterial infection, antibiotics. If the organism causing tonsillitis is a group A beta-hemolytic streptococci, the doctor will usually prescribe penicillin, although another antibiotic may be substituted. (See *Easing the discomfort of tonsillitis.*)

To prevent complications, antibiotic therapy should continue for 10 to 14 days. Chronic tonsillitis or the development of complications (obstructions from swollen tonsils or abscess around the tonsils) may require surgical removal of the tonsils. This operation should take place only after the person has been free of tonsillar or respiratory tract infections for 3 to 4 weeks.

VOCAL CORD NODULES AND POLYPS

What are these conditions?

Nodules and polyps are types of benign growths that may appear on the vocal cords. Both nodules and polyps have good prognoses, unless continued voice abuse causes recurrence, with subsequent scarring and permanent hoarseness.

What causes them?

Vocal cord nodules and polyps usually result from voice abuse, especially in the presence of infection. Consequently, they're most common in teachers, singers, and sports fans, and in energetic children (ages 8 to 12) who continually shout while playing. Polyps are common in adults who smoke, live in dry climates, or have allergies.

What are their symptoms?

Nodules and polyps inhibit the movement of the vocal cords and produce painless hoarseness. The voice may also sound breathy or husky.

How are they diagnosed?

If a person has persistent hoarseness, the doctor may suspect vocal cord nodules and polyps. To confirm the diagnosis, the vocal cords may be visualized using a test called *indirect laryngoscopy.* In a person with vocal cord nodules, laryngoscopy initially shows small red nodes; later, white solid nodes will be seen on one or both cords. In a person with polyps, laryngoscopy reveals polyps of varying size, which may appear anywhere on the vocal cords and may occur on one or both cords.

How are they treated?

Conservative management of small vocal cord nodules and polyps includes humidification, speech therapy (voice rest, training to reduce the intensity and duration of voice production), and treatment of any underlying allergies.

When conservative treatment fails to relieve hoarseness, the doctor will remove nodules or polyps under direct laryngoscopy. The doctor may use microlaryngoscopy for small lesions to avoid injuring the vocal cord surface. (See *Recovering from vocal cord surgery.*)

If nodules or polyps are present on both cords, surgical removal may be performed in two stages so that one cord can heal before polyps are removed from the other cord.

For children, treatment consists of speech therapy. If possible, surgery should be delayed until the child is old enough to benefit from voice training, or until he or she can understand the need to abstain from voice abuse.

 SELF-HELP

Recovering from vocal cord surgery

The following suggestions may help you speed postoperative healing and help prevent vocal cord growths from recurring:

- After surgery, rest your voice for 10 days to 2 weeks while your vocal cords heal. Use an alternative means of communication — Magic Slate, pad and pencil, or alphabet board.
- If you're a smoker, stop smoking entirely or, at the very least, refrain from smoking during recovery from surgery.
- Use a vaporizer to increase room humidity and reduce throat irritation.
- Make sure you receive speech therapy after healing, if necessary, because continued voice abuse will cause a recurrence of growths.

SELF-HELP

What to expect with a tracheotomy

If you're scheduled for a tracheotomy, the procedure will be performed under local anesthesia. Make sure a family member or another caregiver understands the doctor's or nurse's instructions for suctioning, cleaning, and changing your tracheostomy tube after surgery.

After the operation, you'll be able to speak by covering the lumen of the tube with your finger or a tracheostomy plug.

VOCAL CORD PARALYSIS

What is this condition?

Vocal cord paralysis is caused by disease of or injury to one of the nerves that conduct impulses to and from the vocal cord muscles.

What causes it?

Vocal cord paralysis commonly is caused by accidental severing of a nerve during thyroid surgery. Other causes include pressure from an aortic aneurysm or from an enlarged lower heart chamber (in people with a congenital heart disorder called *mitral stenosis*), bronchial or esophageal cancer, enlargement of the thyroid gland, neck injuries, or intubation. Paralysis may also be caused by neuritis from infections or metallic poisoning, or from hysteria.

What are its symptoms?

One-sided paralysis, the most common form, may cause vocal weakness and hoarseness. Paralysis on both sides typically causes vocal weakness and incapacitating airway obstruction if the cords become paralyzed in the adducted position.

How is it diagnosed?

The doctor makes a diagnosis of vocal cord paralysis based on a person's history and symptoms. Diagnosis may be confirmed by a test called *indirect laryngoscopy.* This test shows one or both cords fixed in an adducted or partially abducted position.

How is it treated?

Treatment of one-sided vocal cord paralysis consists of injecting Teflon into the paralyzed vocal cord, under direct laryngoscopy. This procedure enlarges the vocal cord and brings it closer to the other cord, which usually strengthens the voice and protects the airway from aspiration.

In another procedure, an implant is placed through a neck incision. The implant helps establish nerve control of the vocal cord muscles. If a person has bilateral cord paralysis, with the cords pulled toward the center position, he or she may have to undergo tracheotomy. (See *What to expect with a tracheotomy.*)

15

SKIN DISORDERS

ACNE

What do doctors call this condition?
Acne vulgaris

What is this condition?
A person with acne experiences persistent, recurrent blemishes on the skin. Acne primarily affects adolescents, but lesions can appear as early as age 8. Although acne strikes boys more often and more severely, it usually occurs in girls at an earlier age and tends to last longer, sometimes into adulthood. The prognosis is good with treatment.

What causes it?
Acne may be caused by many different factors. Research now centers on clogged skin follicles, production of an oily substance called *sebum* (stimulated by hormones called *androgens*), and a bacterium called *Propionibacterium acnes* as possible primary causes. Theories focusing on dietary influences appear to be groundless.

Certain factors — such as heredity and use of oral contraceptives — increase a person's risk of developing acne. Many women experience an acne flare-up during their first few menstrual cycles after starting or discontinuing oral contraceptives. Certain other drugs also seem to increase a person's risk, including corticosteroids, corticotropin, androgens, iodides, bromides, trimethadione, phenytoin, isoniazid, lithium, and halothane. Other risk factors are injury, rubbing from tight clothing, cosmetics, emotional stress, an unfavorable climate, and exposure to heavy oils, greases, or tars.

What are its symptoms?
The acne plug may appear as a closed comedo, or whitehead (if it doesn't protrude from the follicle and is covered by the epidermis), or as an open comedo, or blackhead (if it does protrude and isn't covered by the epidermis). The black coloration is caused by the melanin (pigment) of the follicle. Rupture or leakage of an enlarged plug into the dermis causes inflammation and characteristic acne pustules and papules or, in severe forms, acne cysts or abscesses. Chronic, recurring lesions produce acne scars. (See *How acne develops*.)

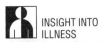

INSIGHT INTO
ILLNESS

How acne develops

Acne is an inflammation of the sebaceous follicles, which are located on the face, back, chest, and upper arms. Numerous large sebaceous glands normally excrete an oily substance called *sebum* through the follicular canal, lubricating the skin. However, during adolescence, a surge of hormones causes the sebaceous glands to make too much sebum and too many skin cells within the hair follicles.

As a result, sebum and dead skin cells combine with bacteria inside the follicles to form plugs called *open comedones (blackheads)* and *closed comedones (whiteheads)*. Rupture of a whitehead causes inflammation, producing papules, pustules, nodules, and cysts.

DISTRIBUTION OF SEBACEOUS FOLLICLES

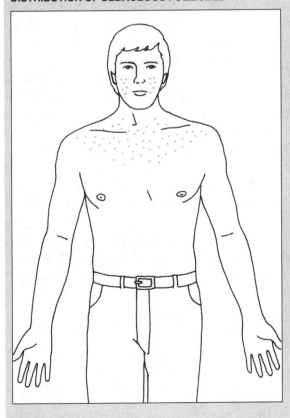

NORMAL SEBACEOUS FOLLICLE

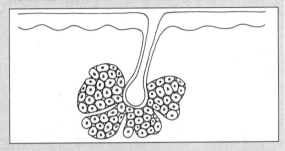

BLACKHEAD

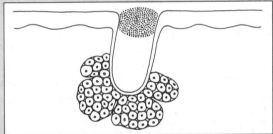

WHITEHEAD

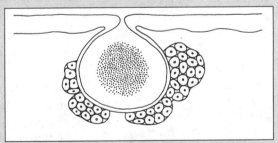

RUPTURED WHITEHEAD

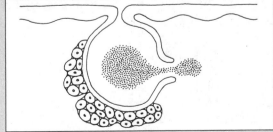

Alleviating acne

The following suggestions can help you get the best results from your acne treatment.

Be good to your skin
- Try to identify any predisposing factors for acne that you can eliminate or modify.
- Continue skin care practices even after acne clears up, which may take years.
- Know that the prescribed treatment is more likely to improve acne than a strict diet and scrubbing with soap and water.

Drug therapy guidelines
- If you're taking Retin-A, apply it at least 30 minutes after washing your face and at least 1 hour before bedtime. Don't use it around your eyes or lips. After treatments, your skin should look pink and dry. If it looks red or starts to peel, the preparation may have to be weakened or applied less often. Avoid exposure to sunlight or use a sunscreen.
- If you're taking Retin-A with benzoyl peroxide, use one preparation in the morning and the other at night to avoid skin irritation.
- Take Achromycin on an empty stomach. Don't take it with antacids or milk, which impair absorption.
- If you're taking Accutane, avoid vitamin A supplements, which can worsen side effects.

How is it diagnosed?

The appearance of characteristic acne lesions, especially in an adolescent, confirms the diagnosis of acne.

How is it treated?

Common therapy for acne includes ointments such as benzoyl peroxide, a powerful antibacterial, or Retin-A. These drugs may be used in combination and may irritate the skin.

Systemic antibiotics, such as Achromycin (tetracycline), Minocin, and Cleocin, may help reduce the effects of acne by decreasing bacterial growth until the person is in remission. (See *Alleviating acne*.) A lower dosage is used for long-term maintenance. Achromycin should not be used during pregnancy because it discolors the teeth of the fetus. E-Mycin is an alternative for pregnant women. If the pustules or abscesses worsen during either type of antibiotic therapy, the doctor will take a culture to identify a possible secondary bacterial infection.

The drug Accutane taken orally effectively combats acne. But because of its severe side effects, use of this drug is limited to those with severe acne who don't respond to conventional therapy. Because this drug is known to cause birth defects, special precautions must be taken when using this drug. For example, women must have a pregnancy test before receiving the drug and the pharmacist is allowed to provide no more than a 30-day supply. Pregnancy testing should be repeated throughout the treatment period, and women should use effective contraception during treatment.

Women may benefit from estrogen administration to inhibit androgen activity. Improvement rarely occurs before 2 months, and exacerbations may follow discontinuation of estrogen therapy. Unfortunately, the high estrogen dosage required presents a major risk of severe side effects.

Other treatments for acne include injection of corticosteroids into lesions, exposure to ultraviolet light (but never when a photosensitizing agent, such as Retin-A, is being used), cryotherapy, and surgery.

CORNS AND CALLUSES

What are these conditions?

Corns and calluses are thickened areas of skin that tend to occur in areas of the body that experience repeated pressure and friction — usually the feet. The prognosis is good with proper foot care.

What causes them?

A corn usually is caused by external pressure, such as that from ill-fitting shoes, or less commonly, from internal pressure, such as that from a protruding underlying bone (due to arthritis, for example).

A callus is an area of thickened skin, generally found on the foot or hand, produced by external pressure or friction. People whose activities or jobs involve repeated trauma (for example, manual laborers or guitarists) commonly develop calluses.

The severity of a corn or callus depends on the degree and duration of trauma.

What are the symptoms?

Both corns and calluses cause pain. Corns contain a central core made up of a protein called *keratin,* are smaller and more clearly defined than calluses, and are usually more painful. The pain they cause may be dull and constant or sharp when pressure is applied. "Soft" corns are caused by pressure from a bony prominence. They appear as whitish thickening and are commonly found between the toes. "Hard" corns are sharply delineated and conical and most often appear on the fifth toe.

Calluses have indefinite borders and may be quite large. They usually produce dull pain on pressure, rather than constant pain. Although calluses commonly appear over plantar warts, they're distinguished from these warts by normal skin markings.

How are they diagnosed?

Diagnosis depends on a careful physical exam of the affected area and on a history that reveals chronic trauma.

How are they treated?

The doctor may perform surgical debridement to remove the nucleus of a corn, usually using a local anesthetic. In intermittent debride-

 SELF-HELP

Treating corns and calluses

Good foot care can often correct corns and calluses. Here are some tips on treatments.

Applying plasters

▪ Make sure you understand your doctor's instructions for applying salicylic acid plasters. The plaster should be large enough to cover the affected area. Place the sticky side down on the foot; then cover the plaster with adhesive tape.

▪ Plasters are usually taken off after an overnight application, but they may be left in place for as long as 7 days. After removing the plaster, soak the area in water and rub off the softened skin with a towel or pumice stone. Then reapply the plaster, and repeat the entire procedure until you've removed all the thickened skin.

▪ Don't remove corns or calluses with a sharp instrument, such as a razor blade.

Other hints

▪ Wear shoes that fit well.
▪ Use toe pads or corn pads to relieve pressure.

Aids for relieving painful pressure

Both toe pads and corn pads can help relieve painful pressure. Commercial products available include, from left to right, a foam toe cap, a foam toe sleeve, a soft corn shield, and a hard corn (fifth toe) shield.

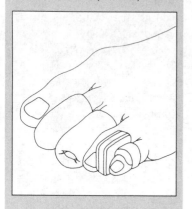

ment, topical drugs called *keratolytics* are applied to affected areas. Keratolytics cause softening and dissolving or peeling of the horny layer of the skin. Injections of corticosteroid drugs beneath the corn may be needed to relieve pain.

The simplest, best treatment is essentially preventive — avoiding trauma. Corns and calluses disappear after the source of trauma has been removed. (See *Treating corns and calluses,* page 547.) Toe pads may redistribute the weight-bearing areas of the foot; corn pads may prevent painful pressure. (See *Aids for relieving painful pressure.*)

People with persistent corns or calluses should see a podiatrist or dermatologist; those with corns or calluses caused by a bony malformation, as in arthritis, should consult an orthopedic specialist.

DERMATITIS

What is this condition?

Dermatitis is an inflammation of the skin that occurs in several forms, including atopic, seborrheic, nummular (coin-shaped), contact, chronic, localized neurodermatitis, exfoliative, and stasis. The discussion below focuses on atopic dermatitis. (For information on contact dermatitis, see *Uncovering the cause of contact dermatitis.*)

Atopic dermatitis (also called *infantile eczema*) is a chronic skin inflammation that affects about 9 out of every 1,000 people. It's often associated with allergy-related diseases, such as bronchial asthma and allergic rhinitis. It usually develops in infants and toddlers ages 1 month to 1 year — typically in those with a strong family history of allergy-related disease.

Atopic dermatitis typically flares up and subsides repeatedly before finally resolving during adolescence. However, it can persist into adulthood. It can lead to viral, fungal, or bacterial infections and can even cause eye disorders.

What causes it?

The cause of atopic dermatitis is unknown, but there's a genetic predisposition, which is worsened by food allergies, infections, irritating chemicals, extremes in temperature and humidity, and emotions. Approximately 10% of childhood cases are caused by allergies to certain foods — especially eggs, peanuts, milk, and wheat. Atopic der-

SELF-HELP

Uncovering the cause of contact dermatitis

Contact dermatitis is caused by a reaction to substances that touch the skin. Once you find out what's causing or aggravating your dermatitis, you've won half the battle. But finding the trigger may take some detective work.

First, think of the things you come in contact with daily — at work, at home, and outside. Don't overlook your toiletries and cosmetics. Sometimes you can suddenly develop an allergy to something you've been using for years. Besides, manufacturers commonly change product formulas.

Mark the substances that you suspect from the following list.

Allergic to something at work?
Depending on your occupation, your skin may react to animal bites, anesthetics, arsenic, benzene, carbon paper, cement, chrome, cleaners, dry-cleaning fluid, dyes, fabric finishes, or formaldehyde. Also consider glue, grease, ink, jewelers' rouge, lacquers, lead, nickel, oil, paints, plastics, rubber, solvents, or turpentine.

Allergic to something at home?
Your skin may react to animal hairs, antibiotics, antiseptics, bleaches, detergents, disinfectants, feathers, insecticides, jewelry, laundry products, polishes, or raw meats. Consider what you wear: fur, silk, or wool.

Allergic to something outside?
Whether you do yard work or just admire nature, you may find you're allergic to flowers, such as chrysan-
themums and geraniums, or to fertilizers, grasses, pesticides, or trees. You may also be allergic to insect bites or stings or to certain plants, especially poison ivy, oak, and sumac. Also consider extreme weather, ivy, fungi, mites, and molds.

Allergic to cosmetics?
Cosmetics and toiletries are among the worst offenders. They contain many substances that can cause rashes. Read labels. Even some "hypoallergenic" preparations contain ingredients that cause allergic reactions. Look for formaldehyde, lanolin, PABA, parabens, quaternium-15, 3-diol (Bronopol), 2-bromo-2-nitropropane-1, ureas, and wool wax.

Contact with the following products may cause dermatitis:
- bath products: astringents, deodorants, antiperspirants, bubble bath, lotions, moisturizers, oils, perfumes, powders, and soaps
- eye products: false eyelashes and glue, eyeliners, mascara, pencils, and shadows
- face products: blushers, creams, foundations, masks, and powders
- hair products: dyes, rinses, shampoos, sprays, and tonics
- lip products: glosses, lipliners, lipsticks, and lotion
- nail products: conditioners, cuticle removers, false fingernails and glue, hardeners, and polishes
- shaving products: after-shave lotions, creams, and depilatories
- other products: douches, suntan lotions, sunscreens, and topical anesthetics.

matitis tends to flare up with increased sweating, psychological stress, and extremes in temperature and humidity. (See *Recognizing plants that cause dermatitis,* pages 550 and 551.)

Irritation is an important secondary cause of atopic dermatitis. It seems to change the skin surface structure, which eventually leads to chronic skin irritation.

SELF-HELP

Recognizing plants that cause dermatitis

Although many plants can cause allergic reactions in sensitive people, three plants cause them in almost everyone. These are poison ivy, poison oak, and poison sumac.

All three of these plants produce urushiol, a strong allergy-causing oil. Poison ivy, in fact, produces this oil year-round, even in the winter when the leaves dry up.

If you're sensitive, you can get dermatitis without even touching these plants. For instance, you can get a rash simply from contact with the airborne particles of these plants in the smoke from burning brush. Or you can break out from touching pets, sports equipment, or gardening tools that have come in contact with urushiol.

By far the most common way to contract dermatitis from these plants is by touching them. Your best defense is to get to know them — and then avoid them.

Poison ivy

Remember the old saying about poison ivy: "Leaves of three, quickly flee." Watch for a small, harmless-looking plant, vine, or low shrub with shiny green leaflets that grow in groups of three. Waxy, yellow-green flowers and, later, greenish berries decorate the leaf stems. In the fall, look for the leaves to turn red.

Poison ivy grows everywhere in the United States, except California and parts of adjacent states. It flourishes in the eastern and central states.

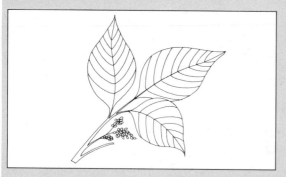

Poison oak

The leaves of poison oak also grow in groups of three. Shaped like oak leaves, they have hairy, light green undersides and darker green surfaces. Poison oak shrubs or vines that bear fruit (not all do) have clustered greenish or creamy white berries. This plant is common in most of the United States.

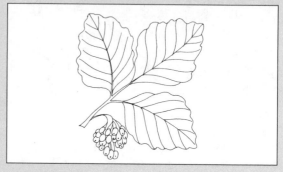

Poison sumac

With 7 to 13 long, smooth, paired leaves, the poison sumac branch is topped with a single velvety leaf. Bright orange in springtime, the leaf surfaces later turn a glossy dark green with a pale green underside, only to change to reddish orange in the fall. Poison sumac has drooping clusters of green berries; nonpoisonous sumac has upright red berries.

If you're in the eastern United States, you can't miss these colorful woody shrubs. They grow from 5 to 25 feet (1.5 to 8 meters) tall and thrive in swampy areas.

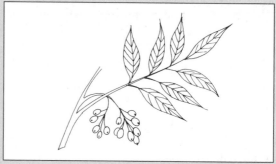

Recognizing plants that cause dermatitis *(continued)*

If you're exposed

Even if you've never had a reaction to poison ivy, oak, or sumac, you're not home free. Some people become allergic to them only after years of repeated exposure. Here's how to protect yourself:

- Immediately after contact, wash the affected skin with soap and cold water. (Hot water may make you itch.) Use yellow or brown laundry soap if you have some; use nonperfumed bath soap if you don't. Lather several times, rinsing the area in running water after each sudsing.
- Use your hands to create the lather. Don't use a brush that could scratch your skin.
- If you're in the woods far from modern plumbing, try to find a brook or stream. Washing your hands and skin in this naturally running water should do the job.

- Wash, rewash, and thoroughly rinse any clothing that touched a plant containing urushiol.
- Wash any pet that touched the plant, too. But first put on rubber gloves so you don't come in contact with your pet's fur. Throw away the gloves when you're finished.

If you get a rash

If preventive measures fail and you notice a mild rash developing, apply cool compresses soaked in water or Burow's solution (available in drugstores). Spread calamine lotion or another preparation with calamine in it, such as Caladryl, over the rash to help dry the area and relieve the itching. If you get a severe rash, don't treat it yourself. Ask your doctor for advice.

What are its symptoms?

The skin lesions of atopic dermatitis start as reddened areas on very dry skin. They typically appear on the forehead, cheeks, knees, elbows, legs, and neck. During flare-ups, itching and scratching cause swelling, crusting, and scaling. Eventually, chronic lesions lead to numerous areas of dry, scaly skin with white, firm, raised, intensely swollen lesions, which become thick and hard.

Intense itching may cause swelling and unusual darkening of the upper eyelids, with a double fold appearing under the lower lids. In rare cases, atopic cataracts (clouding of the eye lens) may develop between ages 20 and 40.

How is it diagnosed?

To diagnose atopic dermatitis, the doctor examines the person's skin and checks for a family history of allergies and chronic inflammation. To rule out other inflammatory skin conditions, such as diaper rash, seborrheic dermatitis, and chronic contact dermatitis, the doctor checks for typical distribution of skin lesions.

How is it treated?

The person with atopic dermatitis must eliminate known allergens and avoid irritants, extreme temperature changes, and other triggers.

SELF-HELP

Coping with dermatitis

The following guidelines can help you minimize the effects of dermatitis:

• Be aware that taking antihistamines to relieve daytime itching may make you drowsy.

• If nighttime itching interferes with sleep, try inducing sleep naturally — for example, by drinking a glass of warm milk.

• Establish a schedule and plan for daily skin care. Bathe in plain, tepid water (96° F [35.6° C]) and use a special nonfatty soap. However, *don't use any soap when lesions are acutely inflamed.* Lubricate your skin after a tub bath.

• Shampoo your hair often and apply a steroid solution to your scalp afterward, if prescribed.

• Keep your fingernails short to prevent scratching, which could injure your skin and cause a secondary infection.

• Try to avoid emotional stress and irritants, such as detergents and wool, which can worsen atopic dermatitis.

To relieve itching and inflammation, the doctor may prescribe a topical steroid ointment such as Cortaid, which can be especially effective when applied after bathing. Between steroid doses, the person should use a moisturizing cream to help the skin retain moisture. Oral steroids should be reserved for extreme flare-ups.

Weak tar preparations and ultraviolet B light therapy may be used to thicken the skin's outer layer. If the doctor determines that a bacterial agent is involved, he or she may prescribe an antibiotic. (See *Coping with dermatitis.*)

FOLLICULITIS, BOILS, AND CARBUNCULOSIS

What are these conditions?

Folliculitis is a bacterial infection of the hair follicle that causes formation of a pustule — a collection of pus beneath the outer skin layer. The infection can be superficial or deep. (See *Forms of bacterial skin infection.*)

Folliculitis may also lead to the development of furuncles (furunculosis), commonly known as boils, or carbuncles (carbunculosis). The prognosis depends on the severity of the infection and on the person's physical condition and ability to resist infection.

What causes them?

The most common cause of folliculitis, boils, or carbunculosis is a bacterium called *Staphylococcus aureus.* Factors that increase a person's risk of developing these conditions include an infected wound, poor hygiene, debilitation, diabetes, cosmetics that clog pores, tight clothes, friction, exposure to chemicals, and treatment of skin lesions with tar or with occlusive therapy, using steroids. Boils often follow folliculitis that's exacerbated by irritation, pressure, friction, or perspiration. Persistent infection and boils may lead to carbunculosis.

What are their symptoms?

Pustules of folliculitis usually appear on the scalp, arms, and legs in children; on the face of bearded men; and on the eyelids. Deep folliculitis may be painful.

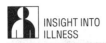

INSIGHT INTO
ILLNESS

Forms of bacterial skin infection

In bacterial skin infections, the degree of hair follicle involvement ranges from superficial redness and a pustule of a single follicle to deep abscesses (carbuncles) involving several follicles.

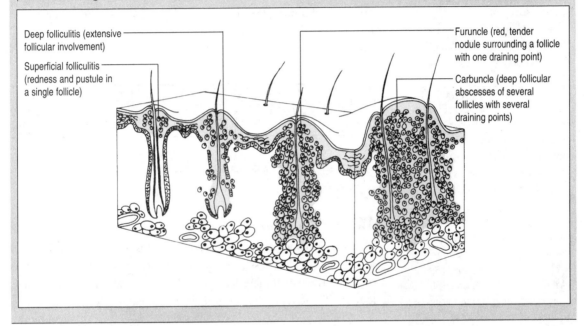

Deep folliculitis (extensive follicular involvement)

Superficial folliculitis (redness and pustule in a single follicle)

Furuncle (red, tender nodule surrounding a follicle with one draining point)

Carbuncle (deep follicular abscesses of several follicles with several draining points)

Folliculitis may progress to hard, painful boils, which commonly develop on the neck, face, underarms, and buttocks. These boils enlarge for several days and then rupture, discharging pus and necrotic material. After they rupture, pain subsides, but redness and swelling may persist for days or weeks.

Carbunculosis is marked by extremely painful, deep abscesses that drain through many openings onto the skin surface, usually around several hair follicles. Fever and malaise may accompany these lesions.

How are they diagnosed?

The presence of characteristic skin lesions confirms folliculitis, boils, or carbunculosis. A wound culture performed in a lab reveals the infecting organism. In carbunculosis, the person's history reveals pre-existent boils. A complete blood count may show an elevated number of white blood cells.

Precautions for people with boils

These guidelines can help reduce the spread of boils:
- *Never* squeeze a boil because that may cause it to rupture into the surrounding area.
- To avoid spreading bacteria to family members, don't share towels and washcloths. These items should be laundered in hot water before being reused.
- Change your clothes and bedsheets daily, and wash them in hot water.
- Change dressings frequently and discard them promptly in paper bags.
- If you have recurrent boils, get a physical because you may have an underlying disease such as diabetes.

How are they treated?

Treatment of folliculitis consists of cleaning the infected area thoroughly with soap and water; applying warm, wet compresses to promote drainage from the lesions; topical antibiotics, such as Bactroban ointment; and in extensive infection, systemic antibiotics (E-Mycin or Dynapen). Boils may also require incision and drainage of ripe lesions after application of warm, wet compresses, and topical antibiotics after drainage. (See *Precautions for people with boils.*) Carbunculosis is treated with systemic antibiotics.

HAIR LOSS

What do doctors call this condition?

Alopecia

What is this condition?

Hair loss usually occurs on the scalp; hair loss elsewhere on the body is less common and less conspicuous. In the nonscarring form of this disorder, the hair follicle can generally regrow hair. But scarring hair loss usually destroys the hair follicle, making hair loss irreversible.

What causes it?

The most common form of nonscarring hair loss is male-pattern hair loss, which appears to be related to androgen levels and aging. Genetic predisposition commonly influences time of onset, degree of baldness, speed with which hair loss spreads, and pattern of hair loss. Women may experience diffuse thinning over the top of the scalp.

Other forms of nonscarring hair loss include:
- *physiologic hair loss* — sudden hair loss in infants, loss of straight hairline in adolescents, and diffuse hair loss after childbirth; usually temporary
- *alopecia areata* — patchy hair loss that is generally reversible and self-limiting (in rare cases alopecia areata can lead to complete hair loss); occurs most frequently in young and middle-aged adults of both sexes
- *trichotillomania* — compulsive pulling out of one's own hair; most common in children.

Other causes of nonscarring hair loss include radiation, many types of drug therapies and reactions to drugs, bacterial and fungal infections, psoriasis, seborrhea, and endocrine disorders, such as thyroid, parathyroid, and pituitary dysfunctions.

Scarring hair loss may be caused by physical or chemical trauma or chronic tension on a hair shaft, as occurs in braiding.

Diseases that produce hair loss include destructive skin tumors, granulomas, lupus, scleroderma, inflammatory skin disease involving the hair follicles, and severe fungal, bacterial, or viral infections, such as tinea infection, folliculitis, or herpes simplex infection.

What are its symptoms?

Male-pattern hair loss occurs gradually and usually affects the thinner, shorter, and less pigmented hairs of the front and side of the scalp. In women, hair loss is generally more diffuse; completely bald areas are uncommon but may occur.

Alopecia areata usually affects small patches of the scalp but may also occur as alopecia totalis, which involves the entire scalp, or as alopecia universalis, which involves the entire body. Although mild redness may occur initially, affected areas of the scalp or skin appear normal. "Exclamation point" hairs (loose hairs with dark, rough, brushlike tips on narrow, less pigmented shafts) occur at the periphery of new patches. Regrowth initially appears as fine, white, downy hair, which is replaced by normal hair.

In trichotillomania, patchy areas of hair loss and many broken hairs appear on the scalp and possibly on other areas, such as the eyebrows.

How is it diagnosed?

A physical exam is usually sufficient to confirm hair loss. In trichotillomania, an occlusive dressing can establish the diagnosis by allowing new hair to grow, revealing that the hair is being pulled out. Diagnosis must also include tests to identify any underlying disorder.

How is it treated?

Topical application of minoxidil, a drug more commonly used to treat high blood pressure, has had limited success in treating male-pattern hair loss. (The topical form of this drug is known as *Rogaine*.) An alternative treatment is surgical redistribution of hair follicles by autografting.

Be good to your hair

Regular care and grooming can keep your remaining hair and any new growth healthy. Here are some tips:

- Don't use harsh hair chemicals, such as permanent wave solutions, hair bleaches, or dyes. These can damage hair, causing splitting and shedding.
- Avoid burning hair with devices such as curling irons and hair dryers at high settings.
- Try smooth rather than toothed rollers and avoid hot curlers.
- Change hairstyles if hair loss results from traction caused by tight braids or ponytails.

In alopecia areata, Rogaine is more effective, although treatment is often unnecessary because spontaneous regrowth is common. The doctor may administer corticosteroid injections into the affected areas; this is beneficial for small patches and may produce regrowth in 4 to 6 weeks. Hair loss that persists for over a year is unlikely to grow back.

In trichotillomania, use of an occlusive dressing may protect the person's hair and allow normal growth. Long-term treatment may include behavior modification therapy. Treatment of other types of hair loss varies according to the underlying cause.

What can a person with hair loss do?

- If you're a woman with female-pattern hair loss, know that it doesn't lead to total baldness. Consider restyling your hair to mask thinning areas or consider wearing a wig. (See *Be good to your hair*.)
- If you have alopecia areata, be aware that complete regrowth is possible.

HIRSUTISM

What is this condition?

Hirsutism is the excessive growth of body hair in women and children. Usually, hair grows in an adult male distribution pattern. This condition commonly occurs spontaneously but may be associated with various underlying diseases. The prognosis varies with the cause of the disorder and the effectiveness of treatment.

What causes it?

Primary hirsutism probably stems from a hereditary trait. In most cases, the person has a family history of the disorder.

Causes of secondary hirsutism include endocrine abnormalities, such as dysfunction of the pituitary gland (acromegaly, precocious puberty) or dysfunction of the adrenal gland (Cushing's disease, Cushing's syndrome, or congenital adrenal hyperplasia). It may also be related to ovarian lesions (such as polycystic ovary disease) and to use of certain drugs, such as Loniten, androgen steroids, or testosterone.

What are its symptoms?

Hirsutism typically causes enlarged hair follicles as well as enlargement and excessive pigmentation of the hairs themselves. People usually seek medical help because of excessive facial hair growth.

The pattern of hirsutism varies widely, depending on the person's race and age. An elderly woman, for example, commonly shows increased hair growth on the chin and upper lip. In secondary hirsutism, other signs of masculinization may appear — deepening of the voice, increased muscle mass, increased size of genitalia, menstrual irregularities, and decreased breast size.

How is it diagnosed?

To diagnose primary hirsutism, the doctor may look for a family history of hirsutism, menstrual abnormalities, and signs of masculinization. Results of a pelvic exam are normal.

Tests for secondary hirsutism depend on symptoms that suggest an underlying disorder.

How is it treated?

At the person's request, treatment of primary hirsutism consists of eliminating excess hair by scissors, shaving, depilatory creams, or removal of the entire hair shaft with tweezers or wax. Bleaching with hydrogen peroxide also may be satisfactory. Electrolysis, a slow and expensive process, can destroy hair bulbs permanently, but it works best when only a few hairs need to be removed.

Hirsutism from elevated androgen levels may require low-dose Decadron, oral contraceptives, or antiandrogens. These drugs vary in effectiveness.

Treatment of secondary hirsutism varies depending on the nature of the underlying disorder.

Electrolysis, a slow and expensive process, can destroy hair bulbs permanently, but it works best when only a few hairs need to be removed. In some cases, bleaching hair may be satisfactory.

IMPETIGO

What is this condition?

Impetigo is a contagious, superficial skin infection marked by patches of tiny blisters that erupt, exposing the skin beneath. It can occur almost anywhere but usually appears in the area around the nose and mouth.

ADVICE FOR CAREGIVERS

Caring for a child with impetigo

To help your child recover from this condition, follow these guidelines:

- Don't allow your child to scratch because this spreads impetigo. Cut his or her fingernails.
- Make sure your child continues taking prescribed medications for 7 to 10 days, even after lesions have healed.
- To prevent further spread of this highly contagious infection, make sure your child bathes frequently using a bactericidal soap. Don't let other family members share the child's towels, washcloths, or bed linens. Have the child wash his or her hands often and thoroughly.

This disorder, which usually occurs in the late summer or early fall, spreads most easily among infants, young children, and the elderly. Certain risk factors — such as poor hygiene, anemia, malnutrition, and a warm climate — may increase the likelihood of an outbreak of this infection. Impetigo can complicate chickenpox, eczema, or other skin conditions marked by open lesions.

What causes it?

Impetigo is caused by bacterial infection. Types of bacteria that produce this disorder include *Staphylococcus aureus* and, less commonly, group A beta-hemolytic streptococci.

What are its symptoms?

Common *nonbullous impetigo* typically begins with a small red macule that turns into a pus-filled vesicle. When the vesicle breaks, a thick yellow crust forms from the discharge. Smaller lesions may appear around the original lesion. Other features include itching, burning, and swollen lymph nodes in the affected region.

A rare but serious complication of streptococcal impetigo is a kidney infection called *glomerulonephritis.* Infants and young children may develop impetigo in the ear or an external ear infection; the lesions usually clear without treatment in 2 to 3 weeks, unless an underlying disorder such as eczema is present.

In *bullous impetigo,* a thin-walled vesicle opens, and a thin, clear crust forms from the discharge. The lesion consists of a central clearing surrounded by an outer rim. It commonly appears on the face or other exposed areas.

Both forms usually produce painless itching; they may appear simultaneously and be clinically indistinguishable.

How is it diagnosed?

When diagnosing impetigo, the doctor looks for characteristic lesions. In the lab, microscopic examination of the causative organism usually confirms bacterial infection and justifies antibiotic therapy. Culture and sensitivity testing of fluid or denuded skin may indicate the most appropriate antibiotic. Lab studies may also reveal that the person's white blood cell count is elevated.

How is it treated?

Generally, the doctor will prescribe systemic antibiotics (usually penicillin, a cephalosporin, or E-Mycin) for 10 days. A topical antibiotic such as Bactroban ointment may be used for minor infections. Therapy also includes removal of the discharge by washing the lesions two or three times a day with soap and water or, for stubborn crusts, warm soaks or compresses of a salt water or diluted soap solution. (See *Caring for a child with impetigo.*)

LICE

What do doctors call this condition?
Pediculosis

What is this condition?
Lice are small, wingless, bloodsucking insects that infest various parts of the human body. Head lice infest the scalp or, rarely, the eyebrows, eyelashes, and beard. Body lice infest the skin, and crab lice infest the pubic hair region.

Lice feed on human blood and lay their eggs (nits) in body hairs or clothing fibers. After the nits hatch, they must feed within 24 hours or die; they mature in 2 to 3 weeks. When a louse bites, it injects a toxin into the skin that causes mild irritation and an itchy spot. Repeated bites sensitize the person to the toxin, leading to more serious inflammation. Treatment can effectively eliminate lice.

What causes it?
Head lice infestations are caused by overcrowded conditions and poor personal hygiene. Common in children, especially girls, they spread by shared clothing, hats, combs, and hairbrushes.

Body lice live in the seams of clothing, next to the skin, leaving only to feed on blood. Common causes of these infestations include wearing the same clothing for days at a time (as might occur in cold climates), overcrowding, and poor personal hygiene. Body lice spread through shared clothing and bedsheets.

Crab lice are found mainly in pubic hairs but may extend to the eyebrows, eyelashes, and underarm or body hair. They spread through sexual intercourse or by contact with clothes, bedsheets, or towels.

Body lice live in the seams of clothing, next to the skin, leaving only to feed on blood. Crab lice are found mainly in pubic hairs but may extend to the eyebrows, eyelashes, and underarm or body hair.

What are its symptoms?

Symptoms of head lice include severe itching with scratching; matted, foul-smelling, lusterless hair (in severe cases); swollen glands in the neck and at the back of the head; and a rash on the trunk.

Body lice at first cause small, red, solid, raised skin lesions, usually on the shoulders, trunk, or buttocks. Later, raised, firm lesions with intense swelling may appear. Untreated body lice may lead to vertical scratches and ultimately to dry, discolored, thickly encrusted, scaly skin, with bacterial infection and scarring. In severe cases, headache, fever, and an overall ill feeling may accompany skin symptoms.

Crab lice cause skin irritation from scratches, which are usually more obvious than the bites. Small gray-blue spots may appear on the thighs or upper body.

How is it diagnosed?

The doctor examines the person for visible lice. With head lice, the doctor finds oval grayish nits that can't be shaken loose like dandruff. Body lice are diagnosed from characteristic skin lesions and nits found on clothing. With crab lice, nits are attached to pubic hairs, which feel coarse and grainy to the touch.

How is it treated?

To treat head lice, the doctor prescribes Elimite cream rinse, which the person rubs into the hair and rinses out after 10 minutes. A single treatment is usually sufficient. Alternatives include Rid and Kwell shampoo.

To remove nits from hair, the person should use a fine-tooth comb dipped in vinegar; washing hair with ordinary shampoo removes crustations.

To remove body lice, the person must bathe with soap and water. A person with severe infestation may need to use Kwell cream. Lice may be removed from clothes by washing them in hot water, ironing, or dry-cleaning. Storing clothes for more than 30 days or placing them in dry heat of 140° F (60° C) also kills lice. If clothes can't be washed or changed, applying 10% DDT or 10% lindane powder is effective.

To treat crab lice, the person must use Kwell shampoo in affected areas. The person leaves it on for 4 minutes, and then repeats the treatment in 1 week. To prevent reinfestation, clothes and bedsheets must be laundered.

What can a person with lice do?

Be sure to follow your doctor's instructions on using prescribed creams, ointments, powders, or shampoos.

MASK OF PREGNANCY

What do doctors call this condition?

Melasma, chloasma

What is this condition?

In this disorder, patches of skin become discolored because of excessive deposits of melanin, the pigment in skin and hair. Mask of pregnancy, a folk name for a condition not always related to pregnancy (it sometimes occurs in men), poses a serious cosmetic problem. Although it tends to occur equally in all races, the light-brown color it produces is most evident in dark-skinned whites. Mask of pregnancy may be chronic but is never life-threatening.

What causes it?

The cause of mask of pregnancy is unknown, but it may be related to the increased hormonal levels associated with pregnancy, ovarian cancer, or use of oral contraceptives. Use of other drugs, such as Dilantin and Mesantoin, may also contribute to this disorder. Exposure to sunlight stimulates mask of pregnancy, but the disorder may develop without any apparent predisposing factor.

What are its symptoms?

Typically, this disorder produces large, brown, irregular patches, symmetrically distributed on the forehead, cheeks, and sides of the nose. Less commonly, these patches may occur on the neck, upper lip, and temples.

How is it diagnosed?

Observation of characteristic dark patches on the face usually confirms mask of pregnancy. The doctor will review the person's history to uncover the presence of risk factors.

Minimizing the mask of pregnancy

To minimize the effects of this condition, take the following steps.

Treatment options
- Avoid sun exposure by using sunscreens and wearing protective clothing.
- Ask your doctor or dermatologist about using bleaching agents. Keep in mind that you may need repeated treatments to maintain the desired effect.
- Use cosmetics to mask deep pigmentation.

Remission possible
Though distressing, the mask of pregnancy may fade after childbirth or after you stop taking oral contraceptives. It may even fade spontaneously if you protect your skin from sunlight.

How is it treated?

Treatment consists primarily of applying bleaching agents containing 2% to 4% hydroquinone to inhibit melanin synthesis. This medication is applied twice daily for up to 8 weeks. Additional measures include avoiding exposure to sunlight, using sunscreens, and discontinuing oral contraceptives. (See *Minimizing the mask of pregnancy*.)

PHOTOSENSITIVITY REACTIONS

What are these conditions?

Photosensitivity reactions are skin eruptions that occur in response to light alone or to light and chemicals. A *phototoxic reaction* is a dose-related toxic response, which means that the severity of the reaction is directly related to the amount of exposure to light. A *photoallergic reaction* is an uncommon, acquired immune response that isn't dose-related — even slight exposure can cause a severe reaction.

What causes them?

Exposure to certain chemicals may lead to a photosensitivity reaction. Such chemicals include dyes, coal tar, furocoumarin compounds found in plants, and drugs such as phenothiazines, sulfonamides, sulfonylureas, tetracycline, griseofulvin, and thiazides.

Berlock dermatitis, a specific photosensitivity reaction, is caused by use of oil of bergamot — common in perfumes and colognes.

What are their symptoms?

Immediately after exposure, a phototoxic reaction causes a burning sensation followed by redness, swelling, peeling skin, and skin discoloration.

Berlock dermatitis causes reddened vesicles that later become deeply pigmented.

Photoallergic reactions may take one of two forms. A polymorphous light eruption develops 2 hours to 5 days after light exposure and produces redness, papules, vesicles, hives, and eczematous lesions on exposed areas; itching may persist for 1 to 2 weeks. Solar urticaria begins minutes after exposure and lasts about an hour; redness and wheals follow itching and burning sensations.

SELF-HELP

How to treat a sunburn

A bad case of sunburn doesn't have to get worse.

Use ointments
Apply a first-aid ointment containing a local anesthetic, or use a sunburn spray or cream. *Caution:* Read labels carefully. Avoid using any preparation that contains agents your skin is sensitive to.

Apply compresses
Apply cool compresses of Burow's Solution, Domeboro Powder (both are in drugstores), witch hazel, or baking soda. Dissolve the powder in tepid water according to directions. Use the compresses for 15 minutes several times a day.

Bathe or shower
Take cool baths or showers to reduce pain and possibly reduce blistering. Consider adding baking soda to the bath water. This may relieve stinging or itching from sunburn. After bathing, keep your skin well moisturized.

Take pain medication
Take aspirin to relieve swelling, redness, and pain. If you can't take aspirin, try an aspirin substitute — for example, Tylenol (or another drug containing acetaminophen) — to relieve some discomfort. However, Tylenol won't reduce swelling and redness.

Prevent other problems
Drink plenty of fluids to replace those lost through perspiration. This helps prevent dehydration.

Stay out of the sun until your skin heals completely. Sunburned skin is more susceptible to a second serious burn.

If you're not feeling better in 2 or 3 days, see your doctor, who may prescribe a medicine to help.

How are they diagnosed?

The doctor will suspect a photosensitivity reaction if a person experiences skin eruptions after recent exposure to light or certain chemicals. A photopatch test for ultraviolet A and B light may aid diagnosis and identify which light wavelength is causing the reaction.

How are they treated?

For many people, treatment involves a sunscreen, protective clothing, and minimal exposure to sunlight. For others, progressive exposure to sunlight can thicken the skin and produce a tan that interferes with photoallergens and prevents further eruptions. (See *How to treat a sunburn.*)

Antimalarial drugs, beta-carotene, and PUVA (psoralens and ultraviolet A light) therapy may be used to treat a polymorphous light eruption. PUVA therapy may also be used to treat solar urticaria. Although hyperpigmentation usually fades in several months, drugs known as hydroquinone preparations may be used to hasten the pro-

Examining your skin: It could save your life

Because persistent photosensitivity reactions can lead to skin cancer, it's a good idea to examine your skin every month. See your doctor if you notice suspicious-looking changes in the size, texture, or color of a mole or if you have a sore that doesn't heal. If detected early, most skin cancers are curable.

Check your skin right after a bath or shower. Stand before a full-length mirror in a well-lighted room. Keep a small mirror handy for seeing behind you and for examining hard-to-see spots. Note any freckles, moles, blemishes, and birthmarks, and remember where they are and what they look like. Then proceed according to the steps below.

1 Standing unclothed in front of the mirror, check the front of your body. Turn to each side and look over your shoulder to see behind you. Use your hand mirror, too. Then lift your arms and examine the sides of your body.

2 Inspect your arms and hands. Check the backs of your hands, your palms, your fingers, and both sides of your forearms and upper arms.

3 Examine your legs, checking the fronts, backs, and sides. Look between your buttocks and around the genital area.

4 Next, move close to the mirror to look carefully at your neck, face, lips, eyes, ears, nose, and scalp. Part your hair with a comb to see better.

5 Now, sit down. Bend your knees to bring your feet close to you. Examine your soles, insteps, ankles, and between your toes.

cess. To prevent reactions, the person should avoid prolonged exposure to light. (See *Examining your skin: It could save your life*.)

PRESSURE SORES

What do doctors call this condition?
Decubitus ulcers

What is this condition?
Pressure sores are localized areas of damaged tissue that occur most often in the skin and tissue over bony prominences. These sores may be superficial, caused by local skin irritation, or deep, originating in underlying tissue. Deep lesions often go undetected until they penetrate the skin. By then they've usually caused tissue damage.

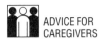

ADVICE FOR
CAREGIVERS

Danger sites for pressure sores

Pressure sores are most likely to develop at pressure points, the parts of the body that must bear the most weight or are exposed to the most friction. To help prevent pressure sores, a person who is confined to a bed or wheelchair should be repositioned frequently. His or her skin should be checked carefully for any changes.

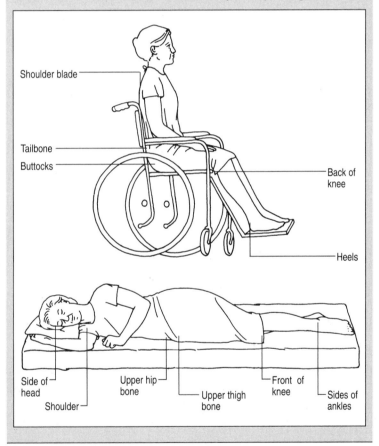

What causes them?

Pressure, particularly over bony prominences, interrupts normal circulatory function and causes most pressure sores. The severity of the sore depends on the intensity and duration of the pressure. Damage to skin and small blood vessels may eventually lead to destruction of

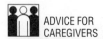

Tools for preventing pressure sores

If you're caring for someone who is at risk for developing pressure sores, such as a person confined to a bed or a wheelchair, ask the doctor or nurse about the use of the devices described below.

Gel flotation pads

These pads disperse pressure over a greater skin surface area. Gel flotation pads are convenient and adaptable for home and wheelchair use.

Water mattress

A water mattress distributes body weight equally but is heavy and awkward. "Mini" water beds may be crafted from partially filled rubber gloves or plastic bags. These may help in small areas, such as heels.

Alternating pressure mattress

This type of mattress contains tubelike sections, running lengthwise, that deflate and reinflate, changing areas of pressure. This mattress should be used with a single untucked sheet because layers of linen decrease the effectiveness of the mattress.

Egg Crate mattress

An Egg Crate mattress uses alternating areas of depression and elevation to minimize the area of skin pressure. Soft, elevated foam areas cushion the skin; depressed areas relieve pressure. This mattress should be used with a single loosely tucked sheet and can be adapted for home and wheelchair use. If the person is incontinent, the mattress should be covered with the provided plastic sleeve.

Spanco mattress

This type of mattress has polyester fibers with silicone tubes to decrease pressure without limiting the person's position. It has no weight limitation.

Sheepskin

Soft, dry, absorbent, and easy to clean, sheepskin can be kept in direct contact with the person's skin. It's available in sizes to fit elbows and heels and can be adapted for home use.

tissue cells. In turn, dead tissue may be invaded by bacteria and become infected.

Anyone who is confined to a bed or wheelchair for a long time risks developing pressure sores. The risk is greater if movement is restricted or sensation is impaired. Pressure sores occur on those parts of the body that bear the weight of the body or rub constantly against the bedclothes. The most common sites are the elbows, knees, shoulder blades, spine, and buttocks.

Other factors that increase the risk of pressure sores include inadequate nutrition (leading to weight loss and subsequent reduction of tissue and muscle bulk), swelling, incontinence, fever, disease, and obesity. (See *Danger sites for pressure sores,* page 565.)

What are the symptoms?

Early features of superficial pressure sores are shiny, red changes over the compressed area. Superficial redness progresses to small blisters or erosions and, ultimately, to necrosis (death of tissue cells) and ulceration.

An inflamed area on the skin's surface may be the first sign of underlying damage when pressure is exerted between deep tissue and bone. Bacteria in a compressed site cause inflammation and, eventually, infection, which leads to further necrosis. A foul-smelling, pus-laden discharge may seep from a lesion that penetrates the skin from beneath.

How are they diagnosed?

Pressure sores are obvious during a physical exam. In the lab, wound culture and sensitivity testing of any discharge can identify the infecting organisms.

How are they treated?

Successful treatment must relieve pressure on the affected area, keep the area clean and dry, and promote healing. (See *Tools for preventing pressure sores* and *Preventing and treating pressure sores*.) Antibiotics may be use to eliminate any bacterial infection.

PSORIASIS

What is this condition?

Psoriasis is a chronic, recurrent skin disease in which the skin's outermost layer is abnormally overgrown. Red patches form and are covered by thick, dry, silvery scales. These lesions vary widely in severity and distribution.

Psoriatic skin cells have an abnormally short life cycle — 4 days as opposed to 28 days for normal skin cells. Four days isn't enough time for skin cells to mature. As a result, the outermost skin layer becomes thick and flaky.

Typically, the disease goes through partial remissions and flare-ups. Flare-ups are often related to specific factors but may be unpredictable. They can usually be controlled with therapy.

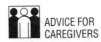

ADVICE FOR CAREGIVERS

Preventing and treating pressure sores

If you're caring for someone who's bedridden, the following advice may help you prevent and treat pressure sores.

Positioning

To help prevent pressure sores, reposition the person at least every 2 hours around the clock. Use a footboard, and don't raise the head of the bed to an angle that exceeds 60 degrees. Keep the person's knees slightly flexed for short periods. Use pressure-relief aids, such as special mattresses and bed pads.

Skin care

Provide meticulous skin care. Keep the person's skin clean and dry without using harsh soaps. To promote healing, gently massage the skin *around* the affected area — not *on* it. Thoroughly rub moisturizing lotion into the skin. Change bed linens often if the person sweats profusely or is incontinent.

Nutrition

Encourage adequate intake of food and fluids to help the person maintain weight and promote healing. If the person is debilitated, provide frequent, small meals that include protein- and calorie-rich supplements. Help a weak person with meals.

Psoriasis affects about 2% of the population in the United States. The incidence is higher among whites than other races. Although this disorder is most common in young adults, it may strike at any age, including infancy.

What causes it?

The tendency to develop psoriasis is genetic. Recent research suggests that the disease may be linked to an immune disorder. Environmental factors influence its onset.

Factors that contribute to psoriasis include:

- infections, which may cause a flare of teardrop-shaped lesions
- pregnancy
- hormonal changes
- climate (cold weather tends to worsen psoriasis)
- emotional stress.

What are its symptoms?

The most common symptom of psoriasis is itching; occasionally, pain from dry, cracked, encrusted lesions may occur. These lesions are red and usually form well-defined patches (also called *plaques*), which sometimes cover large areas of the body. They're most common on the scalp, chest, elbows, knees, back, and buttocks.

The patches consist of silver scales that either flake off easily or can thicken, covering the lesion. If the scales are removed, fine points of bleeding may occur. Occasionally, small teardrop-shaped lesions appear, either alone or with plaques. Typically, these lesions are thin and red, with few scales. Widespread shedding of scales is common in exfoliative (inflammatory) psoriasis and may also develop in chronic psoriasis.

Pustular psoriasis is a rare, severe form of the disorder marked by bright red patches and small, raised areas that contain pus.

In about 30% of cases, psoriasis spreads to the fingernails, producing small indentations and yellow or brown discoloration. In severe cases, buildup of thick, crumbly debris under the nails causes them to separate from the nailbed.

Some people with psoriasis develop arthritic symptoms, usually in one or more joints of the fingers or toes, or sometimes in the joints of the lower back. Some people suffer morning stiffness. People with joint symptoms experience remissions and flare-ups similar to those of rheumatoid arthritis.

How is it diagnosed?

Diagnosis is based on the person's medical history, an examination of the lesions and, if needed, skin biopsy results.

How is it treated?

Treatment depends on the type of psoriasis, the extent of the disorder, the person's response to it, and the effect of the disorder on the person's lifestyle. No permanent cure exists; treatment can only reduce symptoms.

Scale removal

To remove psoriatic scales, the doctor may instruct the person to apply ointments, such as Vaseline, salicylic acid preparations, or preparations containing urea. These medications soften the scales; the person then removes them by scrubbing them carefully with a soft brush while bathing.

Ultraviolet light treatment

To retard rapid skin cell production, the doctor may recommend exposure to light (either ultraviolet B or natural sunlight) to the point of minimal skin redness. Ultraviolet B light exposure is the most common treatment for generalized psoriasis. (See *What to expect during UV light treatments.*)

The person may apply tar preparations or crude coal tar to affected areas about 15 minutes before exposure, or may leave these preparations on overnight and wipe them off the next morning. Exposure time can increase gradually. Outpatient or day treatment with ultraviolet B light avoids long hospitalizations and prolongs remission.

Steroid therapy

Steroid creams and ointments are useful to control psoriasis. A potent fluorinated steroid works well (except on the face and areas where two skin surfaces come into contact). These creams must be applied twice daily, preferably after bathing to promote absorption; overnight, the person covers the areas with occlusive dressings, such as plastic wrap, plastic gloves or booties, or a vinyl exercise suit (under direct medical or nursing supervision). Small, stubborn plaques may require steroid injections into the lesions.

Anthralin

Anthralin, combined with a paste mixture, may be used to treat well-defined plaques, but it must not be applied to unaffected areas

SELF-HELP

What to expect during UV light treatments

The doctor may prescribe ultraviolet (UV) light therapy to relieve and control psoriasis.

Length of treatment
You'll have brief daily treatments for 1 to 3 weeks.

Method of treatment
You'll stand inside a body-sized UV light chamber or use a small light chamber for your hands, feet, or other body parts. For the body-sized chamber, you'll remove any clothing that covers the plaques and expose them to the banks of fluorescent lights surrounding you. You'll wear special goggles to protect your eyes.

Exposure is timed to ensure safety; the first session usually lasts 15 to 30 seconds.

Effects of treatment
Because a mild sunburn produces the best response, exposure time will gradually increase until the light turns your skin pink. If you have dark skin, minimal color changes will be hard to observe. Try to recall whether you felt a mild sunburn after your last treatment.

SELF-HELP

Daily skin care for psoriasis

To prevent infection and promote healing, you'll need to observe a daily skin care routine. Follow the doctor's instructions, and review the tips below.

Soaking in the tub

A daily tub soak will help to remove scales and relieve itching. Add an oatmeal preparation (such as Aveeno) or a tar gel (such as AquaTar, Estar Gel, or psoriGel) to bath water to soothe your skin.

Once you've added a small amount of the bath product to the water, relax and soak for about 20 minutes. Soaking adds moisture to your skin and promotes absorption of tar gels.

While you soak, use a soft brush to gently loosen scales.

After bathing, pat tender skin dry with a soft towel. Remember to pat *gently* to avoid injury and prevent irritation.

Shampooing

If psoriasis affects your scalp, the doctor may recommend a daily shampoo with a tar-based medicine. If so, work the shampoo into your scalp and leave it on for at least 10 minutes before rinsing your hair. After shampooing, remove the scales with a fine-toothed comb.

Tip: If you have severe scaling, apply mineral oil or a prescribed medicine overnight to help loosen the scales so that you can remove them during your morning shampoo.

Applying medicine

Once you're dried off, apply your prescribed medicine. If you notice any unusual redness or burning, stop using it and notify the doctor.

Memorize the directions on your medicine label — especially if you need to apply the medicine two or three times a day.

If you're applying a topical corticosteroid, you can increase its absorption by using an occlusive dressing. Depending on the site and size of the treated area, you may cover up with plastic gloves, plastic wrap, or a vinyl exercise suit.

Apply your medicine at bedtime. Then cover the area with the plastic dressing and secure the dressing with tape. You'll remove the dressing the next morning.

If you're using a tar-based product, never use a plastic dressing. This could cause a severe burn.

If the doctor recommends a combination of tar and a topical corticosteroid (for increased effectiveness), apply one on top of the other. Again, avoid using a plastic dressing.

because it causes injury and stains normal skin. Vaseline should be applied around the affected skin before anthralin is applied.

Anthralin is often used in conjunction with steroid therapy. It's applied at night while steroids are used during the day.

Calcipotriene

Calcipotriene ointment, a vitamin D_3 analogue, is a new topical agent used to treat psoriasis.

Therapy for severe psoriasis

For someone with severe chronic psoriasis, the doctor may prescribe the Goeckerman regimen, which combines tar baths and ultraviolet

SELF-HELP

Coping with psoriasis

For most people, psoriasis is a long-term condition with no permanent cure. The following guidelines will help you live with this condition and its treatment. For more information and support, contact the National Psoriasis Foundation, which has local chapters.

Follow the treatment plan
- Make sure you understand prescribed treatments, including how to apply prescribed ointments, creams, and lotions. For example, you should apply a steroid cream in a thin film and rub it gently into your skin until it disappears. Apply all topical medications, especially those containing anthralin and tar, with a downward motion to avoid rubbing them into the follicles.
- Always wear gloves to apply topical medications because anthralin stains and injures the skin. After application, you may dust yourself with powder to keep anthralin from rubbing off on your clothes.
- When seeking to remove anthralin, try using mineral oil, then soap and water. Avoid scrubbing your skin vigorously. If you've applied a medication to the scales to soften them, use a soft brush to remove them. Never put an occlusive dressing over anthralin.

- Watch for drug side effects, especially allergic reactions to anthralin, skin shrinkage and acne from steroids, and burning, itching, nausea, and squamous cell growths from PUVA therapy.
- If you're receiving PUVA therapy, stay out of the sun on the day of treatment and protect your eyes with sunglasses that screen ultraviolet A light for 24 hours after treatment. Wear goggles during exposure to this light.
- If you're taking Rheumatrex, report for medical evaluation weekly, then monthly.

Learn about your condition
- Be aware that psoriasis isn't contagious and that exacerbations are controllable with treatment. However, understand that there's no cure.
- Because stressful situations tend to worsen psoriasis, learn techniques for coping with stress.
- Know that except for arthritis-like symptoms, psoriasis doesn't causes systemic disturbances.

B light treatments. This therapy may induce remission and clear the skin in 3 to 5 weeks. The Ingram technique, a variation of the Goeckerman regimen, uses anthralin instead of tar.

In a therapy called PUVA, the person first receives psoralens (an agent that promotes the action of ultraviolet light) and then is exposed to high-intensity ultraviolet A light.

As a last resort, a drug that inhibits cell proliferation — usually Rheumatrex — may help to relieve severe psoriasis that's unresponsive to conventional treatment.

Other measures
Low-dose antihistamines, oatmeal baths, emollients, and open wet dressings may help to relieve itching. The drug Tegison may be effective in treating extensive psoriasis.

Aspirin and local heat reduce the pain of psoriatic arthritis; severe cases may require nonsteroidal anti-inflammatory drugs.

For psoriasis of the scalp, the doctor may recommend a tar shampoo, followed by a steroid lotion.

No effective treatment exists for psoriasis of the nails. (See *Daily skin care for psoriasis,* page 570, and *Coping with psoriasis,* page 571.)

SCABIES

What is this condition?

In scabies, the skin is infested by parasitic itch mites (also known as *Sarcoptes scabiei* var. *hominis*). Scabies occurs worldwide but is most common in areas that are overcrowded or where hygiene is poor.

What causes it?

Scabies develops when the microscopic itch mites enter a human host and provoke a sensitivity reaction. Mites can live their entire lives in human skin, causing chronic infection. The female mite burrows into the skin to lay her eggs, from which larvae emerge to copulate and then reburrow under the skin.

Scabies is transmitted through skin or sexual contact. The adult mite can survive without a human host for only 2 or 3 days.

What are its symptoms?

Typically, scabies causes itching that intensifies at night. Sometimes the burrows of the scabies mite can be seen as tiny white lines in the skin, and red lumps may also appear in this area. Common sites of infestation include the hands, wrists, waistline, nipples in women, and genitalia in men. In infants, the burrows (lesions) may appear on the head and neck.

Intense scratching can lead to severe excoriation and secondary bacterial infection. Itching may become generalized secondary to sensitization.

How is it diagnosed?

Your doctor may be able to detect the itch mite by closely examining the contents of the scabies burrow. If not, a drop of mineral oil placed over the burrow, followed by superficial scraping and examination of the scraped material under a microscope, may reveal mite eggs or feces.

If diagnostic tests offer no positive identification of the mite and if scabies is still suspected (for example, if family members and close contacts of the person also report itching), the person may be given a therapeutic trial of a pediculicide (a lice-killing drug). If his or her skin clears, the diagnosis is confirmed.

How is it treated?

Generally, scabies is treated by applying a pediculicide — Nix or Kwell cream — in a thin layer over the entire skin surface and leaving it on for 8 to 12 hours. To make sure all areas have been treated, this application should be repeated in approximately 1 week. Another pediculicide, Eurax cream, may be applied on 4 consecutive nights. (See *Tips for treating scabies*.)

Infants and pregnant women may receive an alternative therapy, which consists of a 6% to 10% solution of sulfur applied for 3 consecutive days. A person with widespread bacterial infections may require systemic antibiotics.

Persistent itching may develop from repeated use of pediculicides. An antipruritic emollient or topical steroid can reduce itching; steroids injected into the lesions may resolve reddened nodules.

STAPHYLOCOCCAL SCALDED SKIN SYNDROME

What is this condition?

Staphylococcal scalded skin syndrome (SSSS) is a severe skin disorder in which the skin develops a scalded appearance marked by redness, peeling, and necrosis (tissue cell death). This condition is most common in infants ages 1 to 3 months but may develop in children. It's uncommon in adults.

SSSS progresses in a consistent pattern, but most people recover fully. Mortality is 2% to 3%, with death usually resulting from complications of fluid and electrolyte loss, severe infection, and involvement of other body systems.

SELF-HELP

Tips for treating scabies

Along with your doctor's instructions, the following suggestions can help you eliminate scabies and avoid complications of treatment:

- Apply Nix or Kwell cream from the neck down, covering your entire body. Wait 15 minutes before dressing, and avoid bathing for 8 to 12 hours. Wash contaminated clothing and linens in hot water or dry-clean them.
- Don't apply Kwell cream if your skin is raw or inflamed. If skin irritation or an allergic reaction develops, notify your doctor immediately, stop using the cream, and wash it off your skin thoroughly.
- Encourage family members and other close personal contacts to get checked for scabies.

To diagnose SSSS, the doctor must carefully observe the disorder's three-stage progression. Then microscopic examination or cultures of skin lesions confirm the diagnosis.

What causes it?

The organism that causes SSSS is called Group II *Staphylococcus aureus*. Factors that may increase a person's risk of developing the disorder include impaired immunity and kidney function. Both risk factors are present to some extent in normal newborns because their immune system and kidneys are not fully developed.

What are its symptoms?

An upper respiratory infection, possibly accompanied by itchy conjunctivitis, may precede development of SSSS. Skin changes pass through three stages:

- *Erythema:* Redness becomes visible, usually around the mouth and other orifices, and may spread in widening circles over the entire body surface. The skin becomes tender; Nikolsky's sign (sloughing of the skin when friction is applied) may appear.
- *Exfoliation* (24 to 48 hours later): In the more common, localized form of this disease, superficial erosions and minimal crusting occur, generally around orifices, and may spread to exposed skin areas. In the more severe forms, large, flaccid, fluid-filled blisters erupt and may spread over extensive areas of the body. These blisters eventually rupture, revealing sections of denuded skin.
- *Desquamation:* In this final stage, affected areas dry up and powdery scales form. Normal skin replaces these scales in 5 to 7 days.

How is it diagnosed?

To diagnose SSSS, the doctor must carefully observe the disorder's three-stage progression. Microscopic examination of peeled skin may help to distinguish SSSS from other disorders. Isolation of the causative organism in cultures of skin lesions confirms the diagnosis.

How is it treated?

Treatment includes systemic antibiotics — usually penicillinase-resistant penicillin — to treat the underlying infection as well as measures to maintain fluid and electrolyte balance. Complications are rare and residual scars are unlikely.

TINEA

What do doctors call this condition?
Dermatophytosis

What is this condition?
Tinea is a fungal infection that may affect the scalp (tinea capitis), body (tinea corporis), nails (tinea unguium), feet (tinea pedis), groin (tinea cruris), and bearded skin (tinea barbae). Tinea infections are common in the United States. With effective treatment, the cure rate is very high, although about 20% of infected people develop chronic tinea.

What causes it?
Tinea infections are caused by the fungi *Trichophyton, Microsporum,* and *Epidermophyton.* Transmission can occur directly through contact with infected lesions or indirectly through contact with contaminated articles, such as shoes, towels, or shower stalls.

What are its symptoms?
Lesions vary in appearance and duration.

Tinea of the scalp
This type of fungal infection mainly affects children and is characterized by small, spreading papules on the scalp, causing patchy hair loss with scaling. These papules may progress to inflamed, pus-filled lesions.

Tinea of the body
This tinea infection produces flat lesions on the skin at any site except the scalp, bearded skin, or feet. These lesions may be dry and scaly or moist and crusty; as they enlarge, their centers heal, producing the classic ring-shaped appearance that gives this infection the common name ringworm.

Tinea of the nails
Infection typically starts at the tip of one or more toenails (fingernail infection is less common) and produces gradual thickening, discoloration, and crumbling of the nail, with buildup of debris under it. Eventually, the nail may be destroyed completely.

SELF-HELP

Treating tinea

Depending on which type of tinea you have, the doctor will probably prescribe drugs and, possibly, some other measures. Here are some general treatment guidelines.

Tinea of the scalp
Be aware that topical therapy is ineffective for this form of tinea; oral Fulvicin or Grisactin for 1 to 3 months is the treatment of choice. If your condition worsens, stop taking the medication and notify the doctor.

Wash your hands thoroughly and often. To help prevent spread of the infection to others, wash your towels, bedclothes, and combs frequently in hot water and avoid sharing them. Encourage family members to get checked for tinea.

Tinea of the body
If you have a lot of abdominal fat, the doctor may want you to use abdominal pads between skin folds; these pads should be changed frequently. Check yourself daily for any new areas of raw, open skin. If the involved area is moist, the doctor may instruct you to apply open wet dressings two or three times daily to ease inflammation and help remove scales.

Tinea of the nails
Keep your nails short and straight. Gently remove debris under them with an emery board. Be aware that

therapy for tinea of the nails is prolonged, and Fulvicin or Grisactin may cause such side effects as headache, nausea, vomiting, and photosensitivity.

Tinea of the feet
Expose your feet to the air whenever possible, and wear sandals or leather shoes and clean cotton socks. Wash your feet twice daily and, after drying them thoroughly, apply an antifungal cream followed by antifungal powder to absorb perspiration and prevent abrasion.

Tinea of the groin
Dry the affected area thoroughly after bathing, and apply antifungal powder evenly after applying the topical antifungal agent. Wear loose-fitting clothing, which should be changed frequently and washed in hot water.

Tinea of bearded skin
Let your beard grow. Trim whiskers with scissors, not a razor. If you must shave, use an electric razor instead of a blade.

Tinea of the feet
This tinea infection, commonly known as athlete's foot, causes scaling and blisters between the toes. Severe infection may lead to inflammation, with severe itching and pain on walking. A dry, scaly inflammation may affect the entire sole.

Tinea of the groin
Commonly known as jock itch, this infection produces red, raised, sharply defined, itchy lesions in the groin that may extend to the buttocks, inner thighs, and external genitalia. Warm weather and tight clothing encourage fungus growth.

Tinea of bearded skin
This uncommon infection affects the bearded area of the face in men.

How is it diagnosed?
To confirm tinea infection, scrapings from lesions are examined under a microscope. Other diagnostic procedures include Wood's light examination (which is useful in only about 5% of cases of tinea of the scalp) and culture of the infecting organism.

How is it treated?
Tinea infections usually respond to topical agents, such as ketoconazole cream. Other antifungals used to treat tinea include Naftin, Loprox, Lamisil, Halotex, and Tinactin. Topical treatments should continue for 2 weeks after lesions resolve. Alternatively, the doctor may prescribe the oral drug Fulvicin, which is especially effective in tinea infections of the skin, hair, and nails.

Supportive measures include applying open wet dressings, removing scabs and scales, and applying drugs known as *keratolytics* to soften and remove lesions of the heels or soles. (See *Treating tinea.*)

VITILIGO

What is this condition?
Vitiligo is caused by destruction and loss of pigment cells. It's marked by stark-white skin patches that may cause a serious cosmetic problem.

This condition affects about 1% of the U.S. population, usually people between ages 10 and 30, with peak incidence around age 20. It shows no racial preference, but the distinctive patches are most prominent in blacks. Vitiligo doesn't favor one sex; however, women tend to seek treatment more often than men.

What causes it?
The cause of vitiligo is unknown. Inheritance seems to play an important role; about 30% of people with vitiligo have family members with the same condition. Other theories point to problems with the immune system or nervous system.

SELF-HELP

Understanding vitiligo therapy

Depending on the extent of your vitiligo, the doctor may recommend either repigmentation or depigmentation therapy. Here are some suggestions to follow if you're undergoing one of these therapies.

Repigmentation therapy
- Use psoralens medications three or four times weekly, as prescribed. Take systemic psoralens 2 hours before exposure to the sun; apply topical solutions 30 to 60 minutes before exposure.
- Be sure to use a sunscreen (SPF 8 to 10) to protect both affected and normal skin during exposure, and wear sunglasses after taking the medication. If you need to expose the area around your eyes, keep your eyes closed during treatment.
- Remember that exposure to sunlight also darkens normal skin. After being exposed to ultraviolet light for the prescribed amount of time, apply a sunscreen if you plan to be exposed to sunlight as well. If sunburn occurs, discontinue therapy temporarily

and apply open wet dressings (using thin sheeting) to affected areas for 15 to 20 minutes, four or five times daily or as necessary for comfort. After applying wet dressings, allow your skin to air-dry. Apply a soothing lubricating cream or lotion while your skin is still slightly moist.

Depigmentation therapy
- During this therapy, wear protective clothing and use a sunscreen (SPF 15). Realize that the results of depigmentation therapy are permanent and that you must thereafter protect your skin from the adverse effects of sunlight.
- Don't buy commercial cosmetics or dyes without trying them first because some may not be suitable.

Some link exists between vitiligo and several other disorders that it often accompanies. These disorders are thyroid dysfunction, pernicious anemia, Addison's disease, aseptic meningitis, diabetes, sensitivity of the eyes to light, hearing defects, alopecia areata (a form of hair loss), and halo nevi (a type of skin lesion).

Outbreaks of vitiligo may be brought on by a stressful physical or psychological event — for example, severe sunburn, surgery, pregnancy, loss of a job, bereavement, or some other source of distress. Chemical agents, such as phenols and catechols, may also cause this condition.

What are its symptoms?
Vitiligo produces depigmented or stark-white patches on the skin. On fair-skinned whites, these patches are almost imperceptible.

The patches are usually bilaterally symmetrical with sharp borders. They generally appear over bony prominences, around orifices (such as the eyes and mouth), within body folds, and at injury sites. The hair within them may also turn white.

How is it diagnosed?

Diagnosis requires an accurate history of onset and of associated illnesses, family history, and observation of characteristic lesions. Other skin disorders, such as tinea versicolor, must be ruled out.

In fair-skinned people, Wood's light examination detects patches resulting from vitiligo. If autoimmune or endocrine disturbances are suspected, the person may undergo lab tests.

How is it treated?

The most common treatment for vitiligo is repigmentation therapy. During this therapy, a person uses systemic or topical psoralens compounds and undergoes periodic exposure to sunlight or artificial ultraviolet A light. New pigment rises from hair follicles and appears on the skin as small freckles, which gradually enlarge and coalesce. Body parts containing few hair follicles (such as the fingertips) may resist this therapy. (See *Understanding vitiligo therapy.*)

During therapy, normal skin turns darker than usual. This may enhance the contrast between normal skin and affected white skin. Use of sunscreen on normal skin may help minimize this problem as well as prevent sunburn. (See *Helping a child undergoing repigmentation therapy.*)

If vitiligo affects over 50% of the body surface, a person may undergo depigmentation therapy. A cream containing 20% monobenzone permanently destroys pigment cells in unaffected skin areas and produces a uniform skin tone. Eventually, the entire skin may be depigmented to achieve a uniform color. Depigmentation is permanent and causes extreme sensitivity to sunlight.

ADVICE FOR CAREGIVERS

Helping a child undergoing repigmentation therapy

If your child is having repigmentation therapy to treat vitiligo, here's one way to modify the treatment regimen to avoid unnecessary restrictions: Give the initial dose of psoralens medication at 1 p.m. and then let your child go out to play as usual. After this, give the medication 30 minutes earlier each day of treatment, provided that his or her skin doesn't turn more than slightly pink from exposure.

If marked redness develops, stop the treatment and notify the doctor. Eventually, your child should be able to take the medication at 9:30 a.m. and play outdoors the rest of the day without side effects. Make sure your child wears clothing that permits areas of vitiligo to get maximum exposure to the sun.

Warts

What do doctors call this condition?

Verrucae

What is this conditions?

Warts are common, benign, viral infections of the skin and nearby mucous membranes. Although they most commonly occur in children and young adults, they may appear at any age.

Some warts disappear readily with treatment. Others require more vigorous and prolonged therapy.

What causes them?

Warts are caused by infection with the human papillomavirus, a family of viruses that contain DNA. They probably spread by direct contact but can also spread from one part of a person's body to another.

What are the symptoms?

Symptoms depend on the type of wart and its location.

- *Common warts* have a rough, rounded surface and are found mostly on hands and fingers of children and young adults.
- *Filiform warts* appear as a single threadlike projection on the face and neck.
- *Periungual warts* are rough and found around the edges of fingernails and toenails. A big one can lift the nail and cause pain.
- *Flat warts* can appear in clusters of up to several hundred. They're smooth and appear on most body parts, more commonly in children than adults. When spread by scratching or shaving, flat warts may appear in a line.
- *Plantar warts* are flat or slightly elevated. They occur singly or in large clusters, mainly at pressure points of the feet.
- *Digitate warts* are fingerlike, horny growths that jut out from a pea-shaped base. They appear on the scalp or near the hairline.
- *Condyloma acuminatum* (venereal warts) are usually small, pink to red, moist, and soft. They may occur singly or in cauliflower-like clusters on the penis, scrotum, vulva, or anus.

How are they diagnosed?

To confirm the diagnosis, the doctor examines the lesion, checking distinguishing features to identify the type of wart. To diagnose recurrent anal warts, the doctor may perform sigmoidoscopy, inserting a tube into the rectum and colon to directly visualize the lesions.

How are they treated?

Treatment of warts varies with the location, size, number, pain level (present and projected), history of therapy, the person's age, and compliance with treatment. Most people eventually develop an immune response that causes warts to disappear on their own and require no treatment.

Removing warts by electrosurgery

1 The area under and around the wart (but not the wart itself) is injected with 1% to 2% lidocaine.

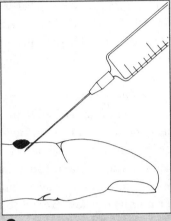

2 The doctor applies an electric current to dry up the wart.

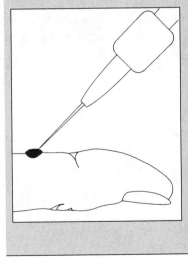

3 The doctor removes wart tissue with a curette and small, curved scissors.

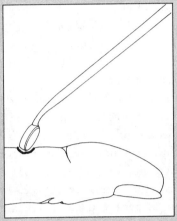

4 The doctor uses another, weaker electric current to the area to control bleeding and prevent recurrence.

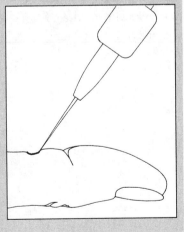

Treatment for warts may include the following:

■ *Electrodesiccation and curettage:* The doctor uses high-frequency electric current to destroy the wart, then surgically removes dead tissue at the base and applies an antibiotic ointment. The site is covered with a bandage for 48 hours. This method is effective for common, filiform, and occasionally plantar warts. (See *Removing warts by electrosurgery*, page 581.)

- *Cryotherapy:* The doctor uses liquid nitrogen to kill the wart. The resulting dried blister is peeled off several days later. This method is used for periungual warts and for common warts on the face, arms and legs, penis, vagina, or anus.

- *Acid therapy:* The person applies acid drops or plaster patches impregnated with acid every 12 to 24 hours for 2 to 4 weeks. This method isn't recommended for areas of heavy sweating, for parts that are likely to get wet, or for exposed body parts where patches are cosmetically undesirable.

- *25% podophyllin in compound with tincture of benzoin:* This treatment is used for venereal warts. First, nearby unaffected skin is covered with dimethicone or Vaseline to protect it. Then, the podophyllin solution is applied to moist warts, where it dries and is worn for 4 hours or more, then is washed off with soap and water. (In some cases, the solution must be left on for 24 hours or more, depending on the person's tolerance.) Treatment may be repeated every 3 to 4 days. *Note:* Pregnant women shouldn't use podophyllin because it can cause fetal abnormalities.

Other measures

Suggestion and hypnosis occasionally succeed in eradicating warts — especially with children. Also, researchers are investigating the use of antiviral drugs in treating warts.

BLOOD DISORDERS

What is Henoch-Schönlein syndrome?

When an allergic rash mainly affects the digestive tract and causes joint pain, it's called *Henoch-Schönlein syndrome* or *anaphylactoid rash*.

Typically, the syndrome causes stomach pain, rectal spasms, constipation, vomiting, and swelling or bleeding of the mucous membranes of the bowel. Some people have gastrointestinal bleeding, hidden blood in the stools and, possibly, a blocked bowel. These problems may occur before the skin rash appears.

ALLERGIC RASH

What do doctors call this condition?
Allergic purpura

What is this condition?
Allergic rash is an inflammation of the cells that line the blood vessels, accompanied by allergic symptoms. The disorder affects the skin, urinary tract, digestive tract, and the joints. (See *What is Henoch-Schönlein syndrome?*) If allowed to develop fully, allergic rash is persistent and debilitating, and may lead to serious kidney disease. An acute attack of allergic rash may last several weeks, and death may result, usually from kidney failure. However, with appropriate treatment, most people recover from the disease.

Allergic rash affects more males than females and is most common in children ages 3 to 7 years.

What causes it?
The most common cause of allergic rash is thought to be an autoimmune reaction, in which the body's immune system responds to a bacterial infection (such as strep) by attacking the tissues of its own blood vessel walls. Typically, symptoms first appear 1 to 3 weeks after an upper respiratory infection. Other possible causes include allergic reactions to certain drugs and vaccines, insect bites, and foods (such as wheat, eggs, milk, or chocolate).

What are its symptoms?
Typically, the person with allergic rash has small, flat, purple skin blotches of varying size, caused by blood leaking from damaged blood vessels into the skin. These blotches usually appear in symmetrical patterns on the arms and legs and are accompanied by itching, prickling, and tingling. (See *Skin lesions in allergic rash.*) Swelling may sometimes occur elsewhere on the body, such as on the face, hands, feet, or genitals.

In children, the skin blotches tend to be raised, firm, and swollen; they may expand and bleed. Tiny purple or red spots may appear on the legs and buttocks and near the genital and rectal areas.

In about 25% to 50% of cases, allergic rash also causes kidney inflammation, bleeding from the kidney or from the tissues lining the bladder or urethra, or a serious kidney disease called *glomerulonephritis*.

How is it diagnosed?

Because no test clearly identifies allergic rash, the doctor diagnoses the condition by carefully observing symptoms, often during the person's second or third allergic attack. X-rays reveal swollen areas in the small bowel. Tests may also show blood in the urine and stools as well as evidence of kidney problems. Before diagnosing allergic rash, the doctor must rule out other types of rash.

How is it treated?

The doctor will work to manage symptoms. For example, to treat severe allergic rash, he or she may prescribe steroids to relieve swelling and pain relievers to alleviate joint and stomach pain. If allergic rash causes chronic kidney disease, the person may benefit from Imuran, a drug that suppresses the immune system. The doctor will also try to identify any substance that may be causing an allergic reaction. An accurate allergy history is essential.

What can a person with allergic rash do?

- Eliminate known rash-causing foods from your diet.
- After the acute stage, be sure to *immediately* report any recurrence of symptoms (most common about 6 weeks after symptoms first appear). Return for follow-up urinalysis.

APLASTIC OR HYPOPLASTIC ANEMIAS

What are these conditions?

Aplastic or hypoplastic anemias result from injury or destruction of stem cells, which are located in the bone marrow and function to produce new blood cells. These anemias impair production of all blood cell types (*pancytopenia*) or retard bone marrow development (*bone marrow hypoplasia*) and generally progress to fatal bleeding or infection.

INSIGHT INTO ILLNESS

Skin lesions in allergic rash

Lesions in allergic rash, such as those shown on the foot and leg below, typically vary in size.

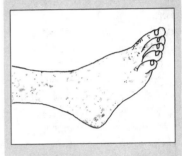

PREVENTION TIPS

Guarding against aplastic and hypoplastic anemias

To help prevent these anemias, take the following steps:

- Keep poisons, such as the solvent benzene, out of the reach of young children.
- If you work with radiation, wear protective clothing and a radiation-detecting badge, and observe safety precautions.
- If you work with benzene, be aware that 10 parts per million is the highest safe level. A delayed reaction may occur.

Understanding blood transfusions

If you have aplastic or hypoplastic anemia, your doctor may want you to have a blood transfusion to help treat the condition.

How will a transfusion help?

A blood transfusion will help your body maintain its normal functions. Keep in mind that blood is composed of red blood cells, white blood cells, and platelets. Also remember that blood carries nutrients, oxygen, and other important substances for growth and repair of your body's tissues.

Your body needs a certain number of red and white blood cells and platelets. When the number of blood cells circulating in your body gets too low, your body can't function properly.

For example, a low red blood cell count impairs your body's ability to carry oxygen, eliminate waste products and poisons, keep warm, and maintain blood pressure. A low white blood cell count affects your ability to fight infection. And if you don't have enough platelets, your blood can't clot properly.

If you develop a deficiency of any of these blood components, your doctor will order a transfusion containing the needed cells. The new blood you receive may contain just one cell type or a mixture.

What happens during a transfusion?

Before your transfusion, a technician will collect a sample of your blood to determine your blood type and match it to donor blood. This may be done the day before the transfusion. On the day of the transfusion, a nurse or another trained specialist will insert an intravenous line in your arm.

Once you're ready for the transfusion, two nurses (or a nurse and a doctor) will carefully check the information on the blood bag to make sure the blood is specifically for you. Then they'll hang the bag above your bed and the transfusion will begin.

Expect to have your temperature, pulse rate, blood pressure, and breathing rate measured before and frequently during the transfusion. A transfusion of red blood cells takes 2 to 4 hours. A platelet transfusion takes 15 to 45 minutes.

What are the risks of a transfusion?

Your greatest risks are infection and an allergic reaction — and these risks are low.

Your risk of infection is low because of careful blood and donor screening procedures. Your chance of getting hepatitis from a blood transfusion is about 1 in 10,000. Your chance of getting AIDS is about 1 in 40,000. (By comparison, your risk of dying in a car accident is 1 in 20,000.)

Occasionally, a transfusion may trigger an allergic reaction. Symptoms include fever, chills, and hives during or after the transfusion. If this happens during the procedure, the nurse will stop the transfusion and return the remaining blood to the blood bank along with a sample of your blood.

If you have an allergic reaction, you'll be given medications such as Tylenol and Benadryl.

Rarely, a reaction to a blood transfusion is severe. If you experience any of the following symptoms during or after your transfusion, tell your doctor or nurse immediately:

- a feeling of warmth or flushing
- redness (especially of your face and chest)
- a rash or itching
- aching muscles
- pain at the transfusion site
- chest pain or a severe headache
- brown urine or pain when you urinate.

What causes them?

Aplastic anemias usually develop when damaged or destroyed stem cells hinder production of red blood cells. Less commonly, they result from damaged vessels in the bone marrow. About half of these anemias result from certain drugs, poisons (such as the solvent benzene and the drug chloramphenicol), or radiation. (See *Guarding against aplastic and hypoplastic anemias,* page 585.) The rest may result from immunologic factors, serious diseases (especially hepatitis), or bone marrow cancers.

What are their symptoms?

Symptoms of aplastic anemias vary with the severity of pancytopenia and often develop gradually.

Anemia, which is a shortage of red blood cells, may cause progressive weakness and fatigue, shortness of breath, headache, pallor and, ultimately, rapid heart rate and congestive heart failure.

A low platelet count leads to red or purple spots on the skin and hemorrhage, especially from the mucous membranes (nose, gums, rectum, vagina) or into the retina or central nervous system.

Neutropenia (deficiency of neutrophils, a type of white blood cell) may lead to infection (fever, oral and rectal ulcers, sore throat) without inflammation.

How are they diagnosed?

To confirm aplastic anemia, the doctor will order a series of blood tests that measure the number and size of red blood cells, the number of white blood cells, iron levels, clotting time, and other factors. Bone marrow aspiration from several sites may provide additional data.

How are they treated?

Effective treatment must eliminate any identifiable cause and provide vigorous supportive measures, including transfusions of specific blood elements. (See *Understanding blood transfusions.*)

Even after the cause is eliminated, recovery can take months. Bone marrow transplantation is the treatment of choice for anemia due to severe aplasia and for people who need continual red blood cell transfusions.

Special infection control precautions are used to prevent infection in people with low white blood cell counts. If an infection develops, it may require antibiotics; however, antibiotics must be administered carefully because they tend to encourage resistant strains of organisms. Some people may need oxygen to help them breathe.

Other treatments include drug therapy with steroids, which are successful in children but not in adults. Drugs that stimulate the bone marrow, such as androgens, are controversial. Antilymphocyte globulin, an experimental drug, may be used. If a person doesn't re-

 SELF-HELP

Advice for a person with aplastic or hypoplastic anemia

If you have one of these anemias, you'll need to take these precautions.

Preventing bleeding
- If your platelet count is low, prevent hemorrhage by using an electric razor and a soft-bristled toothbrush, and using a stool softener and eating the right foods to prevent constipation (which can cause rectal bleeding).
- To detect bleeding early, check for blood in your urine and stools and inspect your skin for tiny purple or red spots.

Warding off infection
- Help prevent infection by eating a nutritious diet high in vitamins and proteins to improve your resistance.
- Brush your teeth often and gargle with an antiseptic mouth wash.
- See your doctor regularly to have nose, throat, urine, rectal, and blood cultures. These tests check for infection.
- If you don't require hospitalization, continue your normal lifestyle, with appropriate restrictions (such as regular rest periods), until remission occurs.

Questions people ask about treating aplastic anemia

Why do I need so many red blood cell and platelet transfusions?

Transfusions help to replenish the blood cells that your bone marrow fails to produce or suppresses. Blood cells are living cells with a limited life span. Red blood cells usually live for 120 days, whereas platelets live for only 8 to 10 days. Normally, bone marrow produces replacements for the cells that die.

Why can't I have a transfusion of white blood cells?

White blood cells have a short life span. They don't survive long enough to be helpful when given by transfusion.

Why can't I just take antibiotics to prevent infections?

Taking antibiotics to prevent an infection may encourage the growth of resistant strains of bacteria. Remember, infections sometimes come from germs existing in your own body. Preventive treatment with antibiotics will kill these normal germs and encourage the growth of bacteria that are resistant to treatment. You're safer practicing standard hygiene (such as washing your hands before eating) and avoiding crowds and people whom you know are sick.

spond to any other therapy, drugs that suppress the immune system may be tried. (See *Advice for a person with aplastic or hypoplastic anemia,* page 587, and *Questions people ask about treating aplastic anemia.*)

DISSEMINATED INTRAVASCULAR COAGULATION

What do doctors call this condition?

Consumption coagulopathy, defibrination syndrome

What is this condition?

This disorder is a complication of conditions that accelerate blood clotting. It causes blockages in the small blood vessels, depletes the body's supply of clotting factors and platelets, and destroys fibrin (a critical component of blood clots). In effect, the disorder causes severe bleeding at multiple sites.

Disseminated intravascular coagulation is generally an acute condition, but it may be chronic in people with cancer. The prognosis depends on early detection and treatment, on the severity of hemorrhaging, and on whether the underlying disease or condition can be treated.

What causes it?

Disseminated intravascular coagulation may result from a variety of disorders, but the reason for this isn't known. (See *Causes of disseminated intravascular coagulation.*)

What are its symptoms?

The most significant symptom is abnormal bleeding in a person who has never had a serious bleeding disorder. The principal signs of such bleeding include oozing from the skin, red or purple skin spots, and hematomas caused by bleeding into the skin. Bleeding from sites of surgical or invasive procedures and from the digestive tract are equally significant, as are bluish, cold hands and feet and kidney problems.

Other possible symptoms include nausea, vomiting, shortness of breath, decreased urination, seizures, coma, shock, failure of major body systems, and severe muscle, back, and abdominal pain.

How is it diagnosed?

Abnormal bleeding in the absence of a known blood disorder suggests disseminated intravascular coagulation. Lab findings that measure blood clotting support the diagnosis. Assessing kidney function may also provide important information.

Final confirmation of the diagnosis may be difficult because many of these test results also occur in other disorders. Additional diagnostic tests determine the underlying disorder.

How is it treated?

Successful management of disseminated intravascular coagulation depends on a prompt diagnosis and adequate treatment of the underlying disorder. Treatment may be supportive (when the underlying disorder is self-limiting, for example) or highly specific. If the person isn't actively bleeding, supportive care alone may reverse the disorder. However, in active bleeding the doctor may order intravenous heparin and transfusions of blood, fresh-frozen plasma, platelets, or packed red blood cells.

ENLARGED SPLEEN

What do doctors call this condition?

Hypersplenism

What is this condition?

In this condition, the spleen aggressively filters the blood and removes any blood cells that are abnormal, aging, or coated with antibodies, even though some may be functionally normal. The overactive spleen may also temporarily withhold normal red blood cells and platelets from the circulation.

What causes it?

An enlarged spleen may have no apparent cause or it may result from another disorder, such as chronic malaria, an abnormal increase in the red blood cell count, or rheumatoid arthritis.

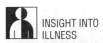 INSIGHT INTO ILLNESS

Causes of disseminated intravascular coagulation

Infection
- Blood poisoning
- Viral, fungal, or rickettsial infection
- Protozoal infection (falciparum malaria)

Obstetric complications
- Amniotic fluid embolism
- Placental abruption
- Retained dead fetus
- Septic abortion
- Eclampsia

Neoplastic disease
- Acute leukemia
- Cancer that has spread

Disorders that produce necrosis
- Extensive burns and injury
- Brain tissue destruction
- Transplant rejection
- Liver necrosis

Other causes
- Heat stroke
- Shock
- Poisonous snakebite
- Cirrhosis of the liver
- Fat embolism
- Incompatible blood transfusion
- Cardiac arrest
- Surgery using cardiopulmonary bypass
- Blood vessel tumor
- Severe blood clot in a vein

What are its symptoms?

Most people with an enlarged spleen have anemia (decreased hemoglobin) or too few circulating white blood cells or platelets. This causes frequent bacterial infections; easy bruising; spontaneous bleeding from the mucous membranes and the digestive or urinary tract; and sores of the mouth, legs, and feet. Fever, weakness, and palpitations are other common symptoms.

How is it diagnosed?

To diagnose the condition, the doctor must find evidence of an enlarged spleen and must determine that the spleen is destroying or trapping red blood cells or platelets.

In the most definitive diagnostic test, the person receives an intravenous infusion of red blood cells or platelets labeled with radioactive chromium; then red blood cells in the spleen and liver are measured.

The doctor also orders a complete blood count, which typically shows decreased hemoglobin, white blood cells, platelets, and immature red blood cells. A spleen scan, spleen biopsy (removal and analysis of tissue), and X-ray studies of the spleen's blood vessels may be useful. However, a biopsy is hazardous and should be avoided if possible.

How is it treated?

If the person doesn't respond to medical therapy and must depend on transfusions, all or part of the spleen is removed. Although spleen removal rarely cures the disorder, it does correct the effects of low blood cell counts. Postoperative complications may include infection and blocked blood vessels.

If spleen enlargement results from an underlying disorder, that disorder must be treated.

FOLIC ACID DEFICIENCY ANEMIA

What is this condition?

Anemia resulting from deficiency of this B vitamin is common and slowly progressive. It occurs most often in infants, adolescents, pregnant and breast-feeding women, alcoholics, the elderly, and in people with cancer or intestinal diseases.

SELF-HELP

Choosing foods high in folic acid

Folic acid, a B vitamin found in most body tissues, is needed for cell growth and reproduction. And recent research suggests that it may prevent certain birth defects.

Although the body stores only small amounts of folic acid, this vitamin is plentiful in most well-balanced diets. Unfortunately, cooking easily destroys folic acid in foods, and about 20% of folic acid is excreted unabsorbed. In fact, if your diet includes less than 50 micrograms per day, you could develop a folic acid deficiency within 4 months. To avoid this condition, make sure your diet includes foods high in folic acid, such as those listed at right.

Food	Folic acid content (Micrograms per 100 grams)
Asparagus spears	109
Beef liver	294
Broccoli spears	54
Collards (cooked)	102
Mushrooms	24
Oatmeal	33
Peanut butter	57
Red beans	180
Wheat germ	305

What causes it?

Folic acid deficiency anemia may result from:
- alcohol abuse
- poor diet (common in alcoholics, elderly people living alone, and infants, especially those with infections or diarrhea)
- impaired absorption (due to various intestinal disorders)
- bacteria, which compete for available folic acid
- excessive cooking, which can destroy a high percentage of folic acids in foods
- prolonged drug therapy (with anticonvulsants or estrogen)
- increased folic acid requirement. (See *When folic acid requirements rise.*)

What are its symptoms?

Folic acid deficiency anemia gradually produces progressive fatigue, shortness of breath, palpitations, weakness, inflammation of the tongue, nausea, loss of appetite, headache, fainting, irritability, forgetfulness, pallor, and slight jaundice.

How is it diagnosed?

Lab tests, such as measuring blood folate levels, are key to diagnosing this disorder. The Schilling test and a therapeutic trial of vitamin B_{12}

SELF-HELP

Recovering from folic acid deficiency anemia

If you have this type of anemia, you'll need to follow these guidelines to help you recover.

Getting enough folic acid

To meet your daily folic acid requirements, include a food from each food group in every meal. If you have a severe folic acid deficiency, be aware that diet only reinforces folic acid supplements and isn't a cure by itself. Be sure to follow your doctor's directions for taking the supplements. And don't stop taking them, even when you begin to feel better.

Taking care of your mouth

If you have a tongue inflammation, practice good oral hygiene. Use a mild or diluted mouthwash and a soft-bristled toothbrush.

Staying rested

Because anemia causes severe fatigue, be sure to schedule regular rest periods once you're able to resume normal activity.

injections distinguish between folic acid deficiency anemia and pernicious anemia (which is more likely to affect the nervous system).

How is it treated?

Your doctor will provide folic acid supplements and work to eliminate underlying causes of the disorder. Supplements may be given orally or by injection into the muscle, skin, or veins (to people who are severely ill, have malabsorption, or cannot take oral medication). Many people respond favorably to a well-balanced diet. (See *Choosing foods high in folic acid,* page 591, and *Recovering from folic acid deficiency anemia.*)

*I*DIOPATHIC THROMBOCYTOPENIC PURPURA

What is this condition?

Idiopathic thrombocytopenic purpura, a low platelet count that results from platelet destruction by the immune system, may be acute or chronic. The acute form usually affects children between ages 2 and 6; the chronic form mainly affects adults under age 50, especially women between ages 20 and 40.

The prognosis for the acute form is excellent; nearly 4 out of 5 people recover without treatment. The prognosis for the chronic form is good; remissions lasting weeks or years are common, especially among women.

What causes it?

Idiopathic thrombocytopenic purpura may be an autoimmune disorder, because antibodies that reduce the life span of platelets have been found in nearly all persons with this disorder. The acute form usually follows a viral infection, such as German measles or chickenpox, and can follow immunization with a live virus vaccine. The chronic form is often linked to immune disorders such as lupus. It's also linked to drug reactions.

What are its symptoms?

Symptoms include red or purple spots on the skin and mucosal bleeding from the mouth, nose, or gastrointestinal tract. Hemorrhage is rare. Purpuric lesions may occur in vital organs, such as the lungs, kidneys, or brain, and may prove fatal.

The acute form usually begins suddenly and without warning, causing easy bruising, nosebleeds, and bleeding gums. The chronic form begins gradually.

How is it diagnosed?

Results of lab tests, including platelet count and bleeding time, suggest the diagnosis. Anemia may be present if bleeding has occurred. Bone marrow studies may also provide important information.

How is it treated?

The acute form may be allowed to run its course without intervention, or it may be treated with glucocorticoids or immune globulin. For the chronic form, corticosteroids may be the initial treatment of choice. People who fail to respond within 1 to 4 months or who need a high dosage are candidates for surgical removal of the spleen. The platelet count typically increases spontaneously after this procedure.

What can a person with idiopathic thrombocytopenic purpura do?

Avoid aspirin and Advil, which can cause bleeding.

IRON DEFICIENCY ANEMIA

What is this condition?

In iron deficiency anemia, a lack of iron in the body causes an array of symptoms, including fatigue, weakness, and abnormally pale skin. When the body's iron stores are low, the red blood cell count falls, and with it the supply of hemoglobin, the iron-containing pigment in red cells that carries oxygen. The blood's oxygen-carrying capacity is thereby diminished.

A common disease worldwide, iron deficiency anemia affects 10% to 30% of adults in the United States. It's most prevalent in premeno-

PREVENTION
TIPS

Guarding against iron deficiency anemia

Here are some steps you can take to avoid this condition.

Diet
- To increase iron in your diet, eat meat, fish, or poultry; whole or enriched grains; and foods high in vitamin C, such as citrus fruits and leafy green vegetables.
- Give children under age 2 supplemental cereals and formulas high in iron.

Supplements and other drugs
- If you're pregnant, take an oral iron supplement as recommended by your doctor.
- Ask your doctor about an iron supplement if you must take pancreatic enzymes and vitamin E, because these preparations may interfere with iron metabolism and absorption.
- Be aware that aspirin, steroids, and certain other drugs may cause gastrointestinal bleeding. To minimize bleeding, take these drugs with meals or milk.

STRAIGHT
TALK

Questions people ask about iron supplements

How long will I have to take iron supplements?
Probably no longer than 6 months. The iron levels in your body will begin to rise shortly after you start taking supplements. However, the replenishing process takes time because the rate of iron absorption decreases as your iron level rises. Your doctor will probably continue therapy for 2 to 4 months after iron levels return to normal.

The first iron pill I took irritated my stomach, so now I'm on enteric-coated supplements. What does this mean?
Enteric-coated tablets or capsules have a special coating that doesn't dissolve until the pill reaches the small intestine. This prevents the iron from being released in the stomach, where it can cause irritation, nausea, and constipation.

Unfortunately, iron isn't absorbed as well in the small intestine, so enteric-coated tablets are less effective. Sometimes, stomach irritation can be avoided by reducing the number of iron tablets you take to one a day. Then you can try gradually adding additional tablets as your tolerance increases. Or trying a different type or brand of iron may help. Ask your doctor about these alternatives.

Is it true that cooking in cast-iron pots will help me get more iron?
Yes, but only when you cook certain types of food and cook them for a long time. Acidic foods like tomato sauce will absorb iron from pots.
The age of your cookware and how well you care for it also affects the amount of iron absorbed by food. Old, rusty pans provide more iron than new ones.

pausal women, infants (especially premature or low–birth-weight infants), children, and adolescents (especially girls).

What causes it?

Iron deficiency anemia may result from:
- too little iron in the diet, as in prolonged unsupplemented breast- or bottle-feeding of infants or during periods of stress, such as rapid growth in children and adolescents
- iron malabsorption, as in chronic diarrhea, surgical removal of the stomach, and malabsorption syndromes
- blood loss caused by heavy menstrual bleeding, injury, gastrointestinal ulcers, cancer, drug-induced gastrointestinal bleeding, or twisted, dilated veins (see *Guarding against iron deficiency anemia,* page 593)
- pregnancy, which diverts the mother's iron supply to the fetus for red blood cell formation
- abnormal presence in urine of free (extracellular) hemoglobin.

SELF-HELP

Choosing iron-rich foods

Although many everyday foods contain large amounts of iron, your body typically absorbs only a small portion of it. So to maintain adequate iron levels, you'll need to eat iron-rich foods.

But which ones should you choose? First, pick foods from all of the four major groups: milk and dairy, meat, bread and cereal, and fruit and vegetables. Then modify the amount from each group by considering your other dietary needs. For instance, if you need to cut back on cholesterol, don't choose liver.

Select wisely
Keep in mind that the iron in grains and vegetables isn't absorbed as readily as the iron in meat, fish, and poultry. On the other hand, eating meat, fish, or poultry *along with* grains and vegetables increases iron absorption. So does eating a food that contains vitamin C — an orange, tomato, or potato, for example. In fact, eating a tomato with a hamburger quadruples iron absorption. (On the other hand, drinking tea with the same meal lowers iron absorption.)

Know how much iron you need
Recommended amounts are 18 milligrams per day for women age 50 and under and 10 milligrams per day for men and women over age 50. Your doctor will tell you exactly how much iron you should consume. Consult the list at right to find the foods highest in iron.

Food	Quantity	Iron (milligrams)
Oysters	3 ounces	13.2
Beef liver	3 ounces	7.5
Prune juice	½ cup	5.2
Clams	2 ounces	4.2
Walnuts	½ cup	3.8
Ground beef	3 ounces	3
Chickpeas	½ cup	3
Bran flakes	½ cup	2.8
Pork roast	3 ounces	2.7
Cashews	½ cup	2.7
Shrimp	3 ounces	2.6
Raisins	½ cup	2.6
Navy beans	½ cup	2.6
Sardines	3 ounces	2.5
Spinach	½ cup	2.4
Lima beans	½ cup	2.3
Kidney beans	½ cup	2.2
Turkey, dark meat	3 ounces	2
Prunes	½ cup	1.9
Roast beef	3 ounces	1.8
Green peas	½ cup	1.5
Peanuts	½ cup	1.5
Potato	1	1.1
Sweet potato	½ cup	1
Green beans	½ cup	1
Egg	1	1
Turkey, light meat	3 ounces	1.0

SELF-HELP

Advice for a person with iron deficiency anemia

- Eat foods high in iron. But be aware that no food in itself contains enough iron to treat iron deficiency anemia; an average-sized person with anemia would have to eat at least 10 pounds of steak daily to receive therapeutic amounts of iron.
- Be aware that milk and antacids interfere with iron absorption but that vitamin C can increase it.
- Drink liquid iron preparations through a straw to prevent tooth stains.
- Don't stop taking prescribed iron supplements, even if you feel better, because replacing iron stores takes time.
- Report any side effects of iron therapy, such as nausea, vomiting, diarrhea, or constipation. These may mean the dosage should be adjusted.
- An iron deficiency may recur, so be sure to get regular medical checkups.

What are its symptoms?

Because iron deficiency progresses slowly, many people have no symptoms at first (except those of any underlying condition). Typically, they don't go to the doctor until anemia is severe. In advanced stages, they may have trouble breathing on exertion, fatigue, weakness, listlessness, pallor, inability to concentrate, irritability, headache, and susceptibility to infection. Also, the heart may pump more blood than usual and the pulse rate may increase.

Chronic iron deficiency anemia causes spoon-shaped and brittle nails, cracks in the corners of the mouth, a smooth tongue, and difficulty swallowing.

How is it diagnosed?

Blood tests and bone marrow studies may confirm iron deficiency anemia. However, test results may be misleading because of complicating factors, such as infection, pneumonia, blood transfusion, or iron supplements. Bone marrow studies may also provide important information about the disorder. The doctor also must rule out other forms of anemia.

How is it treated?

The first goal of treatment is to determine the underlying cause of anemia. Then, iron replacement can begin. (See *Questions people ask about iron supplements,* page 594.) The preferred treatment is an oral iron preparation or a combination of iron and ascorbic acid (which enhances iron absorption). However, some people may need iron injections — for instance, those who need more iron than they can take orally. (See *Choosing iron-rich foods,* page 595, and *Advice for a person with iron deficiency anemia.*)

PERNICIOUS ANEMIA

What is this condition?

This type of anemia is characterized by decreased ability to absorb vitamin B_{12}. The resulting vitamin B_{12} deficiency causes serious neurologic and gastrointestinal abnormalities as well as destruction of red blood cells. Untreated pernicious anemia may lead to permanent neurologic disability and death.

Pernicious anemia primarily affects people of northern European ancestry. In the United States, it's most common in New England and the Great Lakes regions, where many such people have settled. It's rare in children, Blacks, and Asians. The disorder typically begins between ages 50 and 60; its incidence increases with age.

What causes it?

The tendency of this disorder to run in families suggests a genetic predisposition. Pernicious anemia is common in people with certain immune disorders.

What are its symptoms?

Pernicious anemia usually begins gradually but eventually causes these three symptoms: weakness, sore tongue, and numbness and tingling in the arms and legs. The lips, gums, and tongue appear bloodless. Excessive bilirubin in the blood, which is due to destruction of red blood cells, may tint the eyes yellow and cause pale to bright yellow skin. In addition, the person may become highly susceptible to infection, especially of the genitourinary tract.

Other symptoms of pernicious anemia include the following:
- *Digestive tract:* disturbed digestion; nausea; vomiting; loss of appetite; weight loss; gas, diarrhea, and constipation; bleeding gums and tongue inflammation.
- *Nervous system:* neuritis; weakness, numbness, and tingling in the arms and legs; disturbed position sense; poor coordination; ataxia; impaired fine finger movement; light-headedness; double or blurred vision; altered sense of taste; ringing in the ears; optic muscle wasting; loss of bowel and bladder control; and (in males) impotence.
- *Heart and circulation:* weakness, fatigue, and light-headedness due to low hemoglobin levels. The heart works faster to compensate, resulting in palpitations, wide pulse pressure, shortness of breath, difficulty breathing while lying down, faster heart rate, premature beats and, eventually, congestive heart failure.

How is it diagnosed?

A positive family history and results of blood studies, bone marrow aspiration, gastric analysis, and the Schilling test establish the diagno-

SELF-HELP

Coping with pernicious anemia

If you have this condition, you've most likely learned how to self-administer the monthly injections of vitamin B_{12} that are crucial to the treatment. Remember, though, that the vitamin replacement isn't a cure; the injections must be continued for life, even after symptoms subside. Follow this additional advice.

Guard against infection
Promptly report signs of infection, especially those related to the airways, lungs, and urinary tract.

Eat a balanced diet
Your diet should include foods high in vitamin B_{12} (such as meat, liver, fish, eggs, and milk). If a sore tongue and mouth make eating painful, avoid irritating foods.

Be safety-conscious
If you have a sensory deficit, don't use a heating pad; it could burn your skin.

Which drugs lower the platelet supply?

Certain drugs given to treat other illnesses can reduce the body's supply of platelets. These drugs include:

- chlorothiazide (also called Diuril)
- cyclophosphamide (also called Cytoxan)
- heparin
- hydrochlorothiazide (also called HydroDIURIL)
- oxyphenbutazone
- phenylbutazone (also called Butazone)
- quinidine
- quinine
- rifampin (also called Rifadin)
- sulfisoxazole (also called Gantrisin)
- vinblastine (also called VLB or Velban).

sis. Lab tests must rule out other anemias with similar symptoms, such as folic acid deficiency anemia, because treatment differs. The diagnosis must also rule out vitamin B_{12} deficiency due to malabsorption caused by stomach disorders, gastric surgery, radiation, or drug therapy.

How is it treated?

The doctor can prescribe early vitamin B_{12} replacement to reverse pernicious anemia, minimize complications, and possibly prevent permanent nervous system damage. The vitamin is given by injection into the muscle, skin, or veins. An initial high dose of parenteral vitamin B_{12} causes rapid regeneration of red blood cells. Within 2 weeks, the person's condition should markedly improve. Because rapid cell regeneration increases iron and folate requirements, these compounds are given to prevent iron deficiency anemia.

After the person's condition improves, the vitamin B_{12} dosage can be decreased to maintenance levels and given monthly. Because such injections must be continued for life, the person should learn how to give himself or herself the vitamin. (See *Coping with pernicious anemia,* page 597.)

PLATELET SHORTAGE

What do doctors call this condition?

Thrombocytopenia

What is this condition?

Low platelet counts are the most common cause of bleeding disorders. Because platelets play a vital role in blood clotting, this disorder poses a serious threat to the body's ability to control bleeding.

The prognosis depends on how well the person responds to treatment of the underlying cause. For example, in drug-induced platelet shortage the person may recover immediately if the offending drug is withdrawn.

What causes it?

A shortage of platelets may be congenital (present at birth) or, more commonly, acquired. In either case, the condition usually results from decreased or defective production of platelets in the bone marrow (as occurs in leukemia, aplastic anemia, or poisoning with certain drugs) or from increased platelet destruction outside the marrow caused by an underlying disorder (such as cirrhosis of the liver, disseminated intravascular coagulation, or severe infection).

Less commonly, a low platelet count results from sequestration or platelet loss. An acquired low platelet count may result from the use of certain drugs. (See *Which drugs lower the platelet supply?*)

What are its symptoms?

A platelet shortage typically produces a sudden onset of red spots or bruising on the skin or bleeding into any mucous membrane. Nearly all people with this disorder lack other symptoms, although some may complain of malaise, fatigue, and general weakness. In adults, large blood-filled blisters characteristically appear in the mouth. In a severe low platelet count, hemorrhage may lead to rapid heart rate, shortness of breath, loss of consciousness, and death.

How is it diagnosed?

The doctor obtains a history (including a drug history), performs a physical exam, and orders coagulation studies to provide information on platelet count and bleeding time. If increased platelet destruction is causing the low platelet count, bone marrow studies are ordered.

How is it treated?

The preferred treatment is to eliminate the underlying cause or, in a drug-induced platelet shortage, to discontinue the offending drug. Other possible treatments may include giving corticosteroids or immune globulin to increase platelet production. Platelet transfusions are helpful only in treating complications of severe hemorrhage. (See *Precautions for people with platelet shortages.*)

 SELF-HELP

Precautions for people with platelet shortages

Because you don't have enough platelets, you need to take precautions.

Watch your medications
- Avoid aspirin in any form. Also avoid Advil, Nuprin, and other drugs containing ibuprofen.
- If you're on long-term steroid therapy, report any of these symptoms: acne, a moon-shaped face, excessive body hair, thinning arms and legs, swelling, or a humped back. Never abruptly stop taking steroids; these drugs must be discontinued gradually.
- Wear a medical identification bracelet.

Prevent bleeding
- Don't strain during bowel movements and coughing; both can lead to bleeding in the brain. To avoid constipation, use a stool softener.
- Don't engage in activities that may cause bleeding, such as contact sports.
- Wear gloves when gardening.
- Use an electric shaver instead of a razor.
- Use a soft-bristled toothbrush.
- Don't trim calluses and corns.

Coping with polycythemia vera

During daily activities

- Watch for and report symptoms of iron deficiency: pallor, weight loss, lack of energy, and tongue inflammation.
- Stay active and walk, if possible, to prevent blood clots.
- Examine your nose, gums, and skin for signs of bleeding. Report any abnormal bleeding promptly.
- Notify the doctor immediately if you have acute abdominal pain.

During chemotherapy

- If your white blood cell count is low, your resistance to infection is decreased. Avoid crowds and report symptoms of infection such as fever.
- Be aware that Alkeran, Myleran, or Leukeran may cause such side effects as nausea, vomiting, and susceptibility to infection. Also, Myleran, Cytoxan, and Uracil Mustard Capsules can cause hair loss. Cytoxan may cause bladder inflammation; to help prevent this problem, drink plenty of fluids. Watch for and report all side effects.

POLYCYTHEMIA VERA

What do doctors call this condition?

Primary polycythemia

What is this condition?

Polycythemia vera is a chronic bone marrow disorder characterized by increased red blood cell mass, increased white cell production, thrombocytosis, and increased hemoglobin concentration, with normal or increased plasma volume. It usually occurs between ages 40 and 60, most commonly among males of Jewish ancestry. It rarely affects children or Blacks and doesn't appear to run in families.

The prognosis depends on the person's age at diagnosis, the treatment used, and complications. The mortality rate is high if the disease is untreated or is associated with leukemia or other types of cancer.

What causes this condition?

In polycythemia vera, uncontrolled and rapid cell reproduction and maturation cause proliferation of all bone marrow cells. The cause of the uncontrolled cellular activity is unknown. Increased red blood cell mass causes blood thickening, which slows blood flow to small blood vessels. These conditions combine with thrombocytosis to promote blockages in some blood vessels.

What are its symptoms?

In its early stages, polycythemia vera usually produces no symptoms. However, as changes in circulation develop, the person may complain of a vague feeling of fullness in the head, headache, dizziness, and other symptoms, depending on the body system affected. Paradoxically, hemorrhage may occur as a complication of polycythemia vera.

How is it diagnosed?

Lab studies confirm polycythemia vera by showing increased red blood cell mass and other characteristic findings. Bone marrow biopsy (removal and analysis of tissue) reveals increased levels of all bone marrow components.

How is it treated?

Phlebotomy (blood removal therapy) can reduce the red blood cell mass promptly. The frequency of phlebotomy and the amount of blood removed each time depend on the person's condition. Typically, 350 to 500 milliliters of blood can be removed every other day. After repeated phlebotomies, the person develops iron deficiency, which stabilizes red blood cell production and reduces the need for phlebotomy.

For severe symptoms, therapy to depress the bone marrow may be used. In the past, radioactive phosphorus or cancer drugs could usually control the disease. But these agents may cause leukemia and should be reserved for older people and those with problems uncontrolled by phlebotomy. Currently, the preferred myelosuppressive agent is the drug Hydrea. People who've had previous problems with blood clot formation should be considered for myelosuppressive therapy. (See *Coping with polycythemia vera.*)

WHITE BLOOD CELL SHORTAGE

What is this condition?

A shortage of white blood cells may involve granulocytes or lymphocytes. (See *Types of white blood cells.*)

A *low granulocyte count* can occur at any age and can lead to infections and sores in the throat, digestive tract, and other mucous membranes and on the skin. A *low lymphocyte count,* a rare disorder, is a deficiency of white blood cells produced mainly in the lymph nodes.

When the total white blood cell count falls to dangerously low levels, the body is left unprotected against infection. The prognosis depends on the underlying cause and whether it can be treated.

What causes this condition?

A low granulocyte count may result from:
- radiation therapy or cancer drugs
- hypersensitivity to certain antibiotics and heart drugs
- disorders such as aplastic anemia, bone marrow cancer, some hereditary disorders, infectious mononucleosis, and certain viral and bacterial infections
- trapping of blood cells in the spleen.

Types of white blood cells

The blood contains five types of white cells, which function to protect the body against invading bacteria. The cell types compose two major categories.

Granulocytes

These white blood cells have small, beadlike masses in their cytoplasm (cell substance). The three types of granulocytes are basophils, neutrophils, and eosinophils.

Agranulocytes

These white blood cells lack beadlike masses characteristic of granulocytes. The two types of agranulocytes are lymphocytes and monocytes.

A low lymphocyte count may result from:
- a genetic abnormality
- radiation therapy or cancer drugs
- dysfunctional lymphatic vessels in the bowel
- an excess of steroid hormones, caused by use of adrenocorticotropic hormone or steroids, stress, or congestive heart failure
- disorders such as Hodgkin's disease, leukemia, aplastic anemia, sarcoidosis, myasthenia gravis, lupus, protein-calorie malnutrition, kidney failure, terminal cancer, and tuberculosis.

What are its symptoms?

A low granulocyte count typically causes slowly progressive fatigue and weakness followed by sudden onset of overwhelming infection (heralded by fever, chills, rapid pulse, anxiety, headache, extreme exhaustion), mouth and throat sores, ulcers in the colon, pneumonia, and blood infection, possibly leading to mild shock. If the low count results from a drug reaction, infection symptoms develop suddenly, without slowly progressive fatigue and weakness.

A low lymphocyte count causes swollen glands, an enlarged spleen, and enlarged tonsils, along with signs of an associated disease.

How is it diagnosed?

To diagnose a low white cell count, the doctor takes a thorough history and performs a physical exam to look for signs of an underlying disorder, orders appropriate blood cell tests, and, if necessary, obtains biopsy specimens of bone marrow and lymph node tissue for analysis.

How is it treated?

To treat a low granulocyte count, the doctor must find and eliminate the underlying cause, then control infection until the bone marrow can generate more white blood cells. For many people, this means stopping drug or radiation therapy and starting antibiotics immediately, even while awaiting test results. Treatment may also include antifungal preparations. In a newer treatment, the person receives granulocyte colony-stimulating factor or granulocyte-macrophage colony-stimulating factor to stimulate bone marrow production of neutrophils. Generally, white blood cell production in the bone marrow resumes spontaneously within 1 to 3 weeks.

Treatment of a low lymphocyte count aims to eliminate or manage the underlying cause.

CANCER

BASAL CELL CANCER

What do doctors call this condition?
Basal cell epithelioma

What is this condition?
Basal cell cancer is a slow-growing destructive skin tumor. This cancer usually occurs in people over age 40. It's more prevalent in blond, fair-skinned men. In fact, it's the most common malignant tumor in whites.

What causes it?
Prolonged sun exposure is the most common cause of basal cell cancer. Other possible causes include arsenic ingestion, radiation exposure, burns, immunosuppression and, rarely, vaccinations.

Although it's not well known how basal cell cancers develop, some experts suspect they originate when, under certain conditions, undifferentiated skin basal cells become cancerous instead of differentiating into sweat glands, sebum, and hair.

What are its symptoms?
Symptoms vary, depending on which of the three types of basal cell cancer is involved. In one type, lesions develop on the face, particularly the forehead, eyelid margins, and around the nose. The lesions are initially small, smooth, and translucent, later becoming enlarged and ulcerated. In a second type, irregularly shaped, lightly pigmented plaques with clearly defined borders develop on the chest and back. The third type forms indistinct waxy, yellow to white plaques on the head and neck.

How is it diagnosed?
All types of basal cell cancer are diagnosed by clinical appearance, biopsy, and cell microstructure studies.

How is it treated?
Treatment depends on the size, location, and depth of the lesion as well as the individual's age and health. Therapy may involve one or more of the following:
- curettage and electrodesiccation, if the cancer is small

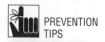

How to minimize sun exposure

The easiest way to prevent skin cancer is to reduce your exposure to the sun. Although most skin cancers occur after age 50, the sun's damaging effects begin in childhood. Fortunately, it's never too late to start protecting yourself from skin cancer. Here's how.

Wear sunscreen

Protect your skin with a lotion or cream containing para-aminobenzoic acid (PABA) or another sunscreen.

Sunscreens are rated in strength according to skin protection factor (SPF), ranging from 2 to 30 or higher. Choose a sunscreen that has an SPF of 15 or higher — especially if you have fair skin and burn easily.

Apply sunscreen at least 15 minutes before you go outside; then reapply it every 2 or 3 hours. Apply sunscreen more often if you perspire heavily or after you swim or exercise. Consider using a water-resistant sunscreen.

Get in the habit of applying sunscreen routinely before you go outside, because the sun's rays can damage your skin whether you're on your way to school or lounging at the pool.

Consider storing your sunscreen in a safe place near your front or back door. Keep an extra container in your car.

Cover up

Wear protective clothing, such as a wide-brimmed hat, long sleeves, and sunglasses. Keep in mind that flimsy, lightweight clothes may not protect against sunburn because the sun's rays can penetrate them.

Don't rely on a shady tree, an umbrella, or a cloudy day to prevent sunburn. Remember that burning ultraviolet rays penetrate overcast skies and a canopy of leaves as well.

Also keep in mind that sun reflected from water, snow, or sand can burn your skin even more intensely than direct sunlight, so carry a coverup with you when you go out.

Adjust your schedule

Avoid outdoor activities when the sun's rays shine their strongest — between 10 a.m. and 3 p.m. (11 a.m. and 4 p.m. daylight saving time). Schedule outdoor activities at other times. For example, play tennis in the early morning or mow the lawn in the late afternoon.

Other tips

- *Remember:* No matter how attractive it may be, a suntan isn't healthful.
- Don't use oils or a reflector device to promote a suntan.
- Check with your doctor or pharmacist about possible phototropic (sensitizing) effects related to any prescription or over-the-counter medicines you take.
- Avoid artificial ultraviolet light. Steer clear of sunlamps, and stay out of tanning parlors or booths.

- chemotherapy, if the cancer is superficial
- microscopically controlled surgery to carefully remove layers of skin until a tumor-free layer is reached
- radiation therapy, for less accessible tumors or if the individual is older or physically unable to endure surgery
- cryotherapy, which freezes and kills cancerous cells
- chemosurgery, if lesions are persistent or recurrent.

What can a person with basal cell cancer do?

If you have basal cell cancer, here are some steps you can take to ease its symptoms and help prevent a recurrence:

▪ If the cancer has invaded the mouth and caused eating problems, substitute egg nog, pureed foods, or liquid protein supplements for solid foods to keep up your nutrition.

▪ To relieve local inflammation from chemotherapy, use cool compresses or a steroid ointment prescribed by your doctor.

▪ If you have facial lesions, wash your face gently when ulcers and crusting occur because scrubbing too vigorously may cause bleeding.

▪ Avoid excessive sun exposure to prevent recurring episodes. (See *How to minimize sun exposure.*)

BLADDER CANCER

What is this condition?

Bladder cancer is a tumor that develops on the surface of the bladder wall or that grows within the bladder wall and quickly invades underlying muscles. Bladder tumors are most common in men over age 50 and occur more often in densely populated industrial areas.

What causes it?

Certain carcinogenic substances can predispose a person to bladder cancer. These include 2-naphthylamine, benzidine, tobacco, and nitrates. So, workers in certain industries — rubber workers, weavers, leather finishers, aniline dye workers, hairdressers, petroleum workers, and spray painters — are at high risk. (See *Answers to questions about bladder cancer,* page 608.)

What are its symptoms?

About 25% of people with bladder cancer have no symptoms during the early stages. Typically, the person first notices blood in the urine. Usually, this is painless, but people with invasive cancers may have pain above the pubic area after urinating. Other symptoms include bladder irritability, frequent urination, nighttime urination, and urine dribbling.

Answers to questions about bladder cancer

My doctor says smoking contributes to bladder cancer. Is this true?
It's almost certain. Cigarette smokers have a two to three times greater risk of developing bladder cancer than do nonsmokers. Even when a person stops smoking, the risk won't drop to the risk level of a person who never smoked.

I was routinely exposed to chemicals while I was working, but that was years ago. Should I be concerned about bladder cancer?
Probably. Bladder cancer may not develop for years (cancer specialists say 18 to 45 years) after exposure to chemicals or other carcinogens.

Even if you weren't exposed to industrial carcinogens, you may have used phenacetin, a popular pain reliever, before it was taken off the market by the Food and Drug Administration because it was highly carcinogenic. To be safe, continue to see your doctor periodically for a cytologic (cell) exam of your urine.

If I have bladder cancer, will the cancer cells show up in a urinalysis?
Not necessarily, although they may be there. If your doctor uses a microscope to detect cancer cells in your urine, he or she will tell you that this method isn't always definitive — especially if you have blood in your urine. An investigational technique called *flow cytometry* may give more accurate results. The test instrument has greater magnifying capability, making it easier to identify abnormal cells.

How is it diagnosed?

To confirm bladder cancer, the doctor will do a biopsy (in which he or she removes some bladder tissue) and will insert an instrument called a *cystoscope* into the urethra to visualize the urinary tract (this procedure is called *cystoscopy*).

The person should have cystoscopy when blood first appears in the urine. The doctor will try to determine if the tumor has invaded the prostate gland or nearby lymph nodes.

Other tests that provide important information about the tumor include urinalysis, X-rays of the urinary system, X-rays of the bladder and blood vessels in the pelvis using contrast dyes, computed tomography scan (commonly called CAT scan), and ultrasound.

How is it treated?

The surgeon will remove a superficial bladder tumor by a procedure called *transurethral resection and fulguration* (electrical destruction). This procedure is adequate if the tumor has not invaded the muscle.

To treat superficial tumors (especially those occurring in many sites) and to help prevent the cancer from recurring, the doctor may

Washing the bladder with drugs

The doctor may treat your bladder cancer by instilling drugs directly into your bladder. Doctors call this procedure *intravesical chemotherapy*, which simply means the use of cancer drugs inside the bladder. Read the information below to learn what you can expect during these treatments. If you have questions, ask your doctor or nurse for more information.

How the medication is delivered
The medication reaches your bladder through a very thin tube called a catheter. The catheter will be inserted in your urethra, which is the opening through which you urinate. First, the urethra will be cleaned with a bacteria-fighting solution, such as povidone-iodine. Then the catheter will be inserted, and the urine that's already in your bladder will be drained into a container. Now you should be ready to receive your medication.

The medication will be instilled through the catheter, and the catheter will remain in place for a certain period of time. During that time, the catheter will be clamped shut so that no medication can escape from the bladder.

Meanwhile, you may be asked to change your position by turning from side to side or walking around. This distributes the medication throughout your bladder.

How the medication is removed
At the end of the scheduled time the clamp on the catheter will be released and the medication will drain out. Then the catheter will be removed. You shouldn't feel any discomfort while this is being done. Try to relax and take a few deep breaths. Afterward, you may wash your genital area.

Understanding side effects
The side effects depend on the kind of medication you receive. For example:
- If you're receiving *thiotepa,* common side effects include fever, chills, a sore throat, hives, itching, bladder spasms, and pain when you urinate.
- If you're receiving *doxorubicin* (also called Adriamycin), you may have pain when you urinate, urinary urgency, and discolored (cherry red) urine.
- If you're receiving *mitomycin* (also called Mutamycin), side effects include pain when you urinate, urinary urgency, and a rash on your palms and buttocks.
- If you're receiving *bacillus Calmette-Guérin* (also called BCG), you may have pain when you urinate, bladder spasms, blood in your urine, fever, chills, and muscle and joint aches.

Ask your doctor, nurse, or infusion therapist how best to relieve these side effects.

---

wash the bladder directly with anticancer drugs. (See *Washing the bladder with drugs.*)

If more tumors develop, fulguration may have to be repeated every 3 months for years. But if the tumors invade the muscle layer or recur frequently, cystoscopy with fulguration is no longer appropriate.

Treating larger tumors
If the tumor is too large to be treated by means of a cystoscope, the surgeon will remove a section of the bladder — provided that the tumor isn't near the bladder neck or the openings of the ureters (the pair of tubes that carry urine from the kidneys into the bladder). To

SELF-HELP

Living with a urinary diversion

Here are some tips to help you care for the urinary stoma, or opening.

- If possible, have your spouse, a friend, or a relative learn about stoma care along with you.
- You may participate in most activities, except for heavy lifting and contact sports.
- For more information, consult an enterostomal therapist.

Handling the pouch

- Know that if you choose a reusable (rather than disposable) pouch, you'll need at least two.
- After you're discharged, remeasure your stoma in case the size has changed. If it has, you'll need a different size pouch — the opening must clear the stoma with a ⅛-inch margin.
- To ensure a good skin seal, use a skin barrier that contains synthetics and little or no karaya (which urine tends to destroy). Check the pouch often to make sure the seal remains intact. A good skin seal with a skin barrier may last for 3 to 6 days, so

change the pouch only that often. To help secure the pouch, you can wear a loose-fitting elastic belt.

- The pouch should have a drainage valve at the bottom. Be sure to empty the pouch when it's one-third full, or every 2 to 3 hours. Be aware that mucus will appear in the draining urine.

Skin care

- Keep the skin around the stoma clean and free of irritation. After you remove the pouch, wash the skin with water and mild soap. Rinse well with clear water to remove soap residue, and then gently pat the skin dry; don't rub. Place a gauze sponge soaked with one part vinegar to three parts water over the stoma for a few minutes to prevent the buildup of uric acid crystals.
- While preparing the skin, place a rolled-up dry gauze sponge over the stoma to collect the draining urine. Coat the skin with a silicone skin protector, and cover it with the collection pouch. If you notice skin irritation or breakdown, apply a layer of antacid precipitate to the clean, dry skin before coating with the skin protector.

help control such tumors, the drug thiotepa may be instilled into the bladder after surgery.

Treating infiltrating tumors

Bladder removal (also called *radical cystectomy*) is the preferred treatment for an infiltrating bladder tumor. The week before the operation, the person may undergo external beam therapy to the bladder. Then, during surgery, the doctor removes the bladder along with adjacent fat, lymph nodes, the urethra, the prostate and seminal vesicles (pouches in the lower part of the bladder surface in males), and the uterus and some nearby structures (in females). The surgeon forms a channel for urine drainage, called a *urinary diversion*. The most common type of channel is called an *ileal conduit*. The person must then wear an external pouch at all times to collect and drain the urine. (See *Living with a urinary diversion*.)

Males are impotent after radical cystectomy and urethrectomy (removal of the urethra or a part of it) because these procedures damage the nerves that control erection and ejaculation. Later, they may desire a penile implant to make sexual intercourse (without ejaculation) possible.

Treating advanced bladder cancer
Treatment for advanced bladder cancer includes surgical removal of the bladder, radiation therapy, and chemotherapy with such drugs as cyclophosphamide, fluorouracil, doxorubicin, and cisplatin. This combination sometimes can halt bladder cancer.

Experimental treatments
Researchers are investigating several treatments, including photodynamic therapy and administration of the drugs interferon alfa and tumor necrosis factor directly into the bladder. In photodynamic therapy, the person receives an intravenous injection of a photosensitizing agent, such as hematoporphyrin ether, which cancer cells readily absorb. Then a cystoscopic laser device delivers laser energy into the bladder, killing the cancer cells. This treatment also causes photosensitivity in normal cells, so the person must avoid all sunlight for about 30 days.

BONE TUMOR

What do doctors call this condition?
Sarcoma of the bone, bone cancer, primary malignant bone tumor

What is this condition?
Most bone tumors are caused by the spread of cancer from another part of the body (secondary tumors).

Tumors that originate in the bones themselves (primary tumors) are rare, accounting for less than 1% of all malignant tumors. Primary tumors are more common in young males, but may affect individuals between ages 35 and 60 as well.

Coping with amputation

If you have cancer in the long bones of your leg and amputation is necessary, here are some steps you can take to speed recovery:
• Cooperate with physical therapy, which typically begins within 24 hours after surgery.
• To promote healing, don't let the stump hang over the edge of the bed or sit with the stump flexed for extended periods.
• Avoid placing a pillow under your hip, knee, or back or between your thighs or lying with your knees flexed.

Phantom limb
You may experience "phantom limb" syndrome, in which you "feel" an itch or tingling in the amputated extremity. This is a normal reaction that can last several hours or continue for years, although it usually subsides.

What causes it?
The causes of a primary malignant bone tumor are unknown. Some researchers suspect that the tumor arises in areas of rapid body growth because children and young adults with such tumors seem to be much taller than average. Additional theories point to heredity, trauma, and excessive radiation therapy.

What are its symptoms?
Bone pain is the most common symptom of a primary malignant bone tumor. Often more intense at night, the pain isn't usually associated with movement. It's dull and usually localized, although it may be referred from the hip or spine and result in weakness or a limp.

Another common sign is a mass or tumor. The tumor site may be tender and swollen; the tumor itself often can be felt. Fractures are common. In late stages, the person may have a fever, impaired mobility, and physical wasting and malnutrition.

How is it diagnosed?
A biopsy is essential for confirming a primary malignant bone tumor. Bone X-rays, radioisotope bone scans, and CAT scans show tumor size.

How is it treated?
Surgical removal of the tumor is the preferred treatment. This may be combined with preoperative chemotherapy using drugs such as doxorubicin, vincristine, cyclophosphamide, cisplatin, and dacarbazine administered through the arteries to the long bones of the legs. In some instances, radical surgery such as amputation is necessary. (See *Coping with amputation*.)

BRAIN TUMOR

What is this condition?
A malignant brain tumor is a cancer of the brain. It's relatively common — slightly more so in men than in women — and may occur at any age. In adults, it most often strikes between ages 40 and 60. In

children, the incidence of malignant brain tumors is generally highest before age 1 and then again between ages 2 and 12.

Malignant brain tumors are classified by the type of cancer cell. In adults, the most common tumors are gliomas and meningiomas. Usually, these tumors are located above the covering of the cerebellum — the area in the back of the brain that coordinates voluntary muscle movements.

What causes it?

The cause of a malignant brain tumor is unknown.

What are its symptoms?

A malignant brain tumor causes changes in the central nervous system (brain and spinal cord) by invading and destroying tissues and causing compression of the brain, cranial nerves, and cerebral blood vessels; brain swelling; and increased intracranial pressure (pressure within the skull). Increased intracranial pressure causes many of this cancer's symptoms, although they vary with the tumor type, its location, and the degree of invasion.

Because symptoms usually develop gradually, brain tumors are commonly misdiagnosed.

How is it diagnosed?

In many cases, a brain tumor is diagnosed by performing a tissue biopsy (removing and analyzing a small portion of brain tissue) during stereotactic surgery. In this procedure, a head ring is affixed to the person's skull, and a device that removes tissue is guided to the tumor by a computed tomography scan (commonly called a CAT scan) or magnetic resonance imaging (commonly known as MRI).

The doctor will also take the person's history and assess his or her neurologic status; the doctor also may order skull X-rays, a brain scan, a CAT scan, MRI, and cerebral angiography (a study of the blood vessels in the brain). A spinal tap shows increased pressure and protein levels, decreased sugar levels and, occasionally, tumor cells in cerebrospinal fluid.

How is it treated?

Treatment seeks to reduce the size of inoperable tumors, reduce brain swelling and increased intracranial pressure, prevent further neurologic damage, and relieve other symptoms. The treatment method

---

Understanding brain surgery

Typically, brain tumors are removed either by craniotomy or craniectomy. To understand what happens during these operations, read the explanations below.

Craniotomy
In this operation, the neurosurgeon makes a large incision in the skull, exposing the cranial (skull) cavity, then forms a bone flap that may be completely removed or may remain attached to muscle during surgery. Next, the surgeon cuts the dura (the outermost membrane covering the brain) and opens it in the opposite direction. Then the surgeon removes the tumor and stitches the dura, skull, and skin flap back into place.

Craniectomy
During this operation, the neurosurgeon removes a tiny skull portion (smaller than a dime or about the size of the little fingertip). If necessary, he or she will enlarge the opening with a bone forceps, then remove the tumor. The surgeon may freeze the detached bone plug for later replacement.

SELF-HELP

How to monitor for brain tumor recurrence

If you've had a brain tumor, stay alert for the signs and symptoms below, which *may* mean that the brain tumor has returned:

- Changes in your breathing pattern
- Decreased alertness or other changes in your mental state (such as unusual drowsiness)
- Dizziness
- Drooping of the face or upper eyelids
- Excessive sleepiness
- Headache
- Hearing loss
- Muscle weakness or paralysis
- Nausea and vomiting
- Personality and behavior changes
- Seizures (convulsions)
- Sensory changes (changes in your senses or sensations)
- Swallowing difficulty
- Tongue protrusion
- Vision changes

Don't panic

Be aware that other conditions may also produce these effects, so there's no need to panic. Just be sure to call your doctor so he or she can investigate further.

depends on the type of tumor, its sensitivity to radiation, and its location.

If the tumor's location permits, surgery is performed to remove the tumor. (See *Understanding brain surgery*.) If the tumor is inoperable, treatment may include some combination of radiation therapy, chemotherapy, and drug therapy.

What can a person with a malignant brain tumor do?

- If you've received chemotherapy drugs called nitrosoureas, such as carmustine (known as BCNU), lomustine (known as CCNU), or procarbazine, you may experience delayed bone marrow suppression. Call your doctor right away if you have a fever or bleeding that appear within 4 weeks after you start chemotherapy.
- Stay alert for signs and symptoms of tumor recurrence. (See *How to monitor for brain tumor recurrence*.)

*B*REAST CANCER

What is this condition?

Breast cancer is the most common form of cancer in women. Although it may develop any time after puberty, it most often arises after age 50. It occurs in men, but rarely.

The survival rate has improved because of earlier diagnosis and the variety of treatments now available. But the death rate hasn't changed in the past 50 years. Breast cancer is the number two killer (after lung cancer) of women ages 35 to 54.

Breast cancer occurs more often in the left breast than the right, and more often in the upper outer quadrant (the upper part of the breast closest to the arm). A woman may not be able to feel a slow-growing breast tumor by touch for up to 8 years, until it has a ³⁄₈-inch (1-centimeter) diameter.

Breast cancer may spread by way of the lymphatic system and bloodstream, through the right side of the heart to the lungs, and eventually to the other breast, chest wall, liver, bone, and brain. (See *Classifying breast cancer*.)

What causes it?

The cause of breast cancer isn't known, but its high incidence in women suggests that estrogen is a cause or contributing factor. Certain predisposing factors are clear, though. Women at *high risk* include those who:

- have a family history of breast cancer
- have long menstrual cycles (began menstruating early or experienced menopause late)
- have never been pregnant
- were first pregnant after age 31
- have had cancer in one breast
- have had endometrial or ovarian cancer
- were exposed to low-level ionizing radiation.

Researchers have looked into many other possible predisposing factors, including estrogen therapy, drugs that lower blood pressure, a high-fat diet, obesity, and fibrocystic breasts.

Women at *lower risk* for breast cancer include those who:

- were pregnant before age 20
- have had more than one pregnancy
- are Indian or Asian.

What are its symptoms?

Warning signs of possible breast cancer include:

- a lump or mass in the breast
- change in the symmetry or size of the breast
- change in the skin, such as thickening or dimpling, scaly skin around the nipple, an orange-peel-like appearance, or ulcers
- change in skin temperature (a warm, hot, or pink area)
- unusual drainage or discharge from the breast
- change in the nipple, such as itching, burning, erosion, or retraction
- pain (with an advanced tumor)
- spread of cancer to the bone, pathologic bone fractures, and increased calcium in the blood
- swelling of the arm.

How is it diagnosed?

The most reliable way to detect breast cancer is by a monthly self-exam, with immediate evaluation of any abnormality. Other tests include mammography (an X-ray of the breast) and biopsy (removal of breast tissue).

Classifying breast cancer

Breast cancer is classified according to cell appearance and tumor location. Your doctor may refer to the following classification terms:

- *Adenocarcinoma,* which occurs in the epithelium (the covering of an organ)
- *Intraductal breast cancer,* which develops within the ducts (narrow tubes carrying secreted or excreted fluids)
- *Infiltrating breast cancer,* which occurs in the tissue of the breast itself (not connective or supporting tissue)
- *Inflammatory breast cancer* (rare) affects the overlying skin, which becomes swollen and inflamed, reflecting rapid tumor growth
- *Lobular carcinoma in situ,* which involves segments of glandular tissue
- *Medullary* or *circumscribed breast cancer,* which refers to a large tumor that grows rapidly.

Classifying the extent of cancer

A staging classification system is also used to provide a clearer understanding of the extent of the tumor. The most commonly used system is called the tumor-node-metastasis (TNM) system.

Options in breast cancer surgery

Fortunately, because of treatment and technological advances, women with breast cancer now have several satisfactory surgical treatment options. Discuss the options offered by the surgeon.

Lumpectomy

The surgeon makes a small incision near the nipple and then removes the tumor, marginal tissue and, possibly, nearby lymph nodes. Typically, the woman undergoes radiation therapy after lumpectomy.

Lumpectomy is used for women with small, well-defined cancers. Currently, fewer than 20% of women with breast cancer have this operation.

In some women, the surgeon freezes the tumor using an instrument called a *cryoprobe*. Then the surgeon thaws the tumor and repeats the procedure four more times. Finally, he or she refreezes the tumor and performs a lumpectomy. Called a *cryolumpectomy,* this cell-destroying, freezing-thawing procedure is recommended only for small, early primary tumors. After cryolumpectomy, the woman may have radiation therapy. The procedure has few complications and may prevent local recurrence.

Partial mastectomy

In this operation, the surgeon removes the tumor along with a wedge of normal tissue, skin, and connective tissue. The lymph nodes under the arms (axillary nodes) may also be removed. Radiation or chemotherapy usually follows in an effort to kill undetected cancer cells in other parts of the breast.

Total mastectomy

In this procedure, also called a *simple mastectomy,* the surgeon removes the entire breast. Typically, this operation is done if the cancer remains confined to breast tissue and no lymph nodes are involved. Radiation or chemotherapy may follow total mastectomy.

Modified radical mastectomy

The surgeon removes the entire breast, axillary nodes, and the lining that covers the chest muscles. If the lymph nodes contain cancer cells, the woman has radiation or chemotherapy after the procedure. Modified radical mastectomy differs from radical mastectomy in that it preserves the woman's pectoral (upper chest) muscles. Modified radical mastectomy has replaced radical mastectomy as the most widely used surgical procedure for treating breast cancer.

Mammography is indicated for a woman with signs or symptoms of breast cancer. Every woman should have a baseline (initial) mammogram between ages 35 and 39. Women ages 40 to 49 should have one every 1 to 2 years; women over age 50, women who have a family history of breast cancer, or those who've had cancer in one breast should have a mammogram every year.

Because mammography can produce a false-negative result in as many as 30% of all tests, most doctors do a fine-needle aspiration or surgical biopsy if the woman has a suspicious mass, even if the mammogram is negative. Ultrasound, which can distinguish a fluid-filled cyst from a tumor, can be used instead of an invasive surgical biopsy.

Bone scans, a computed tomography scan (commonly called a CAT scan), measurement of a substance called *alkaline phosphatase,* liver function studies, and a liver biopsy can detect the spread of cancer to distant sites.

When the doctor recommends a mastectomy

My doctor has recommended that I undergo a modified radical mastectomy. I think I can deal with the operation, but I'm not sure I can deal with my family and friends. What shall I tell them?

Are you wondering if your diagnosis and treatment will change your close relationships? Keep in mind that your family and friends will probably share many of your concerns and feelings — shock, fear, sadness, guilt, anger, and even embarrassment. Your women friends may begin to express fears about their own health.

Your best bet is to be honest. Give accurate information and answer questions if you want to, but don't dwell on the subject — especially if you start to feel uncomfortable. With your closest friends and family members, you might want to be more open about your needs and feelings. In most instances, you'll find that gentle candor enhances communication and strengthens relationships.

My illness and mastectomy have put a lot of stress on my husband and me. Will our relationship ever return to normal?

It can. It might even get better, if you both want it to and if you work on it. Together, look at successful ways you've dealt with stress in the past. Consider using some of these methods now. And keep each other's needs in mind. For instance, console each other if you feel loss and grief. Reassure each other if you feel fearful. Keep your lines of communication open, and give yourself time to adapt to the changes in your life. If you still feel your relationship is on shaky ground, don't be afraid to seek professional counseling or advice from a couples' cancer support group.

I'm worried — how will my mastectomy affect my sex life?

It may slow it down for awhile. You'll have less physical energy because your body's under stress from the surgery and from changes occurring in your system. Fatigue can decrease your sex drive. So make sure to rest when you need to. Take naps and try to schedule sex during your peak energy hours.

Keep in mind that mastectomy will affect your sex life if the surgery alters the way you feel about your sexuality. If you feel you need help in this area, do not hesitate to seek counseling.

Many factors can influence how a trauma like mastectomy can affect a relationship. How comfortable were you and your partner with your sexuality before your surgery? Your answer may predict how comfortable you and your partner will feel afterward. Obviously, you and your partner will need to be open and honest about the changes you're experiencing. Share your feelings and needs, and seek counseling if necessary.

A test called a *hormonal receptor assay* is done to determine if the tumor is estrogen- or progesterone-dependent. This test guides decisions to use therapy that blocks the action of the estrogen hormone, which supports tumor growth.

How is it treated?

Much controversy exists over breast cancer treatments. In choosing therapy, the woman and her doctor should consider the stage of the disease, the woman's age and menopausal status, and the possible disfiguring effects of surgery.

SELF-HELP

Coping with the effects of breast cancer surgery

It's only natural for a woman with breast cancer to dread breast surgery and its aftermath. The guidelines below can help you cope with some of the physical and emotional effects of this operation.

Before mastectomy

- In many cases, reconstructive surgery may be planned before the mastectomy. Ask your doctor about reconstructive surgery or call the local or state medical society for the names of plastic surgeons who regularly perform surgery to create breast mounds.
- Remember — breast cancer surgery doesn't interfere with sexual function. You may resume sexual activity as soon as you desire after surgery.
- For information on breast prostheses, contact the American Cancer Society's Reach to Recovery program. This program offers caring and sharing groups to help women with breast cancer in the hospital and at home. Their members can provide instruction, emotional support and counseling, and a list of area stores that sell prostheses.

After mastectomy

- Look at your incision as soon as feasible, perhaps when the first dressing is removed. Encourage your partner to look at it, too.
- If your axillary (armpit) lymph nodes were removed during a mastectomy, be sure to follow the doctor's instructions on ways to avoid lymphedema (swelling) of the affected arm after you leave the hospital. For example, you'll probably be instructed to exercise your hand and arm regularly and to avoid activities that might cause infection in this hand or arm (infection increases the chance of developing lymphedema). Such prevention is very important because lymphedema can't be treated effectively.
- You may become depressed or experience "phantom breast syndrome" — a tingling or pins-and-needles sensation in the area of the removed breast tissue. For help in dealing with these problems, contact your doctor, nurse, or the American Cancer Society's Reach to Recovery program.

A woman with breast cancer may undergo one or any combination of the following treatments:

- *Surgery* involves either *lumpectomy* (removal of the tumor only) or *mastectomy* (removal of all or part of the breast). (See *Options in breast cancer surgery*, page 616, and *When the doctor recommends a mastectomy*, page 617.)
- *Chemotherapy* is used either as the main treatment or as an auxiliary to the main treatment (known as *adjuvant therapy*), depending on such factors as the tumor stage and estrogen receptor status. The most commonly used drugs are cyclophosphamide, fluorouracil, methotrexate, doxorubicin, vincristine, paclitaxel, and prednisone.
- A treatment called *peripheral stem cell therapy* may be used for a woman with advanced breast cancer. In this treatment, blood is removed from a large vein. Certain cells undergo purification and are frozen and eventually reinfused.

- *Primary radiation therapy* before or after tumor removal is effective for small tumors in early stages that haven't spread to distant sites. It's also used to prevent or treat local recurrence. Also, a woman with inflammatory breast cancer may undergo radiation before surgery to make the tumor easier to remove. (See *Coping with the effects of breast cancer surgery*.)

CERVICAL CANCER

What is this condition?

Cancer of the cervix is the third most common cancer of the female reproductive system. It's classified as either preinvasive or invasive.

Preinvasive cervical cancer ranges from minimal abnormal changes in the cervix to a type of cancer in which the full thickness of the cervical covering contains abnormally proliferating cells. Preinvasive cancer is curable 75% to 90% of the time with early detection and proper treatment. If untreated, it may progress to invasive cervical cancer.

In *invasive cervical cancer,* cancer cells penetrate the deepest layer of cervical tissue and can spread directly to certain pelvic structures or indirectly to distant sites by the lymphatic system. Almost all cases of invasive cervical cancer are what's called *squamous cell carcinoma.* Usually, invasive carcinoma occurs between ages 30 and 50; rarely, before age 20.

What causes it?

Although the cause of cervical cancer is unknown, researchers have identified some predisposing factors: sexual intercourse before age 16, multiple sex partners, multiple pregnancies, and herpesvirus II and other bacterial or viral sexually transmitted infections.

What are its symptoms?

Preinvasive cervical cancer causes no symptoms or other changes that would be obvious to a doctor. Early invasive cervical cancer causes abnormal vaginal bleeding, persistent vaginal discharge, and pain and bleeding after intercourse. In advanced stages, it causes pelvic pain, vaginal leakage of urine and feces from a fistula, appetite loss, weight loss, and anemia.

Who should have a Pap smear?

A Pap smear, a microscopic study of cervical tissue, can detect cancer cells at a curable stage — quickly and painlessly. The National Cancer Institute has established the following guidelines to help women and their doctors determine when and how often a Pap smear should be done:

- All women age 18 or older and all sexually active females under age 18 should have an annual Pap smear and pelvic exam.
- After a woman has had three or more consecutive normal exams, she may have the test less frequently, at her doctor's discretion.

- Women who've had a hysterectomy (uterus removal) for a noncancerous disease should have a Pap smear at least every 3 years.
- Mature women (no age limit) should have a Pap smear as often as recommended by the doctor.

When to have it

For reliable results, schedule your Pap smear 5 or 6 days before or after your menstrual period. The Pap smear can't be done during a period, because cells from the menstrual flow may falsify the findings. Also, don't douche or insert any vaginal medicines for 24 hours before the test because these measures also may alter the test results.

How is it diagnosed?

A microscopic exam of cervical cells (called a *Pap smear*) can detect cervical cancer before the disease causes signs and symptoms. (See *Who should have a Pap smear?*) An abnormal Pap smear routinely calls for colposcopy, a diagnostic test that can detect the presence and extent of preclinical cancers requiring biopsy and cell examination. Other studies can detect cancer spread.

How is it treated?

Appropriate treatment depends on accurate clinical staging. A woman with preinvasive cervical cancer may undergo a total excisional biopsy, cryosurgery (tumor destruction by means of extreme cold), laser destruction, or conization or cone biopsy (removal of a cone of cervical tissue) with frequent Pap smear follow-up. (See *Living with the effects of cervical cancer biopsy and treatment.*) In a few cases, hysterectomy (removal of the uterus) is performed.

Women with invasive squamous cell carcinoma may undergo radical hysterectomy (removal of the entire uterus and other surrounding structures) and radiation therapy (which may be internal, external, or both).

STRAIGHT
TALK

Living with the effects of cervical cancer biopsy and treatment

I recently had a cone biopsy. The doctor says I'm doing well but I might have difficulty with pregnancy. Does this mean I'll never have a baby?

No. It just means that a cone biopsy — or conization — may interfere with your ability to become pregnant or carry the baby to term. If scar tissue forms after the procedure, the cervical canal may become blocked, preventing sperm from reaching the egg. Or the procedure may weaken the cervix, which can cause miscarriage or premature labor. Bear in mind that these complications seldom occur. However, if you continue to feel concerned, talk with your doctor again.

My doctor feels confident that all of my cancer was removed during the hysterectomy. What are my chances for a complete cure?

If your cancer was diagnosed and treated early, before it spread to the lymph nodes or other organs, your chances for full recovery are very good. If the disease progresses, however, treatment becomes more difficult, and the survival odds dip. The American Cancer Society estimates that the 5-year survival rate for all women with cervical cancer (regardless of detection time) is 66%.

Can I have a normal sex life after treatment?

In most cases, you'll be able to resume sexual relations, but you may need to make some changes. For instance, if you've had radiation therapy, your vagina may have less natural lubrication than before. To solve this problem, try using a water-soluble vaginal lubricant, such as K-Y Jelly, available in drug stores. Radiation therapy also may cause scar tissue to form in the vagina, making it narrower. Frequent sexual intercourse will help to widen the vagina. Also talk to the doctor about a dilator, an internal device to expand the vagina. If you've had a hysterectomy or other pelvic surgery, check with the doctor before resuming sexual intercourse.

What can a woman with cervical cancer do?

- If you're scheduled for a biopsy, be aware that you may feel pressure, minor abdominal cramps, or a pinch from the punch forceps. However, pain will be minimal because the cervix has few nerve endings.
- During cryosurgery, you may experience abdominal cramps, headache, and sweating — but you'll feel little, if any, pain.
- With laser therapy, you may have abdominal cramps.
- After excisional biopsy, cryosurgery, and laser therapy, you should expect vaginal discharge or spotting for about 1 week. Don't douche, use tampons, or have sexual intercourse during this time. Watch for and report signs of infection to the doctor. Be sure to have a follow-up Pap smear and pelvic exam within 3 to 4 months after these procedures and from time to time thereafter.
- If you're scheduled for internal radiation therapy, you'll stay in a private room in the hospital for 2 or 3 days. The doctor will implant an applicator containing radioactive material (such as radium or cesium) in the operating room under general anesthesia. While the im-

plant is in place, be sure to lie flat and limit movement. The nurse will help you do range-of-motion arm exercises (leg exercises and other body movements could dislodge the implant). Because of the radiation implant, your visitors will have to take safety precautions, which should be listed on the door to your room.

- If you're going to receive external radiation therapy, be aware that it may make you more vulnerable to infection. Avoid people with obvious infections during this treatment.

COLON CANCER

What do doctors call this condition?
Doctors may also call it colorectal cancer.

What is this condition?
Colon cancer refers to cancer of the colon — the second of the three portions of the large intestine. It affects equal numbers of men and women. Colorectal cancer refers to cancer in the colon and the rectum.

Colon cancer tends to progress slowly and remain localized (not spreading to other parts of the body) for a long time. This makes it potentially curable in 75% of people — provided that early diagnosis allows surgery before the cancer spreads to the lymph nodes. Thanks to better diagnosis, the overall 5-year survival rate is nearing 50%.

What causes it?
Although the exact cause of colon cancer is unknown, studies suggest that it's linked to diets high in animal fat (particularly beef) and low fiber. Also, your risk tends to be higher if you are over age 40 or have a history of digestive tract disease, ulcerative colitis, or familial polyposis (multiple polyps in the colon).

What are its symptoms?
Symptoms of colon cancer result from local intestinal blockages and, in later stages, from direct spread of the cancer to adjacent organs (bladder, prostate, ureters, vagina, sacrum) and distant spread (usually to the liver).

In the early stages, symptoms may be vague and variable, depending on the tumor's location and the function of the intestinal segment involved. Later symptoms may include pallor, general ill health, malnutrition, weakness, emaciation, fluid buildup in the abdomen, an enlarged liver, and dilation of the lymphatic vessels.

On the right side of the colon, early tumor growth may cause black, tarry stools; anemia; and aches, pressure, or dull cramps in the stomach. As the disease progresses, symptoms such as weakness, fatigue, shortness of breath on exertion, and vertigo develop. Eventually the individual experiences diarrhea, obstipation (extreme and persistent constipation), loss of appetite, weight loss, vomiting, and other symptoms of intestinal blockage.

A tumor on the left side of the colon causes signs of blockage even in early stages. Signs typically include rectal bleeding, intermittent abdominal fullness or cramping, and pressure in the rectum. As the disease progresses, constipation continues and diarrhea or "ribbon" or pencil-shaped stools occur. Typically, bowel movements or expelling gas relieves the pain. In later stages, bleeding from the colon becomes obvious, with dark or bright red blood and mucus in or on the stools.

With a rectal tumor, the first symptom is a change in bowel habits, often starting with an urgent need to defecate on arising ("morning diarrhea") or constipation alternating with diarrhea. Other signs are blood or mucus in the stools and a sense of incomplete bowel evacuation. Late in the disease, pain begins as a feeling of rectal fullness that later becomes a dull, and sometimes constant, ache confined to the rectum or lowest part of the spine.

Colon cancer tends to spread slowly and remain localized, which makes it potentially curable in most people.

How is it diagnosed?

Only a biopsy of the tumor can verify colon cancer, but these other tests help detect it:

- *Digital (manual) examination* can detect almost 15% of colon cancers.
- *Hemoccult* test can detect blood in stools. (See *Testing for blood in your stools*, page 624.)
- *Proctoscopy* (insertion of a special instrument called a *proctoscope* to examine the rectum and lower portion of the colon) or *sigmoidoscopy* (insertion of an instrument called a *sigmoidoscope* to examine the mucous membrane lining the colon) can detect up to 66% of colon cancers.
- *Colonoscopy* (insertion of an instrument called a *colonoscope* to examine the entire colon) permits visual inspection (and photographs) of the colon and provides access for surgical removal of polyps and biopsies of suspected tumors.

SELF-HELP

Testing for blood in your stools

A home fecal occult blood test is an easy, inexpensive way to detect blood in your stools. For accurate results, follow the directions given by your doctor or nurse, read the instructions included with the test kit, and review these steps.

How to get ready

Don't eat red meat or raw fruits and vegetables for 3 days before you take the test or during the test period. Also avoid diet supplements containing iron or vitamin C and painkillers containing aspirin or ibuprofen (for example, Advil or Nuprin) for 3 days before the test or during the test period. All of these substances can affect test results.

Increase your intake of high-fiber foods, such as whole-grain breads and cereals. Your doctor may also ask you to eat popcorn or nuts.

How to perform the test

- Make sure all your supplies are in one place. These may include your test cards (or slides), a chemical developer, a wooden applicator, and a watch with a second hand.
- Obtain a stool specimen from the toilet bowl. Use the applicator to smear a thin film of the specimen onto the slot marked "A" on the front of the test card. Smear a thin film of a second specimen from *a different area of the same stool* onto the slot marked "B" on the same side of the card.
- *If the doctor or a lab will be analyzing the test specimens,* close slots A and B. Put your name and the date on the test kit, and return the card (or slide) to the doctor or lab as soon as possible.
- *If you're doing the test yourself,* turn the card over and open the back window. Apply 2 drops of the chemical developer to the paper covering each sample. Wait 1 minute, then read the results.

- *If either slot has a bluish tint,* the test results are positive for blood in the stools. *If neither slot looks blue,* the test results are normal. Write down the results.
- Repeat the test on your next two bowel movements. Report the results of all the tests to the doctor. Even if only one of the six test results is positive, the doctor may recommend other tests.
- Discard any unused supplies when you've completed all of the tests.

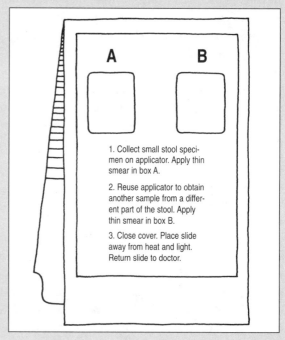

A   B

1. Collect small stool specimen on applicator. Apply thin smear in box A.

2. Reuse applicator to obtain another sample from a different part of the stool. Apply thin smear in box B.

3. Close cover. Place slide away from heat and light. Return slide to doctor.

- *Computed tomography scan* (commonly called a CAT scan) helps to detect cancer spread.
- *Barium X-ray* can locate tumors that are undetectable on manual examination or visually.

How is it treated?

The most effective treatment for colon cancer is surgery to remove the tumor, adjacent tissues, and any lymph nodes that may contain cancer cells. The type of surgery depends on the tumor location.

Chemotherapy should be performed if the cancer has spread to other regions, if some cancer cells persist after surgery, or if the tumor is recurrent and inoperable. Drugs used in such treatment commonly include fluorouracil with levamisole, leucovorin, methotrexate, or streptozocin. If the tumor has extended to regional lymph nodes, the person may receive fluorouracil and levamisole for 1 year after surgery.

Radiation therapy shrinks the tumor and may be used before or after surgery or combined with chemotherapy.

What can a person with a colostomy do?

- If you're having a colostomy, be aware that the stoma will be red, moist, and swollen and that postoperative swelling will eventually subside.
- After surgery, try to look at the stoma and participate in stoma care as soon as possible.
- If you have a sigmoid colostomy, you may be able to do your own stoma irrigation soon after surgery. Try to schedule irrigation for the time of day when you normally moved your bowels before surgery. You may need to irrigate every 1 to 3 days to stay regular.
- After several months, you may be able to establish control with irrigation and no longer need to wear a pouch. A stoma cap or gauze sponge placed over the stoma protects it and absorbs secretions. Before achieving such control, you can resume physical activities, including sports, as long as there's no threat of injury to the stoma or surrounding abdominal muscles. (See *Coping with lifestyle changes after a colostomy*, page 626.) However, avoid lifting heavy objects because this could cause a hernia or other problems related to your weakened stomach muscles. The doctor may put you on a structured, gradually progressive exercise program to strengthen your abdominal muscles.
- Be aware that anyone who has had colon cancer is at increased risk for another primary cancer. You should have yearly screening and testing and eat a high-fiber diet.

STRAIGHT TALK

Coping with lifestyle changes after a colostomy

How can I take a bath or shower?
You can bathe or shower with or without your pouch. Soap and water won't hurt the stoma, and water can't flow into the opening. Be sure to rinse well, though, because soap residue will interfere with pouch adhesion. If you shower, don't let the water hit your stoma directly.

If you decide to keep your pouch on, apply extra tape around the edge of the skin barrier.

Will I be able to exercise?
Having a colostomy shouldn't prevent you from exercising regularly. Check with your doctor first, though, who will probably tell you to avoid weight lifting and rough contact sports like football.

If you swim, ask the doctor or enterostomal therapist about using a stoma plug. This soft foam plug fits into your stoma to block drainage for up to 24 hours. It can't be seen under a bathing suit, and it filters gas without noise or odor.

If you're very active and perspire heavily, you may need to change your pouch more frequently and increase your fluid intake.

Can I go on business trips?
With a little advance preparation, you can travel for business and pleasure. Take along enough colostomy supplies for the entire trip, or call ahead to order replacements if necessary. Always pack your supplies and any prescription medicines (especially for diarrhea or constipation) in your carry-on luggage so that you can care for yourself if your luggage gets lost.

And remember, use only safe drinking water to irrigate your colostomy.

ESOPHAGEAL CANCER

What is this condition?
This type of cancer attacks the esophagus — the canal extending from the throat to the stomach. The tumor is usually infiltrating. There's no known cure yet.

What causes it?
The cause is unknown, but predisposing factors include chronic irritation caused by heavy smoking and excessive alcohol use, stasis-induced inflammation, and nutritional deficiency.

What are its symptoms?
Swallowing difficulty and weight loss are the most common initial symptoms. Swallowing difficulty is mild and intermittent at first but soon becomes constant. Pain, hoarseness, coughing, and esophageal obstruction follow. Physical wasting and malnutrition may develop.

How is it diagnosed?

X-rays of the esophagus, with barium swallow and motility studies, reveal structural and filling defects and reduced peristalsis. An endoscopic examination of the esophagus, biopsies, and cytologic tests confirm esophageal tumors.

How is it treated?

Whenever possible, treatment includes surgical removal of the tumor to maintain a passageway for food. This may require radical surgery. Some people can undergo only palliative surgery, which relieves some symptoms but doesn't cure the disease. Other therapies may consist of radiation, chemotherapy with cisplatin, or insertion of prosthetic tubes to bridge the tumor and alleviate swallowing difficulty. Treatment complications may be severe.

GALLBLADDER AND BILE DUCT CANCER

What is this condition?

Gallbladder cancer is rare, accounting for fewer than 1% of all cancers. The disease occurs mostly in women over age 60. It progresses rapidly and has a poor prognosis because it's usually diagnosed late.

Bile duct cancer accounts for approximately 3% of all cancer deaths in the United States. It occurs in both men and women between ages 60 and 70. Typically, the cancer spreads to local lymph nodes as well as the liver, lungs, and peritoneum.

What causes it?

Many doctors consider gallbladder cancer a complication of gallstones, although this theory is based on circumstantial evidence — 60% to 90% of people with gallbladder cancer also have gallstones.

At diagnosis, the doctor often finds that the cancer has spread to the lymph nodes. Direct spread to the liver is common, and direct spread to both the cystic and common bile ducts, stomach, colon, duodenum, and jejunum also occurs, causing blockages. The cancer also spreads to the peritoneum, ovaries, and lower lung lobes.

The cause of bile duct cancer isn't known; however, statistics show an unexplained increased incidence of this cancer in people with ulcerative colitis. This link may result from a common cause — perhaps an immune mechanism or chronic use of certain drugs by people with colitis.

What are its symptoms?

The symptoms of gallbladder cancer are almost indistinguishable from those of gallbladder inflammation: pain in the upper middle or upper right part of the abdomen, weight loss, loss of appetite, nausea, vomiting, and jaundice. However, chronic, progressively severe pain in someone without a fever suggests cancer. In people with simple gallstones, pain is sporadic. Another telling clue to cancer is a palpable gallbladder with obstructive jaundice. Some people may also have an enlarged liver and spleen.

Progressive profound jaundice is commonly the first sign of obstruction due to extrahepatic bile duct cancer. The jaundice is usually accompanied by chronic pain in the upper middle or upper right part of the abdomen, radiating to the back. Other common symptoms include itching, skin problems, loss of appetite, weight loss, chills, and fever.

How is it diagnosed?

No one test can diagnose gallbladder cancer. However, lab tests support this diagnosis when they suggest liver problems and extrahepatic biliary obstruction.

How is it treated?

Surgery relieves symptoms but doesn't cure the disease. It includes various procedures, such as gallbladder removal, common bile duct exploration, tube drainage, and wedge excision of liver tissue. Surgery should normally be performed to relieve obstruction and jaundice that result from extrahepatic bile duct cancer.

Other measures to help relieve symptoms include radiation, radiation implants (mostly used for local and incisional recurrences), and chemotherapy (with combinations of fluorouracil, doxorubicin, and lomustine). All of these treatment measures have limited effects.

What can a person undergoing surgery do?

▪ After biliary surgery, you'll probably want to take shallow breaths. To improve your breathing, you may receive pain relievers and be

Many doctors consider gallbladder cancer a complication of gallstones, although this theory is based on circumstantial evidence — 60% to 90% of people with gallbladder cancer also have gallstones.

instructed to splint your abdomen with a pillow or an abdominal binder.

- Be aware that you'll have a nasogastric tube in place for 24 to 72 hours after surgery to relieve distention, as well as a T tube.

HODGKIN'S DISEASE

What is this condition?

Hodgkin's disease is a type of cancer in which the lymph nodes and spleen enlarge painlessly and progressively as certain lymphoid tissues and cells multiply abnormally. Thanks to recent treatment advances, a person who gets treated in time can potentially be cured, even if the disease is advanced.

What causes it?

Experts don't know the cause of Hodgkin's disease. The disease is most common in young adults, affecting more men than women. It occurs in all races but is slightly more common in whites. Its incidence peaks in two age-groups: ages 15 to 38 and after age 50 — except in Japan, where it occurs only among people over 50.

What are its symptoms?

The first sign of Hodgkin's disease is usually a painless swelling of one of the cervical lymph nodes — the "glands" in the neck. But sometimes other lymph nodes, such as those in the armpit or groin, are the first to swell.

In older people, the first symptoms may be vague — persistent fever, night sweats, fatigue, weight loss, and malaise. In a few people, the disease first affects the chest, causing respiratory symptoms.

Another early symptom of Hodgkin's disease is itching. Mild at first, it becomes acute as the disease progresses. Other symptoms depend on whether — and to what degree — the disease involves the body as a whole.

Lymph nodes may enlarge rapidly, causing pain and blockages, or they may enlarge slowly and painlessly for months or years. It's not unusual to see the lymph nodes wax and wane (grow alternately larger and smaller), but they usually don't return to normal. (See *Signs of advanced Hodgkin's disease*, page 630.)

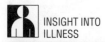

Signs of advanced Hodgkin's disease

Sooner or later, most people with Hodgkin's disease develop signs of whole-body involvement, including the following:
- swelling of the lymph nodes in the stomach
- cancerous masses in the spleen, liver, and bones
- swelling of the face and neck
- progressive anemia
- possible jaundice
- nerve pain
- increased susceptibility to infection.

How is it diagnosed?

After taking a thorough medical history and performing a complete physical exam, the doctor will order a lymph node biopsy to check for Reed-Sternberg cells — abnormal cells characteristic of Hodgkin's disease — and abnormal changes in the lymph nodes. The doctor also may order biopsies of the bone marrow, liver, chest, lymph nodes, and spleen, along with a routine chest X-ray, an abdominal computed tomography scan (commonly called a CAT scan), a lung scan, a bone scan, and lymphangiography (X-rays of the lymphatic system), to detect lymph node or organ involvement.

To stage the disease (determine the period in its development), the person will have a lymph node biopsy and laparoscopy. In laparoscopy, the doctor inserts a fiber-optic tube through a small incision in the abdomen to examine the abdominal cavity.

Typically, blood tests show anemia and abnormal levels of certain white blood cells. Before diagnosing Hodgkin's disease, the doctor must rule out other disorders that enlarge the lymph nodes.

How is it treated?

With correct and timely treatment, many people with Hodgkin's disease can be cured. The choice of treatment depends on the disease stage, cell and tissue analysis, and the person's symptoms.

Radiation therapy is used alone for people with stage I and stage II Hodgkin's disease. Those with stage III disease usually get chemotherapy combined with radiation. Chemotherapy is used for stage IV, sometimes bringing a complete remission.

Certain chemotherapy protocols (combinations) have been especially successful. A person receiving anticancer drugs may also need to take antinausea medication, sedatives, and antidiarrhea medication to combat the side effects.

New treatments for Hodgkin's disease include high-dose chemotherapy with bone marrow transplantation or transfusions of peripheral blood stem cells.

What can a person with Hodgkin's disease do?

If you'll receive radiation or chemotherapy as an outpatient, take the following precautions:
- Watch for and promptly report side effects of radiation and chemotherapy — particularly appetite loss, nausea, vomiting, diarrhea, fever, and bleeding.

How cancer treatment can affect your life

Will I become bald during treatment?
That depends on the treatment you receive. If you get radiation therapy, you'll lose some or all of the hair in the treatment area. You'll lose hair on your head if you receive mantle radiation, which extends into the back of the neck to include all the lymph nodes. Some people report that their roots ache a few days before the hair starts to fall out. After treatment, your hair will grow back slowly but may never completely return.

If you undergo chemotherapy, you'll lose hair on your head and possibly your eyelashes, eyebrows, and body hair. It may fall out slowly or rapidly 1 to 2 weeks after your first treatment. Once chemotherapy ends, and occasionally before, the hair starts growing back, possibly in a slightly different color or texture.

Consider shopping for a wig, hat, scarf, or turban before treatment begins.

Will I still be able to have children after treatment?
Some men who undergo radiation therapy and chemotherapy remain fertile and produce healthy sperm. Others become sterile.

Men who undergo pelvic radiation or chemotherapy may stop producing sperm. So you may want to consider banking sperm before treatment. Unfortu-nately, men with Hodgkin's disease sometimes have a low sperm count. Ask your doctor to evaluate whether sperm banking is feasible.

Treatment also may impair fertility in women. Pelvic radiation can cause sterility. Techniques used to protect the ovaries include shielding them with custom blocks and ovariopexy, an operation to move the ovaries out of the treatment field. Chemotherapy may cause ovarian dysfunction, which is usually temporary.

Not every woman becomes sterile during treatment, so be sure to use a reliable form of birth control during treatment. If you were to become pregnant, the fetus could have severe defects.

Will radiation harm my skin?
After therapy, irradiated skin may feel sore or sensitive. Don't apply soap, deodorant, lotion, perfume, topical medication, or extreme heat or cold to the area. Avoid rubbing the affected skin and, if necessary, use an electric razor to shave it.

Shield the affected skin from the sun by wearing soft, lightweight clothing, and apply a sunscreen with the doctor's permission. Limit activities that might irritate the area or that cause clothing to rub against it.

- To reduce the side effects of radiation therapy, maintain proper nutrition, for example, by eating small, frequent meals of favorite foods. Drink plenty of fluids. Pace your activities to combat fatigue, and keep the skin in irradiated areas dry.
- If you get mouth sores, control pain and bleeding by using a soft toothbrush, a cotton swab, or an anesthetic mouthwash such as viscous lidocaine. (Ask your doctor to prescribe this for you.) Avoid astringent mouthwashes. Also, try applying Vaseline to your lips.
- If you're a woman of childbearing age, delay getting pregnant until you've been in prolonged remission, because radiation and chemo-

SELF-HELP

How to examine your lymph nodes

Examining the lymph nodes in your armpit, neck, and groin will help you find any enlargements early in their development. Usually, you won't be able to feel normal lymph nodes. Keep in mind, however, that enlarged nodes don't necessarily signal the return of Hodgkin's disease — nodes may become enlarged for other reasons.

To examine a lymph node, move your fingers slowly, in a circular motion, over the area. Feel with the pads of your middle three fingers.

Armpit nodes

To check the lymph nodes in your armpits, keep one arm hanging at your side, and put the opposite hand in your armpit and press firmly but gently. Using proper technique, feel down to the ribs. Repeat the examination on the other side of your body.

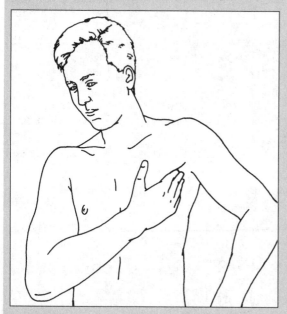

Neck nodes

Check these lymph nodes by pressing your fingers in front of and behind your ears, and into the indentation at the base of your skull. Next, feel along your jawbone and chin. Press along the neck muscles under the ear, feeling all the way down to the collarbone.

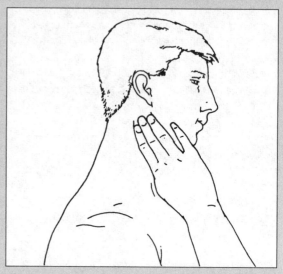

Groin nodes

Press your fingers along the crease between your hip bone and groin, feeling for any hard, painless swelling. Check both sides of your groin.

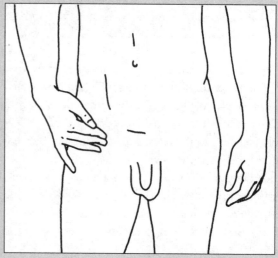

therapy can cause genetic mutations and miscarriages. (See *How cancer treatment can affect your life,* page 631.)

- If you're in remission, the doctor may instruct you to examine your lymph nodes from time to check for return of the disease. (See *How to examine your lymph nodes.*)

KAPOSI'S SARCOMA

What is this condition?

Kaposi's sarcoma is a type of cancer affecting the walls of certain lymphatic cells. Until the 1980s, doctors viewed it as a rare sarcoma (soft-tissue cancer) of the blood vessels, occurring mostly in elderly Italian and Jewish men. But the incidence of Kaposi's sarcoma has risen dramatically along with the incidence of AIDS. Currently, it's the most common AIDS-related cancer.

Kaposi's sarcoma causes both structural and functional damage. When associated with AIDS, it has an aggressive course, involving the lymph nodes, internal organs, and possibly the digestive tract.

What causes it?

The exact cause of Kaposi's sarcoma is unknown, but the disease may be related to suppression of the immune system. Genetic or hereditary predisposition is also suspected.

What are its symptoms?

The first sign of Kaposi's sarcoma is one or more obvious skin lesions. These lesions vary in shape and size, and their color may range from red-brown to dark purple. They are most common on the skin, inside of the cheek or mouth, lips, gums, tongue, tonsils, eyes, and eyelids. Besides the skin, Kaposi's sarcoma may affect the lungs, gastrointestinal tract, and other areas.

When the disease advances, the lesions may join, becoming one large plaque, or patch. Untreated lesions may look like large, craterlike masses. Other signs and symptoms include:

- pain (if the sarcoma advances beyond the early stages or if a lesion breaks down or presses on nerves or organs)
- swelling caused by clogged lymphatic channels

The incidence of Kaposi's sarcoma has risen dramatically along with the incidence of AIDS. Currently, it's the most common AIDS-related cancer.

- shortness of breath or difficulty breathing (if the disease affects respiratory structures), wheezing, slow and shallow breathing, and respiratory distress
- digestive problems.

How is it diagnosed?

The doctor performs a tissue biopsy (removal and analysis of tissue from the lesion) to identify the type and stage of the lesion. Then the person may undergo a computed tomography scan (commonly called a CAT scan) to detect and evaluate possible disease spread.

How is it treated?

Treatment isn't indicated for all cases of Kaposi's sarcoma. But if the disease is progressing quickly and the lesions are cosmetically offensive or painful or if they're blocking vital functions, the person should get treatment.

Treatment options include radiation therapy, chemotherapy, and biotherapy (administration of drugs called *biological response modifiers*). Radiation therapy eases symptoms, including pain from obstructing lesions in the mouth, throat, arms, or legs and swelling caused by lymphatic blockage. It may also be used to improve the person's appearance.

Chemotherapy includes combinations of the drugs doxorubicin, vinblastine, vincristine, and etoposide (VP-16).

Biotherapy with interferon alfa-2b may be prescribed for AIDS-related Kaposi's sarcoma. This treatment reduces the number of skin lesions but isn't effective in advanced disease.

KIDNEY CANCER

What do doctors call this condition?

Nephrocarcinoma, renal cell carcinoma, hypernephroma, Grawitz's tumor

What is this condition?

Kidney cancer usually occurs in older adults. About 85% of the tumors arise in the kidneys; others result from cancer spread from other primary sites. Certain types of kidney cancer (renal pelvic tumors and Wilms' tumor) occur mainly in children.

Most kidney tumors are large, firm, nodular, enclosed, and solitary and affect only one kidney. They can be classified as clear cell, granular, or spindle cell type.

Depending on the disease stage, some people with kidney cancer can live 5 years or longer.

What causes it?

The causes of kidney cancer aren't known. However, this cancer is being seen more often, possibly because of exposure to environmental carcinogens and increased longevity. Even so, this cancer accounts for only about 2% of all adult cancers. Kidney cancer affects twice as many men as women and usually strikes after age 40.

Kidney cancer is being seen more often, possibly because of increased exposure to environmental carcinogens and greater longevity.

What are its symptoms?

The three classic symptoms of kidney cancer are blood in the urine, pain, and a mass that can be felt. But any one of these may be the first sign of cancer. All three findings coexist in only about 10% of people with kidney cancer.

Constant stomach or flank pain may be dull or, if the cancer causes bleeding or blood clots, acute and colicky. The mass generally is smooth, firm, and nontender.

Other symptoms include fever, increased blood pressure, increased calcium in the bloodstream, and urine retention. People with advanced disease often lose weight and have swelling in the legs, nausea, and vomiting.

How is it diagnosed?

Studies to identify kidney cancer usually include a computed tomography scan (commonly called a CAT scan), X-rays of the kidney and urinary tract, ultrasound, and nephrotomography (a specialized type of kidney X-ray) or renal angiography (X-rays of blood vessels using a contrast medium). The doctor also may order blood tests.

How is it treated?

The surgeon will remove the kidney in an operation called *radical nephrectomy.* Because the disease resists radiation, radiation therapy is used only if the cancer spreads to other regions or the lymph nodes, or if the primary tumor or sites of cancer spread can't be fully removed. In these cases, high radiation doses are used.

Chemotherapy has had only limited success against kidney cancer. Biotherapy (lymphokine-activated killer cells with recombinant interleukin-2) shows promise but causes side effects. Interferon is somewhat effective in advanced disease.

LARYNGEAL CANCER

The goal of treatment for laryngeal cancer is to eliminate the cancer and preserve speech.

What is this condition?

Laryngeal cancer is cancer of the larynx — the "voice box." It is nine times more common in males than in females and usually strikes between ages 50 and 65.

Intrinsic laryngeal cancer, which originates in a pair of folds called the *true vocal cords,* rarely spreads because underlying connective tissues lack lymph nodes. *Extrinsic laryngeal cancer,* which originates outside these structures, tends to spread early.

Laryngeal cancer is classified according to its location:
- supraglottic (false vocal cords)
- glottic (true vocal cords)
- subglottic (downward extension from the vocal cords).

What causes it?

Major factors that can lead to laryngeal cancer include smoking and alcoholism. Minor factors include chronic inhalation of noxious fumes and familial tendency.

What are its symptoms?

In intrinsic laryngeal cancer, the primary and earliest symptom is hoarseness that lasts more than 3 weeks. In extrinsic cancer, it's a lump in the throat or pain or burning in the throat when drinking citrus juice or hot liquid.

If the disease spreads to other sites, the person may have trouble swallowing, shortness of breath or difficulty breathing, a cough, enlarged lymph nodes in the neck, and pain radiating to the ear.

Understanding laryngeal cancer surgery

For most people with laryngeal cancer, treatment means surgery. The information below will help you understand the purpose, extent, and effects of the different types of surgery for this cancer.

Removing a small tumor with a laser
This procedure, performed during laryngoscopy, uses a laser beam to remove a glottic tumor that's confined to a small area — usually a single true vocal cord. The laser beam will effectively eliminate the cancerous growth. You'll retain your voice, and you can resume your usual activities shortly after the procedure, as the doctor permits.

Removing a larger tumor in one vocal cord
A laryngofissure removes larger glottic tumors confined to a single vocal cord. The surgeon makes an incision in the thyroid cartilage and removes the diseased vocal cord.

After surgery, you'll have a temporary tracheostomy and your voice may be hoarse. But the hoarseness will subside as scar tissue replaces the vocal cord.

Removing one side of the larynx
This procedure removes a widespread tumor. It involves excision of about half the thyroid cartilage and the subglottic cartilage, one false vocal cord, and one true vocal cord. Then the surgeon rebuilds the area with strap muscles.

You won't have a laryngectomy stoma but will have a temporary tracheostomy. Postoperative hoarseness will subside as scar tissue replaces the vocal cord.

Removing the top half of the larynx
This operation removes a large supraglottic tumor. The surgeon removes the top of the larynx (epiglottis, hyoid bone, and false vocal cords), leaving the true vocal cords intact.

Although you won't have a laryngectomy stoma, you will have a temporary tracheostomy to ensure a patent airway until swelling subsides. You won't lose your voice, but you may have trouble swallowing without the epiglottis.

Removing the entire larynx
A total laryngectomy removes the true vocal cords, false vocal cords, epiglottis, hyoid bone, cricoid cartilage, and two or three tracheal rings. The surgeon also may remove neighboring areas, depending on the tumor's extent. Besides treating cancer of the larynx, this operation is also performed to remove a large glottic or supraglottic tumor attached to the vocal cord.

Because the surgeon must create a permanent tracheostomy and a laryngeal stoma, you'll lose your ability to speak.

Performing radical neck dissection
When cancer spreads to surrounding tissues and glands, the surgeon extends the supraglottic or total laryngectomy to remove the lymph nodes in the neck, the sternomastoid muscle, the fascia, and the internal jugular vein.

After this operation, you'll have little muscle control and support for your head and neck. However, certain exercises will help to strengthen your accessory support muscles. This operation also causes some disfigurement of the face and neck.

How is it diagnosed?

Anyone who is hoarse for more than 2 weeks should have laryngoscopy, a procedure in which the doctor directly visualizes the larynx after inserting an instrument called an *endoscope.*

Firm diagnosis also requires xeroradiography (a special X-ray technique), biopsy, laryngeal tomography (an X-ray showing a detailed

How to strengthen your neck after surgery

Here are some exercises to help you strengthen the muscles in your neck, shoulders, and arms after surgery. You can do most of them sitting down. Try to do them twice a day, or as often as your doctor directs.

Head turns
Turn your head as far to the right as you can. Then turn it as far to the left as you can.

Head tilts
Tilt your head to the left and then to the right. Straighten your head. Next, tilt it forward and then backward.

Head circles
Tilt your head forward and try to touch your chin to your chest. Then slowly rotate your head in a circle, passing your left ear over your left shoulder, tilting your head over your back, and then passing your right ear over your right shoulder, until your chin touches your chest again. Repeat the rotation in the opposite direction.

Shoulder rolls
First, sit straight in a chair. Now roll your shoulders forward and then backward.

Shoulder lifts
Still sitting in the chair, grasp each elbow with the opposite hand. Use your hand to lift your shoulder toward your ear. Repeat with the opposite shoulder.

Arm swings and circles
Place the hand of your unaffected arm on a table or chair back for support. Let the arm on your affected side hang loosely. Now swing your affected arm forward and backward from your shoulder.
    Then swing it in a circle. Make sure that the motion comes from your shoulder joint and not from your elbow.

cross-section of the larynx), a computed tomography scan (commonly called a CAT scan), or laryngography (an X-ray of the larynx after instillation of a radiopaque substance). These studies define the tumor borders. To detect cancer spread, the doctor will take chest X-rays.

How is it treated?

Early tumors are treated with surgery or radiation; advanced tumors with surgery, radiation, and chemotherapy. Surgical procedures vary with tumor size. (See *Understanding laryngeal cancer surgery*, page 637.)

Drugs used in chemotherapy may include methotrexate, cisplatin, bleomycin, fluorouracil, and vincristine.

The treatment goal is to eliminate the cancer and preserve speech. If speech can't be preserved, the person may receive a special speech or prosthetic device. (Surgical techniques to construct a new voice box are still experimental.)

What can a person with laryngeal cancer do?

- If you're scheduled for a partial or total laryngectomy, the doctor or nurse will help you choose a temporary nonspeaking communication method (such as writing) before surgery. Be aware that right after the operation, you'll breathe through your neck and won't be able to speak. You also won't be able to smell, blow your nose, whistle, gargle, sip, or suck on a straw.

- After a partial laryngectomy, you won't be permitted to use your voice at all until the doctor allows it (usually 2 to 3 days after surgery). Then you'll be told to whisper until healing is complete.

- After a total laryngectomy, speech rehabilitation may help you to speak again. For support, contact the International Association of Laryngectomees.

- After radical neck dissection, you can do special exercises to strengthen your neck, arm, and shoulder muscles. (See *How to strengthen your neck after surgery.*)

LEUKEMIA, ACUTE

What is this condition?

In acute leukemia, white blood cell precursors called blasts multiply abnormally in the bone marrow or lymph tissue, accumulating in the peripheral blood, bone marrow, and body tissues. With treatment, some people with acute leukemia — especially children — can survive for years. For example, in acute lymphoblastic leukemia, treatment induces remissions in 90% of children and 65% of adults. Children between ages 2 and 8 have the best survival rate with intensive therapy.

What causes it?

Research suggests some predisposing factors for acute leukemia — some combination of viruses, genetic and immunologic factors, and exposure to radiation and certain chemicals.

Although experts don't know exactly how the disease comes about, they've determined that immature, nonfunctioning white blood cells seem to accumulate first in the tissue where they originate. These immature cells then spill into the bloodstream and from there infiltrate other tissues, eventually causing organ malfunction.

Answers to questions about donating bone marrow

What determines whether I can be a donor?
Tissue compatibility, for one thing. Poorly matched marrow could make the recipient gravely ill by triggering a rejection reaction in his or her immune system. Before you can donate marrow, a sample of your blood cells will be mixed and grown in a special solution with a sample of blood cells from the recipient. If cell destruction results, your tissues aren't compatible. If the cells remain healthy, they're compatible, indicating that you may be a suitable donor.

Is the procedure risky?
The risk of serious complications is quite small. And no irreversible complications or deaths have been reported among bone marrow donors. To protect your-self from a blood-borne disease, you may want to bank 1 or 2 units of your own blood. These could be used in the unlikely event of complications.

Will I have any bone marrow left?
Yes. In fact, the doctor removes only about 5% of your bone marrow cells. Your body makes marrow cells quickly, so the amount you donate will be replaced within a few weeks. Just a few days after the procedure, you should feel like your old self again.

Will the procedure hurt?
You'll probably feel some stiffness and tenderness for a day or two, but you'll receive medications to relieve it.

Acute leukemia is more common in males than in females, in whites (especially people of Jewish descent), in children (between ages 2 and 5), and in people living in urban and industrialized areas.

What are its symptoms?

Typically, the person has a sudden high fever with abnormal bleeding, such as nosebleeds, bleeding gums, tiny purple or red spots, easy bruising after minor trauma, and prolonged menstrual periods. Vague symptoms, such as low-grade fever, weakness, and lack of energy, may persist for days or months before visible symptoms appear. The person also may be pale and have chills and recurrent infections. In addition, certain types of acute leukemia may cause shortness of breath, anemia, fatigue, malaise, a rapid heart rate, palpitations, a heart murmur, and stomach or bone pain.

How is it diagnosed?

The doctor diagnoses acute leukemia from the person's history, physical examination findings, and analysis of a bone marrow sample that indicates proliferation of immature white blood cells. If this sample is free of leukemic cells, a bone marrow biopsy (removal and analysis of a bone marrow sample) is performed.

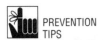
PREVENTION
TIPS

How to avoid infection

If you or someone you know has leukemia, the simple steps described below will help protect against infection.

Follow your doctor's directions
- Take all medications exactly as prescribed. Don't discontinue your medication unless your doctor tells you to do so.
- Keep all medical appointments so that your doctor can monitor your progress and the drug's effects.
- If you need to go to another doctor or to a dentist, be sure to explain that you're receiving an immunosuppressant drug.
- Wear a medical identification bracelet that states you take an immunosuppressant drug.

Avoid sources of infection
- To minimize your exposure to infections, avoid crowds and people who have colds, flu, chicken pox, shingles, or other contagious illnesses.
- Don't receive any vaccinations without checking with your doctor, especially live-virus vaccines such as the polio vaccine. These contain weakened but living viruses that can cause illness in anyone who's taking

an immunosuppressant drug. Similarly, avoid contact with anyone who has recently been vaccinated.
- Examine your mouth and skin daily for lesions, cuts, or rashes.
- Wash your hands thoroughly before preparing food. To avoid ingesting harmful organisms, thoroughly wash and cook all food before you eat it.

Recognize hazards
- Learn to recognize the early signs and symptoms of infection: sore throat, fever, chills, or a tired or sluggish feeling. Call your doctor *immediately* if you think you're coming down with an infection.
- Treat minor skin injuries with triple antibiotic ointment. If the injury is a deep one or if it becomes swollen, red, or tender, call your doctor at once.

Perform routine hygiene
- Practice good oral and personal hygiene, especially hand washing. Report any mouth sores or ulcerations to your doctor.
- Don't use commercial mouthwashes because their high alcohol and sugar content may irritate your mouth and provide a medium for bacterial growth.

The doctor will order blood studies, which typically show too few platelets (blood cells that allow clotting) and too few neutrophils (a type of white blood cell). To see if the meninges are involved, the doctor may do a spinal tap.

How is it treated?

The doctor will recommend chemotherapy to kill leukemic cells and induce remission. Chemotherapy varies with the type of leukemia present.

A bone marrow transplant may be possible. (See *Answers to questions about donating bone marrow.*) Treatment also may include antibiotic, antifungal, and antiviral drugs and injections of granulocytes (a type of white blood cell) to control infection. Some people also get transfusions of platelets to prevent bleeding and of red blood cells to prevent anemia.

What can a person with acute leukemia do?

▪ Watch for and report symptoms of infection (fever, chills, cough, sore throat) and abnormal bleeding (bruising, tiny purple or red spots). If bleeding occurs, apply pressure or ice compresses to the area. (See *How to avoid infection,* page 641.)

▪ Eat and drink high-calorie, high-protein foods and beverages to maintain good nutrition during treatment. However, be aware that chemotherapy and prednisone may cause weight gain.

▪ To prevent constipation, drink plenty of fluids, use stool softeners if needed, and walk regularly.

▪ If you get mouth sores, use a soft toothbrush and avoid hot, spicy foods and use of commercial mouthwashes.

LEUKEMIA, CHRONIC GRANULOCYTIC

What do doctors call this condition?

Doctors also call this condition chronic myelogenous leukemia and chronic myelocytic leukemia.

What is this condition?

In chronic granulocytic leukemia (CGL), precursors to certain white blood cells called *granulocytes* multiply abnormally in the bone marrow, blood, and body tissues. It is most common in young and middle-aged adults (rare in children) and is slightly more common in men than women. In the United States, CGL accounts for roughly 20% of all diagnosed cases of leukemia.

There are two distinct phases of the disease: an *insidious chronic phase,* with anemia and bleeding abnormalities, and an *acute phase* (blastic crisis), in which myeloblasts (the most primitive granulocytic precursors) multiply rapidly. No cure exists for this disease — at least not yet.

What causes it?

Experts believe that this disease is caused by an unidentified virus. It is notable that most people with CGL have a chromosomal abnormality called the *Philadelphia chromosome,* which may be caused by radiation and carcinogenic chemicals.

What are its symptoms?

Typical symptoms include:

- anemia (marked by fatigue, weakness, decreased exercise tolerance, pallor, shortness of breath, rapid heart rate, and headache)
- a low platelet count, with resulting bleeding and clotting disorders such as retinal hemorrhage, blood in the urine, black tarry stools, bleeding gums, nosebleeds, and easy bruising
- an enlarged liver and spleen, with abdominal discomfort and pain.

Other common symptoms include tenderness in the ribs and sternum, low-grade fever, weight loss, loss of appetite, gouty arthritis, occasional prolonged infection and ankle swelling and, rarely, prolonged or constant erection of the penis.

How is it diagnosed?

Lab tests, including chromosomal analysis, confirm a diagnosis of CGL. Blood tests usually reveal changes in white blood cells and other abnormalities. A test called *bone marrow aspiration* shows the effect of the disorder on bone cells. A computed tomography scan (commonly called a CAT scan) may identify the organs affected by leukemia.

How is it treated?

Even with chemotherapy, doctors have had little success in producing remissions in people with CGL. The goal of treatment during the chronic phase is to control the proliferation of white blood cells and platelets by giving drugs. The most commonly used oral drugs are busulfan and hydroxyurea. Aspirin is commonly given to prevent stroke if the person's platelet count is especially high.

Other potentially helpful treatments include:

- radiation therapy of the spleen or removal of the spleen to increase the platelet count and limit the complications of spleen enlargement
- leukapheresis (selective leukocyte removal) to reduce the white blood cell count
- allopurinol, a drug that helps prevent excess uric acid in the blood, or colchicine, a drug that relieves gout caused by elevated uric acid levels
- prompt treatment of infections (chemotherapy may cause bone marrow suppression, which can lead to infection).

During the acute phase of CGL, lymphoblastic or myeloblastic leukemia may develop. Treatment is similar to that for acute lymphoblastic leukemia. A bone marrow transplant may produce long peri-

SELF-HELP

Advice for the person with chronic granulocytic leukemia

Avoid complications

• To help prevent lung problems, perform coughing and deep-breathing exercises as instructed by your doctor.

• Call your doctor if you have symptoms of an infection: any fever over 100° F (37.8° C), chills, redness or swelling, sore throat, and cough.

• Be sure to get adequate rest to reduce fatigue.

• If you're receiving chemotherapy, eat a high-calorie, high-protein diet.

Reduce your risk of bleeding

• Don't take aspirin and aspirin-containing products because they increase the risk of bleeding.

• To minimize bleeding, use a soft-bristle toothbrush and an electric razor.

• Immediately apply ice and pressure to any bleeding site.

ods without symptoms in the early phase of illness but has been less successful in the acute phase. (See *Advice for the person with chronic granulocytic leukemia*.)

LEUKEMIA, CHRONIC LYMPHOCYTIC

What is this condition?

Chronic lymphocytic leukemia (CLL) is a generalized, progressive cancer marked by an uncontrollable spread of abnormal, small lymphocytes (a type of white blood cell) in lymphoid tissue, blood, and bone marrow. Older males have the highest risk (almost all cases involve men over age 50). According to the American Cancer Society, CLL accounts for almost one-third of new leukemia cases annually.

What causes it?

Although the cause of CLL is unknown, researchers suspect hereditary factors (a higher incidence has been recorded within families), still-undefined chromosome abnormalities, and certain immunologic defects. The disease doesn't seem to be associated with radiation exposure.

What are its symptoms?

CLL is the most benign and the most slowly progressing form of leukemia. In early stages, people usually complain of fatigue, malaise, fever, and lymph node enlargement. They're particularly susceptible to infection.

In advanced stages, they may experience severe fatigue and weight loss, with liver or spleen enlargement, bone tenderness, and swelling from lymph node blockage. Pulmonary infiltrates may appear when lung tissue is involved. Skin spots and nodules occur in about 50% of people with CLL.

As the disease progresses, bone marrow involvement may lead to anemia, pallor, weakness, shortness of breath, an increased heart rate, palpitations, bleeding, and infection. Opportunistic fungal, viral, and bacterial infections commonly occur in late stages.

How is it diagnosed?

Typically, CLL is an incidental finding during a routine blood test that reveals numerous abnormal lymphocytes. In early stages, the white blood cell count is mildly but persistently elevated. A reduced level of granulocytes (a type of white blood cell) is typical, but the white blood cell count climbs as the disease progresses. Also, bone marrow biopsy shows lymphocytic invasion.

How is it treated?

Chemotherapy includes alkylating agents, usually chlorambucil or cyclophosphamide, and sometimes steroids (prednisone). When CLL causes obstruction or organ impairment or enlargement, local radiation treatment can be used to reduce organ size. (See *Advice for the person with chronic lymphocytic leukemia*.)

LIVER CANCER

What do doctors call this condition?

Primary or metastatic hepatic carcinoma

What is this condition?

Liver cancer is more common in men (particularly those over age 60) than women and its incidence increases with age. Primary tumors (those arising in the liver itself) are called *hepatomas*. However, most cases of liver cancer are the result of metastasis (the spread of cancer from another area) from the intestine, rectum, stomach, pancreas, esophagus, lung, breast, or skin. In the United States, metastatic liver cancer is 20 times more common than primary liver cancer.

No cure exists at this time.

What causes it?

The cause of primary liver cancer is unknown, but it may be a congenital disease in children. In adults, it may result from exposure to environmental carcinogens and possibly androgens and oral estrogens.

Notably, 30% to 70% of people with hepatomas also have cirrhosis, a chronic degenerative liver disease. (Hepatomas are 40 times more likely to develop in a cirrhotic liver than in a normal one.) Researchers aren't sure if cirrhosis is a precancerous state or if alcohol and malnutrition predispose a person to develop hepatomas.

Another risk factor is exposure to the hepatitis B virus, although this risk will probably decrease with the availability of the hepatitis B vaccine.

What are its symptoms?

Liver cancer may cause:

- weight loss, weakness, appetite loss, fever
- a mass in the right upper part of the abdomen
- tenderness in the liver that the examiner can feel on examination
- severe pain in the center or right upper part of the abdomen
- an abnormal sound, such as a hum or rubbing sound, heard by the examiner (if the tumor involves a large part of the liver)
- jaundice or fluid buildup in the abdomen
- swelling of the feet or legs.

How is it diagnosed?

To confirm liver cancer, the doctor will remove and analyze some liver tissue — a procedure called a *liver biopsy*. If cirrhosis is present, liver cancer can be hard to diagnose; however, your doctor may order the following lab tests to aid confirmation:

- *Liver function tests* indicating abnormal liver function.
- *Alpha-fetoprotein* (a protein normally produced in the liver) at abnormally high levels.
- *Chest X-ray* may rule out cancer spread.
- *Liver scan* may show certain defects.
- *Arteriography* (a type of X-ray that visualizes arteries) may define large tumors.

Other blood tests may indicate sodium retention (causing functional kidney failure), low blood sugar, increased calcium, increased white blood cell count, or decreased cholesterol.

How is it treated?

Liver cancer is often advanced at the time of diagnosis, which means the tumor can't be removed surgically. (Only a single tumor in one liver lobe can safely be removed—if the person doesn't have cirrhosis, jaundice, or fluid buildup in the abdomen.) In this case, radiation therapy is usually done to relieve symptoms. Unfortunately, the liver has a low tolerance for radiation, so this therapy has not increased survival to date.

> *Researchers aren't sure if cirrhosis is a precancerous state or if alcohol and malnutrition predispose a person to develop liver cancer.*

Another treatment option is chemotherapy. Some people have pumps implanted in the body for long-term infusion of chemotherapy drugs on an outpatient basis.

If cancer has spread to the liver from another site, the surgeon may remove the organ or the person may get chemotherapy. For some people, liver transplantation is now an alternative.

What can a person with liver cancer do?
- Follow your prescribed diet carefully. The doctor will instruct you to restrict salt, fluids, and protein. You can't drink alcohol.
- Don't take Tylenol or other drugs that contain acetaminophen — your liver can't metabolize it.

LUNG CANCER

What is this condition?
Lung cancer usually develops within the wall or lining of the bronchial tree, the system of branching air passages within the lungs. Some people have survived for 5 years or more with diagnosed lung cancer; however, the general prognosis is poor. Although it is largely preventable, lung cancer is the most common cause of cancer death in men and is fast becoming the most common cause in women.

What causes it?
Medical experts agree that lung cancer is caused by inhalation of carcinogenic pollutants. Pollutants in tobacco smoke cause progressive damage to lung cells.

Who is most susceptible to lung cancer? Any smoker over age 40, especially if he or she began to smoke before age 15, has smoked a whole pack or more per day for 20 years, or works with or near asbestos. (See *Smoking: The chief risk factor*, page 648, and *Lung cancer: Danger in the workplace*, page 649.)

What are its symptoms?
Because lung cancer rarely causes symptoms in its early stage, this disease is often advanced at diagnosis. Late-stage respiratory symptoms typically include "smoker's cough," hoarseness, wheezing,

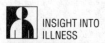

Smoking: The chief risk factor

There's no argument over smoking any longer. Study after study has confirmed that smoking dramatically increases a person's risk of lung cancer.

The hard facts

- Lung cancer is 10 times more common in smokers than in nonsmokers.
- 80% of people with lung cancer are smokers.
- The risk of lung cancer is determined by the number of cigarettes smoked daily, the depth of inhalation, how early in life a smoker started the habit, and the nicotine content of cigarettes.

Other risk factors

Two other factors can make a person more vulnerable to lung cancer:

- exposure to cancer-causing industrial and air pollutants, such as asbestos, uranium, arsenic, nickel, iron oxides, chromium, radioactive dust, and coal dust
- a family history of lung cancer.

shortness of breath, coughing up blood, chest pain, fever, weakness, weight loss, appetite loss, and shoulder pain.

Lung cancer may spread to any part of the body, most commonly to the brain and spinal cord, liver, and bone. The effects of cancer spread vary greatly depending on tumor size and location.

Hormonal effects

Lung tumors may alter the production of hormones that regulate body functions. Possible problems include:

- breast enlargement in males
- bone and joint pain from cartilage erosion due to abnormal production of growth hormone
- Cushing's syndrome (overproduction of certain steroid hormones) and carcinoid syndrome (diarrhea, cramps, flushing, skin lesions, labored breathing)
- increased calcium levels in the blood.

How is it diagnosed?

The person's symptoms and physical exam findings may strongly suggest lung cancer, but firm diagnosis requires further evidence.

- *Chest X-ray* usually shows an advanced tumor, but it can detect a tumor up to 2 years before symptoms appear. It also indicates tumor size and location.
- *Sputum cytology* (the analysis of cells in the sputum), which is 75% reliable, requires a specimen coughed up from the lungs.
- *Computed tomography scan* (commonly called a CAT scan) of the chest may help determine the tumor's size and whether it affects surrounding structures.
- *Bronchoscopy* (visual exam of the lungs using an instrument called a bronchoscope) can locate the tumor site. Specimens taken during this test provide material for cell and tissue analysis.
- *Needle biopsy* of the lungs can detect tumors in the outer portion of the lungs. This procedure allows firm diagnosis in 80% of people with lung cancer.
- *Tissue biopsy* (removal and analysis of affected tissue) can be done if the site of cancer spread is accessible.
- *Thoracentesis* (draining of fluid from the chest) allows chemical and cell analysis of pleural fluid.

Other tests to detect cancer spread include bone scan, bone marrow biopsy (removal of some bone marrow for analysis), and CAT scan of the brain or abdomen.

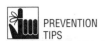
PREVENTION
TIPS

Lung cancer: Danger in the workplace

Almost everyone knows that cigarette smoking is a risk factor for lung cancer. But not everyone knows that other airborne pollutants are villains, too. In particular, exposure to industrial carcinogens can cause lung cancer, especially among smokers.

The list below can help you identify and avoid (or at least avoid exposure to) these known workplace carcinogens.

Acrylonitrile
Fiber mills (blankets, carpets, clothing, draperies, synthetic furs, and wigs)

Arsenic
Copper smelting and metallurgical industries, mines, insecticide and pesticide plants (and products), tanning factories

Asbestos
Asbestos factories (and asbestos removal work sites); insulation, rubber, and textile plants; mines and shipyards

Beryllium
Beryllium plants and electronic-parts and missile-parts factories

Cadmium
Cadmium factories; battery, chemical, jewelry, paint and pigment plants; electroplating and metallurgical industries

Coal tar pitch volatiles
Foundries, steel mills

Coke oven emissions
Coke plants, steel mills

Dimethylsulfate
Chemical, drug, and dye plants

Epichlorohydrin
Chemical plants

Hematite
Hematite mines

Mineral oils, soot, and tars
Construction sites, roofing plants (and roofs), chimney sweep businesses, heavy industry

Nickel
Nickel refineries

Vinylchloride
Plastics and vinylchloride polymer plants

Also, the doctor will stage the tumor to determine the extent of the disease, help plan treatment, and make a prognosis.

How is it treated?

Treatment — which consists of combinations of surgery, radiation, and chemotherapy — may improve the prognosis and prolong survival.

Surgery may be performed for certain types of lung cancer. It may include partial or total removal of the lung. (See *Learning about lung surgery*, page 650.)

Learning about lung surgery

If you're scheduled for surgery to remove a lung tumor, the surgeon may perform one of four procedures.

Pneumonectomy
The surgeon removes an entire cancerous lung.

Lobectomy
The surgeon removes a cancerous lobe (portion) from the lung.

Segmentectomy
By removing one or more lung segments, the surgeon attempts to preserve as much functional, healthy tissue as possible.

Wedge resection
The surgeon removes lung tissue without regard to segmental planes. This operation is reserved for small lung tumors in people with poor respiratory function.

Before surgery, the person may undergo radiation therapy to help reduce the tumor's size. Chemotherapy before radiation helps improve the person's response to radiation. Chemotherapy may involve combinations of certain drugs.

Radiation therapy may also be performed after surgery. Generally, radiation therapy is delayed until 1 month after surgery to let the wound heal. Then, radiation is directed at the part of the chest where the tumor is most likely to spread.

Radiation treatments may be the main form of treatment when surgery is not possible. Radiation implants are another possible treatment.

In laser therapy, still largely experimental, a laser beam is directed through a bronchoscope to destroy local tumors.

What can a person with lung cancer do?

If you're receiving chemotherapy and radiation, take the following steps:

- Eat soft, nonirritating foods that are high in protein. To maintain proper nutrition, eat high-calorie snacks between meals.
- To conserve your energy, alternate activity with rest periods.
- If you're receiving outpatient radiation therapy, avoid tight clothing, sun exposure, and harsh ointments on your chest. As instructed, perform exercises to help prevent shoulder stiffness.

MALIGNANT LYMPHOMAS

What do doctors call this group of conditions?

Non-Hodgkin's lymphomas, lymphosarcomas

What is this group of conditions?

Malignant lymphomas are a group of malignant diseases originating in lymph nodes and other lymphoid tissue. Nodular lymphomas have a better prognosis than the diffuse form of the disease, but in both, the prognosis is worse than in Hodgkin's disease.

What causes them?

The cause of malignant lymphoma is unknown, although some theories suggest a viral source. Up to 35,000 new cases appear annually in the United States. Malignant lymphomas are two to three times more common in men than women and occur in all age-groups (median age is 50; rare in children). Also, incidence is higher for whites, particularly people with Jewish ancestry.

What are their symptoms?

Usually, the first indication of malignant lymphoma is swelling of the lymph nodes, enlarged tonsils and adenoids, and painless, rubbery nodes in and around the neck. In children, the disease causes shortness of breath and coughing.

As the lymphoma progresses, the person develops symptoms specific to the area involved and systemic complaints of fatigue, malaise, weight loss, fever, and night sweats.

How are they diagnosed?

Biopsies of lymph nodes, tonsils, bone marrow, liver, bowel, or skin help the doctor diagnose this disorder. (Biopsy differentiates malignant lymphoma from Hodgkin's disease.)

Other tests include bone and chest X-rays, lymphangiography, liver and spleen scan, computed tomography scan (commonly called CAT scan) of the abdomen, and intravenous pyelography. Common lab tests include a complete blood count, uric acid, blood calcium, blood protein, and liver function studies.

How are they treated?

Radiation therapy is used mainly in the early localized stage of the disease. Total irradiation of lymph nodes is often effective.

Chemotherapy is most effective when combinations of drugs are used. For example, one drug protocol, called the *CHOP protocol,* includes cyclophosphamide, doxorubicin, vincristine, and prednisone.

MALIGNANT MELANOMA

What is this condition?

Malignant melanoma is a relatively rare cancer that arises from melanocytes, the skin cells that produce the pigment melanin. There are three types: *superficial spreading melanoma, nodular malignant mela-*

Usually, the first indication of malignant lymphoma is swelling of the lymph nodes, enlarged tonsils and adenoids, and painless, rubbery nodes in and around the neck.

noma, and *lentigo maligna melanoma.* Melanoma spreads through the lymphatic and vascular systems to regional lymph nodes, skin, liver, lungs, and the central nervous system.

Melanoma is slightly more common in women than in men and is rare in children. Peak incidence occurs between ages 50 and 70, although the incidence in younger age-groups is increasing.

The prognosis varies with tumor thickness and can be unpredictable. Recurrence and spread may occur 5 years or more after surgical removal of a primary lesion. Generally, surface lesions are curable; deeper lesions tend to spread. The prognosis is better for a tumor on an arm or leg than for a lesion on the head, neck, or trunk.

What causes it?

Several factors seem to influence the development of melanoma:

■ *Excessive exposure to sunlight.* Melanoma is most common in sunny, warm areas and usually develops on parts of the body that are exposed to the sun.

■ *Skin type.* Most people who get melanoma have blond or red hair, fair skin, and blue eyes; are prone to sunburn; and are of Celtic or Scandinavian ancestry. Melanoma is rare among blacks. When it does develop in blacks, it usually arises in lightly pigmented areas (the palms, soles of the feet, or mucous membranes).

■ *Hormonal factors.* Pregnancy may increase the risk and speed the growth of melanomas.

■ *Family history.* Melanoma occurs slightly more often within families.

■ *Past history of melanoma.* A person who's had one melanoma has a greater risk of developing a second.

What are its symptoms?

Common sites for melanoma are the head and neck in men, the legs in women, and the backs of people exposed to excessive sunlight. Up to 70% of cases arise from a preexisting mole. Suspect melanoma when any skin lesion or mole enlarges, changes color, becomes inflamed or sore, itches, ulcerates, bleeds, shows changes in texture, or shows signs of surrounding discoloration. Melanoma rarely appears in the eye, pharynx, mouth, vagina, or anus. (See *How to check for melanomas.*)

SELF-HELP

How to check for melanomas

How can you tell whether the spot on your skin is a malignant melanoma or a harmless mole or keratosis? Using the *ABCD* system of melanoma may help you understand the differences. Always check with your doctor if you have a suspicious lesion.

Signs of melanoma

A is for asymmetry. One half of the lesion doesn't match the other half in shape.

B is for border irregularity. The lesion's edges look ragged, uneven, or blurred.

C is for color. The color is mixed, with shades of tan, brown, and black. Dashes of red, white, and blue may add to the mottled appearance.

D is for diameter. Lesions usually grow wider than 6 millimeters (or bigger than the tip of a pencil eraser).

The lesion may be tender, itchy, or painful. Other characteristics include scaling, oozing, and bleeding.

Normal mole

Most moles are harmless, evenly colored spots, ranging from pink to dark brown. They may be flat or raised, hairy or hairless. Most moles appear in adolescence and fade with age.

Keratosis

Not a mole or a melanoma, a keratosis comes with age, growing slowly after age 40. Raised, with a waxy, crusted surface, it looks like it's stuck on the skin — commonly the back and chest and occasionally the face.

Tan, brown, or black, a keratosis rarely grows larger than 1 inch (2.5 centimeters) in diameter.

MELANOMA

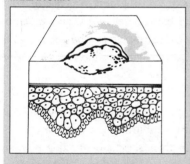

MOLE

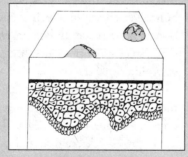

KERATOSIS

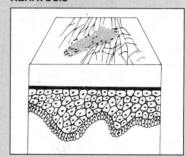

How is it diagnosed?

Skin biopsy is used to distinguish malignant melanoma from a harmless mole or other lesion and to determine tumor thickness. Physical exam (especially of lymph nodes) helps the doctor anticipate spread.

Typical lab studies include blood tests, liver function studies, and urinalysis. Depending on the tumor's depth and spread, other tests may include chest X-ray and computed tomography scans (commonly called CAT scans) of the chest, abdomen, or brain. A bone scan may be ordered if there are signs of spread to the bone.

How is it treated?

Surgical removal of the lesion is the most common treatment. If necessary, one or more regional lymph nodes may be removed as well. Deep primary lesions may require chemotherapy and biotherapy as well to eliminate or reduce the number of tumor cells. Radiation therapy is usually reserved for melanoma that has spread.

Regardless of the treatment method, melanomas require long-term follow-up care to detect any spread or recurrence.

MULTIPLE MYELOMA

What do doctors call this condition?

Doctors also call this condition malignant plasmacytoma, plasma cell myeloma, and myelomatosis.

What is this condition?

Multiple myeloma is a disseminated cancer of marrow plasma cells that infiltrates bone to produce lesions throughout the skeleton (flat bones, vertebrae, skull, pelvis, and ribs). These lesions cause destruction of bone tissue. In late stages, cancer infiltrates the body organs (liver, spleen, lymph nodes, lungs, adrenal glands, kidneys, skin, and gastrointestinal tract).

Multiple myeloma strikes about 10,000 people yearly — mostly men over age 40. Usually, the prognosis is poor because diagnosis is often made after the disease has already infiltrated the vertebrae, pelvis, skull, ribs, clavicles, and sternum. By then, skeletal destruction is widespread and, without treatment, leads to vertebral collapse. However, early diagnosis and treatment prolong the lives of many people by 3 to 5 years.

What are its symptoms?

The earliest symptom of multiple myeloma is severe, constant back pain that increases with exercise. Arthritic symptoms may also occur: achiness, joint swelling, and tenderness, possibly from compression of the vertebrae. Other effects include fever, malaise, slight evidence of peripheral neuropathy (such as tingling in the fingers or toes), and pathologic fractures.

As multiple myeloma progresses, symptoms of vertebral compression may become acute, accompanied by anemia, weight loss, chest deformities (ballooning), and loss of body height — 5 inches (13 centimeters) or more—due to vertebral collapse. Kidney complications such as inflammation may occur. Severe, recurrent infection, such as pneumonia, may follow damage to nerves associated with respiratory function.

How is it diagnosed?

After the physical exam and careful review of the individual's medical history, the doctor orders diagnostic tests of blood, urine studies, and bone marrow. Additional studies that help confirm a diagnosis of multiple myeloma include serum electrophoresis, intravenous pyelography (to investigate kidney involvement), and X-rays of the skull, pelvis, and spine.

How is it treated?

Long-term treatment of multiple myeloma consists mainly of chemotherapy to suppress plasma cell growth and control pain. Local radiation given in addition to chemotherapy reduces acute lesions, such as collapsed vertebrae, and relieves localized pain.

Other treatments usually include a combination of melphalan and prednisone as well as analgesics for pain. For spinal cord compression, the person may require an operation to remove part of the affected vertebrae; for kidney complications, dialysis.

Because the person may have bone demineralization and may lose large amounts of calcium into the blood and urine, he or she is a prime candidate for kidney stones, nephrocalcinosis, and, eventually, kidney failure due to excessive calcium in the blood. To decrease calcium levels in the blood, the person may be given fluids, diuretics, corticosteroids, oral phosphate, and intravenous mithramycin.

The prognosis for multiple myeloma is poor; however, early diagnosis and treatment prolong the lives of many people by 3 to 5 years.

OVARIAN CANCER

What is this condition?

This cancer attacks the ovaries, the organs in women that produce the hormones estrogen and progesterone. There are three main types of ovarian cancer: primary epithelial tumors (accounting for 90% of all ovarian cancers), germ cell tumors, and sex cord (stromal) tumors.

Prognosis depends on the type of cancer cell and the disease stage. Unfortunately, there are few early warning signs and the disease is often advanced by the time it's diagnosed. About 40% of women with ovarian cancer survive for 5 years.

What causes it?

The exact cause of ovarian cancer isn't known. Risk factors include a family history of ovarian, breast, or uterine cancer; infertility; celibacy; exposure to asbestos, talc, or industrial pollutants; and a high-fat diet.

Ovarian cancer spreads rapidly throughout the abdominal cavity and, occasionally, through the lymphatic system and the bloodstream. Generally, when it spreads outside the abdomen, it enters the chest cavity, where it may cause abnormal fluid buildup in the lungs. Spread to other sites is rare.

What are its symptoms?

Typically, symptoms vary with tumor size. Some women with early-stage disease experience vague stomach upset. As the cancer develops, symptoms become more distinct, including frequent urination, constipation, pelvic discomfort, and weight loss. In advanced disease fluid builds up in the abdomen. If the tumor ruptures or becomes twisted or infected, it may cause pain. In young women, this pain may be mistaken for appendicitis. Some older women experience postmenopausal bleeding and pain.

Some types of tumors cause feminizing effects, such as bleeding between periods in premenopausal women; other types cause masculinizing effects, such as developing masculine secondary sex characteristics. Ovarian cancer that has spread to other sites may cause different symptoms.

How is it diagnosed?

The doctor performs a pelvic exam and takes a complete history. Before surgery, the doctor will take a Pap smear (although this is positive in few women with ovarian cancer) and will order many different diagnostic tests. For example, a woman may undergo abdominal ultrasound, a computed tomography scan (commonly called a CAT scan), or X-rays. A test called *lymphangiography* (a special X-ray of the lymphatic system) helps to investigate lymph node involvement. Mammography may be used to rule out primary breast cancer.

Usually, a surgeon performs exploratory surgery, taking cell and tissue samples for analysis.

How is it treated?

Treatment involves a combination of surgery, chemotherapy and, in rare cases, radiation therapy — depending on the woman's age and the disease stage. In most cases, treatment is aggressive: the surgeon removes the uterus, both fallopian tubes, both ovaries, the omentum (part of the abdominal wall lining), and the appendix. If the tumor has matted around other organs or spread to other vital organs, complete removal of the tumor is impossible.

In rare instances, for example — a young woman with an encapsulated tumor in one ovary — the surgeon may elect to remove only the diseased ovary.

Chemotherapy can prolong life in most women with ovarian cancer, but in those with advanced disease, it can only relieve symptoms. However, prolonged remissions are being achieved in some women.

Radiation therapy is generally not used for ovarian cancer because it depresses the bone marrow, which could make chemotherapy less effective. Radioisotopes have been used as secondary therapy, but they can cause intestinal problems such as blockages.

Intravenous administration of drugs called *biological response modifiers* — interleukin-2, interferon, and monoclonal antibodies — is currently being investigated.

> *With the help of chemotherapy, some women with ovarian cancer are achieving prolonged remissions.*

What can a woman with ovarian cancer do?

If you are premenopausal and must have both ovaries removed, be aware that you'll have an early menopause and may experience hot flashes, headaches, palpitations, insomnia, depression, and excessive perspiration.

PANCREATIC CANCER

What do doctors call this condition?

Pancreatic carcinoma

What is this condition?

This cancer strikes the pancreas — the gland in the back of the abdomen that secretes insulin and digestive enzymes. Fish-shaped, the pancreas is divided into segments known as the *head, body,* and *tail.* It also contains about 1 million cell clusters called the *islets of Langerhans*, which produce insulin and glucagon.

Pancreatic cancer progresses rapidly. Most pancreatic tumors arise in the head of the pancreas. Rarely, they arise in the body, tail, and islet cells.

Pancreatic cancer occurs most commonly in men between ages 35 and 70. The incidence is highest in Israel, the United States, Sweden, and Canada.

What causes it?

Experts believe pancreatic cancer may be linked to inhalation or absorption of the following carcinogens, which are then excreted by the pancreas:

- cigarettes
- foods high in fat and protein
- food additives
- industrial chemicals, such as benzidine and urea.

Possible predisposing factors are chronic pancreatitis (inflammation of the pancreas), diabetes, and chronic alcohol abuse.

What are its symptoms?

The most common symptoms of pancreatic cancer are weight loss, pain in the stomach or lower back, jaundice, and diarrhea. Other generalized effects include fever, skin lesions (usually on the legs), and emotional disturbances, such as depression, anxiety, and premonition of fatal illness.

How is it diagnosed?

Confirming a diagnosis of pancreatic cancer involves exploratory surgery and biopsy (tissue removal for analysis). Additional lab studies of blood, urine, and stools help confirm a diagnosis. Other common diagnostic tests include:

- *ultrasound* to identify an abdominal mass
- *computed tomography scan* (commonly called a CAT scan), which shows greater detail than ultrasound
- *angiography* (a special X-ray of the heart and blood vessels) to determine the tumor's blood supply
- *endoscopic retrograde cholangiopancreatography* (X-ray examination of the bile ducts and pancreas), which permits visual inspection and specimen biopsy
- *magnetic resonance imaging* (commonly called MRI) to help determine tumor size and location.

Experts suspect pancreatic cancer is linked to inhalation or absorption of various carcinogens — including cigarettes, foods high in fat and protein, food additives, and certain industrial chemicals — which are then excreted by the pancreas.

How is it treated?

Pancreatic cancer is hard to treat because it is usually widespread by the time it's diagnosed. Treatment involves surgery and, in some cases, radiation therapy and chemotherapy. Surgical options include:
- removing the entire pancreas (may improve survival)
- joining the gallbladder and common bile duct with portions of the small intestine (rather than removing the entire pancreas), which prevents side effects of jaundice and severe itching
- Whipple's operation (rare) to remove the head of the pancreas, the duodenum, and portions of the body and tail of the pancreas, stomach, jejunum, pancreatic duct, and portions of the bile duct
- linking the stomach to part of the small intestine, if total pancreas removal isn't recommended and the doctor expects duodenal blockage to develop later.

Although pancreatic cancer generally responds poorly to chemotherapy, recent studies using combinations of fluorouracil, streptozocin, ifosfamide, and doxorubicin show a trend toward prolonging survival time. (See *Drugs used in the fight against pancreatic cancer.*)

Radiation therapy is usually ineffective except to aid chemotherapy or relieve symptoms.

What can a person with pancreatic cancer do?

This disease may cause pronounced itching. To prevent skin scratches, keep your nails clipped and wear cotton gloves.

PITUITARY TUMORS

What causes this condition?

Pituitary tumors are abnormal growths in the pituitary gland — a small gland within the brain that secretes various hormones. These tumors, which make up 10% of cancers in the skull, originate most often in the front of the pituitary (called the *adenohypophysis*). They occur in adults of both sexes, usually during the third and fourth decades of life. The prognosis is fair to good, depending on the extent of tumor spread.

Drugs used in the fight against pancreatic cancer

In addition to chemotherapy drugs, the following medications may be prescribed for patients with pancreatic cancer.

Antibiotics
Oral, intravenous, or intramuscular antibiotics may be used to prevent infection and relieve symptoms.

Anticholinergics
These drugs help to decrease gastrointestinal spasms and motility and reduce pain and secretions.

Antacids
Given by mouth or nasogastric tube, antacids help to limit damage to the stomach lining.

Diuretics
These drugs help to remove fluid in the abdomen.

Insulin
The insulin supply needs a boost after pancreas removal.

Narcotics
If analgesics fail to relieve pain, narcotics may be administered.

Pancreatic enzymes
These agents help to improve digestion of proteins, carbohydrates, and fats.

Advice for a person with a pituitary tumor

- Be aware that you'll need life-long evaluations and, possibly, hormone replacement.
- Know that altered sexual drive, impotence, infertility, loss of hair, and emotional lability typically disappear with treatment.
- If your vision has been affected, be aware that you'll probably recover your sight.
- If you've had transsphenoidal surgery, expect to lose your sense of smell.
- Buy and wear a medical identification bracelet or necklace that identifies your hormone deficiencies and their proper treatment.

What causes it?

Although the exact cause is unknown, a predisposition to pituitary tumors may be inherited.

What are its symptoms?

As a pituitary adenoma grows, it enlarges the sella turcica, which contains the pituitary gland. Symptoms reflect the tumor's effect on both neurologic and endocrine function.

Neurologic symptoms

- Headache
- Blurred vision progressing to visual field defects and then blindness in one eye
- Eye or gaze deviation, double vision, nystagmus, ptosis, limited eye movement
- Increased pressure inside the skull
- Personality changes or dementia
- Seizures
- Runny nose
- Hemorrhage in the pituitary gland, possibly causing both cardiovascular and adrenocortical collapse

Endocrine symptoms

- Cessation of menses, reduced sex drive, impotence, discolored or waxy skin or fewer wrinkles, loss of armpit and pubic hair, lack of energy, weakness, easily fatigued, cold intolerance, constipation
- Addisonian crisis precipitated by stress and resulting in nausea, vomiting, low blood sugar, decreased blood pressure, circulatory collapse
- Diabetes insipidus
- Galactorrhea, acromegaly, and Cushing's syndrome

How is it diagnosed?

- *Skull X-rays* with tomography show enlargement of the sella turcica or erosion of its floor; if growth hormone secretion predominates, X-rays show enlarged paranasal sinuses and mandible, thickened cranial bones, and separated teeth.
- *Carotid angiography* shows displacement of the anterior cerebral and internal carotid arteries if the tumor is enlarging; it also rules out intracerebral aneurysm.
- *Computed tomography scan* (commonly called a CAT scan) may confirm the existence of the adenoma and accurately depict its size.

- *Cerebrospinal fluid analysis* may show increased protein levels.
- *Endocrine function tests* may contribute helpful information, but results are often ambiguous and inconclusive.

How is it treated?

Surgical options include transfrontal removal of a large tumor impinging on the optic apparatus and transsphenoidal resection for a smaller tumor confined to the pituitary fossa.

Radiation is the primary treatment for small, nonsecretory tumors that don't extend beyond the sella turcica or for people who may be poor surgical risks; otherwise, it's used as an adjunct to surgery.

Postoperative treatment includes hormone replacement with cortisone, thyroid hormone, and sex hormones; correction of electrolyte imbalances; and insulin therapy as needed.

Drug therapy may include bromocriptine, which shrinks prolactin-secreting and growth hormone-secreting tumors, and cyproheptadine, which can reduce corticosteroid levels in the person with Cushing's syndrome.

Adjuvant radiation therapy is used when only partial removal of the tumor is possible. Freezing the area with a probe inserted transsphenoidally is a promising alternative to surgical dissection of the tumor. (See *Advice for a person with a pituitary tumor.*)

PROSTATE CANCER

What is this condition?

This cancer affects the prostate — the chestnut-sized gland in males that surrounds the neck of the bladder and urethra (the structure that drains urine from the bladder). Prostate cancer is the second most common cancer in men over age 50.

Most prostate cancers arise in the rear portion of the prostate gland; the rest originate near the urethra. Prostate cancer rarely results from the benign enlargement that commonly develops around the prostatic urethra in older men.

Prostate cancer accounts for about 18% of all cancers. It's most common in Blacks and least common in Asians. Its incidence increases with age more rapidly than any other cancer.

What you should know about prostate surgery

Before surgery

A nurse or other staff member will teach you how to do perineal exercises 1 to 10 times an hour. In these exercises, you squeeze the buttocks together, hold this position for a few seconds, then relax. You should do perineal exercises within 24 to 48 hours after surgery.

After surgery

▪ You'll have a urinary catheter. Take care not to pull on it because this could cause kinks and blockages.

▪ Be aware that you may be impotent and incontinent.

What causes it?

Researchers haven't found a definite link between prostate cancer and increased levels of androgens (male hormones), although androgens regulate prostate growth and function and may speed tumor growth.

What are its symptoms?

Prostate cancer seldom causes symptoms until it's advanced. Symptoms include difficulty starting a urine stream; urine dribbling or retention; urinary pain, frequency, or urgency; and, rarely, blood in the urine.

How is it diagnosed?

The doctor will perform a manual rectal exam, which may reveal a small, hard mass, or nodule. The American Cancer Society advises a yearly rectal exam for men over age 40, a yearly blood test to detect prostate-specific antigen (PSA) in men over age 50, and ultrasound if results are abnormal.

Biopsy confirms the diagnosis. Magnetic resonance imaging (commonly called MRI), a computed tomography scan (commonly called a CAT scan), and special X-rays of the urinary tract may also aid diagnosis.

How is it treated?

The preferred treatment depends on symptoms, the person's tolerance for therapy and expected life span, and the disease stage. Care is taken when choosing a treatment method, because older men (commonly affected) typically have other disorders, such as high blood pressure, diabetes, or heart disease.

Generally, treatment includes surgery to remove the prostate, and occasionally one or both testicles, radiation therapy, and hormone therapy. Radiation therapy is also used to cure some invasive tumors and to relieve pain from cancer spread to bone.

If hormone therapy, surgery, and radiation therapy aren't feasible or successful, chemotherapy may be tried. However, current drug therapy offers limited benefit. Combining several treatment methods may be most effective. (See *What you should know about prostate surgery*.)

SPINAL TUMOR

What is this condition?

The spinal cord is the cord of nervous tissue that extends from your brain down your back through a canal inside your vertebrae. A spinal tumor can occur anywhere along the length of the spinal cord or its roots. If untreated, it can eventually cause paralysis.

A primary spinal tumor may originate within the cord itself, the vertebrae, or the cord's protective layers. A tumor that's located within the cord is called an *intramedullary* tumor and one that's located outside the spinal cord is called an *extramedullary* tumor. An extramedullary tumor produces symptoms by pressing on the nerve roots, the spinal cord, and the spinal vessels.

A spinal tumor can also occur when a primary tumor from another site, such as the breasts, lungs, or prostate, spreads to the spine.

What causes it?

Spinal tumors are rare. Their cause is not yet known.

What are its symptoms?

The precise symptoms depend on what part of the spinal cord and which nerves are damaged by the tumor. Symptoms common to all spinal cord tumors include:
- pain — most severe directly over the tumor; radiates around the trunk or down the limb on the affected side, and is unrelieved by rest
- spastic muscle weakness, decreased muscle tone, exaggerated reflexes
- loss of the sensations of pain, temperature, and touch on the side of the body opposite the tumor (Brown-Séquard syndrome)
- constipation
- incomplete emptying of the bladder or difficulty with the urinary stream (an early sign of spinal cord compression)
- urine retention (an inevitable late sign with spinal cord compression)
- loss of bladder and bowel control with some tumors.

How is it diagnosed?

Tests to confirm a diagnosis of a spinal cord tumor include spinal tap to investigate spinal fluid flow and spinal X-rays to assess distortions in the cord and changes in vertebrae. Myelography determines the anatomic relationship of the tumor to the cord and the dura (the cord's outermost membrane). Computed tomography scan (commonly called a CAT scan) reveals cord compression and tumor location. Radioisotope bone scan is used to confirm spread of the cancer to the vertebrae. Frozen section biopsy, performed during surgery, helps identify the type of tumor.

How is it treated?

Treatment of a spinal tumor generally includes decompression or radiation. Laminectomy (an operation that relieves spinal cord compression) may be performed for a primary tumor. If the tumor is slowly progressive or if it's treated before the cord degenerates, symptoms may disappear, and the person may achieve complete restoration of function.

Tumors that spread to the cord from other sites may be controlled with radiation, analgesics and, in the case of hormone-mediated tumors (breast and prostate), appropriate hormone therapy.

Transcutaneous electrical nerve stimulation may control spinal root pain from spinal tumors and is a useful alternative to narcotics. In this procedure, an electrical charge is applied to the skin to stimulate large-diameter nerve fibers and thereby inhibit transmission of pain impulses through small-diameter nerve fibers.

Transcutaneous electrical nerve stimulation may control pain from spinal tumors and is a useful alternative to narcotics.

SQUAMOUS CELL CANCER

What do doctors call this condition?

Squamous cell carcinoma

What is this condition?

Squamous cell cancer of the skin is an invasive tumor with the potential to spread. It occurs most often in fair-skinned white men over age 60. Outdoor employment and residence in a sunny, warm climate (southwestern United States and Australia, for example) greatly increase the risk of developing squamous cell cancer.

What causes it?

Predisposing factors include overexposure to the sun's ultraviolet rays, the presence of premalignant lesions (such as actinic keratosis or

Bowen's disease), X-ray therapy, ingestion of herbicides containing arsenic, chronic skin irritation and inflammation, exposure to local carcinogens (such as tar and oil), and hereditary diseases (such as xeroderma pigmentosum and albinism). (See *How to lessen your risk of squamous cell cancer.*) Rarely, squamous cell cancer may develop on the site of smallpox vaccination, psoriasis, or chronic discoid lupus.

What are its symptoms?

Squamous cell cancer commonly develops on the skin of the face, the ears, the back of the hands and forearms, and other sun-damaged areas. Lesions on sun-damaged skin tend to be less invasive and less likely to spread than lesions on unexposed skin. Notable exceptions to this tendency are squamous cell lesions on the lower lip and the ears. These are almost always invasive spreading lesions with a generally poor prognosis.

Transformation from a premalignant lesion to squamous cell cancer may begin with hardening and inflammation of the preexisting lesion. When squamous cell cancer arises from normal skin, the nodule grows slowly on a firm, hard base. If untreated, this nodule eventually ulcerates and invades underlying tissues. It may spread to the regional lymph nodes, causing characteristic symptoms of pain, malaise, fatigue, weakness, and appetite loss.

How is it diagnosed?

An excisional biopsy (tissue removal and analysis) provides a definitive diagnosis of squamous cell cancer. Other appropriate lab tests depend on symptoms.

How is it treated?

The size, shape, location, and invasiveness of a squamous cell tumor and the condition of the underlying tissue determine the treatment method used. A deeply invasive tumor may require a combination of techniques.

All the major treatments have excellent rates of cure; generally, the prognosis is better with a well-differentiated lesion than with a poorly differentiated one in an unusual location. Depending on the lesion, treatment may consist of:

- wide surgical excision
- micrographic surgery (see *What you should know about Mohs' surgery*, page 666.)
- electrodesiccation and curettage (offer good cosmetic results for small lesions)

PREVENTION TIPS

How to lessen your risk of squamous cell cancer

Overexposure to the sun can predispose a person to squamous cell cancer. The following guidelines may help you avoid getting this disease.

Care under the sun

- Avoid excessive sun exposure.
- Wear protective clothing (such as hats and shirts with long sleeves).
- Use strong sunscreen agents containing PABA, benzophenone, and zinc oxide. Apply them 30 to 60 minutes before sun exposure.
- Use lipscreens to protect your lips from sun damage.

Periodic exams

Periodically examine your skin for precancerous lesions; if you find any, have them removed promptly.

What you should know about Mohs' surgery

If you have squamous cell or basal cell cancer, the doctor may perform Mohs' micrographic surgery to remove cancerous tissue one thin section at a time until only healthy tissue remains. With this surgery, cure rates for both of these cancers exceed 90%. Scarring is minimal, the risk of recurrence decreases, and the technique can be done in the doctor's office.

What to expect during surgery

The doctor removes the visible lesion and nearby normal-looking skin. A map of the defect is drawn while the tissue is cut into sections and analyzed. After reading the results, the doctor marks on the map the sections that hold cancerous tissue, then removes additional tissue from those areas, repeating the steps until all microscopically examined tissue appears cancer-free.

The procedure takes hours, most of them spent waiting for results. Numerous excisions are common. Electrocautery, which controls bleeding, leaves a burning odor. The doctor either sutures the wound or leaves it open to heal. In some situations, the doctor may recommend plastic surgery.

Post-procedure care

- Be sure to leave the dressing in place for 24 hours.
- Call the doctor if the wound shows signs of infection, such as redness, warmth, or extreme tenderness at the incision site.
- If the wound bleeds, reinforce the dressing and apply direct pressure to the wound for 20 minutes. If the bleeding continues, call the doctor.
- To prevent bleeding and promote healing, avoid alcohol, aspirin, other anticoagulants, and excessive exercise for 48 hours after surgery.
- Be sure to make and keep follow-up appointments to monitor your progress or to investigate reconstructive surgery.

- radiation therapy (generally for older or debilitated people)
- chemosurgery (reserved for resistant or recurrent cancers).

STOMACH CANCER

What do doctors call this condition?

Gastric carcinoma

What is this condition?

Stomach cancer is common throughout the world and affects all races. But for unknown reasons, it's more likely to be fatal to people in Japan, Iceland, Chile, and Austria.

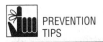

The link between stomach cancer and diet

Foods and other substances may play a role in increasing or decreasing a person's chances for stomach cancer.

The bad foods
Offenders include pickled vegetables, salted fish and meat, smoked foods, and chocolate. High salt consumption is also a common link among people with stomach cancer.

Other culprits include food preservatives — especially the nitrates added to vegetables and cured meats and found in drinking water. Nitrites are suspected, too. Bear in mind that most nitrites in the body result from the body's conversion of nitrates to nitrites, although they're consumed with some foods.

Coffee and alcohol aren't associated with stomach cancer unless they're consumed excessively or on an empty stomach.

The good foods
Foods associated with a reduced risk of stomach cancer include whole milk, fresh vegetables, fibers and grains, citrus fruits, and other foods rich in vitamin C.

A positive development
Refrigeration, which decreases the need for nitrates and other preservatives, may be one reason for declining stomach cancer rates in the United States.

In the United States, the incidence of stomach cancer has decreased 50% during the past 25 years and the death rate is one-third what it was 30 years ago. Some people believe (although without proof) that the decrease in stomach cancer is due to the balanced American diet and to refrigeration, which reduces nitrate-producing bacteria in food.

Stomach cancer is more common in men over age 40. It spreads rapidly to regional lymph nodes, the omentum (part of the peritoneum, the lining of the abdominal wall), liver, and lungs.

What causes it?
The cause of stomach cancer is unknown, but this cancer is often associated with gastritis (inflammation of the stomach lining) accompanied by stomach shrinkage. Predisposing factors include environmental influences, such as smoking and high alcohol intake. Genetic factors are also suspected. It's more common in people with a family history of stomach cancer.

Diet also seems to be related. Experts suspect a link between stomach cancer and certain types of food preparation, the physical properties of some foods, and certain methods of food preservation — especially smoking, pickling, and salting. (See *The link between stomach cancer and diet.*)

What are its symptoms?

Early symptoms of stomach cancer are chronic stomach upset and discomfort. In later stages, people lose weight and may experience appetite loss, a feeling of fullness after eating, anemia, and fatigue. If the cancer is in the cardia (where the stomach joins the esophagus), the first symptom may be difficulty swallowing; later, vomiting may occur (the vomit may look like coffee grounds). The person also may have blood in the stools.

Stomach cancer may have a sudden or slow onset. Many people treat themselves with antacids until the symptoms of advanced stages appear.

How is it diagnosed?

The doctor thoroughly investigates any persistent or recurring gastrointestinal changes and complaints. To rule out other conditions causing similar symptoms, the doctor will order lab tests of the person's blood, stools, and stomach fluid. Additional tests typically include:

- *Barium X-rays of the digestive tract* reveal changes in the stomach's shape, loss of flexibility and ability to enlarge, and abnormalities in the stomach's mucous membrane lining.
- *Gastroscopy* (visual inspection of the stomach using a *gastroscope*, which is inserted through the esophagus) helps rule out other abnormalities of the stomach's mucous membrane lining.

Studies that help determine if cancer has spread to other organs include computed tomography scans (commonly called CAT scans), chest X-rays, liver and bone scans, and liver biopsy.

How is it treated?

Surgery is often the preferred treatment. In many cases, the surgeon can remove the tumor successfully. For people whose disease isn't surgically curable, tumor removal relieves symptoms and improves their response to chemotherapy and radiation therapy.

The tumor's cell type, location, and development determine which type of surgery is appropriate. The surgeon may remove all or part of the stomach, sometimes including the duodenum (a part of the small intestine). If the cancer has spread, he may remove the omentum and spleen as well. (See *Learning about stomach surgery.*)

If cancer has spread to the liver, peritoneum, or lymph glands, the surgeon may perform palliative surgery to temporarily relieve vomiting, nausea, pain, and swallowing problems while allowing normal eating.

Learning about stomach surgery

The names of stomach (gastric) surgeries usually refer to the stomach portion removed. Many procedures combine two surgery types. *Ostomy* means "an opening into." Two prefixes preceding ostomy indicate anastomosis — joining. For example, in *gastroduodenostomy*, the surgeon attaches a stomach (gastro-) remnant to a small intestine (duodeno-) segment.

The illustrations and information below will help you understand stomach surgery. (Note that the dotted lines represent the areas removed.)

Gastroduodenostomy

Also called a *Billroth I*, gastroduodenostomy may be performed to remove a stomach tumor in or near the pylorus — one of the three main sections of the stomach. The surgeon removes one-third to one-half of the stomach and joins the remaining stomach portion to the duodenum (the first section of the small intestine).

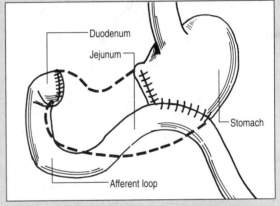

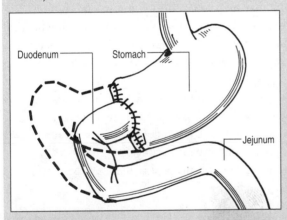

Partial gastric resection

If a tumor lies in a defined area of the stomach, the surgeon removes the diseased stomach portion and attaches the remaining stomach portion to the jejunum.

Gastrojejunostomy

Also called a *Billroth II*, this operation is used for a stomach tumor located in the pyloric region or antrum (the passage from the esophagus to the stomach). The surgeon removes a portion of the antrum, joins the remaining stomach to the jejunum (the second section of the small intestine), and then closes the duodenal stump.

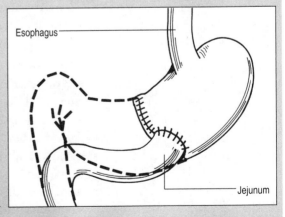

(continued)

Learning about stomach surgery *(continued)*

Total gastrectomy

A person with a tumor in the cardia (near the opening of the esophagus) or high in the fundus (the enlarged portion of the stomach) may need a total gastrectomy. In this operation, the surgeon removes the entire stomach and attaches the lower end of the esophagus to the jejunum at the entrance to the small intestine.

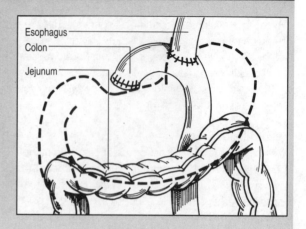

Chemotherapy may help to control symptoms and prolong survival. The doctor may prescribe drugs to control nausea, which increases as the cancer advances. For advanced disease, the doctor may prescribe sedatives and tranquilizers to control anxiety and narcotics to relieve pain.

Radiation has been particularly useful when combined with chemotherapy in people with inoperable or partially inoperable tumors. However, radiation shouldn't be given before surgery because it may damage internal organs and impede healing.

Treatment with antacids and drugs that reduce spasms may help relieve gastrointestinal distress.

What can a person with stomach cancer do?

- If you're scheduled for a partial gastric resection (removal of part of the stomach), be aware that you may eventually be able to eat normally.
- You may develop vitamin deficiencies from gastrointestinal blockages, diarrhea, or an inadequate diet. Ask the doctor about taking ascorbic acid, thiamine, riboflavin, nicotinic acid, and vitamin K supplements. Maintain good nutrition because this promotes weight gain, strength, independence, a positive outlook, and tolerance for surgery, radiation therapy, or chemotherapy. The doctor may prescribe steroids or antidepressants or suggest that you drink wine or brandy to boost your appetite.

TESTICULAR CANCER

What is this condition?

Cancer of the testicles primarily affects young to middle-aged men. In children, it's rare.

Most testicular cancers originate in gonadal cells. About 40% are seminomas — uniform, undifferentiated cells resembling primitive gonadal cells. The remainder are nonseminomas — tumor cells showing various degrees of differentiation.

The prognosis varies with the cell type and disease stage. When treated with surgery and radiation, almost all men with localized disease live more than 5 years.

What causes it?

The cause of testicular cancer isn't known, but the incidence peaks between ages 20 and 40. It's highest in men with cryptorchidism (failure of one or both testicles to descend) — even when surgically corrected — and in men whose mothers used the drug diethylstilbestrol (also called DES) during pregnancy.

Testicular cancer is rare in nonwhite men and accounts for fewer than 1% of male cancer deaths. This cancer spreads to the lymph nodes and possibly to the lungs, liver, viscera, and bone.

What are its symptoms?

The first sign is usually a firm, painless, and smooth testicular mass, varying in size and sometimes producing a sense of testicular heaviness. When such a tumor causes production of certain hormones, gynecomastia (abnormal breast enlargement) and nipple tenderness may result.

In advanced stages, signs and symptoms include obstruction of the ureters (the tubes that bring urine from the kidneys to the bladder), abdominal mass, cough, coughing up of blood, shortness of breath, weight loss, fatigue, pallor, and sluggishness.

How is it diagnosed?

Two effective ways to detect a testicular tumor are regular self-examinations and testicular palpation during a routine physical exam. A technique called *transillumination* can distinguish between a tumor (which doesn't transilluminate) and a hydrocele or spermatocele

Sex after testicular cancer surgery

You're bound to feel anxious about your future after learning you have testicular cancer — and you may be afraid that you'll lose sexual function after orchiectomy (surgery to remove one or both testicles). Understanding how orchiectomy affects sexual activity will help you overcome these fears.

If one testicle is removed
Unilateral orchiectomy doesn't cause sterility or impotence. Most surgeons remove only the testicle, leaving the scrotum. A gel-filled prosthesis, which weighs and feels like a normal testicle, can be implanted in the scrotum. Once the incision heals, you can resume sexual activity.

If both testicles are removed
Bilateral testicular cancer (cancer in both testicles) is rare. If both testicles will be removed, you'll be sterile. But remember: A loss of fertility doesn't equal a loss of masculinity. The doctor will prescribe synthetic hormones to replace or supplement depleted hormone levels.

(which does). Follow-up measures should include an exam for gynecomastia and abdominal masses.

Lab tests are performed to measure levels of alpha-fetoprotein and beta-human chorionic gonadotropin in the blood, which indicates testicular tumor activity. These tests provide a baseline for measuring response to therapy and determining the prognosis.

Surgical excision and biopsy of the tumor and testicle permits the doctor to verify the tumor cell type — essential for effective treatment. Examination of the groin determines the extent of lymph node involvement.

How is it treated?

The extent of surgery, radiation, and chemotherapy varies with the tumor cell type and stage. Surgery includes orchiectomy (testicle removal) and retroperitoneal lymph node dissection. Most surgeons remove the testicle, not the scrotum (to allow for a prosthetic implant). Hormone replacement therapy may be needed if a bilateral orchiectomy (removal of both testicles) is performed.

Radiation therapy to the retroperitoneal and homolateral iliac lymph nodes follows removal of a seminoma. All positive nodes receive radiation after removal of a nonseminoma. Men with retroperitoneal extension of the cancer receive preventive radiation to the mediastinal and supraclavicular nodes.

Chemotherapy is essential for tumors beyond stage 0. Chemotherapy and radiation followed by autologous bone marrow transplantation may help people with unresponsive tumors.

What can a man with testicular cancer do?

- Be aware that removal of one testicle does not always cause sterility and impotence, that synthetic hormones can restore hormonal balance, and that most surgeons don't remove the scrotum. In many cases, a testicular prosthesis can correct anatomic disfigurement. (See *Sex after testicular cancer surgery.*)
- After surgery, you'll wear an athletic supporter to minimize pain when moving.

THYROID CANCER

What do doctors call this condition?
Thyroid carcinoma

What is this condition?
Cancer of the thyroid gland — an endocrine gland in the front of the neck — occurs in all age-groups, especially in persons who have had radiation treatment to the neck area.

Papillary and follicular carcinoma are the most common types of thyroid cancer. *Papillary carcinoma* is the least aggressive form of thyroid cancer. *Follicular carcinoma* is less common but more likely to recur and spread to regional lymph nodes and through blood vessels into the bones, liver, and lungs. *Giant* and *spindle cell cancers* are seldom curable with surgery. These tumors tend to resist radiation and spread rapidly.

What causes it?
Predisposing factors include radiation exposure, prolonged stimulation of thyroid-stimulating hormone (a substance secreted by the pituitary gland) through radiation or heredity, family predisposition, and chronic goiter (enlarged thyroid).

What are its symptoms?
The most common signs and symptoms of thyroid cancer are a painless nodule (mass), a hard nodule in an enlarged thyroid gland, or lymph nodes that can be felt by palpation (touch), and an enlarged thyroid. Eventually, the pressure of such a nodule or enlargement causes hoarseness, difficulty swallowing, shortness of breath, and pain on palpation. If the tumor is large enough to destroy the gland, thyroid hormone deficiency follows, accompanied by symptoms of low metabolism — mental apathy and sensitivity to cold. However, if the tumor causes excessive production of thyroid hormone, symptoms include sensitivity to heat, restlessness, and hyperactivity.

Other symptoms of thyroid cancer include diarrhea, appetite loss, irritability, and inability to speak (from vocal cord paralysis).

How is it diagnosed?

The first clue to thyroid cancer is usually an enlarged node that you can feel in the thyroid gland, neck, lymph nodes of the neck, or vocal cords. The doctor also will ask if the person has a history of radiation therapy or a family history of thyroid cancer because these factors support the diagnosis.

Before confirming thyroid cancer, the doctor must rule out noncancerous thyroid enlargements, which are much more common. A thyroid scan can determine if the node is functional (which is rarely malignant) or hypofunctional (which is commonly malignant).

Other tests include needle biopsy (removal and analysis of thyroid tissue), computed tomography scan (commonly called a CAT scan), ultrasound, chest X-ray, and certain lab tests (such as serum alkaline phosphatase and serum calcitonin assay).

The first clue to thyroid cancer is usually an enlarged node in the thyroid gland, neck, lymph nodes of the neck, or vocal cords.

How is it treated?

Treatment of thyroid cancer may consist of total or partial removal of the thyroid and removal of some lymph nodes. In some cases, the surgeon also must remove some neck tissue. Following thyroid surgery, a person may lose his or her voice and be hoarse for several days.

External radiation therapy is given to people with inoperable cancer and sometimes after surgery.

To increase a person's tolerance of surgery and radiation, the doctor may prescribe drugs that suppress the thyroid, along with an adrenergic blocking agent such as Inderal.

Chemotherapy is given to some people whose symptoms suggest that the cancer has spread to other areas.

UTERINE CANCER

What is this condition?

This cancer affects the endometrium — the mucous membrane lining of the uterus. It's the most common gynecologic cancer.

Uterine cancer most commonly strikes postmenopausal women between ages 50 and 60. It's uncommon between ages 30 and 40 and extremely rare before age 30. An average of 33,000 new cases of uterine cancer are reported each year. Most premenopausal women who develop uterine cancer have a history of menstrual cycles without ovulating or other hormonal imbalances.

What causes it?

Experts have linked uterine cancer with these predisposing factors:
- low fertility and lack of ovulation
- abnormal uterine bleeding
- obesity, high blood pressure, or diabetes
- family tendency
- history of uterine polyps (growths) or abnormal endometrial cell growth
- estrogen therapy (this is still controversial).

Uterine cancer typically spreads late — usually from the endometrium to the cervix, ovaries, fallopian tubes, and other structures in the abdominal cavity. It may spread to distant organs, such as the lungs and brain, through the blood or lymphatic system. Lymph nodes also may be involved.

What are its symptoms?

Typically, uterine cancer causes an enlarged uterus with persistent and unusual premenopausal bleeding. (Any postmenopausal bleeding typically suggests this type of cancer.) At first, the discharge may be watery and blood-streaked, but it gradually becomes more bloody. Other symptoms, such as pain and weight loss, don't appear until the cancer is well advanced.

How is it diagnosed?

Unfortunately, a Pap smear, so useful for detecting cervical cancer, doesn't dependably detect early-stage uterine cancer. To diagnose uterine cancer, the doctor will biopsy (remove and analyze) endometrial, cervical, and endocervical tissue. Negative biopsies call for a fractional dilatation and curettage (commonly known as a D & C) to determine the diagnosis. (See *What to expect with an endometrial biopsy,* page 676.)

If the woman has a positive diagnosis, the doctor will perform a complete physical exam and do other tests to determine the stage of the tumor's development and obtain baseline information.

What to expect with an endometrial biopsy

If the doctor suspects uterine cancer, he or she will want you to have an endometrial biopsy. This test helps diagnose disorders of the endometrium (a layer of tissue lining the inside of the uterus). In this procedure, the doctor will remove a small sample of cells from the endometrium for examination under a microscope.

Getting ready
Before the test, you'll be asked to empty your bladder and remove your clothes from the waist down.

During the procedure
You'll lie on your back on an examination table. The nurse will give you a sheet to cover you, and you'll place your feet in stirrups. (This is the same position as the one used when you're having a Pap smear.)

First, the doctor will perform a pelvic exam and insert an instrument called a *speculum* into your vagina. The speculum holds the vagina open and allows a clear view of the vagina and the cervix (the lowest part of the uterus that protrudes into the vagina). Then the doctor will clean the vagina and cervix with an antiseptic solution.

Next, the doctor will gently insert a hollow plastic tube called a cannula into the uterus. The cannula is attached to a syringe. The doctor uses the syringe to irrigate the endometrial tissue with a saline solution. After the solution returns through the cannula to the syringe, the doctor will withdraw the cannula and disconnect the syringe, then send the specimen in the syringe to the lab for microscopic analysis.

How does it feel?
The instruments may feel cold. You may also experience some cramping as the speculum is inserted into your uterus.

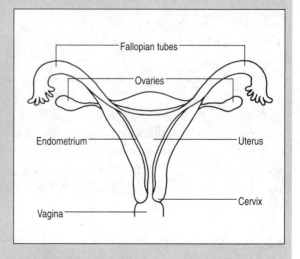

What to expect afterward
After the test, you may have mild cramping for an hour and vaginal spotting for a day or two.

Plan to rest for the remainder of the day. You may resume your normal activities the next day.

Make sure to call the doctor if you experience:
- heavy bleeding
- fever over 100° F (37.8° C)
- foul-smelling vaginal discharge.

Avoid sexual intercourse, tampons, and douching for a week. Use sanitary pads for bleeding. Note that your next two menstrual periods may be heavier than usual.

How is it treated?
Treatment varies, depending on the extent of the disease.
- *Surgery.* Surgery, which rarely cures the disease, generally involves removal of the uterus, ovaries, and fallopian tubes and sometimes other pelvic structures and lymph nodes. In some cases, the surgeon removes all pelvic organs, including the vagina. Removal of the ovaries will induce menopause in a premenopausal woman.

- *Radiation therapy.* Some women undergo radiation therapy, which may be external, internal, or a combination. When given 6 weeks before surgery, radiation therapy may reduce the risk of tumor recurrence and prolong survival. (See *What you should know about radiation therapy*.)
- *Hormonal therapy.* Synthetic progesterones, such as megestrol or medroxyprogesterone, may be administered if the cancer has spread to other organs. The drug tamoxifen (which has a 20% to 40% response rate) may be given as an auxiliary treatment.
- *Chemotherapy.* Varying combinations of anticancer drugs are usually tried when other treatments have failed.

VULVAR CANCER

What is this condition?

This cancer affects the vulva — the external female genitalia. The most common type is squamous cell carcinoma. Vulvar cancer, which accounts for about 5% of all gynecologic cancers, can occur at any age, even in infants; however, peak incidence is in the mid-60s.

Early diagnosis increases the chance of effective treatment and survival. If lymph nodes are not involved, the 5-year survival rate is 85%; if lymph nodes are involved, it's less than 75%.

What causes it?

Although the cause of vulvar cancer is unknown, several factors seem to predispose woman to this disease. For example, about 25% of affected women have *leukoplakia*, white lesions on the vulva. Other predisposing factors include a history of venereal disease; chronic itching of the vulva, with friction, swelling, and dryness; irradiation of the skin; herpes simplex or genital warts; high blood pressure; diabetes; and not having children.

What are its symptoms?

About half the time, vulvar cancer begins with vulvar itching, bleeding, or a small vulvar mass, which may start as a small ulcer on the surface and eventually become infected and painful. Therefore, these symptoms call for immediate diagnostic evaluation. Less common signs include a mass in the groin and abnormal urination or defecation.

What you should know about radiation therapy

Internal radiation

If you'll be receiving an internal radiation implant, know that this usually requires a 2- to 3-day hospital stay in a private room. The radioactive source may be implanted in your vagina by the doctor, or it may be implanted by a member of the radiation team while you're in your room. You must limit your movements while the implant is in place (certain body movements could dislodge it). To help you relax and remain still, you may receive a tranquilizer.

External radiation

If you'll be receiving external radiation, be aware that this treatment is usually given 5 days a week for 6 weeks. Take care not to scrub body areas marked for treatment, because it's important to direct treatment to exactly the same area each time. To minimize skin breakdown and reduce the risk of skin infection, keep the treatment area dry, avoid wearing clothes that rub against the area, and avoid using heating pads, alcohol rubs, or any skin creams.

How is it diagnosed?

Typical symptoms along with a Pap smear that reveals abnormal cells strongly suggest vulvar cancer. Firm diagnosis requires a biopsy (removal and analysis) of abnormal tissue.

Other diagnostic studies include a complete blood count, X-rays, an electrocardiogram, and a thorough physical (including pelvic) exam. Occasionally, a computed tomography scan (commonly called a CAT scan) may pinpoint lymph node involvement.

How is it treated?

Depending on the disease stage, vulvar cancer usually calls for radical or simple vulvectomy (removal of all or part of the vulva) or, for some small tumors, laser therapy. Radical vulvectomy requires bilateral dissection of superficial and deep inguinal lymph nodes. Depending on how far the cancer has spread, the surgeon also may remove the urethra, vagina, and bowel, leaving an open perineal wound until healing occurs, in about 2 to 3 months. Plastic surgery may be done later.

Small, confined tumors with no lymph node involvement may require a simple vulvectomy or a hemivulvectomy (without pelvic node dissection). Personal considerations (young age, active sex life) may also call for such conservative management. However, a simple vulvectomy requires careful postoperative follow-up because it leaves the woman at higher risk for developing a new tumor.

If extensive cancer spread, advanced age, or fragile health rules out surgery, radiation therapy helps to relieve symptoms.

What can a woman with vulvar cancer do?

- Be aware that sensation in your vulva will return eventually, after the nerve endings heal.
- Know that you'll probably be able to have sexual intercourse 6 to 8 weeks after surgery. You and your partner may want to try different sexual techniques, especially if your clitoris has been removed.

18

IMMUNE DISORDERS

ACQUIRED IMMUNODEFICIENCY SYNDROME (AIDS)

What is this condition?

One of the most widely publicized diseases, AIDS is marked by progressive weakening of the immune system, which makes a person vulnerable to opportunistic infections and unusual cancers. The syndrome was first defined by the Centers for Disease Control and Prevention in 1981. Since then, the agency has revised its definition of AIDS, most recently in 1993.

Homosexual and bisexual men who are sexually active with many partners have the highest risk for contracting AIDS. Other high-risk groups include intravenous drug users and hemophiliacs, especially those who've been treated with Factor VIII (one of the blood clotting factors) concentrate. Most recently, heterosexual partners and children of persons with AIDS or of those in high-risk groups and persons receiving multiple blood transfusions have been added to the high-risk category. Drug therapy and prevention and treatment of common opportunistic infections can delay the natural progression of HIV infection and prolong survival.

To reduce the risk of contracting AIDS, public health advocates recommend following safe sex practices, such as condom use.

What causes it?

AIDS is caused by a retrovirus called *human immunodeficiency virus* (HIV). The retrovirus strikes cells bearing a substance called the *CD4* antigen. This antigen serves as a receptor for HIV and lets it enter the cell. HIV prefers to infect CD4$^+$ cells, which are white blood cells that are sometimes called *helper cells*. But it may also infect other cells, including certain digestive tract cells, uterine cervical cells, and neuroglial cells, a type of nerve cell.

After HIV invades a cell, it reproduces. Recent research shows that in the first weeks after infection, HIV is extremely active. It eventually causes profound illness by hindering the immune system's ability to fight disease.

The infection process takes three forms:

- immunodeficiency — opportunistic infections and unusual cancers
- autoimmunity — the body's reaction against its own tissues

- neurologic problems — AIDS dementia, a brain condition known as *HIV encephalopathy*, and peripheral nerve disorders.

Transmission modes

HIV is transmitted by intimate sexual contact, especially during rectal intercourse that injures the mucous membranes; by transfusion of contaminated blood or blood products (this risk has diminished thanks to routine testing of all blood products); by sharing of contaminated needles; and by transmission from an infected mother to her fetus (by cervical or blood contact at delivery and in breast milk). Mounting evidence suggests that HIV is *not* transmitted by casual household or social contact. (See *Caring for a person with AIDS at home,* pages 682 and 683.)

What are its symptoms?

Some people with AIDS lack symptoms until they suddenly develop an opportunistic infection or the purple skin lesions of Kaposi's sarcoma, one of the cancers associated with AIDS.

But more often, they have nonspecific signs and symptoms, such as fatigue, afternoon fevers, night sweats, weight loss, diarrhea, or cough. Soon after these appear, they typically develop several infections at the same time.

In children with AIDS, the time between exposure to HIV and appearance of symptoms seems to be shorter (an average of 8 months). Signs and symptoms resemble those of adults with AIDS, except for those related to sexually transmitted disease. Finally, in children, the most common manifestation and cause of death isn't *Pneumocystis carinii* pneumonia, as in adults, but diffuse interstitial pneumonitis.

How is it diagnosed?

According to the Centers for Disease Control and Prevention, a diagnosis of AIDS is confirmed by the presence of an opportunistic infection with lab evidence of HIV infection and a CD4$^+$ T-cell count of less than 200 cells per microliter.

How is it treated?

Currently, no cure exists for AIDS. However, the drug Retrovir (known as *AZT*) is used alone or along with other drugs, such as Hivid, to inhibit HIV reproduction. Videx may be used if a person can't tolerate AZT or no longer responds to it.

HIV is transmitted primarily by sexual contact, contaminated needles, and from an infected mother to her child at delivery. Mounting evidence says HIV is not transmitted by casual household contact or social contact.

Caring for a person with AIDS at home

You can care for a person with AIDS at home without exposing yourself or other family members to the virus and without giving the person a new infection. How? By ensuring that no one comes into contact with the person's blood, semen, or vaginal secretions. Although the virus that causes AIDS may be detected in saliva, urine, feces, mucus, perspiration, or other body secretions, no one has developed AIDS by touching these body fluids.

The precautions below take time and planning, but they'll soon become second nature. Remember, though, precautions shouldn't be so exaggerated that the person feels isolated.

To prevent AIDS transmission at home, follow these guidelines.

Hand washing

Use soap and water to wash your hands, arms, and any other body surfaces that touch the person before and after all contact with him or her, and before preparing food or eating.

Don't touch your own body or your mouth when providing care. Also remind the person to wash his or her hands frequently, especially before eating and after using the bathroom.

Gloves, gowns, and masks

Protective clothing isn't needed for general care or during casual contact, such as when bathing intact skin or feeding a person with AIDS. However, you should wear it in the following instances.

Use *gloves* when touching body secretions or excretions (for example, during mouth, wound, or nose care) or when caring for a woman who's menstruating or who's just given birth.

Also wear gloves when handling soiled diapers, sheets, or clothing; when the person with AIDS has vomited or been incontinent; or when caring for the person's rectal or genital lesions (sores or blisters). Remember to wash your hands after removing gloves.

Wear a *gown* if you may be splattered with body fluids. Wear a *mask* if the person with AIDS has *Mycobacterium tuberculosis* and is coughing. Wear a *mask* and *protective eyewear* to prevent vomit or saliva from splashing into your eyes, nose, or mouth.

Eating utensils

Wash dishes used by a person with AIDS in hot, soapy water, and dry them after washing. You needn't keep his dishes separate from other dishes.

Kitchen and bathroom facilities

A person with AIDS doesn't need separate kitchen and bathroom facilities. He may use the same toilet as other family members without special precautions, unless he is incontinent or has diarrhea or herpes lesions.

If he does, disinfect the toilet with a 1:10 solution of bleach and water after each use. Wait 10 minutes; then rinse with clear water.

Cleanups

If blood, urine, or other body fluids spill, clean them up promptly with hot, soapy water. Then disinfect the washed surface with a 1:10 bleach solution, and rinse with clear water after 10 minutes.

Soak sponges or mops used to clean up body fluids in a 1:10 bleach solution for 5 minutes. Don't rinse them in sinks where food is prepared, and don't use them to clean food-preparation areas.

Empty the mop water into the toilet.

Clean the kitchen and bathroom. Wash surfaces frequently with soap and water and scouring powder. Clean the refrigerator regularly, and mop the floors at least once a week.

Disinfect the bathroom and shower floor with a 1:10 solution of bleach and water. Pour a small amount of full-strength bleach down the toilet. Clean up spills as soon as they occur, and don't use the same sponge to clean the bathroom and kitchen.

Caring for a person with AIDS at home *(continued)*

Laundry

Wear gloves when handling soiled items. Always launder towels and washcloths after the person with AIDS uses them. Seal laundry soiled with body fluids in heavy-duty, double plastic bags until you can wash them. Soak items soiled with body fluids in cold water and an enzymatic detergent; then wash in hot water, detergent, and 1 cup of bleach. Machine dry on the hot setting. Wash all the person's laundry separately.

Disposable items

Place soiled disposable gloves, diapers, linen-saver pads, tissues, and other items in sealed, heavy-duty, double plastic bags before discarding. Regular trash pickup is usually adequate, but follow your community's regulations for disposal.

Injection needles

Dispose of used needles immediately in a sealed, rigid, puncture-proof plastic or metal can. Never recap or break needles. Follow your community's regulations for disposal.

Personal items

Never share the person's toothbrush, razor, or other personal items that might be contaminated with blood.

Glass thermometers can be shared if they are cleaned thoroughly first. Wash them with soap and cold water, soak them in 70% to 90% ethyl alcohol for 30 minutes, then rinse under running water.

Supportive measures aim to reduce the person's risk of infection, treat existing infections and cancers, maintain adequate nutrition, and provide emotional support.

Additional drug treatment

Although drugs can eliminate many of the organisms that cause opportunistic infections, these infections tend to recur once drug treatment stops. The drug of choice for *P. carinii* pneumonia is oral or intravenous Bactrim or Septra. If this treatment fails or if toxicity occurs, the person may be given NebuPent or Pentam 300. However, this drug may cause liver problems, a rapid pulse, low blood pressure, low blood sugar, and rashes.

To treat Kaposi's sarcoma, the person may receive chemotherapy drugs, such as Oncovin and VePesid. Unfortunately, aggressive treatment of this cancer makes infection more likely. An interferon alfa drug is also being used to treat Kaposi's sarcoma. Radiation and laser therapy can relieve, but not cure, local Kaposi's lesions.

To treat retinitis, the person may receive Foscavir or Cytovene.

ALLERGIES

What are these conditions?

Allergies are reactions to airborne (inhaled) allergens — substances that can produce hypersensitivity reactions such as a runny nose and eye inflammation. Some allergies, such as hay fever, are seasonal. Others occur year-round (perennial allergies).

Allergies affect over 20 million Americans. They're most prevalent in young children and adolescents but occur in people of all ages.

What causes them?

Hay fever is a hypersensitivity response brought about by antibodies called *immunoglobulin E*. In most cases, hay fever is induced by wind-borne pollens: in the spring, by tree pollens; in the summer, by grass pollens; and in the fall, by weed pollens. Occasionally, allergy to fungal spores induces hay fever.

In year-round allergies, the allergens provoke responses year-round. Major year-round allergens and irritants include dust mites, feather pillows, mold, cigarette smoke, upholstery, and animal danders. A seasonal pollen allergy may worsen the symptoms of year-round allergies.

What are their symptoms?

In seasonal allergies, the main signs and symptoms are sneezing spells, a runny nose with profuse watery discharge, nasal congestion, and itching of the nose and eyes. The person usually has swollen nasal passages, reddened eyes with swollen eyelids, excessive tearing, and headache or sinus pain. Some allergy sufferers also complain of an itchy throat and a general ill feeling called *malaise*.

Year-round allergies usually cause only a runny nose and nasal congestion. But they can cause chronic nasal blockage, which then blocks the auditory tube that extends from the middle ear to the throat (called the *eustachian tube*). Blocked eustachian tubes are especially common in children with year-round allergies.

In both seasonal and year-round allergies, "allergic shiners" (dark circles) may appear under the eyes. The severity of signs and symptoms may vary from season to season and from year to year.

How are they diagnosed?

With allergies, the person's sputum and nasal discharge usually contain large amounts of a type of white blood cell active in hypersensitivity responses called *eosinophils*. Blood tests show normal or elevated immunoglobulin E antibody levels.

For a firm diagnosis, the doctor takes a personal and family history of allergies and considers physical exam findings. To pinpoint the responsible allergens, he or she may order skin testing and assess the person's responses to environmental stimuli.

To rule out a common cold, which mimics an allergy, the doctor checks for typical cold symptoms, such as fever, sore throat, beet-red nasal mucous membranes, and nasal discharge without eosinophils. In a child, the doctor checks for a foreign body in the nose, such as a bean or a button, which can cause allergy-like symptoms.

How are they treated?

Treatment aims to control allergy symptoms by eliminating environmental allergens, if possible, and by drug therapy and a special treatment called *immunotherapy*. (See *Identifying allergens year-round*, page 686.)

Drug therapy

Antihistamines may be given, although these commonly cause sedation, dry mouth, nausea, dizziness, blurred vision, and nervousness. Newer antihistamines, such as Seldane, have fewer side effects and are less likely to cause sedation. However, an overdose of these drugs may cause irregular heartbeats.

Some people get relief from inhaled intranasal steroids, which reduce inflammation without causing the systemic side effects of antihistamines. The most commonly used intranasal corticosteroids are Nasalide, Beconase, and Vancenase. Unfortunately, during acute allergy attacks, these drugs rarely give relief. Nasal decongestants and oral antihistamines may be needed instead.

Immunotherapy

For long-term allergy management, the doctor may recommend immunotherapy. In this treatment, the person receives increasingly large doses of the offending allergens to gradually develop immunity. The doses are administered before or during allergy season or year-round.

For long-term allergy management, the doctor may recommend immunotherapy. In this treatment, you receive increasingly large doses of the offending allergens to help you gradually develop immunity.

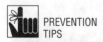

PREVENTION
TIPS

Identifying allergens year-round

Watch for a seasonal pattern in your allergy symptoms. The information below can help you identify and avoid the offending allergens.

Seasonal patterns for tree and grass pollens vary throughout the country and somewhat from year to year. If you're allergic to more than one substance, you may have trouble figuring out exactly what's causing your symptoms. For a definitive diagnosis, see an allergist.

Spring allergens

If your symptoms worsen a month or so before new leaves unfold, you may be allergic to tree pollens. Elm, maple, oak, sycamore, ash, pecan, mountain cedar, and walnut trees are potential culprits.

Summer allergens

If you suffer more from June to August, you may be hypersensitive to grass pollen. Bermuda grass is a common offender, with sheep sorrel, English plantain, and other pollen-producing grasses and plants running close behind.

Fall allergens

Ragweed pollen, the most notorious fall allergen, causes symptoms from August to October, depending on the region. Sagebrush, Russian thistle, and other pollen-shedding plants also may trigger fall allergies.

Year-round allergens

If you sniff and sneeze year-round, you may be allergic to dust mites, animal dander, cigarette smoke, or other allergens in your environment. Mold spores also may cause perennial allergy, but this occurs more commonly in summer and fall.

What can a person with allergies do?

- If the doctor has prescribed intranasal corticosteroids, use them regularly, as directed, for optimal effectiveness.
- If you're taking Nasalcrom, be aware that although this drug can help prevent allergies, it may take up to 4 weeks to work. Also, you must take it regularly during allergy season.
- Call the doctor if you have a delayed reaction to immunotherapy.
- To reduce your exposure to airborne allergens, sleep with the windows closed, and use air conditioning to filter allergens. (See *Allergy-proofing your surroundings*.)
- If you have severe and resistant allergies, you may have to consider drastic lifestyle changes, such as moving to a pollen-free area, either seasonally or year-round.

SELF-HELP

Allergy-proofing your surroundings

Here's an inexpensive, safe, and effective treatment for an allergy: Simply avoid the things that cause your symptoms. Maybe you can't remove all of them from your environment, but by limiting your exposure, you can minimize your symptoms.

In your bedroom
- Remove dust catchers, such as knickknacks, stuffed animals, wall hangings, and books.
- If you're allergic to animal dander, keep furry pets (dogs, cats, gerbils, and hamsters) out of the bedroom.
- Use blankets made of synthetic materials rather than wool.
- Replace feather pillows and comforters with those filled with Dacron, nylon, or other polyester fibers.
- Encase your mattress and boxspring in airtight vinyl covers.
- Remove plants or an aquarium from the room because these may increase mold spores in the air.

Throughout your house
- Dust at least two or three times weekly. Use a damp mop or cloth instead of a broom, which can raise dust.
- Use an electronic air cleaner to remove mold, house dust, and pollens from the air. Be sure to wash or replace the filter periodically.
- In warm weather, close the windows and use an air conditioner.
- Clean air-conditioner and heat outlet filters regularly.
- Remove heavy rugs and draperies that catch and hold dust. Replace them with washable curtains and cotton throw rugs.
- Keep humidity low to reduce mold spores. Use a dehumidifier. Clean bathrooms frequently.
- Cover upholstered furniture with vinyl sheeting or slipcovers that can be washed frequently.
- Ban smoking and the use of aerosol or scented products in your home.

Outdoors
- Don't landscape your home with pollen-bearing trees, such as elm, maple, birch, poplar, ash, oak, walnut, sycamore, or cypress.
- Rake fallen leaves so that mold won't grow on them. Wear a dust mask when you rake.
- Wear a dust mask when you cut the grass.
- Plan vacations to avoid major allergy seasons. Remember that when allergy season is in full swing, pollen counts are usually lower in urban areas.

ANAPHYLAXIS

What is this condition?

Anaphylaxis is a dramatic, acute allergic reaction marked by the sudden onset of rapidly progressive hives and respiratory distress. A severe reaction may precipitate vascular collapse, leading to systemic shock and sometimes death.

What causes it?

Anaphylactic reactions are caused by eating or other systemic exposure to sensitizing drugs or other substances. Such substances may include serums (usually horse serum), vaccines, allergen extracts, enzymes, hormones, penicillin and other antibiotics, sulfonamides, local anesthetics, salicylates, polysaccharides, diagnostic chemicals (such as radiographic contrast dye), foods (legumes, nuts, berries, seafood, and egg albumin) and sulfite-containing food additives, insect venom (honeybees, wasps, hornets, yellow jackets, fire ants, mosquitoes, and certain spiders) and, rarely, a ruptured hydatid cyst.

Penicillin is a common cause of anaphylaxis. It induces anaphylaxis in 1 to 4 of every 10,000 people treated with it. Penicillin is most likely to induce anaphylaxis after parenteral administration or prolonged therapy and in people with allergies to other drugs or foods.

An anaphylactic reaction requires previous sensitization or exposure to the specific substance that causes the allergic reaction (called an *antigen*), which results in the production of specific immunoglobulin E antibodies by plasma cells. This antibody production takes place in the lymph nodes and is enhanced by helper T cells. Immunoglobulin E antibodies then bind to membrane receptors on mast cells (found throughout connective tissue) and basophils.

On reexposure, the antigen binds to adjacent immunoglobulin E antibodies or receptors, causing a series of cellular reactions that trigger degranulation — the release of powerful chemical mediators from mast cell stores. Immunoglobulin G or immunoglobulin M enters into the reaction and activates the release of complement fractions.

At the same time, two other chemical mediators (bradykinin and leukotrienes) induce blood vessel collapse by stimulating contraction of certain groups of smooth muscles and by increasing blood vessel permeability. In turn, this increased permeability decreases peripheral resistance and plasma leakage from the circulation to extravascular tissues (which lowers blood volume, causing low blood pressure, shock, and heart failure).

What are its symptoms?

Anaphylactic reaction produces physical distress within seconds or minutes after exposure to an allergen; a delayed or persistent reaction may occur for up to 24 hours. The reaction's severity is inversely related to the interval between exposure to the allergen and the start of symptoms. Usually, the first symptoms include a feeling of impending doom or fright, weakness, sweating, sneezing, shortness of breath, nasal itching, hives, and angioedema, followed rapidly by symptoms in one or more target organs.

Cardiovascular symptoms include low blood pressure, shock, and sometimes irregular heartbeats, which, if untreated, may cause circulatory collapse. Respiratory symptoms can occur at any level in the respiratory tract and commonly include nasal mucosal swelling, profuse watery nasal discharge, itching, nasal congestion, and sudden sneezing attacks. Early signs of acute respiratory failure, which can be fatal, include swelling in the upper respiratory tract that obstructs the throat and larynx, with hoarseness, stridor (a harsh, high-pitched, breathing sound) and shortness of breath. Gastrointestinal and genitourinary symptoms include severe stomach cramps, nausea, diarrhea, and urinary urgency and incontinence.

How is it diagnosed?

Anaphylaxis can be diagnosed by the rapid onset of severe respiratory or cardiovascular symptoms after ingestion or injection of a drug, vaccine, diagnostic agent, food or food additive, or after an insect sting. If these symptoms occur without a known allergic stimulus, other possible causes of shock (acute heart attack, status asthmaticus, heart failure) must be ruled out.

How is it treated?

Anaphylaxis is always an emergency. It requires an *immediate* injection of Adrenalin, repeated every 5 to 20 minutes, as needed.

In the early stages of anaphylaxis, when the person has not lost consciousness and has normal blood pressure, Adrenalin is given intramuscularly or under the skin; the injection site is massaged to help the drug circulate faster. In severe reactions, when the person has lost consciousness and has low blood pressure, Adrenalin is given intravenously.

An open airway is maintained. The person is observed for early signs of laryngeal swelling (stridor, hoarseness, and shortness of breath), which typically requires endotracheal tube insertion or a tracheotomy and oxygen therapy.

In case of cardiac arrest, treatment includes CPR (including closed-chest heart massage), assisted breathing, and sodium bicarbonate. Other therapy depends on clinical response.

The person is monitored for low blood pressure and shock. Circulatory volume is maintained with volume expanders (plasma, plasma expanders, saline, and albumin) as needed. Blood pressure is stabi-

Anaphylaxis is always an emergency. It requires an immediate injection of Adrenalin — if the person is still conscious — and the injection site is massaged to help the drug circulate faster.

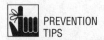

Avoiding common antigens

If you've had a severe reaction to one *antigen* (a substance that can cause an allergic reaction), you'll react to this antigen in all forms. For example, if you've had an anaphylactic reaction to a penicillin tablet, you'll also have one after a penicillin shot. If peanuts produce an anaphylactic response, watch out for peanut butter hidden in other foods.

Review the following list of the most common antigens and then make your own list of antigens to avoid.

Food
- Beans, including soybean products
- Chocolate
- Eggs
- Fruit, especially strawberries and citrus fruits
- Milk
- Nuts and seeds
- Seafood, especially shellfish

Drugs
- Pain relievers, such as aspirin and Indocin
- Antibiotics, especially penicillin and drugs derived from it
- Diuretics

- Insulin and other hormones
- Iodine-based radiographic contrast dye
- Serum proteins such as gamma globulin
- Vaccines

Other antigens
- Animal dander
- Bites and stings from insects (such as ants, bees, hornets, and wasps), jellyfish, snakes, and spiders
- Grass and ragweed pollens
- Mold spores
- Tartrazine (yellow dye number 5), used to color foods and drugs

lized with the intravenous vasopressors Levophed and Intropin. Blood pressure, central venous pressure, and urine output are monitored.

After the initial emergency, other drugs are given. These may include Adrenalin given under the skin; longer-acting Adrenalin, corticosteroids, and Benadryl given intravenously for long-term management; and Aminophyllin given intravenously for bronchospasm.

What can a person who's susceptible to anaphylaxis do?

- To prevent anaphylaxis, avoid exposure to known allergens. (See *Avoiding common antigens.*) If you have a food or drug allergy, avoid that food or drug in all its forms. If you're allergic to insect stings, avoid open fields and wooded areas during the insect season and carry an anaphylaxis kit (which contains Adrenalin, an antihistamine, and a tourniquet) whenever you must go outdoors.

Medic Alert service

If you've suffered anaphylaxis, your doctor or nurse has probably told you about Medic Alert. In an emergency, this nonprofit, 24-hour medical identification service alerts caregivers to a subscriber's special medical needs.

How the service works

A person wears a Medic Alert necklace or bracelet to identify a special health condition, for example, allergies. The engraved emblem (available in stainless steel, silver, or gold) contains the person's personal identification number and Medic Alert's 24-hour hot line number.

By calling the hot line and identifying the person by his identification number, the caregiver has access to crucial medical information. The service also records the names and phone numbers of the doctor and people to contact in a crisis.

Who needs medical identification?

People with:
- allergies to drugs, venoms, or other substances
- conditions, such as diabetes, heart disease, or asthma
- drug regimens, such as insulin for diabetes
- devices, such as contact lenses or a pacemaker
- special instructions (organ donation, for example).

How to obtain medical identification

You can get more information by writing or calling:
Medic Alert
Turlock, CA 95381-1009
1-800-ID-ALERT

- Wear a Medic Alert bracelet identifying your allergy or allergies. (See *Medic Alert service.*)
- If you must receive a drug to which you're allergic, you can avoid a severe reaction through careful desensitization. To do this, your caregiver will administer gradually increasing doses of the antigen or give you corticosteroids beforehand.

ANKYLOSING SPONDYLITIS

What do doctors call this condition?

Rheumatoid spondylitis

What is this condition?

A chronic, usually progressive inflammatory disease, ankylosing spondylitis affects the spine and adjacent soft tissue. Typically, the disease begins in the lower back and progresses up the spine to the neck. Deterioration of bone and cartilage can lead to fibrous tissue formation and eventual fusion of the spine or peripheral joints.

SELF-HELP

Coping with ankylosing spondylitis

Although some deformities are inevitable with this disease, you can slow their progress by taking these steps.

Minimize back stress
- Avoid any physical activity that places undue stress on your back, such as lifting heavy objects.
- Stand upright. Sit upright in a high, straight chair. Avoid leaning over a desk.
- Sleep in a prone position on a hard mattress. Avoid using pillows under your neck or knees.
- Avoid prolonged walking, standing, sitting, or driving.
- Seek vocational counseling if your work requires standing or prolonged sitting at a desk.
- Do regular stretching and deep-breathing exercises. Swim regularly, if possible.

Watch for changes
- Have your height measured every 3 to 4 months to detect any tendency toward kyphosis (curvature of the spine).
- Contact your local Arthritis Foundation chapter to find a support group.

Ankylosing spondylitis is diagnosed more often in men, but may be equally prevalent in both sexes. Diagnosis is often overlooked or missed in women, who tend to show more peripheral joint involvement.

What causes it?

Recent evidence strongly suggests a familial tendency in ankylosing spondylitis. The presence of human leukocyte antigen B27 (found in over 90% of people with this disease) and circulating immune complexes suggests immunologic activity.

What are its symptoms?

The first is intermittent low back pain that's usually most severe in the morning or after inactivity. Other symptoms depend on the disease stage and may include:
- stiffness and limited motion of the lumbar spine
- pain and limited chest expansion caused by involvement of the costovertebral joints
- arthritis involving shoulders, hips, and knees
- kyphosis (curvature of the spine) in advanced stages, caused by chronic stooping to relieve symptoms
- hip deformity with limited range of motion
- tenderness over the inflammation site
- mild fatigue, fever, loss of appetite or weight; occasional inflammation of the iris; aortic regurgitation and enlarged heart; upper lobe pulmonary fibrosis (which mimics tuberculosis).

These symptoms progress unpredictably, and the disease can disappear temporarily or permanently or flare up at any stage.

How is it diagnosed?

Typical symptoms, family history, and blood tests showing human leukocyte antigen B27 strongly suggest ankylosing spondylitis. However, confirmation requires additional blood tests as well as X-rays.

How is it treated?

No treatment reliably stops progression of this disease, so management aims to delay further deformity by enforcing good posture, stretching and deep-breathing exercises and, in some people, wearing braces and lightweight supports. (See *Coping with ankylosing spondylitis.*)

Anti-inflammatory pain relievers, such as aspirin, Indocin, Azulfidine, and Clinoril, control pain and inflammation.

Severe hip involvement usually requires hip replacement surgery. Severe spinal involvement may require a spinal wedge osteotomy (surgical cutting of bone) to separate and reposition the vertebrae. This surgery is performed only on selected people because of the risk of spinal cord damage and the long convalescence involved.

Asthma

What is this condition?

Asthma is a reversible lung disease in which the breathing passages become narrow or blocked, are typically inflamed, and overrespond to various types of stimulation. Asthma may stop on its own or with treatment. Symptoms range from mild wheezing and labored breathing to life-threatening respiratory failure. Between acute attacks, the person may have symptoms of bronchial airway obstruction.

What causes it?

Although this common condition can strike at any age, half of all cases first occur in children under age 10; in this age-group, asthma affects twice as many boys as girls.

Asthma can be extrinsic or intrinsic. *Extrinsic asthma* is caused by sensitivity to specific external allergens (substances that can produce hypersensitivity reactions). In *intrinsic asthma,* the allergen isn't obvious. Many people have both intrinsic and extrinsic asthma.

Allergens that cause extrinsic asthma include pollen, animal dander, household dust or mold, kapok or feather pillows, food additives containing sulfites, and any other sensitizing substance. Extrinsic asthma usually starts in childhood and is accompanied by related disorders, such as eczema and allergies.

In intrinsic asthma, no external allergen can be identified. Usually, a severe respiratory infection precedes intrinsic asthma attacks. Irritants, emotional stress, fatigue, harmful fumes, and endocrine, temperature, and humidity changes may aggravate intrinsic asthma attacks.

Several drugs and chemicals may also provoke an asthma attack. Examples of these include aspirin, various nonsteroidal anti-inflammatory drugs (such as Indocin and Ponstel), and the yellow food dye tartrazine.

Exercise also may trigger an asthma attack. In exercise-induced asthma, heat and moisture loss in the upper respiratory airways cause bronchospasm, or smooth-muscle contraction, causing acute airway narrowing and obstruction.

What are its symptoms?

An asthma attack may begin dramatically, with the person experiencing many severe symptoms at once. But sometimes it begins slowly, causing gradually increasing respiratory distress. Typically, the person becomes increasingly short of breath, with worsening cough, wheezing, and chest tightness or some combination of these symptoms.

During an acute attack, the cough sounds tight and dry. As the attack subsides, thick, sticky sputum is produced (except in young children). The lungs overinflate, causing use of accessory breathing muscles, particularly in children. An increased pulse, abnormally fast breathing, and profuse sweating are also common. In severe attacks, the person may be unable to speak more than a few words without pausing for breath. A bluish skin discoloration, confusion, and sluggishness signal the start of respiratory failure.

How is it diagnosed?

In people with asthma, lab tests often show these abnormalities:
- *Pulmonary function studies* reveal signs of airway obstruction. (However, between attacks, these studies may be normal.)
- *Pulse oximetry* may reveal decreased arterial oxygen saturation.
- *Arterial blood gas analysis* provides the best indication of an attack's severity. In acutely severe asthma, the partial pressure of arterial oxygen measures less than 60 millimeters of mercury, the partial pressure of arterial carbon dioxide is 40 millimeters of mercury or more, and pH usually decreases.
- *Complete blood count with white blood cell differential* reveals an increased eosinophil count.
- *Chest X-rays* may show overinflated lungs with areas of collapsed air sacs.

Before ordering tests for asthma, the doctor rules out other causes of airway obstruction and wheezing. In children, such causes include cystic fibrosis, chest tumors, and acute viral bronchitis. In adults, other causes include obstructive pulmonary disease, heart failure, and epiglottitis.

How is it treated?

Treatment of acute asthma aims to ease bronchoconstriction, reduce bronchial airway swelling, and improve pulmonary ventilation. After

> *An asthma attack may begin dramatically, with many severe symptoms at once — an increased pulse rate, abnormally fast breathing, and profuse sweating are common. The person may be unable to speak more than a few words without pausing for breath.*

an acute episode, treatment includes avoiding or removing factors that trigger asthma, such as environmental allergens or irritants.

If the person knows which substances trigger the asthma, he or she may receive limited amounts of the offending substance in a series of injections. This desensitizing therapy curbs the person's immune response to the substance. If asthma is caused by an infection, the doctor prescribes antibiotics.

Drug therapy for asthma is most effective when started soon after signs and symptoms begin. It usually includes:

- bronchodilators that open blocked airways; commonly used bronchodilators include methylxanthines (Theo-Dur and Aminophyllin) and beta$_2$-adrenergic agonists (Ventoline and Brethaire)
- corticosteroids (Solu-Cortef, Orasone, Medrol, and Beconase) to reduce inflammation and suppress the immune response, thereby easing airway inflammation and swelling
- Nasalcrom and Tilade to help block the release of the chemical mediators active in asthma
- anticholinergic bronchodilators, such as Atrovent, which block acetylcholine, another chemical mediator of asthma attacks.

For the most part, medical treatment of asthma is tailored to each person. However, the following treatments are generally used:

- *Chronic mild asthma.* A beta$_2$-adrenergic agonist by metered-dose inhaler is used (alone or with Nasalcrom) before exercise and exposure to an allergen to prevent symptoms. The person uses the drug every 3 to 4 hours if symptoms occur.
- *Chronic moderate asthma.* At first, the person receives an inhaled beta-adrenergic bronchodilator, an inhaled corticosteroid, and Nasalcrom. If symptoms persist, the doctor may increase the inhaled corticosteroid dosage and add sustained-release Theo-Dur or an oral beta$_2$-adrenergic agonist (or both). Brief therapy with oral corticosteroids also may be used.
- *Chronic severe asthma.* Initially, the person may need around-the-clock oral bronchodilators with a long-acting theophylline or a beta$_2$-adrenergic agonist. This therapy is supplemented with an inhaled beta$_2$-adrenergic agonist and an inhaled corticosteroid with or without Nasalcrom. In acute attacks, the doctor may add an oral corticosteroid.
- *Acute asthma attack.* Acute attacks that don't respond to self-treatment may require hospital care, inhaled or injected beta$_2$-adrenergic agonists and, possibly, oxygen. The doctor may prescribe intravenous therapy. People who don't respond to this treatment, whose airways remain blocked, and who have increasing breathing difficulty are at

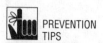

Avoiding asthma triggers

To make it easier for you to live with asthma, try to avoid the following common asthma triggers.

At home
- Such foods as nuts, chocolate, eggs, shellfish, and peanut butter
- Such beverages as orange juice, wine, beer, and milk
- Mold spores; pollens from flowers, trees, grasses, hay, and ragweed (if pollen is the offender, install a bedroom air conditioner with a filter, and avoid long walks when pollen counts are high)
- Dander from rabbits, cats, dogs, hamsters, gerbils, and chickens; consider finding a new home for the family pet, if necessary
- Feather or hair-stuffed pillows, down comforters, wool clothing, and stuffed toys; use smooth (not fuzzy), washable blankets on your bed
- Insect parts, such as those from dead cockroaches
- Medicines, such as aspirin and antibiotics
- Vapors from cleaning solvents, paint, paint thinners, and liquid chlorine bleach
- Fluorocarbon spray products, such as furniture polish, starch, cleaners, and room deodorizers
- Scents from spray deodorants, perfumes, hair sprays, talcum powder, and cosmetics
- Cloth-upholstered furniture, carpets, and draperies that collect dust; hang lightweight, washable cotton or synthetic-fiber curtains; use washable, cotton throw rugs on bare floors
- Brooms and dusters that raise dust; instead, clean your bedroom daily by damp dusting and damp mopping and keep the door closed
- Dirty filters on hot-air furnaces and air conditioners that blow dust into the air
- Dust from vacuum cleaner exhaust

In the workplace
- Dust, vapors, or fumes from wood products (western red cedar, some pine and birch woods, mahogany); flour, cereals, and other grains; coffee, tea, or papain; metals (platinum, chromium, nickel sulfate, soldering fumes); and cotton, flax, and hemp
- Mold from decaying hay

Outdoors
- Cold air, hot air, or sudden temperature changes (when you go in and out of air-conditioned buildings in the summer)
- Excessive humidity or dryness
- Changes in seasons
- Automobile exhaust, smog

Anyplace
- Overexertion, which may cause wheezing
- Common cold, flu, and other viruses
- Fear, anger, frustration, laughing too hard, crying, or any emotionally upsetting situation
- Smoke from cigarettes, cigars, and pipes; don't smoke and don't stay in a room with people who do.

Tips for staying healthy
Remember to:
- drink enough fluids — six eight-ounce glasses daily.
- take all prescribed drugs exactly as directed.
- tell your doctor about any and all drugs you take, even nonprescription ones.
- avoid sleeping pills or sedatives to help you sleep because of mild asthma attacks. These drugs may slow your breathing and make it more difficult to breathe; instead, try propping yourself up on extra pillows while waiting for your antianxiety drug to work.
- schedule only as much activity as you can tolerate. Take frequent rests on busy days.

How to control an asthma attack

Usually, an asthma attack is preceded by warning signs that give you time to take action.

Early warning signs
Be alert for:
- chest tightness
- coughing
- changes in your breathing
- wheezing.

Once you've had a few asthma attacks, you'll have no trouble recognizing these early warning signs. Above all, *do not ignore them.*
- Take your prescribed medicine with an oral inhaler, if directed, to prevent the attack from getting worse.

How to relax
- As your medicine goes to work, try to relax. Although you may be understandably nervous or afraid, remember that these feelings only increase your shortness of breath.

To help relax, sit upright in a chair, close your eyes, and breathe slowly and evenly. Then, begin consciously tightening and relaxing the muscles in your body. First, tighten the muscles in your face and count to yourself "one, 1,000; two, 1,000." Be sure not to hold your breath. Then, relax these muscles and repeat with the muscles in your arms and hands, legs and feet. Finally, let your body go limp.

Helpful breathing techniques
- Regain control of your breathing by doing the pursed-lip breathing exercises you've been taught. *Don't gasp for air.* Continue pursed-lip breathing until you no longer feel breathless.
- If the attack triggers a coughing spell, you'll need to control your cough so that it effectively brings up mucus and helps clear your airways. To do so, lean forward slightly, keeping your feet on the floor. Next, breathe in deeply and hold that breath for a second or two. Cough twice, first to loosen mucus and then to bring it up. Be sure to cough into a tissue.
- If the attack gets worse even after you've followed these steps, call your doctor right away.

risk for a potentially lethal condition called *status asthmaticus.* To maintain their breathing, they may require mechanical ventilation.
- *Status asthmaticus.* A person with status asthmaticus (an acute, severe, prolonged asthma attack) needs aggressive drug therapy. He or she receives a beta$_2$-adrenergic agonist by nebulizer every 30 to 60 minutes. The doctor may also give an Adrenalin injection; intravenous corticosteroids, aminophylline, and fluids; and oxygen. Some people need mechanical ventilation to assist breathing.

What can a person with asthma do?
- Avoid known allergens and irritants. (See *Avoiding asthma triggers.*)
- If you have trouble using a metered-dose inhaler, you may need an extender device to improve drug delivery and lower the risk of yeast infection with orally inhaled corticosteroids.

- If you have moderate to severe asthma, learn how to use a peak flowmeter to measure the degree of airway obstruction. Keep a record of peak flow readings and bring it to medical appointments. Call the doctor at once if the peak flow drops suddenly. (A drop may signal severe respiratory problems.)
- Notify the doctor if you develop a fever above 100° F (37.8° C), chest pain, shortness of breath without coughing or exercising, or uncontrollable coughing. An uncontrollable asthma attack requires immediate attention.
- To manage asthma attacks, learn diaphragmatic and pursed-lip breathing as well as effective coughing techniques. (See *How to control an asthma attack,* page 697.)
- Drink at least 6 eight-ounce glasses of fluids daily to help loosen airway secretions and maintain hydration.

ATOPIC DERMATITIS

What is this condition?

This chronic skin disorder is characterized by superficial skin inflammation and intense itching. Although atopic dermatitis may appear at any age, it typically begins during infancy or early childhood. It may then disappear spontaneously, followed by flare-ups in late childhood, adolescence, or early adulthood. Atopic dermatitis affects approximately 0.7% of the population.

What causes it?

The cause of atopic dermatitis is still unknown. However, several theories attempt to explain its cause. One theory suggests an underlying metabolic- or biochemical-induced skin disorder genetically linked to elevated serum immunoglobulin E levels; another suggests defective T-cell function.

Exacerbating factors of atopic dermatitis include irritants, infections (commonly caused by *Staphylococcus aureus),* and some allergens. Although no reliable link exists between atopic dermatitis and exposure to inhaled allergens (such as household dust and animal dander), exposure to food allergens (such as soybeans, fish, or nuts) may coincide with flare-ups of atopic dermatitis.

What are its symptoms?

Scratching the skin intensifies itching, resulting in red, weeping lesions. Eventually, the lesions become scaly. Usually, they're found on the neck, inside the elbows, and behind the knees and ears. People with atopic dermatitis are prone to unusually severe viral infections, bacterial and fungal skin infections, eye complications, and allergic contact dermatitis.

How is it diagnosed?

Typically, the person has a history of allergies, such as asthma, hay fever, or hives; family members may have a similar history. Lab tests show an increase in the white blood cells active in hypersensitivity responses and elevated serum immunoglobulin E.

How is it treated?

Measures to ease this chronic disorder include meticulous skin care, environmental control of offending allergens, and drug therapy. Because dry skin aggravates itching, frequent application of nonirritating skin lubricants is important, especially after bathing or showering. Minimizing exposure to allergens and irritants, such as wools and harsh detergents, also helps control symptoms.

Drug therapy involves corticosteroids and antipruritics. Active dermatitis responds well to topical corticosteroids such as Synalar and Cordran. These drugs should be applied immediately after bathing for the best penetration. Oral antihistamines, especially the phenothiazine derivatives such as Tacaryl and Temaril, help control itching. A bedtime dose of antihistamines may reduce involuntary scratching during sleep. If secondary infection develops, antibiotics are necessary.

Because this disorder may frustrate the person and strain family ties, counseling may play a role in treatment.

What can a person with atopic dermatitis do?

- Avoid factors that trigger this condition. (See *Avoiding triggers for atopic dermatitis*.)
- Maintain good personal hygiene.
- Be alert for signs and symptoms of secondary infection.

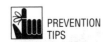 PREVENTION TIPS

Avoiding triggers for atopic dermatitis

If you have atopic dermatitis, you need to discover what triggers these attacks so you can take steps to avoid them. Common triggers include:

- irritants, such as soaps, household cleansers, chemicals, and certain fabrics — for example, wool
- activities that cause sweating
- inhaled or ingested allergens (or both)
- scratching or other skin trauma
- emotional stress
- infections
- environmental temperature changes, heat, and humidity.

BLOOD TRANSFUSION REACTION

What is this condition?

Transfusion reaction accompanies or follows intravenous administration of blood components. Its severity varies from mild (fever and chills) to severe (acute kidney failure or complete vascular collapse and death), depending on the amount of blood transfused, the type of reaction, and the person's general health.

What causes it?

Hemolytic reactions (red blood cell rupture) follow transfusion of mismatched blood. Transfusion with incompatible blood triggers the most serious reaction, marked by intravascular clumping of red blood cells. The recipient's antibodies (immunoglobulin G or M) adhere to the donated red blood cells, leading to widespread clumping and destruction of the recipient's red blood cells and, possibly, the development of disseminated intravascular coagulation and other serious effects.

Transfusion with Rh-incompatible blood triggers a less serious reaction within several days to 2 weeks. Rh reactions are most likely in women sensitized to red blood cell antigens by prior pregnancy or by unknown factors, such as bacterial or viral infection, and in people who have received more than five transfusions.

Allergic reactions are fairly common but only occasionally serious.

Febrile nonhemolytic reactions, the most common type of reaction, apparently develop when antibodies in the recipient's plasma attack antigens.

Bacterial contamination of donor blood, although fairly uncommon, can occur during donor phlebotomy. Also possible is contamination of donor blood with viruses (such as hepatitis), cytomegalovirus, and the organism causing malaria.

What are its symptoms?

Immediate effects of hemolytic transfusion reaction develop within a few minutes or hours after the start of transfusion and may include chills, fever, hives, rapid heartbeat, shortness of breath, nausea, vomiting, tightness in the chest, chest and back pain, low blood pressure, bronchospasm, angioedema, and signs and symptoms of anaphylaxis, shock, pulmonary edema, and congestive heart failure. In a person having surgery under anesthesia, these symptoms are masked, but blood oozes from mucous membranes or the incision.

Delayed hemolytic reactions can occur up to several weeks after transfusion, causing fever, an unexpected decrease in serum hemoglobin, and jaundice.

Allergic hemolytic reactions typically don't cause a fever and are characterized by hives and angioedema, possibly progressing to cough, respiratory distress, nausea and vomiting, diarrhea, abdominal cramps, vascular instability, shock, and coma.

The hallmark of febrile nonhemolytic reactions is a mild to severe fever that may begin when the transfusion starts or within 2 hours after its completion.

Bacterial contamination causes high fever, nausea and vomiting, diarrhea, abdominal cramps and, possibly, shock. Symptoms of viral contamination may not appear for several weeks after transfusion.

How is it diagnosed?

Confirming a hemolytic transfusion reaction requires proof of blood incompatibility and evidence of hemolysis. When such a reaction is suspected, the person's blood is retyped and crossmatched with the donor's blood.

When bacterial contamination is suspected, a blood culture should be done to isolate the causative organism.

How is it treated?

At the first sign of a hemolytic reaction, the transfusion is stopped immediately. Depending on the nature of the person's reaction, the health care team may:
- monitor vital signs every 15 to 30 minutes, watching for signs of shock
- maintain an open intravenous line with normal saline solution, insert an indwelling urinary catheter, and monitor intake and output
- cover the person with blankets to ease chills
- deliver supplemental oxygen at low flow rates through a nasal cannula or hand-held resuscitation bag (called an *Ambu bag*)
- administer drugs such as intravenous medications to raise blood pressure and normal saline solution to combat shock, Adrenalin to treat shortness of breath and wheezing, Benadryl to combat cellular histamine released from mast cells, corticosteroids to reduce inflammation, and Osmitrol or Lasix to maintain urinary function. Parenteral antihistamines and corticosteroids are given for allergic

reactions (anaphylaxis, a severe reaction, may require Adrenalin). Drugs to reduce fever are administered for febrile nonhemolytic reactions and appropriate intravenous antibiotics are given for bacterial contamination.

CHRONIC FATIGUE SYNDROME

What do doctors call this condition?
Chronic fatigue and immune dysfunction syndrome, "yuppie flu"

What is this condition?
In this recently recognized illness, the person typically has overwhelming fatigue, fever, painful glands, and other symptoms that mimic those of chronic mononucleosis. It commonly affects adults under age 45, mostly women.

What causes it?
The cause of chronic fatigue syndrome is unknown, but researchers suspect that it may be found in human herpesvirus type 6 or in other herpesviruses, enteroviruses, or retroviruses. Possibly, this disorder may be a reaction to viral illness that's complicated by a faulty immune response and by other factors, such as sex, age, genetic disposition, prior illness, stress, and environment.

What are its symptoms?
The hallmark of chronic fatigue syndrome is prolonged, often overwhelming fatigue, commonly accompanied by a varying array of other symptoms. To help identify the disease, the Centers for Disease Control and Prevention uses a "working case definition" to group symptoms and their severity. In general, this case definition includes the following symptoms:
- profound or prolonged fatigue, especially after exercise levels that the person would have previously tolerated
- low-grade fever
- painful glands
- muscle weakness

To help identify chronic fatigue syndrome, the Centers for Disease Control and Prevention uses what they call a "working case definition" that groups symptoms and their severity — from profound fatigue to vision problems.

- sleep disturbances (insomnia or increased sleep)
- headaches of a new type, severity, or pattern
- joint pain without joint swelling or redness
- abnormal sensitivity to light
- irritability
- forgetfulness, confusion, difficulty thinking, or poor concentration
- depression
- areas of decreased vision within the visual field.

How is it diagnosed?

The cause and nature of chronic fatigue syndrome are still unknown and no single test clearly confirms it. Therefore, doctors base the diagnosis on the person's history and the Centers for Disease Control and Prevention criteria. However, diagnosis is difficult and uncertain because these criteria are admittedly a working concept that may not include all forms of the disease and are based on symptoms that can result from other diseases.

How is it treated?

No treatment is known to cure chronic fatigue syndrome. Experimental treatments include the antiviral drug Zovirax and selected drugs that adjust the immune response, such as intravenous gamma globulin, Ampligen, and transfer factor.

To treat symptoms, the doctor may prescribe tricyclic antidepressants, histamine$_2$-blocking agents such as Tagamet, and antianxiety agents such as Xanax. In some people, avoiding environmental irritants and certain foods may help to relieve symptoms.

What can a person with chronic fatigue syndrome do?

Contact the Chronic Fatigue and Immune Dysfunction Syndrome Association for information and referral to local support groups.

GOODPASTURE'S SYNDROME

What is this condition?

Goodpasture's syndrome affects the lungs and kidneys. Coughing up blood and rapidly progressive glomerulonephritis follow the deposition of antibody against the alveolar (lung) and glomerular (kidney) basement membranes. This syndrome may occur at any age but is most common in men between ages 20 and 30. The prognosis improves with aggressive immunosuppressants and antibiotic therapy and with dialysis or kidney transplantation.

What causes it?

The cause of Goodpasture's syndrome is unknown. Although some cases have been associated with exposure to hydrocarbons or type 2 influenza, many have no precipitating events. Evidence suggests a genetic predisposition to this syndrome. Abnormal production and deposition of the antibody against glomerular and alveolar basement membranes damages glomerular and alveolar tissues.

What are its symptoms?

Goodpasture's syndrome may initially cause malaise, fatigue, and pallor associated with severe iron deficiency anemia. Pulmonary findings range from slight shortness of breath and cough with blood-tinged sputum to frank pulmonary hemorrhage. Subclinical pulmonary bleeding may precede overt hemorrhage and kidney disease by months or years. Usually, such findings are more subtle, although some people note blood in the urine and peripheral swelling.

How is it diagnosed?

Confirmation of Goodpasture's syndrome requires tests to distinguish Goodpasture's from other lung-kidney syndromes.

Chest X-rays and removal and analysis of lung and kidney tissue, along with blood and urine tests, can help confirm the diagnosis.

How is it treated?

Treatment aims to remove antibody by plasmapheresis (processing of formed blood elements) and to suppress antibody production with immunosuppressants. A person with kidney failure may benefit from dialysis or transplantation. Aggressive ultrafiltration helps relieve pulmonary edema that may aggravate pulmonary hemorrhage. High-dose intravenous corticosteroids also help control pulmonary hemorrhage.

Initially, Goodpasture's syndrome may cause malaise, fatigue, and pallor associated with severe iron deficiency anemia. Pulmonary bleeding may precede overt hemorrhage and kidney disease by months or years.

What can a person with Goodpasture's syndrome do?

- Take steps to conserve your energy.
- Learn what signs and symptoms to expect and how to relieve them.

HIVES

What do doctors call this condition?

Urticaria, angioedema

What is this condition?

Hives refers to two conditions: urticaria and angioedema. *Urticaria* is an episodic, usually self-limiting skin reaction characterized by local wheals surrounded by an area of redness called an *erythematous flare*. *Angioedema* is an eruption on and beneath the skin that produces deeper, larger wheals (usually on the hands, feet, lips, genitalia, and eyelids) and a more diffuse swelling of loose tissue under the skin. Urticaria and angioedema can occur simultaneously, but angioedema may last longer.

What causes it?

Hives are a common allergic reaction that may occur in 20% of the general population. Possible causes include allergy to drugs, foods, insect stings and, occasionally, inhaled allergens (animal danders, cosmetics). When hives are part of an anaphylactic reaction, they almost always persists long after the systemic response has subsided. This occurs because circulation to the skin is the last to be restored after an allergic reaction.

Nonallergic urticaria and angioedema are probably also related to histamine release by some still-unknown mechanism. External physical stimuli, such as cold (usually in young adults), heat, water, or sunlight, may also provoke urticaria and angioedema. *Dermographism urticaria,* which develops after stroking or scratching the skin, occurs in up to 20% of the population. This type of urticaria develops with varying pressure, most often under tight clothing, and is aggravated by scratching.

Several different mechanisms and underlying disorders may provoke hives. These include immunoglobulin E–induced release of me-

Hives are a common allergic reaction that may occur in 20% of the general population. Causes include allergy to drugs, foods, insect stings, and, occasionally, inhaled allergens (such as animal danders and cosmetics).

diators from cutaneous mast cells; binding of immunoglobulin G or immunoglobulin M to an antigen, resulting in complement activation; and disorders such as localized or secondary infection (respiratory infection), connective tissue diseases (lupus), neoplastic diseases (Hodgkin's disease), collagen vascular diseases, and psychogenic disorders.

What are its symptoms?

The characteristic features of urticaria are distinct, raised, transient wheals surrounded by an erythematous flare. These lesions may vary in size. In cholinergic urticaria, the wheals may be tiny and blanched, surrounded by erythematous flares.

Angioedema characteristically produces nonpitted swelling of deep tissue under the skin, usually on the eyelids, lips, genitalia, and mucous membranes. These swellings don't usually itch but may burn and tingle.

How is it diagnosed?

An accurate history can help determine the cause of hives. Such a history should include:
- drug history, including over-the-counter preparations (vitamins, aspirin, antacids)
- frequently ingested foods (strawberries, milk products, fish)
- environmental influences (pets, carpet, clothing, soap, inhalants, cosmetics, hair dye, insect bites and stings).

Diagnosis also requires physical assessment to rule out similar conditions, plus lab tests and chest X-ray to rule out inflammatory infections. Skin testing, an elimination diet, and a food diary (record of the time and amount of food eaten and circumstances) can pinpoint provoking allergens. The food diary may also suggest other allergies. For instance, someone who is allergic to fish may also be allergic to contrast dyes containing iodine.

Recurrent angioedema without urticaria, along with a family history, points to hereditary angioedema. Blood tests can confirm this diagnosis.

How is it treated?

Treatment aims to prevent or limit contact with triggering factors or, if this is impossible, to desensitize the person to them and to relieve symptoms. Once the triggering stimulus has been removed, urticaria usually subsides in a few days except for drug reactions, which may persist as long as the drug is in the bloodstream.

During desensitization, progressively larger doses of specific antigens (determined by skin testing) are injected into the skin.

Atarax or another antihistamine can ease itching and swelling in every kind of urticaria. Corticosteroid therapy also may be necessary for some people.

IMMUNOGLOBULIN A DEFICIENCY

What is this condition?

Selective deficiency of immunoglobulin A is the most common immunoglobulin deficiency, appearing in as many as 1 in 800 persons. Immunoglobulin A, the major immunoglobulin in human saliva, nasal and bronchial fluids, and intestinal secretions, guards against bacterial and viral reinfections. Consequently, immunoglobulin A deficiency leads to chronic sinus and respiratory infections, gastrointestinal diseases, and other disorders. The prognosis is good for people who receive correct treatment, especially if they are free of associated disorders. Such people have been known to survive to age 70.

What causes it?

Immunoglobulin A deficiency is an inherited disorder. It also seems related to autoimmune disorders, because many people with rheumatoid arthritis or lupus are also immunoglobulin A deficient. Some drugs, such as anticonvulsants, may cause temporary immunoglobulin A deficiency.

What are its symptoms?

Some people with immunoglobulin A deficiency have no symptoms, possibly because their bodies compensate for the deficiency. Among people who do develop symptoms, chronic sinus and respiratory infection is most common. Other effects are respiratory allergy, often triggered by infection; gastrointestinal diseases, such as celiac disease, ulcerative colitis, and regional enteritis; autoimmune diseases, such as rheumatoid arthritis, lupus, hemolytic anemia, and chronic hepa-

Immunoglobulin A deficiency leads to chronic sinus and respiratory infections, gastrointestinal diseases, and other disorders. The prognosis is good for people who receive correct treatment. Such people have been known to live to age 70.

titis; and malignant tumors, such as squamous cell cancer of the lungs, reticulum cell sarcoma, and thymoma.

Age of onset varies. Some children with immunoglobulin A deficiency who have recurrent respiratory disease and middle-ear inflammation may begin to synthesize immunoglobulin A spontaneously as recurrent infections subside and their condition improves.

How is it diagnosed?

Blood tests confirm diagnosis. Immunologic analyses show serum immunoglobulin A levels below 5 milligrams per deciliter.

Tests may also indicate autoantibodies and antibodies against immunoglobulin G (rheumatoid factor), immunoglobulin M, and cow's milk.

How is it treated?

Selective immunoglobulin A deficiency has no known cure. Treatment aims to control symptoms of associated diseases, such as respiratory and gastrointestinal infections, and is generally the same as for a person with normal immunoglobulin A, with one exception: A person with immunoglobulin A deficiency must not receive immune globulin because sensitization may lead to anaphylaxis during future administration of blood products.

If transfusion with blood products is necessary, the risk of side effects can be reduced by using washed red blood cells; it can be avoided completely by crossmatching the person's blood with that of a donor who's deficient in immunoglobulin A.

JUVENILE RHEUMATOID ARTHRITIS

What is this condition?

An affliction of children under age 16, juvenile rheumatoid arthritis is an inflammatory disorder of the connective tissues characterized by joint swelling, pain, or tenderness. It may also involve organs such as the skin, heart, lungs, liver, spleen, and eyes, producing signs and symptoms other than those affecting movement.

Juvenile rheumatoid arthritis has three major types: *systemic* (Still's disease or acute feverish type), *polyarticular*, and *pauciarticular*. Depending on the type, this disease can occur as early as age 6 weeks (although rarely before 6 months) with peaks of onset between ages 1 and 3 and ages 8 and 12.

Considered the major chronic rheumatic disorder of childhood, this condition affects an estimated 150,000 to 250,000 children in the United States. Overall incidence is twice as high in girls, with variation among the types.

What causes it?

The cause of juvenile rheumatoid arthritis remains puzzling. Research continues to test several theories, such as those linking the condition to genetic factors or to an abnormal immune response. Viral or bacterial (particularly streptococcal) infection, trauma, and emotional stress may be precipitating factors, but their relationship to juvenile rheumatoid arthritis remains unclear.

What are its symptoms?

Signs and symptoms vary with the type of arthritis.

Systemic juvenile rheumatoid arthritis

Affecting boys and girls almost equally, the systemic disorder accounts for approximately 20% to 30% of cases. The affected children may have mild, transient arthritis or frank polyarthritis associated with fever and rash. Joint involvement may not be evident at first, but the child's behavior may clearly suggest joint pain. Such a child may want to constantly sit in a flexed position, may not walk much, or may refuse to walk at all. Young children with juvenile rheumatoid arthritis are noticeably irritable and listless.

Fever in systemic juvenile rheumatoid arthritis occurs suddenly and spikes to 103° F (39.4° C) or higher, once or twice daily, usually in the late afternoon, and then rapidly returns to normal or subnormal. (This "sawtooth" or intermittent spiking fever pattern helps distinguish juvenile rheumatoid arthritis from other inflammatory disorders.)

When fever spikes, a transient rheumatoid rash often appears, consisting of small, pale, or salmon-pink macules, most commonly on the trunk and proximal extremities and, occasionally, on the face, palms, and soles. Massaging or applying heat intensifies this rash, which is usually most conspicuous where the skin has been rubbed or subjected to pressure, such as from tight-fitting underclothing.

Other signs and symptoms of the systemic type may include an enlarged liver and spleen, disease of the lymph nodes, pleuritis, pericarditis, myocarditis, and nonspecific abdominal pain.

The behavior of a child with juvenile rheumatoid arthritis may clearly suggest joint pain. For instance, he or she may want to constantly sit in a flexed position, may not walk much, or may refuse to walk at all.

Polyarticular juvenile rheumatoid arthritis

This type affects girls three times more often than boys and may be seronegative or seropositive for rheumatoid factor. It involves five or more joints and usually develops insidiously. Most commonly involved joints are the wrists, elbows, knees, ankles, and small joints of the hands and feet. The polyarticular type can also affect larger joints, including the temporomandibular joints and those of the cervical spine, hips, and shoulders. These joints become swollen, tender, and stiff. Usually, the arthritis affects both sides; it may come and go or cause little discomfort. The person may run a low-grade fever with daily peaks. Listlessness and weight loss also can occur, possibly with enlarged lymph nodes, liver, and spleen. Other signs of the polyarticular type include lumps under the skin of the elbows or heels and noticeable developmental retardation.

Seropositive polyarticular juvenile rheumatoid arthritis, the most severe type, usually occurs late in childhood and can cause destructive arthritis that mimics adult rheumatoid arthritis.

Pauciarticular juvenile rheumatoid arthritis

This type involves few joints (usually no more than four) and most often affects the knees and other large joints. It accounts for 45% of cases. Three major subtypes exist:

▪ The first type, *pauciarticular juvenile rheumatoid arthritis with chronic iridocyclitis,* most commonly strikes girls under age 6 and involves the knees, elbows, ankles, or iris. Inflammation of the iris and ciliary body is often without symptoms but may produce pain, redness, blurred vision, and sensitivity to light.

▪ The second subtype, *pauciarticular juvenile rheumatoid arthritis with sacroiliitis,* usually strikes boys over age 8, who tend to be positive for human leukocyte antigen B27. This subtype is characterized by lower extremity arthritis that produces hip, sacroiliac, heel, and foot pain and Achilles tendinitis. These children may later develop the sacroiliac and lumbar arthritis characteristic of ankylosing spondylitis. Some also experience acute iritis, but not as frequently as those with the first subtype.

▪ The third subtype includes people with joint involvement who are negative for antinuclear antibody and human leukocyte antigen B27 and do not develop iritis. These people have a better prognosis than those with the first or second subtype.

Common to all types of juvenile rheumatoid arthritis is joint stiffness in the morning or after periods of inactivity. Growth disturbances may also occur, resulting in overgrowth or undergrowth adjacent to inflamed joints.

How is it diagnosed?

Persistent joint pain and the rash and fever clearly point to juvenile rheumatoid arthritis. Lab tests are useful for ruling out other inflammatory or even malignant diseases that can mimic the condition and for monitoring disease activity and response to therapy.

How is it treated?

Successful management of juvenile rheumatoid arthritis usually involves administration of anti-inflammatory drugs, physical therapy, carefully planned nutrition and exercise, and regular eye exams. Both child and parents must be involved in therapy.

Aspirin is the initial drug of choice, with dosage based on the child's weight. However, other nonsteroidal anti-inflammatory drugs may also be used. If these prove ineffective, gold salts, Plaquenil, and Cuprimine may be tried. Because of side effects, corticosteroids are generally reserved for treatment of systemic complications, such as pericarditis or iritis, that are resistant to nonsteroidal anti-inflammatory drugs. Corticosteroids and mydriatic drugs are commonly used for iridocyclitis. Low-dose cytotoxic drug therapy is currently being investigated.

Physical therapy promotes regular exercise to maintain joint mobility and muscle strength, thereby preventing contractures, deformity, and disability. Good posture, gait training, and joint protection are also beneficial. Splints help reduce pain, prevent contractures, and maintain correct joint alignment.

Regular slit-lamp examinations help ensure early diagnosis and treatment of iridocyclitis. Children with pauciarticular juvenile rheumatoid arthritis with chronic iridocyclitis should be checked every 3 months during periods of active disease and every 6 months during remissions.

Generally, the prognosis for juvenile rheumatoid arthritis is good, although disabilities can occur. Surgery is usually limited to soft-tissue releases to improve joint mobility. Joint replacement is delayed until the child has matured physically and can handle vigorous rehabilitation.

Parents and health care professionals should encourage the child to be as independent as possible and to develop a positive attitude toward school, social development, and vocational planning.

Successful management of juvenile rheumatoid arthritis usually involves giving the child anti-inflammatory drugs, physical therapy, carefully planned nutrition and exercise, and regular eye exams. The parents, too, must be involved in therapy.

LUPUS ERYTHEMATOSUS

What is this condition?

A chronic inflammatory disorder of the connective tissues, lupus erythematosus appears in two forms: *discoid lupus erythematosus*, which affects only the skin, and *systemic lupus erythematosus,* which affects multiple organ systems (as well as the skin) and can be fatal.

Like rheumatoid arthritis, systemic lupus is characterized by recurring remissions and flare-ups, especially common during the spring and summer. The annual incidence of this disorder averages about 27 cases in 1 million whites and 75 cases in 1 million blacks. Systemic lupus strikes women 8 times as often as men, increasing to 15 times as often during childbearing years. Systemic lupus occurs worldwide but is most prevalent among Asians and blacks.

The prognosis improves with early diagnosis and treatment but remains poor for people who develop heart and blood vessel, kidney, or nervous system complications or severe bacterial infections.

What causes it?

The exact cause of systemic lupus remains a mystery, but available evidence points to interrelated immunologic, environmental, hormonal, and genetic factors. An immune dysfunction, such as autoimmunity, is considered the prime causative mechanism. In autoimmunity, the body produces antibodies (such as the antinuclear antibody) against its own cells. The formed antigen-antibody complexes can suppress the body's normal immunity and damage tissues. One significant feature in people with this disorder is their ability to produce antibodies against many different tissue components, such as red blood cells, neutrophils, platelets, lymphocytes, or almost any organ or tissue in the body.

Certain predisposing factors may make a person susceptible to systemic lupus. Physical or mental stress, streptococcal or viral infections, exposure to sunlight or ultraviolet light, immunization, pregnancy, and abnormal estrogen metabolism all may affect the disease's development.

Systemic lupus also may be triggered or aggravated by treatment with certain drugs — for example, Procan SR, Apresoline, antiseizure drugs and, less frequently, penicillins, sulfa drugs, and oral contraceptives.

What are its symptoms?

The onset of systemic lupus may be acute or insidious and produces no characteristic clinical pattern. However, its symptoms commonly include fever, weight loss, malaise and fatigue, as well as rashes and pain in multiple joints.

Systemic lupus may involve every organ system. In 90% of cases, joint involvement is similar to that in rheumatoid arthritis. Skin lesions are most commonly a red rash in areas exposed to light. The classic butterfly rash over the nose and cheeks occurs in fewer than 50% of people with systemic lupus. Ultraviolet rays often provoke or aggravate skin eruptions. Vasculitis can develop (especially in the fingers and toes), possibly leading to infarctive lesions, necrotic leg ulcers, or gangrene of the fingers or toes. Raynaud's phenomenon (decreased blood flow to the fingers and toes, causing numbness and pain) appears in about 20% of cases. Patchy hair loss and painless ulcers of the mucous membranes are common.

Constitutional symptoms of systemic lupus include aching, malaise, fatigue, low-grade or spiking fever, chills, loss of appetite, and weight loss. Lymph node enlargement (diffuse or local, and nontender), abdominal pain, nausea, vomiting, diarrhea, and constipation may occur. Women may experience absent or irregular menstrual periods during the active phase of systemic lupus erythematosus.

About 50% of people with systemic lupus develop signs of cardiopulmonary abnormalities, such as pleuritis, pericarditis, and shortness of breath. Myocarditis, endocarditis, rapid heartbeat, parenchymal infiltrates, and pneumonitis may occur. Kidney effects may include blood, protein, sediment, and cellular casts in the urine and may progress to total kidney failure. Urinary tract infections may be caused by heightened susceptibility to infection. Seizure disorders and mental dysfunction may indicate neurologic damage. Central nervous system involvement may produce emotional instability, psychosis, and organic brain syndrome. Headaches, irritability, and depression also are common.

Systemic lupus may be triggered or aggravated by treatment with some drugs. For example, Procan SR, Apresoline, antiseizure drugs and, less frequently, penicillins, sulfa drugs, and oral contraceptives may be involved.

How is it diagnosed?

Diagnostic tests for people with systemic lupus include a complete blood count with differential, platelet count, erythrocyte sedimentation rate, and serum electrophoresis.

Specific tests include antinuclear antibody, anti-DNA, and lupus erythematosus cell tests, urine studies, blood complement studies, chest X-ray, electrocardiography, and kidney biopsy.

Some people show a positive lupus anticoagulant test and a positive anticardiolipin test. These people are prone to antiphospholipid syndrome (blood clot formation, miscarriage, and low platelet count).

How is it treated?

People with mild systemic lupus require little or no medication. Nonsteroidal anti-inflammatory compounds, including aspirin, control arthritis symptoms in many cases. Skin lesions need topical treatment. Corticosteroid creams, such as Cordran, are recommended for acute lesions.

Refractory skin lesions are treated with intralesional corticosteroids or antimalarials, such as Plaquenil and Aralen. Because these drugs can cause retinal damage, such treatment requires eye exams every 6 months.

Corticosteroids remain the treatment of choice for systemic symptoms of systemic lupus, for acute generalized flare-ups, or for serious disease related to vital organ systems, such as pleuritis, pericarditis, lupus nephritis, vasculitis, and central nervous system involvement. Initial doses equivalent to 60 milligrams or more of Orasone often bring noticeable improvement within 48 hours. As soon as symptoms are under control, corticosteroid dosage is tapered down slowly.

Diffuse proliferative glomerulonephritis, a major complication of this disorder, requires treatment with large doses of corticosteroids. If kidney failure occurs, dialysis or kidney transplant may be necessary. In some people, cytotoxic drugs such as Imuran and Cytoxan may delay or prevent deteriorating kidney status. Antihypertensive drugs and dietary changes may also be warranted in kidney disease.

The light-sensitive person should wear protective clothing (hat, sunglasses, long sleeves, slacks) and use a sunscreen containing para-aminobenzoic acid when outside. (See *Protecting your skin.*) Because systemic lupus usually strikes women of childbearing age, questions associated with pregnancy often arise. The best evidence available indicates that a woman with this disorder can have a safe, successful pregnancy if she has no serious kidney or nervous system impairment. (See *Lupus and pregnancy,* page 716.)

What can a person with lupus do?

▪ Watch for symptoms, such as joint pain or stiffness, weakness, fever, fatigue, and chills. Stay alert for shortness of breath, chest pain, and arm or leg swelling. Check for blood in your urine, scalp hair loss, and bleeding, ulcers, pallor, and bruised skin and mucous membranes.

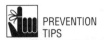

PREVENTION
TIPS

Protecting your skin

Exposure to the sun, or even to fluorescent lights, may make lupus worse. Excessive exposure, in fact, may cause rashes, fever, and arthritis and could even damage the organs inside your body.

But you needn't spend your waking hours in the dark to be safe. Just take the precautions below.

Prepare for going outdoors
Wear a wide-brimmed hat or visor and sunglasses to shield yourself from the sun's rays. Put on a long-sleeved shirt and trousers to filter out harmful rays. In hot weather, choose clothing made of lightweight loosely woven fabrics such as cotton.

Buy a sunscreen containing para-aminobenzoic acid with an SPF of 8 to 15. If you're allergic to para-aminobenzoic acid, choose a product without it that offers equal sun protection.

Before you go outside, rub the sunscreen on unprotected parts of your body, such as your face and hands. Reapply frequently, especially after swimming or perspiring.

Avoid strong sunlight
Try to stay indoors during the most intense hours of sunlight, from 10 a.m. to 2 p.m. The ideal time to garden, take a walk, play golf, or do any other outdoor activity is just after sunrise or just before sunset.

Remove fluorescent lights
At home, replace any fluorescent fixtures or bulbs with incandescent ones. At work, though, avoiding fluorescent light may be difficult. Consider asking your supervisor about moving to a work area closer to a window so that you can use natural light. If you have a fluorescent light above your desk, turn it off and request a lamp that uses incandescent bulbs.

Be careful with soaps and drugs
Certain toiletries, including deodorant soaps, may increase your skin's sensitivity to light.

Try switching to nondeodorant or hypoallergenic soaps. Certain drugs, including tetracyclines and phenothiazines, also make you more sensitive to light.

Always check with your doctor or pharmacist before taking any new drug.

Recognize and report rashes
Be alert for the key sign of a photosensitivity reaction: a red rash on your face or other exposed area. If you discover a suspicious rash or other reaction to light, call your doctor. Remember, prompt treatment can prevent damage to the tissues under the skin.

- Eat a balanced diet. Foods high in protein, vitamins, and iron help maintain optimum nutrition and prevent anemia. However, if you have kidney problems, the doctor will recommend a low-sodium, low-protein diet.
- Get plenty of rest.
- Apply heat packs to relieve joint pain and stiffness. Get regular exercise to maintain a full range of motion and prevent contractures. Perform range-of-motion exercises, as well as body alignment and postural techniques.
- Take prescribed drugs exactly as directed, and watch for side effects, especially if you're taking high doses of corticosteroids.

STRAIGHT
TALK

Lupus and pregnancy

Does becoming pregnant make lupus worse?
In about 25% of women, systemic lupus erythematosus gets worse during pregnancy. For the rest, it stays the same or even improves. After the birth of your baby, there's a small chance that your disease will flare up. Unfortunately, doctors can't predict how pregnancy and childbirth will affect your symptoms. Before pregnancy, you and your spouse need to discuss the possibility that your condition may worsen.

Before I get pregnant, is there anything special I should do?
Ideally, you should try to get pregnant when your disease is in remission or under good medical control. Let your doctor know about your plans well before you try to become pregnant so that he can discontinue any drugs you're taking that could harm a fetus. Birth defects caused by drugs may occur in the first few weeks of pregnancy, long before you know you're pregnant.

Will I need special care during pregnancy?
You'll probably need to see your obstetrician more often than you would normally. Certain problems of pregnancy, such as toxemia, occur more commonly in patients with lupus. To minimize complications, make sure you keep all medical appointments and follow through with recommended blood, urine, and other tests.

What are my chances of having a healthy baby?
It's very unlikely that your baby will be born with systemic lupus erythematosus. Unfortunately, women with lupus face a greater risk of miscarriages and stillbirths. Following your doctor's advice throughout your pregnancy will greatly improve your chances of having a healthy baby.

- If you're receiving Cytoxan, be sure to drink plenty of fluids.
- Use hypoallergenic makeup, if needed, and consult a hairdresser who specializes in scalp disorders.
- Buy drugs in quantity, if possible. Be skeptical about "miracle" drugs for relief of arthritis symptoms.
- Contact the Lupus Foundation of America and the Arthritis Foundation for more information.

POLYMYOSITIS AND DERMATOMYOSITIS

What are these conditions?

Polymyositis and dermatomyositis, widespread, inflammatory diseases of unknown cause, produce symmetrical weakness of striated muscle, primarily muscles of the shoulder and pelvic girdles, neck, and pharynx. In dermatomyositis, such muscle weakness is accompanied by skin involvement.

These diseases usually progress slowly, with frequent flare-ups and remissions. They occur twice as often in women as in men (with the exception of dermatomyositis with malignancy, which is most common in men over age 40).

Generally, the prognosis worsens with age. The 7-year survival rate for adults is approximately 60%, with death often occurring from associated malignancy, respiratory disease, heart failure, or side effects of drug therapy (corticosteroids and immunosuppressants). On the other hand, 80% to 90% of affected children regain normal function if properly treated; but, if untreated, childhood dermatomyositis may progress rapidly to disabling contractures and muscular atrophy.

What causes them?

Although the cause of polymyositis remains puzzling, researchers believe that it may be caused by an autoimmune reaction. Presumably, the person's T cells inappropriately recognize muscle fiber antigens as foreign and attack muscle tissue, causing widespread or localized muscle fiber degeneration. (Regeneration of new muscle cells then follows, producing remission.)

What are their symptoms?

Polymyositis begins acutely or insidiously with muscle weakness, tenderness, and discomfort. It affects proximal muscles (shoulder, pelvic girdle) more often than distal muscles. Muscle weakness impairs performance of ordinary activities. The person may have trouble getting up from a chair, combing his or her hair, reaching into a high cupboard, climbing stairs, or even raising his or her head from a pillow. Other muscular symptoms include inability to move against resistance, regurgitation of fluid through the nose, and a nasal voice.

In dermatomyositis, a red rash usually erupts on the face, neck, upper back, chest, and arms and around the nail beds. A characteristic purplish rash appears on the eyelids, accompanied by swelling around the eyes. Flat-topped violet-colored lesions may appear on the finger joints.

How are they diagnosed?

A biopsy of muscle tissue that shows evidence of necrosis, degeneration, regeneration, and interstitial chronic lymphocytic infiltration confirms the diagnosis. Other lab tests differentiate polymyositis

SELF-HELP

Coping with polymyositis and dermatomyositis

If you have one of these disorders, you know how frustrating the muscle weakness and the resulting activity limitations can be. With dermatomyositis, you may also have to contend with an itchy rash. The following tips can help you cope.

Daily activities

- Feed and dress yourself to the best of your ability, but ask for help when needed.
- Pace your activities to counteract muscle weakness, which is probably temporary.
- If you have a rash, don't scratch; this may cause infection. If your anti-itching drug doesn't bring relief, apply lukewarm sponges or compresses.

Steroid considerations

- If the doctor has prescribed corticosteroids, be aware that these drugs may cause weight gain, increased body hair, swelling, high blood pressure, absence of menstrual periods, purplish skin streaks, sugar in the urine, acne, and easy bruising.
- To help prevent fluid retention while taking corticosteroids, limit your salt intake. Be aware that the weight gain will diminish when you discontinue the drug. Report troubling side effects to the doctor, *but don't abruptly discontinue corticosteroids.*

from diseases that cause similar muscular or skin symptoms, such as muscular dystrophy, advanced trichinosis, psoriasis, seborrheic dermatitis, and systemic lupus.

How are they treated?

High-dose corticosteroid therapy relieves inflammation and lowers muscle enzyme levels. Within 2 to 6 weeks following treatment, serum muscle enzyme levels usually return to normal and muscle strength improves, permitting a gradual tapering down of corticosteroid dosage. If the person responds poorly to corticosteroids, treatment may include cytotoxic or immunosuppressant drugs, such as Cytoxan, given intravenously (intermittent injection) or by mouth. Supportive therapy includes bed rest during the acute phase, range-of-motion exercises to prevent contractures, pain relievers and application of heat to relieve painful muscle spasms, and Benadryl to relieve itching. People over age 40 need thorough assessment for coexisting malignant disease. (See *Coping with polymyositis and dermatomyositis.*)

PSORIATIC ARTHRITIS

What is this condition?

Psoriatic arthritis is a syndrome of rheumatoid-like joint disease associated with psoriasis of nearby skin and nails. It may be difficult to distinguish some symptoms of this disorder from rheumatoid arthritis.

Psoriatic arthritis usually is mild, with intermittent flare-ups. In rare cases, it may progress to a crippling disorder. This disease affects both men and women equally; usually, onset occurs between ages 30 and 35.

What causes it?

Evidence suggests that predisposition to psoriatic arthritis is hereditary. However, onset is usually precipitated by streptococcal infection or trauma.

What are its symptoms?

Psoriatic lesions usually precede the arthritic component, but once the full syndrome is established, joint and skin lesions recur simultaneously. Arthritis may involve one joint or several joints symmetrically. Rarely, spinal involvement may occur. Peripheral joint involvement is most common in the distal joints of the hands, which have a characteristic sausagelike appearance. Nail changes include pitting, transverse ridges, separation, hardening, yellowing, and destruction. The person may experience general malaise, fever, and eye involvement.

How is it diagnosed?

The doctor will suspect psoriatic arthritis if a person exhibits inflammatory arthritis accompanied by psoriatic skin lesions. X-rays confirm joint involvement and show bone erosion and deformity.

Blood tests aid in confirming the diagnosis.

How is it treated?

In mild psoriatic arthritis, treatment is supportive and consists of immobilization through bed rest or splints, isometric exercises, paraffin baths, heat therapy, and aspirin and other nonsteroidal anti-inflammatory drugs. Some people respond well to low-dose systemic corticosteroids; topical steroids may help control skin lesions. Gold salts and Rheumatrex therapy are effective in treating both the ar-

 SELF-HELP

Advice for the person with psoriatic arthritis

As you may know, the skin plaques of psoriasis aren't contagious. Here are some suggestions to help you manage them and help you live with this disorder:

- Get regular exercise — particularly swimming — to maintain your strength and range of motion. Also get regular, but moderate, exposure to the sun.
- Ask your doctor or nurse how to apply skin care products and medications correctly.
- Get adequate rest.
- Protect affected joints.
- Consult the Arthritis Foundation for information about self-help and support groups.

thritic and skin effects of psoriatic arthritis. Antimalarials should not be given because they can provoke exfoliative dermatitis.

(See *Advice for the person with psoriatic arthritis, page 719.*)

REITER'S SYNDROME

What is this condition?

Reiter's syndrome is a self-limiting syndrome associated with polyarthritis (its dominant feature), inflammation of the urethra or penis, conjunctivitis, and lesions on the mucous membranes and skin. It appears to be related to infection, either venereal (sexually transmitted) or enteric (intestinal). This disease usually affects young men (ages 20 to 40); it's rare in women and children.

What causes it?

Although the exact cause of Reiter's syndrome is unknown, most cases follow venereal or enteric infection. Since 75% to 85% of people with Reiter's syndrome are positive for the human leukocyte antigen B27, genetic susceptibility is likely. Reiter's syndrome has followed infections caused by *Mycoplasma, Shigella, Salmonella, Yersinia,* and *Chlamydia* organisms. More common in persons who are HIV positive, it may precede or follow AIDS.

What are its symptoms?

The person with Reiter's syndrome may complain of difficult, urgent, or frequent urination; blood in the urine; and mucus and pus discharged from the penis, with swelling and reddening of the urethral opening. Small painless ulcers may erupt on the tip of the penis and coalesce to form irregular patches that cover the penis and scrotum. The person may also experience suprapubic pain, fever, and loss of appetite with weight loss. This disorder may also cause other genitourinary complications, such as prostatitis and hemorrhagic cystitis.

Arthritic symptoms usually follow genitourinary or intestinal symptoms and often last from 2 to 4 months. Asymmetrical and extremely variable polyarticular arthritis occurs most often and tends to develop in weight-bearing joints of the legs and sometimes in the lower back or sacroiliac joints. The arthritis is usually acute, with warm, reddened, and painful joints; but it may be mild, with minimal synovitis. Muscle wasting is common near affected joints. Fingers and toes may swell and appear sausagelike.

Eye symptoms include mild bilateral conjunctivitis, possibly complicated by inflammation of the cornea, iris, retina, or optic nerve. In severe cases, burning, itching, and profuse discharge of pus and mucus are possible.

In 30% of people, skin lesions develop 4 to 6 weeks after onset of other symptoms and may last for several weeks. These macular to hyperkeratotic lesions often resemble those of psoriasis. They occur most commonly on the palms and soles but can develop anywhere on the trunk, extremities, or scalp. Nails become thick, opaque, and brittle, and a horny debris accumulates under the nails. In many people, painless, transient ulcerations erupt on the mucous membranes of the cheek, palate, and tongue.

How is it diagnosed?

Nearly all people with Reiter's syndrome are positive for human leukocyte antigen B27 and have an elevated white blood cell count and erythrocyte sedimentation rate. Mild anemia also may develop. Cultures of urethral discharge and synovial fluid rule out other causes such as gonococci.

During the first few weeks, X-rays are usually normal and may remain so. If inflammation persists, X-rays may show erosions of the small joints, new bone formation in involved joints, and heel spurs.

How is it treated?

No specific treatment exists for Reiter's syndrome. Most people recover in 2 to 16 weeks. About 50% have recurring acute attacks, whereas the rest follow a chronic course, experiencing continued synovitis and sacroiliitis. In acute stages, limited weight-bearing or complete bed rest may be necessary. (See *Coping with Reiter's syndrome.*)

Anti-inflammatory agents, the primary treatment, can be given to relieve discomfort and fever. Corticosteroids may be used for persistent skin lesions; gold therapy and Rheumatrex or Imuran, for bony erosion. Testing for human immunodeficiency virus (HIV) is needed before initiating corticosteroid therapy. Physical therapy includes range-of-motion and strengthening exercises and the use of padded or supportive shoes to prevent contractures and foot deformities.

Coping with Reiter's syndrome

Following this advice will make it easier to handle Reiter's syndrome:
- Take prescribed drugs with meals or milk to prevent gastrointestinal bleeding.
- Keep up your normal daily activities and get moderate exercise.
- Maintain good posture and body mechanics.
- Sleep on a firm mattress.
- If you have severe or chronic joint impairment, consider seeking occupational counseling.

RHEUMATOID ARTHRITIS

What is this condition?

A chronic, systemic, inflammatory disease, rheumatoid arthritis primarily attacks the joints of the hands, arms, and feet as well as surrounding muscles, tendons, ligaments, and blood vessels. Spontaneous remissions and unpredictable flare-ups mark the course of this potentially crippling disease.

Rheumatoid arthritis usually requires lifelong treatment and, sometimes, surgery. In most people, the disease follows an intermittent course and allows normal activity, although 10% suffer total disability from severe articular deformity or associated extra-articular symptoms, or both. The prognosis worsens with the development of nodules, vasculitis, and high titers of rheumatoid factor.

What causes it?

Rheumatoid arthritis occurs worldwide, striking women three times more often than men. Although the disorder can occur at any age, the peak onset period for women is between ages 30 and 60. It affects more than 6.5 million people in the United States alone.

What causes the chronic inflammation characteristic of rheumatoid arthritis isn't known, but various theories point to infectious, genetic, and endocrine factors. Currently, it's believed that a genetically susceptible person develops abnormal or altered immunoglobulin G antibodies when exposed to an antigen. This altered immunoglobulin G antibody is not recognized as "self," and the individual forms an antibody against it an antibody known as *rheumatoid factor*. By aggregating into complexes, rheumatoid factor generates inflammation. Eventually, cartilage damage by inflammation triggers additional immune responses, including activation of complement. This in turn attracts polymorphonuclear leukocytes and stimulates release of inflammatory mediators that enhance joint destruction.

What are its symptoms?

Rheumatoid arthritis usually develops insidiously and initially produces nonspecific symptoms such as fatigue, malaise, loss of appetite, persistent low-grade fever, weight loss, disease of the lymph nodes, and vague symptoms involving movement. Later, more specific, localized symptoms affecting movement develop, frequently in the fin-

Rheumatoid arthritis occurs worldwide; it affects more than 6.5 million people in the United States alone. The exact cause isn't known.

gers at the proximal interphalangeal, metacarpophalangeal, and metatarsophalangeal joints. These symptoms usually occur bilaterally and symmetrically and may extend to the wrists, knees, elbows, and ankles. The affected joints stiffen after inactivity, most noticeably when the person rises in the morning. The fingers may assume a spindle shape from marked swelling and congestion in the joints. The joints become tender and painful, at first only when the person moves them but, eventually, even at rest. They usually feel hot to the touch. Ultimately, joint function is diminished.

Deformities of the fingers are likely if active disease continues. Carpal tunnel syndrome, resulting from synovial pressure on the median nerve, causes tingling in the fingers.

The most common extra-articular finding is the gradual appearance of rheumatoid nodules — round or oval nontender masses under the skin — usually on pressure areas such as the elbows. Vasculitis can lead to skin lesions, leg ulcers, and multiple systemic complications. Peripheral neuropathy may produce numbness or tingling in the feet or weakness and loss of sensation in the fingers. Stiff, weak, or painful muscles are common. Other common extra-articular effects include pericarditis, pulmonary nodules or fibrosis, pleuritis, and eye inflammation.

Another complication is destruction of the odontoid process, part of the second cervical vertebra. Rarely, cord compression may occur, particularly in people with long-standing, deforming rheumatoid arthritis. Upper motor neuron signs, such as a positive Babinski's sign and muscle weakness, may also develop.

Rheumatoid arthritis can also cause temporomandibular joint disease, which impairs chewing and causes earaches. Other extra-articular findings may include infection, osteoporosis, myositis, cardiopulmonary lesions, lymphadenopathy, and peripheral neuritis.

How is it diagnosed?

Typical clinical features suggest rheumatoid arthritis, but a firm diagnosis relies on lab test results, including blood tests, analysis of synovial fluid, and X-rays.

How is it treated?

Salicylates, particularly aspirin, are the mainstay of rheumatoid arthritis therapy because they decrease inflammation and relieve joint pain. Other useful medications include nonsteroidal anti-inflammatory agents (such as Indocin, Nalfon, and Motrin or Advil), antima-

The lowdown on arthritis treatments

Should I be taking "arthritis-strength" aspirin?
Over-the-counter drugs advertised as "arthritis-strength" contain larger doses of the active ingredient, but that doesn't make them more effective in relieving pain. However, because you need to take fewer tablets per dose, this convenience may be worth the extra cost.

Will I benefit from using ointments and liniments?
Ointments and liniments depend on skin irritants, such as oil of wintergreen, for their effects. When applied, these external pain relievers increase blood flow to the upper layers of your skin, resulting in redness, a warm sensation, and increased skin temperature. They provide brief relief. Be aware that substances contained in these products are absorbed through the skin and can cause problems if used too often.

How effective are the diets advertised to cure my arthritis?
There's no scientific evidence that any diet, food, or vitamin can cure rheumatoid arthritis. If you're overweight and your hips, knees, ankles, or feet are affected by arthritis, then losing weight can help you. You'll feel less pain and reduce stress on weight-bearing joints.

larials (Aralen and Plaquenil), gold salts, penicillamine, and corticosteroids (Orasone). Immunosuppressants such as Imuran are also therapeutic. (See *The lowdown on arthritis treatments.*)

Supportive measures include 8 to 10 hours of sleep every night, frequent rest periods between daily activities, and splinting to rest inflamed joints. A physical therapy program including range-of-motion exercises and carefully individualized therapeutic exercises prevent loss of joint function; application of heat relaxes muscles and relieves pain. (See *Restoring strength and relieving pain,* pages 726 and 727.)

Moist heat (hot soaks, paraffin baths, whirlpool) usually works best for people with chronic disease. Ice packs are effective during acute episodes.

Advanced disease may require synovectomy, joint reconstruction, or total joint arthroplasty. Useful surgical procedures in rheumatoid arthritis include arthrodesis (joint fusion) and osteotomy (the cutting of bone or excision of a wedge of bone). Tendons may also require surgical repair. Tendon transfers may prevent deformities or relieve contractures.

What can a person with rheumatoid arthritis do?

- Be aware that this is a chronic disease that requires major lifestyle changes. There are no miracle cures, despite claims to the contrary.
- Eat a balanced diet but don't look for some special diet to cure rheumatoid arthritis.
- Control your weight; obesity puts added stress on joints.
- Perform activities of daily living, such as dressing and feeding yourself, to the best of your ability. Give yourself enough time to calmly perform these tasks. Whenever possible, buy easy-to-open cartons, lightweight cups, and unpackaged silverware.
- Use dressing aids, such as a long-handled shoehorn, elastic shoelaces, zipper-pull, and buttonhook, and helpful household items, such as easy-to-open drawers, a handheld shower nozzle, handrails, and grab bars. If you have trouble maneuvering your fingers into gloves, wear mittens. Dress while in a sitting position.
- Wear shoes with proper support.
- Pace daily activities, rest for 5 to 10 minutes out of each hour, and alternate sitting and standing tasks.
- To increase your mobility, take pain medication and use moist heat as needed.
- Take hot showers or baths at bedtime or in the morning to reduce your need for pain medication.
- Always stand, walk, and sit correctly: upright and erect. Sit in chairs with high seats and armrests; you'll find it easier to get up from a chair if your knees are lower than your hips. If you don't own a chair with a high seat, put blocks of wood under the legs of a favorite chair. Consider getting an elevated toilet seat.
- Adequate sleep is important, and so is correct sleeping posture. Sleep on your back on a firm mattress. Avoid placing a pillow under your knees, which encourages flexion deformity.
- Avoid putting undue stress on joints. For instance, always use the largest joint available for a given task; support weak or painful joints as much as possible; avoid positions of flexion and promote positions of extension; hold objects parallel to your knuckles as briefly as possible; use your hands toward the center of your body; and slide, don't lift, objects, whenever possible.
- For more information on coping with rheumatoid arthritis, contact the Arthritis Foundation.

Restoring strength and relieving pain

Don't underestimate the benefits of exercise in treating rheumatoid arthritis. Done regularly, it can help you overcome pain and stiffness, restore and maintain strength, and limber up your joints. It can also improve your circulation.

Develop a routine. Perform 5 to 10 repetitions of selected exercises once or twice each day. Move in a slow, steady manner. Don't bounce. If a joint is inflamed, gently move it as much as you comfortably can. Have someone help you, if necessary.

Don't hold your breath during exercise. Instead, slowly breathe in and out. You may count out loud.

Shoulder exercises

Try these two exercises for your shoulders.

1 Lie on your back. Raise one arm over your head, keeping your elbow straight and your arm close to your ear. Then return your arm slowly to your side. Repeat with your other arm.

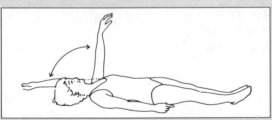

2 While standing, place your hands behind your head. Move your elbows back as far as you can. As you move your elbows back, tilt your head back. Return to the starting position and repeat.

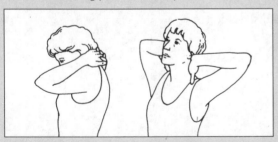

Knee and hip exercises

Try these five exercises for your knees and hips.

1 Lie on your back with one knee bent. Keep the other leg as straight as possible. Now bend the knee of the straight leg and bring it toward your chest. Push the leg into the air, and then lower it to the floor. Repeat, using the other leg.

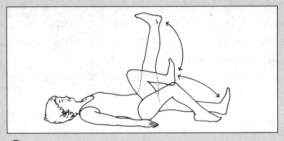

2 Lie on your back with your legs as straight as possible, about 6 inches (15 centimeters) apart. Keep your toes pointed up. Roll one hip and knee from side to side, keeping your knees straight. Repeat with your other hip and knee.

3 While lying on your back with both legs out straight, try to push the back of your knee against the floor. Then tighten the muscle on the front of your thigh. Hold it tight and slowly count to 5. Relax. Repeat with the other knee.

4 Lie on your back with your legs straight and about 6 inches apart. Point your toes up. Slide one leg out to the side and return. Try to keep your toes pointing up. Repeat with your other leg.

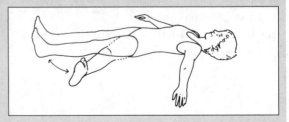

Restoring strength and relieving pain *(continued)*

5 Sit in a chair that's high enough for you to swing your leg. Keep your thigh on the chair and straighten your knee. Hold a few seconds. Then, bend your knee back as far as possible. Repeat with the other knee.

Thumb exercise
Open your hand and straighten your fingers. Reach your thumb across your palm until it touches the base of your little finger. Stretch your thumb out and repeat. Repeat with the other thumb.

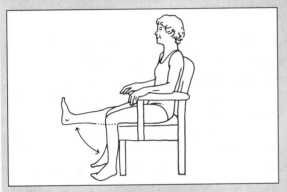

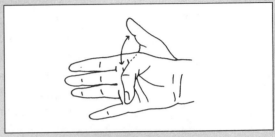

Ankle exercise
While sitting, keep your heels on the floor and lift your toes as high as possible. Then lower your toes to the floor and lift your heels as high as possible. Lower your heels and repeat.

Finger exercise
Open your hand, with fingers straight. Bending all the finger joints except the knuckles, touch the top of your palm with your fingertips. Open your hand and repeat.

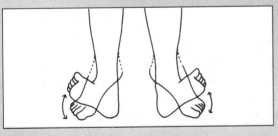

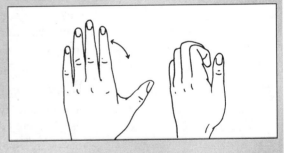

SCLERODERMA

What do doctors call this condition?

Progressive systemic sclerosis, CREST syndrome

What is this condition?

Scleroderma is a diffuse connective tissue disease characterized by fibrotic, degenerative, and occasionally inflammatory changes in skin, blood vessels, synovial membranes, skeletal muscles, and internal organs (especially the esophagus, intestinal tract, thyroid, heart, lungs, and kidneys). It affects women more frequently than men, especially between ages 30 and 50. Approximately 30% of people with scleroderma die within 5 years of onset.

What causes it?

The cause of scleroderma is unknown. This disease occurs in distinctive forms:

- *CREST syndrome:* a benign form characterized by calcinosis, Raynaud's phenomenon, esophageal dysfunction, thickening of the skin of the fingers, and vascular lesions
- *diffuse systemic sclerosis:* characterized by generalized skin thickening and invasion of internal organ systems
- *localized scleroderma:* characterized by patchy skin changes with a droplike appearance known as *morphea*
- *linear scleroderma:* characterized by a band of thickened skin on the face or extremities that severely damages underlying tissues, causing wasting and deformity (most common in childhood).

Other forms include *chemically induced localized scleroderma, eosinophilic myalgia syndrome* (recently associated with ingestion of L-tryptophan), *toxic oil syndrome* (associated with contaminated oil), and *graft-versus-host disease.*

What are its symptoms?

Scleroderma typically begins with Raynaud's phenomenon — blanching, bluish skin discoloration, and erythema of the fingers and toes — in response to stress or exposure to cold. The person may develop ulcerations on the tips of the fingers or toes that may lead to gangrene. His or her fingers may become shortened. Raynaud's phenomenon may precede scleroderma by months or years.

Later symptoms include pain, stiffness, and swelling of fingers and joints. Skin thickening produces taut, shiny skin over the entire hand and forearm. Facial skin also becomes tight and inelastic, causing a masklike appearance and "pinching" of the mouth. As tightening progresses, contractures may develop.

Gastrointestinal dysfunction causes frequent reflux, heartburn, difficulty swallowing, and bloating after meals. These symptoms may cause the person to decrease food intake and lose weight. Other gastrointestinal effects include a swollen abdomen, diarrhea, constipation, and bad-smelling, floating stools.

SELF-HELP

Dealing with the discomforts of scleroderma

One way to reduce the discomfort that comes with your condition is to take an active role in protecting yourself.

Protect yourself from cold
Because exposure to cold can trigger *Raynaud's phenomenon*, be sure to dress warmly before going outside in cool weather (and before going into a cold, air-conditioned building in warm weather). Wear mittens or thermal gloves and fleece-lined boots. You may want to carry an extra sweater with you.

Keep an extra pair of mittens by your refrigerator to wear when you remove ice cubes or other cold items. Use thermal cups to hold cold drinks. In cold weather, ask someone else to bring in the newspaper from outside or to start the car.

Avoid skin infection
Take care to avoid injuring your hands or feet, which may heal more slowly, allowing an infection to start. For the same reason, be cautious when using sharp knives or picking up pieces of broken glass or pottery.

Keep your nails short, and don't pull on hangnails. Protect your feet from injury and infection by avoiding open-toed shoes or sandals. Don't go barefoot or walk around in your stocking feet.

Prevent skin dryness
Help your skin retain moisture by sealing it with unperfumed moisturizing lotions or bath oils. When you wash and dry your skin, always pat or gently massage it; never rub it. After you bathe, apply skin lotions or oils to your damp skin. The lotion will slide on more easily. Consider using a cold-water room humidifier, which also helps to retain skin moisture. Avoid using strong detergent cleansers and solvents, which may irritate your skin. If you must use them, wear heavy rubber gloves.

Reduce stress
Emotional stress plays a role in reducing blood flow. So make it a point to get enough sleep and avoid or resolve situations that make you tense. Set aside time to relax each day. Ask your doctor or nurse to teach you specific relaxation techniques, which relieve stress by promoting deep relaxation. Consider learning biofeedback techniques so you can increase blood flow to your fingers and prevent Raynaud's phenomenon.

Stop smoking
Smoking can trigger attacks of Raynaud's phenomenon by reducing the blood supply to your fingers. If you need help quitting, ask your doctor for help. Or contact your local American Lung Association chapter or the American Cancer Society.

In advanced disease, heart and lung fibrosis produce irregular heartbeats and shortness of breath. Kidney involvement is usually accompanied by malignant high blood pressure, the main cause of death.

How is it diagnosed?
Typical skin changes provide the first clue to diagnosis. Diagnostic tests include blood studies, urinalysis, pulmonary function studies, electrocardiography, and removal and analysis of skin tissue, and X-rays of the hand, chest, and gastrointestinal system.

How is it treated?

Currently, no cure exists for scleroderma. Treatment aims to preserve normal body functions and minimize complications. (See *Dealing with the discomforts of scleroderma, page 729.*) The doctor may prescribe immunosuppressants such as Leukeran. Corticosteroids and Colsalide have been used experimentally and seem to stabilize symptoms; Cuprimine also may be helpful. Blood platelet levels need to be monitored throughout drug therapy.

Other treatments vary according to symptoms:

- *Raynaud's phenomenon:* various vasodilators and drugs to lower blood pressure (such as Aldomet or calcium channel blockers), intermittent cervical sympathetic blockade or, rarely, thoracic sympathectomy
- *chronic digital ulcerations:* a digital plaster cast to immobilize the affected area, minimize trauma, and maintain cleanliness; possibly surgical debridement
- *esophagitis with narrowing:* antacids; Tagamet; a soft, bland diet; and periodic esophageal dilation
- *small-bowel involvement* (diarrhea, pain, malabsorption, weight loss): broad-spectrum antibiotics, such as E-Mycin or Achromycin V, to counteract bacterial overgrowth in the duodenum and jejunum related to hypomotility
- *scleroderma kidney* (with severe high blood pressure and impending kidney failure): dialysis, drugs to lower blood pressure, and calcium channel blockers
- *hand debilitation:* physical therapy to maintain function and promote muscle strength, heat therapy to relieve joint stiffness, and teaching to make performance of daily activities easier.

SEVERE COMBINED IMMUNODEFICIENCY DISEASE

What is this condition?

In severe combined immunodeficiency disease, both T-cell and B-cell immunity are deficient or absent, resulting in susceptibility to infection from all classes of microorganisms during infancy.

At least three types exist:

- *reticular dysgenesis,* the most severe type
- *Swiss-type agammaglobulinemia*
- *enzyme deficiency* such as adenosine deaminase deficiency.

This disorder affects more men than women; its estimated incidence is 1 in every 100,000 to 500,000 births. Most untreated persons die from infection within 1 year of birth.

What causes it?

Severe combined immunodeficiency disease is usually caused by an inherited genetic defect. Less commonly, it is caused by an enzyme deficiency.

What are its symptoms?

An extreme susceptibility to infection becomes obvious in the infant with severe combined immunodeficiency disease in the first months of life. The infant fails to thrive and develops chronic ear infections; sepsis; watery diarrhea; recurrent pulmonary infections; persistent oral candidiasis, sometimes with esophageal erosions; and, possibly, fatal viral infections.

P. carinii pneumonia usually strikes a severely immunodeficient infant in the first 3 to 5 weeks of life. Onset is typically insidious, with gradually worsening cough, low-grade fever, rapid breathing, and respiratory distress. A chest X-ray characteristically shows bilateral pulmonary infiltrates.

How is it diagnosed?

Diagnosis is generally made clinically because most affected infants suffer recurrent overwhelming infections within 1 year of birth. Some infants are diagnosed after a severe reaction to vaccination.

Defective humoral immunity is difficult to detect before an infant is 5 months old. However, severely diminished or absent T-cell number and function and the removal and analysis of lymph node tissue showing an absence of lymphocytes can confirm the diagnosis.

How is it treated?

Treatment aims to restore the immune response and prevent infection. Histocompatible bone marrow transplantation is the only satisfactory treatment available to correct immunodeficiency. Because bone marrow cells must be matched according to human leukocyte antigen and mixed leukocyte cultures, the most common donors are

In the infant with severe combined immunodeficiency disease, extreme susceptibility to infection becomes obvious during the first few months after birth.

Staying close to an infant with immuno-deficiency disease

- Although your infant must remain in strict protective isolation, you may visit often, hold him or her, and bring toys that can be easily sterilized.
- If you can't visit, ask the hospital staff to call you often to report on your child's condition.
- Because this is a genetic disease, seek genetic counseling if you're considering having more children.

histocompatible siblings. But because bone marrow transplant can produce a potentially fatal graft-versus-host disease, researchers are evaluating newer methods of bone marrow transplantation that eliminate graft-versus-host disease.

Fetal thymus gland and liver transplantation have achieved limited success. Administration of immune globulin may also play a role in treatment. Some infants have received long-term protection by being isolated in a completely sterile environment. (See *Staying close to an infant with immunodeficiency disease.*) However, this approach isn't effective if the infant already has had recurring infections. Gene therapy is being used for adenosine deaminase deficiency.

VASCULITIS

What is this condition?

Vasculitis includes a broad spectrum of disorders characterized by inflammation and necrosis of blood vessels. Its clinical effects depend on the vessels involved.

The prognosis is also variable. For example, hypersensitivity vasculitis is usually a benign disorder limited to the skin, but more extensive polyarteritis nodosa can be rapidly fatal.

Vasculitis can occur at any age, except for mucocutaneous lymph node syndrome, which occurs only during childhood. Vasculitis may be a primary disorder or secondary to other disorders, such as rheumatoid arthritis or lupus.

What causes it?

Exactly how vascular damage develops in vasculitis isn't well understood. Current theory holds that it's initiated by excessive levels of antigen in the circulation. This starts a chain of events culminating in the release of enzymes that cause vessel damage and necrosis, which may precipitate blood clot formation, occlusion, hemorrhage, and tissue ischemia.

Vascular damage may also result from the action of intracellular enzymes released by the cell-mediated (T-cell) immune response.

Types of vasculitis

TYPE	SIGNS AND SYMPTOMS
Polyarteritis nodosa	High blood pressure; muscle, joint, and abdominal pain; headache; weakness
Allergic angiitis and granulomatosis (Churg-Strauss syndrome)	Resembles polyarteritis nodosa with hallmark of severe pulmonary involvement
Polyangiitis overlap syndrome	Combines symptoms of polyarteritis nodosa and allergic angiitis and granulomatosis
Wegener's granulomatosis	Fever, pulmonary congestion, cough, malaise, anorexia, weight loss, blood in the urine
Temporal arteritis	Fever, muscle pain, jaw muscle dysfunction, visual changes, headache (associated with polymyalgia rheumatica syndrome)
Takayasu's arteritis (aortic arch syndrome)	Malaise, pallor, nausea, night sweats, joint pain, loss of appetite, weight loss, pain or paresthesia distal to affected area, bruits, loss of distal pulses, fainting and, if carotid artery is involved, double vision and transient blindness; may progress to congestive heart failure or cerebrovascular accident
Hypersensitivity vasculitis	Palpable purpura, papules, nodules, vesicles, bullae, ulcers, or chronic or recurrent urticaria
Mucocutaneous lymph node syndrome (Kawasaki disease)	Fever; nonsuppurative cervical adenitis; swelling; congested conjunctivas; erythema of oral cavity, lips, and palms; and scaly skin on fingertips; may progress to arthritis, myocarditis, pericarditis, heart attack, and an enlarged heart
Behçet's disease	Recurrent oral ulcers; eye, genital, and skin lesions

What are its symptoms and how is it diagnosed?

Clinical effects of vasculitis and laboratory procedures used to confirm diagnosis depend on the blood vessels involved. (For specific signs and symptoms, see *Types of vasculitis*.)

How is it treated?

Treatment of vasculitis aims to minimize irreversible tissue damage associated with decreased blood flow. In primary vasculitis, treatment may involve removal of an offending antigen or use of anti-inflammatory drugs or immunosuppressants. For example, antigenic drugs, food, and other environmental substances should be identified and eliminated, if possible. Drug therapy in primary vasculitis frequently involves low-dose Cytoxan (2 milligrams per kilogram daily by mouth) with daily corticosteroids. In rapidly fulminant vasculitis, Cytoxan dosage may be increased to 4 milligrams per kilogram daily for the first 2 to 3 days, followed by the regular dose. Orasone should be given in a dose of 1 milligram per kilogram daily in divided doses for 7 to 10 days, with consolidation to a single morning dose by 2 to 3 weeks. When the vasculitis appears to be in remission or when prescribed cytotoxic drugs take full effect, corticosteroids are tapered down to a single daily dose and then to an alternate-day schedule that may continue for 3 to 6 months before they are slowly discontinued. In secondary vasculitis, treatment focuses on the underlying disorder.

19

INFECTION

ACTINOMYCOSIS

What is this condition?

Actinomycosis is an infection that produces granulomatous, pus-discharging lesions with abscesses. Common infection sites are the head, neck, chest, and abdomen, but it can also spread to tissues that border each other, causing multiple draining sinuses.

Sporadic and infrequent, actinomycosis affects twice as many males — especially those ages 15 to 35 — as females. It's likely to infect people with dental disease.

What causes it?

Actinomycosis is caused mainly by a bacterium called *Actinomyces israelii*. This bacterium is anaerobic, which means it lives without oxygen, and it occurs as part of the normal bacteria of the throat and mouth. Infection results when this bacterium enters into body tissues following an injury.

What are its symptoms?

Symptoms appear from days to months after injury and may vary depending on the site of infection.

In *cervicofacial actinomycosis* (lumpy jaw), hard, painful swellings appear in the mouth or neck up to several weeks following injury or tooth extraction. They gradually enlarge and form fistulas that open onto the skin. Sulfur granules (yellowish gray masses) appear in the discharge.

In lung infection, the person develops a fever and a cough that becomes productive and occasionally contains blood. Eventually, pus accumulates in the chest cavity, a sinus forms through the chest wall, and blood poisoning may occur.

In gastrointestinal infection, the person may develop abdominal discomfort, fever, a palpable mass, and an external sinus. This follows disruption of the intestinal mucosa, usually by surgery or an inflammatory bowel condition such as appendicitis.

How is it diagnosed?

Lab tests that isolate *A. israelii* in discharge or tissue specimens confirm the diagnosis. Chest X-rays may show unusual lesions.

How is it treated?

High-dose intravenous penicillin or Achromycin therapy precedes surgical excision and drainage of abscesses in all forms of the disease and continues for 3 to 6 weeks. Following this regimen, treatment with oral penicillin or Achromycin may continue for 1 to 6 months.

ASPERGILLOSIS

What is this condition?

Aspergillosis is a fungal infection that occurs in four major forms: *aspergilloma* (which affects the lungs); *allergic aspergillosis* (a hypersensitive asthmatic reaction); *aspergillosis endophthalmitis* (an infection of the eye); and *disseminated aspergillosis* (an acute infection that produces blood poisoning and blood clots).

The organism may infect the ear, cornea, or prosthetic heart valves; it may also cause pneumonia (especially in persons receiving immunotherapy), sinusitis, and brain abscesses. The prognosis varies with each disorder.

> *Aspergillus infects people who are especially vulnerable because of excessive or prolonged use of such drugs as antibiotics and glucocorticoids; radiation; conditions such as AIDS, Hodgkin's disease, leukemia, and alcoholism; and organ transplants.*

What causes it?

Aspergillosis is caused by *Aspergillus* fungi, which occur worldwide, often in fermenting compost piles and damp hay. It's transmitted by inhalation of fungal spores or, in aspergillosis endophthalmitis, by the invasion of spores through a wound or other tissue injury.

Aspergillus infects people who are especially vulnerable because of excessive or prolonged use of antibiotics or other drugs, radiation treatments, organ transplants, or conditions such as AIDS, Hodgkin's disease, leukemia, alcoholism, sarcoidosis, bronchitis, bronchiectasis, or tuberculosis.

What are its symptoms?

The incubation period ranges from a few days to weeks. Symptoms depend on the form of infection.

Aspergilloma

Characteristically, aspergilloma either produces no symptoms or causes a productive cough and blood-tinged sputum, shortness of breath, pus accumulation in the chest cavity, and lung abscesses.

Allergic aspergillosis

This infection causes wheezing, shortness of breath, cough with some sputum production, pleural pain, and fever.

Aspergillosis endophthalmitis

This infection causes clouded vision, eye pain, and reddened conjunctivas. Eventually, it produces a pus-containing discharge.

Disseminated aspergillosis

In this form, *Aspergillus* causes blood clots, infarctions, and the signs of blood poisoning (chills, fever, low blood pressure, delirium), with blood in the urine, urinary tract obstruction, headaches, seizures, bone pain and tenderness, and soft-tissue swelling. This form of aspergillosis is rapidly fatal.

How is it diagnosed?

A chest X-ray may help detect aspergilloma. In aspergillosis endophthalmitis, a history of eye injury or surgery and lab tests showing *Aspergillus* confirm the diagnosis. In allergic aspergillosis, sputum analysis shows eosinophils.

How is it treated?

Aspergillosis doesn't require isolation. Treatment of aspergilloma requires local excision of the lesion and supportive therapy, such as chest physical therapy and coughing, to improve pulmonary function. Allergic aspergillosis requires desensitization and, possibly, steroid drugs. Disseminated aspergillosis and aspergillosis endophthalmitis require a 2- to 3-week course of the intravenous drug Fungizone.

BLASTOMYCOSIS

What do doctors call this condition?

Besides blastomycosis, doctors call this condition North American blastomycosis or Gilchrist's disease.

What is this condition?

Blastomycosis is a fungal condition that usually affects the lungs and produces bronchopneumonia. Less frequently, the fungus may

The fungus that causes blastomycosis is probably inhaled by people who are in close contact with the soil. The incubation period may range from weeks to months.

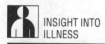

Facts about blastomycosis

A fungus living in the soil

The fungus that causes blastomycosis appears in the soil in North America and is native to the southeastern United States. While no occupational link has been found, people in close contact with the soil, such as farmers and ranchers, should recognize the risk of infection, which probably stems from inhalation of the fungus.

Outlook improves with treatment

Untreated blastomycosis is slow, progressive, and potentially fatal. However, the outlook is good when the individual receives antifungal drugs and supportive treatment.

spread through the blood and cause osteomyelitis and disorders of the central nervous system, skin, and genitalia. The incubation period may range from weeks to months. (See *Facts about blastomycosis*.)

What causes it?

Blastomycosis is caused by the fungus *Blastomyces dermatitidis*.

What are its symptoms?

Initial signs and symptoms of blastomycosis in the lungs include a dry, hacking, or productive cough (occasionally spitting up blood), pleuritic chest pain, fever, shaking, chills, night sweats, malaise, and appetite and weight loss.

Blastomycosis of the skin causes small, painless, nonitching, and nondistinctive macules or papules on exposed skin. These lesions become raised and reddened and occasionally progress to draining skin abscesses or fistulas.

Spread of the fungus to the bone causes soft-tissue swelling, tenderness, and warmth over bony lesions, which generally occur in the thoracic, lumbar, and sacral regions of the spine; the long bones of the legs; and, in children, the skull.

Spread of the fungus to the genitalia produces painful swelling of the testicles, the epididymis, or the prostate; deep perineal pain; and pus and blood in the urine.

If the fungus affects the nervous system, it causes meningitis or cerebral abscesses with resultant decreased level of consciousness, lack of energy, and change in mood or demeanor. Spread of the fungus to other areas may result in Addison's disease (adrenal insufficiency), pericarditis, and arthritis.

How is it diagnosed?

Diagnosis of blastomycosis requires:

- *culture* of *B. dermatitidis* from skin lesions, pus, sputum, or lung secretions
- *microscopic examination* and analysis of tissue removed from the skin or the lungs, or of bronchial washings, sputum, or pus
- *immunologic tests* to detect antibodies to the fungus.

In addition, the doctor may order a chest X-ray if he or she suspects lung infection.

How is it treated?

All forms of blastomycosis respond to Fungilin. Nizoral or Diflucan are alternatives. Care is mainly supportive.

BOTULISM

What is this condition?

A life-threatening paralytic illness, botulism results from an exotoxin produced by the anaerobic bacterium *Clostridium botulinum*. The death rate from botulism is about 25%; death most often results from respiratory failure during the first week of illness.

What causes it?

Botulism usually results from ingestion of poorly cooked, contaminated foods, especially those with low acid content, such as home-canned fruits and vegetables, sausages, and smoked or preserved fish or meat. Rarely, it results from wound infection with *C. botulinum*.

Botulism occurs worldwide and affects adults more often than children. Incidence had been declining, but the current trend toward home canning has caused an upswing (approximately 250 cases annually in the United States) in recent years.

What are its symptoms?

Symptoms usually appear within 12 to 36 hours (the range is 6 hours to 8 days) after contaminated food is eaten. Severity varies with the amount of poison ingested and the person's degree of immunocompetence. Generally, early onset (within 24 hours) signals critical and potentially fatal illness. Initial symptoms include dry mouth, sore throat, weakness, vomiting, and diarrhea. The cardinal sign of botulism, though, is cranial nerve impairment (drooping eyelid, double vision, slurred speech), followed by descending weakness or paralysis of muscles in the arms, legs, or trunk, and shortness of breath from respiratory muscle paralysis. Such impairment doesn't affect mental or sensory processes and isn't associated with fever.

Infant botulism usually afflicts infants between 3 and 20 weeks of age and can produce floppy infant syndrome, characterized by constipation, feeble cry, depressed gag reflex, and inability to suck. Cra-

PREVENTION
TIPS

Avoiding the hazards of botulism

Ingesting even a small amount of botulism-contaminated food can kill you. Here's how you can prevent this deadly illness.

For yourself
- Always use safe techniques of processing, preparing, and storing food. Read and follow food labels for directions on refrigeration.
- Don't even taste food from a bulging can or food that has a peculiar odor.
- Boil any utensil that comes in contact with food that you suspect is contaminated.

For your family
- If a family member exhibits symptoms, check to see if other family members have similar symptoms and have eaten the same foods.
- If a member of the family is hospitalized for botulism poisoning, watch closely when he returns home for signs of weakness, blurred vision, or slurred speech. Take him back to the hospital immediately if any of these signs appear.

nial nerve deficits also occur in infants and are manifested by a limp facial expression, drooping eyelid, and paralysis of the eye muscles. Infants also develop generalized muscle weakness, decreased muscle tone, and lack of normal reflexes. Loss of head control may be striking. Respiratory arrest is likely.

How is it diagnosed?

Identification of the offending poison in the person's blood, stools, stomach contents, or the suspected food confirms the diagnosis. The diagnosis also must rule out other diseases often confused with botulism.

How is it treated?

Treatment consists of intravenous or intramuscular administration of botulinum antitoxin (available through the Centers for Disease Control and Prevention). (See *Avoiding the hazards of botulism*.)

CANDIDIASIS

What do doctors call this condition?

Besides candidiasis, doctors call this condition candidosis or moniliasis.

What is this condition?

Candidiasis is usually a mild, superficial fungal infection caused by the genus *Candida*. Most often, it infects the nails, skin (diaper rash), or mucous membranes, especially the oropharynx, vagina, esophagus, and gastrointestinal tract. The prognosis varies, depending on the person's resistance.

What causes it?

Most cases of *Candida* infection result from *C. albicans*. These fungi are part of the normal bacteria and fungi found in the gastrointestinal tract, mouth, vagina, and skin. Infection occurs when a change in the body encourages fungal growth.

The most common predisposing factor is the use of broad-spectrum antibiotics. Other predisposing factors include rising sugar levels in diabetes, lowered resistance due to disease (such as cancer), treatment with immunosuppressive drugs or radiation, aging, or

HIV infection. Infection also may be introduced by intravenous lines or urinary catheters, drug abuse, tube feeding, or surgery.

An infant of a mother with vaginal moniliasis can contract oral thrush while passing through the birth canal. The incidence of candidiasis is rising because of wider use of intravenous therapy and a greater number of people with immune system problems, especially people with HIV infection.

What are its symptoms?

Symptoms of superficial candidiasis correspond to the site of infection:

- *Skin:* scaly, red, papular rash, sometimes covered with discharge, appearing below the breast, between the fingers, under the arms, and at the groin and navel. In diaper rash, papules appear at the edges of the rash.
- *Nails:* red, swollen, darkened nail bed; occasionally, a pus-containing discharge and the separation of a nail from the nail bed
- *Mouth and pharynx:* cream-colored or bluish white patches of discharge (called thrush) on the tongue, mouth, or pharynx that reveal bloody engorgement when scraped. The patches may swell, causing respiratory distress in infants. They are only occasionally painful but cause a burning sensation in the throats and mouths of adults.
- *Esophagus:* difficult swallowing, pain below the sternum, regurgitation and, occasionally, scales in the mouth and throat
- *Vagina:* white or yellow discharge, with itching and local abrasion; white or gray raised patches on vaginal walls, with local inflammation; and painful intercourse.

Generalized infection produces chills; high, spiking fever; low blood pressure; prostration; and occasional rash. The person may develop other symptoms depending on the site of infection; for example, infection of the lungs may produce fever and a cough, or possibly even a bloody cough.

How is it diagnosed?

The diagnosis of superficial candidiasis depends on evidence of *Candida* on a Gram stain of skin, vaginal scrapings, pus, or sputum. Systemic (generalized) infections require specimen collection for a blood or tissue culture.

How is it treated?

Treatment first aims to improve the underlying condition that predisposes the person to candidiasis, such as controlling diabetes or discontinuing antibiotic therapy and catheterization, if possible.

The incidence of candidiasis is rising partly because of a greater number of people with immune system problems, especially people with HIV infection.

SELF-HELP

Getting over candidiasis

Follow these tips to ensure that you recover from candidiasis:
- If the doctor has prescribed Nilstat solution, swish it around in your mouth for several minutes before you swallow it.
- Use a nonirritating mouthwash to loosen thick secretions and a soft toothbrush to avoid mouth irritation.
- If you have slight difficulty swallowing, chew foods thoroughly so that you don't choke. If you have a great deal of trouble swallowing, eat soft foods.
- If you're overweight, apply cornstarch or dry padding in skin folds to prevent irritation.
- If you're pregnant, be examined for vaginal candidiasis to protect your infant from infection at birth.

Nilstat is an effective antifungal for superficial candidiasis. Mycelex, Diflucan, Nizoral, and Monistat are effective in mucous-membrane *Candida* infections. Nizoral or Diflucan is the treatment of choice for chronic candidiasis of the mucous membranes. Treatment for systemic infection consists of intravenous Fungizone or Diflucan. (See *Getting over candidiasis*.)

CHICKENPOX

What is this condition?

Chickenpox is a common, acute, and highly contagious infection. It can occur at any age, but it's most common in children ages 2 to 8.

Congenital chickenpox may affect infants whose mothers had acute infections during their first or early second trimester. Infection in newborns is rare. So are second attacks.

Chickenpox occurs throughout the world and is especially common in large cities. The disease occurs in all races and affects both sexes equally. Outbreaks are sporadic, usually in areas with large groups of susceptible children. In regions with temperate climates, the incidence is higher during late autumn, winter, and spring.

Most children recover from chickenpox completely. But life-threatening complications may occur in children receiving certain drugs (such as drugs that suppress the system) and in those with cancer or deficient immune systems. The disease may also have severe effects in adults and in babies born with it.

What causes it?

Chickenpox is caused by the herpesvirus varicella-zoster — the same one that causes shingles (herpes zoster). It spreads by direct contact (mainly with respiratory secretions; less often, with skin lesions) and indirect contact (through the air).

Symptoms generally appear about 13 to 17 days after exposure. Chickenpox is probably contagious from 1 day before the characteristic lesions erupt until 6 days after blisters form. It's most contagious in the early stages of the skin lesions' eruption.

What are its symptoms?

The most distinctive symptom is an itchy rash. At onset, the person has a slight fever, a general ill feeling, and appetite loss. Within 24 hours, the rash typically begins as small, reddish blemishes on the trunk or scalp that eventually develop into clear blisters. The blisters become cloudy and break easily; then scabs form. The rash spreads to the face and, rarely, to the arms and legs. New blisters continue to appear for 3 or 4 days. Occasionally, shallow ulcers appear on the mucous membranes of the mouth, eyes, and genitals.

Severe itching may cause the person to scratch, which can lead to infection, scarring, and other problems.

How is it diagnosed?

The doctor diagnoses chickenpox from its characteristic symptoms.

How is it treated?

A person with chickenpox must be kept in strict isolation until all the blisters and most of the scabs disappear (usually for 1 week after the rash appears). However, children can go back to school if just a few scabs remain because the disease is no longer contagious at that stage. A baby born with chickenpox doesn't require isolation.

Generally, the person is treated with anti-itching drugs, cool baths containing baking soda, calamine lotion, or another antihistamine. Antibiotics aren't needed unless a bacterial infection occurs. (See *Caring for a child with chickenpox*.)

In March of 1995, the Food and Drug Administration approved a chickenpox vaccine. The American Academy of Pediatrics recommends the vaccine for all children (and adolescents and adults) who haven't had the disease. The vaccine prevents chickenpox in 70% to 90% of recipients.

CHOLERA

What is this condition?

This acute infection causes severe diarrhea, vomiting, massive fluid loss, and possibly death. Untreated cholera may kill up to 50% of infected people. Even with prompt diagnosis and treatment, cholera

ADVICE FOR CAREGIVERS

Caring for a child with chickenpox

If your child has chickenpox, itching will be a big problem. And you'll have to try to stop your child from scratching the skin. Because the need to scratch may be overwhelming, make sure to keep your child's fingernails trimmed or tie mittens on the hands. Ask your doctor or nurse how to apply anti-itching drugs.

Prevent infection

To prevent the skin from getting infected, keep your child clean throughout the illness. Also, call your doctor right away if your child gets symptoms of complications — for instance, severe skin pain and burning. These symptoms may signal a serious secondary infection.

Don't give a dangerous drug

You've probably taken aspirin for aches and fevers. That's okay. But you must never give this usually beneficial drug to a child with chickenpox for any reason. That's because aspirin has been linked to Reye's syndrome, a potentially deadly illness, in children who've had chickenpox.

Instead, give your child Tylenol (or another drug containing acetaminophen), if needed. Or ask your doctor for another safe medication.

TRAVELER'S
ADVISORY

Avoiding cholera infection

Cholera is a fact of life in many areas of the world. If you're traveling to one of these areas, you must boil all drinking water and avoid eating uncooked vegetables and unpeeled fruits. Check with your doctor about a cholera vaccination. If you get one, you'll need a booster 3 to 6 months later for continued protection.

Danger zones

Cholera is most common in Africa, southern and Southeast Asia, and the Middle East, although outbreaks have occurred in Japan, Australia, and Europe. A new epidemic is now occurring in western South America and parts of Central America.

Cholera occurs during the warmer months and is most prevalent among lower socioeconomic groups. In India, it's common among children ages 1 to 5, but in other endemic areas, it's equally distributed among all age-groups.

is fatal in up to 2% of infected children; in adults, it's fatal in fewer than 1%.

What causes it?

Cholera is caused by the bacterium *Vibrio cholerae*. It's transmitted through food and water contaminated with fecal material from disease carriers or people with active infections.

What are its symptoms?

After an incubation period ranging from several hours to 5 days, cholera produces acute, painless, profuse, watery diarrhea and effortless vomiting (without preceding nausea). As the number of stools increases, the stools contain white flecks of mucus. Because of massive fluid and electrolyte loss from diarrhea and vomiting, cholera causes intense thirst, weakness, loss of skin tone, wrinkled skin, sunken eyes, pinched facial expression, muscle cramps (especially in the extremities), bluish skin discoloration, inadequate urine production, rapid heart rate and breathing, thready or absent peripheral pulses, falling blood pressure, fever, and inaudible, insufficiently active bowel sounds.

People with cholera usually remain oriented but apathetic, although small children may become stuporous or develop seizures.

If complications don't occur, the symptoms subside within a week of treatment.

How is it diagnosed?

In areas that are native to the organism or during epidemics, typical clinical features strongly suggest cholera. A culture of *V. cholerae* from feces or vomit indicates cholera, but definite diagnosis requires additional lab tests.

How is it treated?

Improved sanitation and the administration of cholera vaccine to travelers to areas where the organism is prevalent can control this disease. Unfortunately, the vaccine now available confers only 60% to 80% immunity and is effective for only 3 to 6 months. If you're traveling abroad, see *Avoiding cholera infection*.

Treatment requires rehydration by rapid intravenous infusion of large amounts of normal saline solution, alternating with isotonic sodium bicarbonate or sodium lactate. To avoid this disease, family members of a person with cholera should take Achromycin as directed by the doctor.

COMMON COLD

What is this condition?

The common cold is an acute viral infection that causes inflammation of the upper respiratory tract. It accounts for more time lost from school or work than any other cause and is the most common infectious disease. Although benign and self-limiting, it can lead to secondary bacterial infections.

The common cold is more prevalent in children than in adults, in adolescent boys than in girls, and in women than in men. In temperate zones, it occurs more often in the colder months; in the tropics, during the rainy season.

Although benign and self-limiting, the common cold can lead to secondary bacterial infection.

What causes it?

About 90% of colds stem from a viral infection of the upper respiratory passages. Over a hundred different viral strains can cause the common cold. Colds are spread through the air, through contact with contaminated objects, and by hand-to-hand transmission. Children get new strains from their schoolmates and pass them on to family members. Fatigue and drafts *don't* make a person more susceptible. A cold is contagious for 2 to 3 days after symptoms first appear.

What are its symptoms?

About 1 to 4 days after being exposed to a cold virus, the person gets a sore throat, nasal congestion, runny nose, headache, and burning, watery eyes. Children may get a fever. Other symptoms may include chills, muscle and joint aches, malaise, lack of energy, and a hacking, nonproductive, or nighttime cough.

As the cold progresses, the symptoms get worse. After about a day, the person has a feeling of fullness with nasal discharge that often irritates the nose, adding to the discomfort.

About 3 days after onset, major symptoms diminish, but the "stuffed-up" feeling may last for a week. Reinfection with a productive (sputum-producing) cough is common. Fortunately, complica-

SELF-HELP

Treating a cold

It may be a cliché, but getting plenty of rest and drinking fluids really *is* the best medicine for a cold. For the first few days, stay in bed as much as possible. Drink lots of fluids to prevent dehydration, and eat light meals. Here are some other tips for fighting a cold.

Relieving your symptoms
- Apply a lubricant to your nostrils if they're sore from a runny nose and constant blowing.
- If your throat is sore, suck on hard candy or cough drops.
- To relieve aches and pains, take warm baths or use heating pads.

Taking medications
- To get rid of mucus secretions, you may be tempted to take an over-the-counter expectorant such as Robitussin. However, these drugs haven't been proven effective. A better bet may be a hot or cold steam vaporizer.

- Nose drops or sprays may relieve a runny nose and nasal congestion, but don't use them for more than a few days because you may get rebound congestion. Use them only as directed.
- Unless your symptoms suggest a more serious illness, don't expect the doctor to prescribe an antibiotic — antibiotics can't cure the common cold.

Keeping it to yourself
To avoid spreading your cold to others, wash your hands often and cover your mouth when you cough or sneeze. Don't share towels and drinking glasses.

tions, such as sinus inflammation, ear infection, and lower respiratory tract infection, are rare.

How is it diagnosed?

There's no diagnostic test that can isolate the specific organism causing the common cold. So diagnosis rests on the typically mild, localized upper respiratory symptoms without fever.

The doctor will rule out allergies, measles, German measles, and other disorders that cause similar early symptoms. With certain symptoms — such as a temperature above 100° F (37.7° C), severe malaise, appetite loss, a rapid heart rate, a distinctive coating on the tonsils or throat, tiny purple or red spots on the skin, and tender lymph nodes — the doctor may do more tests to rule out a more serious problem.

How is it treated?

The common cold can't be cured, but there are ways to relieve symptoms: taking aspirin or Tylenol (or another drug containing acetaminophen), drinking plenty of fluids, and getting plenty of rest. Aspirin or Tylenol eases muscle ache and headache, fluids help loosen respiratory secretions and prevent dehydration, and rest combats fatigue and weakness. *Important:* In a child with a fever, Tylenol is the drug of choice.

The doctor may also recommend decongestants to relieve congestion, throat lozenges to relieve sore throat, and steam treatments to help expel secretions. Nasal douching, sinus drainage, and antibiotics aren't necessary unless the person has complications or chronic illness. (See *Treating a cold.*)

If the person has a severe cough, the doctor may recommend a cough suppressant. But these are inadvisable for productive coughs, when cough suppression is harmful. The role of vitamin C in fighting colds remains controversial. In infants, giving saline (saltwater) nose drops and suctioning mucus with a bulb syringe may be beneficial.

Currently, no known measure can prevent the common cold. Researchers are investigating vitamin therapy, interferon administration, and ultraviolet irradiation.

CRYPTOCOCCOSIS

What is this condition?
Cryptococcosis usually starts as a lung infection without symptoms but spreads to other body regions, usually the central nervous system. It also can spread to the skin, bones, prostate gland, liver, or kidneys. With appropriate treatment, the prognosis is good. However, central nervous system infection can be dangerous.

Cryptococcosis is especially likely to develop in people with compromised immune systems, such as people with AIDS.

What causes it?
Cryptococcosis is caused by the fungus *Cryptococcus neoformans.* Transmission is through inhalation of *C. neoformans* in particles of dust contaminated by pigeon feces that harbor this organism. Therefore, cryptococcosis is primarily an urban infection. It's most prevalent in men, usually those between ages 30 and 60, and is rare in children.

Cryptococcosis is especially likely to occur in immunocompromised people, such as those with Hodgkin's disease, sarcoidosis, leukemia, or lymphoma, as well as those taking drugs that suppress the immune system. People with AIDS are by far the most commonly affected group.

What are its symptoms?

Typically, cryptococcosis in the lungs produces no symptoms. Skin involvement produces red facial papules and other skin abscesses, with or without ulcerations; bone involvement produces painful bony lesions of the long bones, skull, spine, and joints.

Onset of brain and spinal cord involvement is gradual. It causes progressively severe frontal and temporal headache, blurred and double vision, dizziness, lack of muscle coordination, loss of speech, vomiting, "ringing in the ears," memory changes, inappropriate behavior, irritability, psychotic symptoms, seizures, and fever. If untreated, symptoms progress to coma and death, usually a result of cerebral swelling or "water on the brain."

How is it diagnosed?

Although a routine chest X-ray may help detect cryptococcosis in the lungs, the disorder is difficult to diagnosis until it spreads. Firm diagnosis requires identification of *C. neoformans* by culture of sputum, urine, prostatic secretions, bone marrow aspirate or biopsy (removal and analysis of tissue), or pleural biopsy and, in central nervous system infection, by cerebrospinal fluid culture.

How is it treated?

People with pulmonary cryptococcosis require close medical observation for a year after diagnosis. Treatment is unnecessary unless extrapulmonary lesions develop or pulmonary lesions progress.

Treatment of disseminated infection calls for intravenous Fungizone or Diflucan. People with AIDS also need long-term therapy, usually with oral Diflucan.

CYTOMEGALOVIRUS INFECTION

What do doctors call this condition?

Generalized salivary gland virus, cytomegalic inclusion disease

What is this condition?

Cytomegalovirus infection is a disease that occurs worldwide and is transmitted by human contact. About 80% of people over age 35 have been infected with cytomegalovirus, usually during childhood or early adulthood. In most of these people, the disease is so mild that it's often overlooked. However, infection during pregnancy can be hazardous to the fetus.

What causes it?

This infection is caused by the cytomegalovirus, a virus related to herpesviruses.

Cytomegalovirus has been found in the saliva, urine, semen, breast milk, feces, blood, and vaginal and cervical secretions of infected persons. Infected secretions can harbor the virus for months or even years. It may be transmitted by contact with infected secretions, sexual contact, or across the placenta of a pregnant woman.

Immunosuppressed people, especially those who have received transplanted organs, run a 90% chance of contracting cytomegalovirus infection. Recipients of blood transfusions from donors with antibodies to cytomegalovirus are at some risk.

What are its symptoms?

Cytomegalovirus often produces inflammatory reactions in the lungs, liver, gastrointestinal tract, eyes, or central nervous system.

Most people with this infection have mild, nonspecific complaints, or none at all. In these individuals, the disease is usually self-limiting. However, people with immunodeficiencies and those receiving immunosuppressive drugs may develop pneumonia or other secondary infections. In people with AIDS, disseminated cytomegalovirus infection may cause chorioretinitis (resulting in blindness), colitis, or encephalitis. Infected infants ages 3 to 6 months usually appear to lack symptoms but may develop liver dysfunction, liver and spleen enlargement, spider angiomas (tumors made up of blood or lymph vessels), pneumonitis, and lymph node disease.

When infection is present at birth, it's seldom immediately apparent. About 1% of all newborns have cytomegalovirus infection.

The virus can cause brain damage that may not show up for months after birth. It can also produce a newborn illness characterized by jaundice, petechial rash, enlarged liver and spleen, low platelet count, hemolytic anemia, microcephaly (an abnormally small head), psychomotor retardation, mental deficiency, and hearing loss. Occasionally, this form is rapidly fatal.

About 80% of people over age 35 have been infected with cytomegalovirus, usually during childhood or early adulthood. In most of these people, the disease is so mild that it's often overlooked.

How is it diagnosed?

Although virus isolation in urine is the most sensitive lab method, the diagnosis can also rest on virus isolation from saliva, throat, cervix, white blood cell, and biopsy specimens.

How is it treated?

Treatment aims to relieve symptoms and prevent complications. In the immunosuppressed person, the infection is treated with Zovirax, Cytovene and, possibly, Foscavir. Most important, parents of children with severe cytomegalovirus infection that's present at birth need support and counseling to help them cope with the possibility of brain damage or death.

What can a person with cytomegalovirus infection do?

- Wash your hands thoroughly to prevent spreading it. This is especially important for young children.
- To help *prevent* this infection, immunosuppressed people and pregnant women should avoid exposure to confirmed or suspected cytomegalovirus infection.

DIPHTHERIA

What is this condition?

Diphtheria is a serious, highly contagious infection that's rare in the United States and many other parts of the world — thanks to effective immunization. Most people who do get diphtheria are children under age 15. Diphtheria is fatal in about 10% of people who get it. Children must get immunizations at the appropriate times.

What causes it?

Diphtheria is caused by *Corynebacterium diphtheriae,* a bacterium that usually infects the respiratory tract, primarily involving the tonsils, nasopharynx, and larynx.

Transmission usually occurs through intimate contact or by airborne respiratory droplets from apparently healthy carriers or convalescing people. Diphtheria is more prevalent during the colder months because of closer person-to-person contact indoors. But it may be contracted at any time during the year. It is also most likely to occur in areas of crowding and poor sanitation.

What are its symptoms?

Most infections go unrecognized, especially in partially immunized individuals. After an incubation period of less than a week, diphtheria infection causes a thick, patchy, grayish green membrane over the mucous membranes of the pharynx, larynx, tonsils, soft palate, and nose; fever; sore throat; and a rasping cough, hoarseness, and other symptoms similar to croup. Attempts to remove the membrane usually cause bleeding. If this membrane causes airway obstruction, symptoms include rapid breathing; a harsh, high-pitched breath sound; possibly bluish skin discoloration; retractions above the sternum; and suffocation, if untreated. In skin diphtheria, skin lesions resemble impetigo.

Complications may include myocarditis, nervous system involvement, kidney involvement, and lung involvement.

How is it diagnosed?

The doctor will make a diagnosis based on an exam of the person. Throat culture or a culture of other suspect lesions confirm this diagnosis. However, treatment can't wait for confirmation by a culture.

How is it treated?

Standard treatment includes diphtheria antitoxin administered intramuscularly or intravenously and antibiotics, such as penicillin or Pediazole. The person may need to undergo strict isolation to prevent spread of the disease. Family members should ask their doctor whether they need treatment with diphtheria toxoid.

Thanks to effective immunization, diphtheria is rare in many parts of the world, including the United States.

FLU

What do doctors call this condition?

Besides flu, doctors call this condition influenza or grippe.

What is this condition?

The flu is an acute, highly contagious infection of the respiratory tract that affects all age-groups, although its incidence peaks in schoolchildren. It's most severe and most dangerous in the very young, the elderly, and people with chronic diseases.

The flu occurs sporadically or in epidemics (usually during the colder months). Epidemics tend to peak within 2 to 3 weeks after the first cases occur and subside within a month.

What causes it?

The flu results from three different types of the virus *Myxovirus influenzae*. A person can catch it by inhaling respiratory droplets through the air from an infected person or by indirect contact such as by using a contaminated drinking glass. The virus invades the respiratory tract, causing inflammation. There are three flu virus strains:

- *Type A*, the most prevalent, strikes every year, undergoing major changes that cause epidemics every 3 years.
- *Type B* also strikes annually, but only causes epidemics every 4 to 6 years.
- *Type C* causes only sporadic cases.

A subgroup of the myxoviruses, the paramyxoviruses, causes a variety of milder, self-limiting upper and lower respiratory infections collectively called *parainfluenza*. Most adults become immune to paramyxoviruses following childhood infections and subsequent multiple exposures. Symptoms of parainfluenza resemble those of other respiratory diseases: sudden fever, nasal discharge, reddened throat (with little or no discharge), chills, and muscle pain.

One of the remarkable features of the myxovirus (flu) virus is its ability to change in subtle or major ways. This leads to infection by flu strains to which the population at risk has little or no resistance. Minor changes may occur yearly or every few years; major changes can lead to major outbreaks called *pandemics*. (See *How flu viruses multiply*.)

What are its symptoms?

Symptoms appear about 24 to 48 hours after a person is exposed to the flu virus. They include sudden onset of chills, a temperature of 101° to 104° F (38.3° to 40° C), headache, malaise, muscle ache (particularly in the back and limbs), a nonproductive cough and, occasionally, laryngitis, hoarseness, eye inflammation, runny nose, and nasal congestion. These symptoms usually subside in 3 to 5 days, but a cough and weakness may persist. Fever is usually higher in children

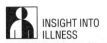

INSIGHT INTO
ILLNESS

How flu viruses multiply

Do you know how the flu invades the body? The answer lies in the flu virus's makeup.

Classified as type A, B, or C, a flu (influenza) virus contains only a portion of nucleic acid (RNA or DNA) on which are strung the genes that carry the instructions for the virus to replicate. The fragmentation of the genetic material accounts for its ability to undergo genetic mutations.

Having only a partial genetic component, the virus can't reproduce or carry out chemical reactions on its own. It needs a host cell. And once you inhale this airborne virus, it seeks this necessary host.

Inside the respiratory tract

Here, the flu virus attaches itself to a healthy host cell. In an attempt to destroy the invader, the healthy cell engulfs the virus and sends chemicals to dissolve the virus cell's wall. This attempt at destruction releases the virus's genetic material into the healthy cell.

Inside the host cell

Here, the genes of the virus find fertile conditions in which to replicate, arranging themselves into identical bundles. These new viruses — up to 1,000 reproduced within 6 hours — burst forth to invade other healthy cells. The viral invasion destroys the host cells, impairing respiratory defenses and predisposing the person to secondary bacterial infection.

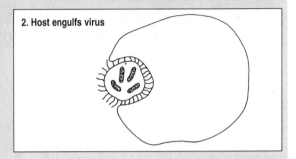

2. Host engulfs virus

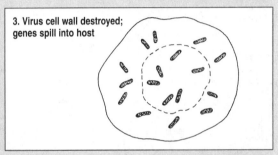

3. Virus cell wall destroyed; genes spill into host

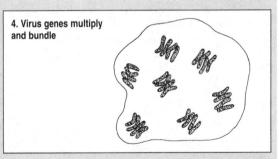

4. Virus genes multiply and bundle

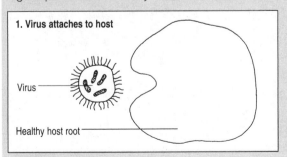

1. Virus attaches to host

Virus

Healthy host root

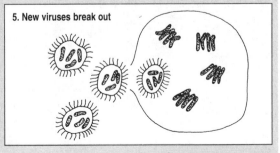

5. New viruses break out

What you should know about flu shots

During flu season, you may hear people discussing the pros and cons of flu shots. As a result, you may wonder whether you should have a flu shot. The following information can help answer your questions.

Do flu shots really work?
Yes. The Centers for Disease Control and Prevention reports that the vaccine reduces your chance of coming down with the flu by 60% to 80%. Even if you were to catch the flu, you would experience fewer and milder symptoms.

Should I get a flu shot?
Depending on the specific flu virus and the risk of a widespread flu outbreak, your doctor will probably recommend vaccination if you:
- are over age 65.
- have a chronic lung disease, such as asthma or emphysema.
- have heart disease, kidney disease, diabetes, or severe anemia.
- have cancer or take a drug that interferes with the body's immune system.
- run a high risk of exposure to the flu virus.
- are pregnant and due to deliver in the winter months.

Flu shots are also recommended for children and teenagers who are taking long-term aspirin therapy and may be at risk for Reye's syndrome if they get the flu.

When's the best time to get a flu shot?
In the fall. Immunization usually consists of one dose of vaccine. Children under age 9 who've never been vaccinated may need two injections, given 1 month apart.

Immunity develops about 2 weeks after vaccination and lasts for 1 year only. This is because the flu virus changes, and different strains usually are responsible for epidemics from year to year.

I'm allergic to eggs. Can I still get a flu shot?
That depends on your symptoms when you eat eggs. Because the vaccine may contain egg protein, you shouldn't have a flu shot if eggs or egg-containing foods cause swelling in your face or tongue, hives, or wheezing.

However, if you get only stomach cramps or gas after eating eggs, you can probably receive the vaccine safely.

Can a flu shot give me the flu?
No. The vaccine contains inactive or weakened virus, so it can't produce the flu. When you receive the vaccine, your body responds by creating antibodies to the virus. These antibodies then fight the virus when you're exposed to it.

About 30% of the people vaccinated experience mild soreness and swelling at the injection site. A few others suffer from muscle and joint aches and a low fever (less than 100° F [37.7° C]).

than in adults. Some people (especially elderly people) may have fatigue and loss of energy for several weeks.

A fever that persists more than 3 days may signal complications; the most common one is pneumonia. The flu may also worsen chronic obstructive lung disease and cause other serious illness.

How is it diagnosed?

At the start of a flu epidemic, early cases are usually mistaken for other respiratory disorders. Because signs and symptoms of the flu are not highly distinctive, isolation of the causative virus in the nasal secretions of infected people is essential at the first sign of an epidemic. Nose and throat cultures and increased serum antibody titers help confirm this diagnosis.

After these measures confirm a flu epidemic, a diagnosis requires only observation of signs and symptoms.

How is it treated?

Treatment of uncomplicated flu includes bed rest, adequate fluids, aspirin or Tylenol (in children) to relieve fever and muscle pain, and an expectorant to relieve nonproductive coughing. Preventive antibiotics aren't recommended because they have no effect on the flu virus. (See *What you should know about flu shots.*)

Symmetrel, an antiviral agent, can reduce the duration of signs and symptoms in influenza A infection. If the flu is complicated by pneumonia, the person may need fluid and electrolyte supplements, oxygen, and mechanical ventilation. If the person also has a bacterial infection, the doctor will prescribe antibiotics.

What can a person with the flu do?

Use mouthwashes and increase your fluid intake. Warm baths or heating pads may relieve muscle ache. Take pain relievers and fever-reducing drugs (such as aspirin or Tylenol) as directed by your doctor.
- To prevent others from catching the flu, discard used tissues properly and wash your hands often and thoroughly.
- To avoid getting the flu, talk to your doctor about getting a flu shot.

GAS GANGRENE

What is this condition?

Gas gangrene results from local infection with a bacterium called *Clostridium perfringens*. This bacterium is anaerobic, which means it doesn't need oxygen to survive. It infects tissue damaged by injury or surgery. It's most often found in deep wounds, usually in the extremities, the abdomen, and, less frequently, the uterus.

This rare infection has a high risk of death unless therapy begins immediately. However, with prompt treatment, 80% of people with gas gangrene of the extremities survive. The prognosis is poorer for gas gangrene in other sites, such as the abdominal wall or the bowels.

What causes it?

C. perfringens inhabits the gastrointestinal and female genital tracts without causing problems; it's also prevalent in soil. Infection results from entry of organisms during injury or surgery.

What are its symptoms?

Gas gangrene causes inflammation of the muscle and the layer of tissue under the skin. Most signs of infection develop within 72 hours of an injury or surgery. The hallmark of gas gangrene is crepitation (a crackling sound), which results from carbon dioxide and hydrogen accumulation in dying tissues.

Other typical symptoms are severe localized pain, swelling, and skin discoloration (often dusky brown or reddish), with formation of blisters and localized tissue death within 36 hours from onset of symptoms. Soon the skin over the wound may rupture, revealing dark red or black dying muscle tissue; a foul-smelling, watery or frothy discharge; blood clots; and evidence that the infection has spread.

In addition to these local symptoms, gas gangrene produces early signs of sepsis (blood poisoning) and low fluid volume (rapid heart rate, rapid breathing, and low blood pressure), with moderate fever usually not above 101° F (38.3° C). Although pale, prostrate, and motionless, most people remain alert and oriented and are extremely apprehensive.

Usually death occurs suddenly, often during surgery for removal of dead tissue. Less often, death is preceded by delirium and coma, and is sometimes accompanied by vomiting, profuse diarrhea, and circulatory collapse.

How is it diagnosed?

A history of recent surgery or a deep puncture wound and the rapid onset of pain and crepitation around the wound suggest this diagnosis. It is confirmed by cultures of wound drainage which reveal

Gas gangrene results from compromised arterial circulation following injury or surgery. With prompt treatment, 80% of people with gas gangrene of the extremities survive.

C. *perfringens*. X-rays may reveal gas in tissues. Blood studies show the effects of infection.

How is it treated?

Treatment should begin immediately upon the appearance of signs of inflammation of muscle and of tissues under the skin. Measures include surgical removal of all affected tissues and dead muscle (delayed or inadequate surgery can be a fatal mistake) and administration of high-dose penicillin. The person may also undergo high-pressure oxygen therapy in a hyperbaric chamber, if available.

GERMAN MEASLES

What do doctors call this condition?

Besides German measles, doctors call this condition rubella.

What is this condition?

German measles is an acute, mildly contagious viral disease that causes a distinctive 3-day rash and swollen glands. It occurs most often among children ages 5 to 9, adolescents, and young adults.

The disease is self-limiting, and the prognosis is excellent. However, if a pregnant woman gets this infection — especially during the first trimester — her baby may have severe birth defects.

Occurring worldwide, German measles flourishes during the spring (particularly in big cities). Major outbreaks occur sporadically.

What causes it?

The German measles virus is spread through contact with the blood, urine, stools, or nasal or throat secretions of an infected person, and possibly from contact with contaminated articles of clothing. It can also be transmitted through the placenta to an embryo or fetus.

German measles is contagious from about 10 days before until 5 days after the rash appears.

What are its symptoms?

In children, a rash of elevated, reddish spots erupts suddenly, about 16 to 18 days after exposure to the virus. In adolescents and adults,

Should you get the German measles vaccine?

German measles is a relatively mild illness that rarely causes complications. But in an embryo or fetus, it can lead to serious birth defects. That's why women of childbearing age who haven't yet had the disease should get vaccinated. However, for at least 3 months after vaccination, they must use an effective means of birth control to avoid getting pregnant.

Who shouldn't get the vaccine?

If you're pregnant — or think you may be — *don't* get the vaccine. Nor should you get the vaccine if you have a depressed immune system or an immunodeficiency disease (such as AIDS), if you're taking steroids or other drugs that suppress the immune system, or if you're receiving radiation therapy. Instead, ask your doctor about getting immune serum globulin to help prevent or reduce infection.

Getting over the side effects

You may get a mild fever, slight rash, joint aches (if you're a teenager), or arthritis (if you're elderly) after receiving the vaccine. For fever and joint aches, take aspirin or Tylenol (or another drug containing acetaminophen).

To help your body absorb the vaccine, apply warmth to the injection site for 24 hours after getting the shot. If the site is still swollen after the first 24 hours, apply a cold compress.

warning symptoms — headache, malaise, appetite loss, slight fever, runny nose and congestion, swollen glands, and sometimes conjunctivitis (an eye inflammation) — appear first.

Typically, the rash starts on the face and spreads rapidly, often covering the trunk, arms, and legs within hours. Small, red spots on the inside of the mouth may precede or accompany the rash. By the end of the second day, the facial rash begins to fade, but the spots on the trunk may merge and be mistaken for scarlet fever.

The rash continues to fade in the order in which it appeared. Generally, it disappears on the third day but may persist for 4 or 5 days — sometimes accompanied by mild runny nose and conjunctivitis. The rash's rapid appearance and disappearance distinguishes it from the measles. (German measles can occur without a rash, but this is rare.)

A slight fever may accompany the rash (99° to 101° F [37.2° to 38.3° C]), but this usually disappears after the first day of the rash. Rarely, a person's temperature may reach 104° F (40° C).

Complications seldom occur in children, but when they do, they often appear as bleeding problems. Young women, however, often experience transient joint pain or arthritis, usually just as the rash is fading. Fever may then return. These complications usually disappear within 5 to 30 days.

How is it diagnosed?

In a person with the distinctive rash, swollen glands, other characteristic signs, and a history of exposure, the doctor can diagnose the disease without doing lab tests. However, cell cultures of the throat, blood, urine, and cerebrospinal fluid can confirm the disease.

How is it treated?

Because the German measles rash is self-limiting and causes only mild itching, it doesn't require topical or systemic medication. Treatment consists of aspirin for fever and joint pain. Bed rest isn't necessary, but the person should be isolated until the rash disappears.

To prevent German measles, people can be immunized with live virus vaccine RA 27/3 — the only German measles vaccine available in the United States. This vaccine should be given with measles and mumps vaccines at age 15 months to decrease the cost and the number of injections needed. (See *Should you get the German measles vaccine?*)

GIARDIASIS

What do doctors call this condition?

Besides giardiasis, doctors call this condition giardia enteritis or lambliasis.

What is this condition?

Giardiasis is an infection of the small bowel. A mild infection may not produce intestinal symptoms. In untreated giardiasis, symptoms wax and wane; with treatment, recovery is complete. (See *Facts about giardiasis,* page 762.)

What causes it?

Giardiasis is caused by the protozoan *Giardia lamblia.* Ingestion of *G. lamblia* cysts in fecally contaminated water or the fecal-oral transfer of cysts by an infected person results in giardiasis.

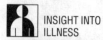

Facts about giardiasis

Occurs worldwide
Giardiasis occurs worldwide but is most common in developing countries and other areas where sanitation and hygiene are poor.

Travelers and campers at risk
In the United States, giardiasis is most common in travelers who've recently returned from areas where the infecting organism is prevalent. It also strikes campers who drink unpurified water from contaminated streams.

Affects children
Probably because of frequent hand-to-mouth activity, children are more likely to become infected with giardiasis than adults.

Reinfection possible
Giardiasis doesn't confer immunity, so reinfections may occur.

What are its symptoms?

Attachment of *G. lamblia* to the intestinal lining causes superficial mucosal invasion and destruction, inflammation, and irritation. All of these destructive effects decrease food transit time through the small intestine and result in malabsorption. Such malabsorption produces chronic gastrointestinal complaints — such as abdominal cramps, nausea, and frequent bowel movements (2 to 10 daily) producing pale, loose, greasy, bad-smelling stools. Stools may contain mucus but not pus or blood. Chronic giardiasis may produce fatigue and weight loss in addition to the typical signs and symptoms.

How is it diagnosed?

Giardiasis should be suspected when travelers who have visited endemic areas or campers who may have drunk unpurified water develop symptoms.

Actual diagnosis requires lab examination of fresh stool specimens. A barium X-ray of the small bowel may show mucous membrane swelling and barium segmentation.

How is it treated?

Giardiasis responds readily to a 10-day course of Flagyl or a 7-day course of Atabrine and oral Furoxone. Severe diarrhea may require parenteral fluid replacement to prevent dehydration if oral fluid intake is inadequate.

What can a person with giardiasis do?

■ If you're taking Flagyl, be aware of the expected side effects of this drug: commonly headache, loss of appetite, and nausea and less commonly vomiting, diarrhea, and abdominal cramps. Don't drink alcoholic beverages, because these may provoke a reaction similar to Antabuse. If you are or think you may be pregnant, tell the doctor; Flagyl is prohibited during pregnancy.

■ Use good personal hygiene, especially proper hand-washing technique.

■ To help prevent giardiasis, don't drink the water or eat uncooked and unpeeled fruits or vegetables when traveling to endemic areas. (Fruits and vegetables may have been rinsed in contaminated water.) Preventive drug therapy isn't recommended. When camping, purify all stream water before drinking it.

HAEMOPHILUS INFLUENZAE
INFECTION

What is this condition?

Haemophilus influenzae is a small, aerobic bacterium that appears in exudates. It causes disease in many organ systems but most frequently attacks the respiratory system. It's a common cause of epiglottitis, laryngotracheobronchitis, pneumonia, bronchiolitis, otitis media, and meningitis.

Less often, it causes bacterial endocarditis, conjunctivitis (an eye inflammation), facial cellulitis (inflammation of tissues under the skin), septic arthritis, and osteomyelitis (bone inflammation).

H. influenzae pneumonia is an increasingly common nosocomial (hospital-related) infection. It infects about half of all children before age 1 and virtually all children by age 3, although a new vaccine given at ages 2, 4, and 6 months has reduced this number.

To prevent infection in children up to age 6, have them vaccinated.

What are its symptoms?

H. influenzae provokes a characteristic tissue response — acute suppurative (pus-discharging) inflammation. When *H. influenzae* infects the larynx, the trachea, and the bronchial tree, it leads to swelling of the mucous membranes and a thick discharge; when it invades the lungs, it leads to bronchopneumonia. In the pharynx, *H. influenzae* usually produces no remarkable changes, except when it causes epiglottitis, which generally affects both the laryngeal and the pharyngeal surfaces. The mucous membranes of the pharynx may be reddened and, rarely, produce a soft yellow discharge. More likely, however, it appears normal or shows only slight diffuse redness, even while severe pain makes swallowing difficult or impossible. These infections typically cause high fever and generalized malaise.

How is it diagnosed?

Isolation of the organism confirms *H. influenzae* infection, usually with a blood culture. Other lab findings include high white blood cell count, low white blood cell count in young children with severe infection, and *H. influenzae* bacteremia, found frequently in people with meningitis.

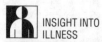

Facts about hantavirus

Rodent risk

Hantavirus infections have occurred in people whose activities bring them into contact with rodents, such as farming, hiking or camping in rodent-infested areas, and occupying rodent-infested dwellings.

Transmission trends

Infection may result from inhalation, ingestion (of contaminated food or water, for example), contact with rodent excrement, or rodent bites. So far, there's no evidence that the virus is spread by personal contact or by mosquitos, fleas, or other insects.

How is it treated?

H. influenzae infections usually respond to a 2-week course of Omnipen (resistant strains are becoming more common), cephalosporins, or Chloromycetin. Discomfort can be eased by using a room humidifier or breathing moist air from a shower or bath. To prevent infection in children up to age 6, get the *H. influenzae* vaccine.

HANTAVIRUS PULMONARY SYNDROME

What is this condition?

Hantavirus pulmonary syndrome is a new viral disease first reported in May 1993. It occurs mainly in the southwestern United States but isn't confined to that area. Potentially fatal, this syndrome rapidly progresses from flulike symptoms to respiratory failure.

What causes it?

Caused by *Hantavirus,* the disease is spread by contact with the feces, urine, and saliva of infected rodents. Deer mice are the main source but pinon mice, brush mice, and western chipmunks living near humans in rural areas are also sources.

What are its symptoms?

Fluid in the lungs is the hallmark of hantavirus pulmonary syndrome. Common symptoms include muscle ache, fever, headache, nausea and vomiting, and cough. Respiratory distress, such as shortness of breath, typically follows the onset of a cough. The breathing rate and pulse may rise. After being hospitalized, a person typically develops a fever and may have severely low blood pressure.

How is it diagnosed?

Doctors are trying to identify the clinical features and laboratory results that distinguish hantavirus pulmonary syndrome from other infections with similar features. For now, the doctor diagnoses it from the infected person's history and physical exam, along with a protocol developed by the Centers for Disease Control and Prevention with the Council of State and Territorial Epidemiologists. The Centers for Disease Control and Prevention and state health departments can perform definite testing for hantavirus exposure and antibody formation.

Lab tests usually show an elevated white blood cell count with certain white cells predominating, an elevated hematocrit, a decreased platelet count, an elevated partial thromboplastin time, and a normal fibrinogen level. Usually, tests show only minor abnormalities in kidney function. Chest X-rays eventually show characteristic lung changes.

How is it treated?

Treatment consists of maintaining the person's respirations and breathing, monitoring vital signs, and intervening to stabilize the heart rate and blood pressure.

The person may receive intravenous fluids and drugs that increase blood pressure, such as Dopastat or Primatene Mist. Researchers are investigating the use of the drug Virazole.

HERPES SIMPLEX

What is this condition?

Herpes simplex is a recurrent viral infection that occurs in two types. Type 1, spread by oral and respiratory secretions, causes cold sores and fever blisters in the skin and mucous membranes. Type 2 mainly affects the genital area and is spread by sexual contact.

Herpes is equally common in males and females. It's found worldwide and is most prevalent among children in lower socioeconomic groups living in crowded environments.

What causes it?

Herpes simplex is caused by Herpesvirus hominis, a widespread virus transmitted by contact with saliva, stools, skin lesions, eye discharge, and urine. After the first infection, the person carries the virus permanently and is vulnerable to recurrent herpes infections. Such conditions as fever, menstruation, stress, heat, and cold may trigger recurrences.

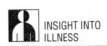 INSIGHT INTO ILLNESS

Herpes in infants and children

Primary herpes simplex virus is the leading cause of gingivostomatitis (mouth and gum sores) in children ages 1 to 3. The virus can pass from mother to fetus and, in early pregnancy, may cause a miscarriage or premature birth.

Infection in newborns

Symptoms usually appear a week or two after birth. They range from skin sores to widespread infection of such organs as the liver, lungs, or brain. Complications may include seizures, mental retardation, blindness, and spastic muscles. Widespread infection may be life-threatening.

Infection in children

Primary infection in childhood may be generalized or localized. About 2 to 12 days after exposure to the virus, generalized infection begins with fever, sore throat, skin redness, and swelling. After brief tingling and itching, typical sores erupt in the form of blisters on a reddened base. Eventually, these burst and leave a painful ulcer, followed by a yellowish crust. Painful mouth sores may lead to severe dehydration. Healing starts 7 to 10 days after the first symptoms appear and is complete in 3 weeks.

SELF-HELP

Sex and genital herpes

Genital herpes can cause long-term sexual problems. If you have herpes, you may fear that you're a danger to your sexual partner. You may retreat from revealing your condition to your partner or may hesitate to initiate a relationship. To compound the problem, a herpes-free partner runs the risk of getting the disease through sexual intercourse.

But you *can* have a meaningful sex life without transmitting herpes. Here are a few guidelines to help you deal with this dilemma.

When to avoid sex
Don't have sex from the disease's warning stage until 10 days after the lesions heal. Though herpes can be transmitted at any time, transmission probably is less likely during symptom-free periods.

What condoms can and can't do
Using a condom doesn't guarantee protection against herpes. But it does increase safety.

How to break the news
Approach relationships with honesty, but avoid shocking revelations like, "I have something terrible to tell you." Instead, broach the subject of herpes with discretion at a convenient time. Use neutral words and terms. For instance, think of herpes as intermittently limiting rather than incurable.

What are its symptoms?

About 85% of all initial herpes simplex infections cause no obvious symptoms. The rest cause localized lesions. Blisters may form on any part of the mouth, especially the tongue, gums, and inside of the cheeks.

Generalized infection causes blisters, along with swelling of the lymph nodes under the jaw, increased salivation, appetite loss, and a fever of up to 105° F (40.5° C). Generalized infection usually runs its course in 4 to 10 days. (See *Herpes in infants and children*, page 765.)

Genital herpes

Genital herpes usually affects adolescents and young adults. The first attack, typically painful, produces fluid-filled blisters that ulcerate and heal in 1 to 3 weeks. Fever, swollen lymph nodes, and painful urination may also occur.

Usually, herpetic keratoconjunctivitis (herpes of the eye) occurs just in one eye and causes only local symptoms: conjunctivitis (eye inflammation), regional lymph node swelling, and eyelid ulcers. Other eye symptoms may include excessive tearing, swollen lids, light sensitivity, and a puslike discharge.

How is it diagnosed?

Typical skin sores may suggest herpes simplex, but to confirm the disease, the doctor may take cultures from a sore and do a biopsy (removal and analysis of tissue).

How is it treated?

The person with herpes simplex needs symptomatic and supportive treatment. For a generalized primary infection, the doctor usually prescribes aspirin or Tylenol (or another drug containing acetaminophen) to reduce fever and relieve pain. Anesthetic mouthwashes such as liquid Xylocaine may reduce the pain of mouth sores so the person can eat and avoid dehydration.

To relieve the pain of genital lesions, the doctor may recommend applying a drying agent, such as calamine lotion. Zovirax ointment may bring relief, too; this drug also is used to treat herpes skin infections in people with impaired immune systems. With more severe infection, Zovirax is given intravenously.

A person with a herpetic eye infection must see an ophthalmologist, who may prescribe such drugs as Stoxil, 1% Viroptic Ophthalmic Solution, and Vira-A Ophthalmic.

What can a person with herpes simplex do?

- If you have genital herpes, apply warm compresses to the lesions, take sitz baths several times a day, and use a drying agent such as povidone-iodine solution. Increase your fluid intake, and avoid all sexual contact during the active stage of the virus. (See *Sex and genital herpes*.)
- If you're pregnant and have genital herpes, get weekly viral cultures of the cervix and external genitalia, starting at 32 weeks' gestation.
- If you have cold sores, don't kiss infants or people with eczema. (See *Relieving cold sores*.) People with genital herpes pose no risk to infants if they use meticulous hygiene.

 SELF-HELP

Relieving cold sores

Although there's no cure for a cold sore caused by herpes simplex, these measures may relieve the discomfort:
- Apply cool compresses to the sore.
- Take aspirin or other pain medication as directed.
- Avoid irritating food and beverages, such as grapefruit juice, which has a high acid content.
- Use an over-the-counter cold sore remedy recommended by your doctor, such as Campho-Phenique or Blistex.
- Call your doctor if the cold sore doesn't heal in 10 days or if symptoms recur frequently.

HISTOPLASMOSIS

What is this condition?

Histoplasmosis is a fungal infection. In the United States, it occurs in three forms: *primary acute histoplasmosis, progressive disseminated his-*

toplasmosis (acute disseminated or chronic disseminated disease), and *chronic pulmonary (cavitary) histoplasmosis,* which produces cavitations in the lung similar to those in pulmonary tuberculosis.

The prognosis varies with each form. The primary acute disease is benign; the progressive disseminated disease is fatal in approximately 90% of infected people; and without proper chemotherapy, chronic pulmonary histoplasmosis is fatal in 50% of infected people within 5 years.

What causes it?

Histoplasmosis is caused by *Histoplasma capsulatum,* which is found in the feces of birds and bats or in soil contaminated by their feces. Histoplasmosis occurs worldwide, especially in the temperate areas of Asia, Africa, Europe, and North and South America. In the United States, it's most prevalent in the central and eastern states, especially in the Mississippi and Ohio River Valleys.

Transmission is through inhalation of *H. capsulatum* spores or through the invasion of spores after minor skin injury. Probably because of occupational exposure, histoplasmosis is more common in adult males. Fatal disseminated disease, however, is more common in infants and elderly men.

The incubation period is from 5 to 18 days, although chronic pulmonary histoplasmosis may progress slowly for many years.

What are its symptoms?

Symptoms vary with each form of this disease. Primary acute histoplasmosis may produce no symptoms, or it may cause symptoms of a mild respiratory illness similar to a severe cold or the flu. Typical clinical effects may include fever, malaise, headache, muscle pain, loss of appetite, cough, and chest pain.

Progressive disseminated histoplasmosis causes an enlarged liver and spleen, general lymph node disease, loss of appetite, weight loss, fever, and possibly ulceration of the tongue, palate, epiglottis, and larynx, with resulting pain, hoarseness, and difficulty swallowing. It may also cause endocarditis, meningitis, pericarditis, and adrenal insufficiency.

Chronic pulmonary histoplasmosis mimics pulmonary tuberculosis and causes a productive cough, shortness of breath, and occasional coughing up of blood. Eventually, it produces weight loss, extreme weakness, breathlessness, and bluish skin coloration.

Symptoms of histoplasmosis vary with each form of this disease. Primary acute histoplasmosis may produce no symptoms or may cause symptoms similar to a severe cold or the flu. Chronic pulmonary histoplasmosis mimics tuberculosis.

How is it diagnosed?

A history of exposure to contaminated soil in an area that's native to the organism, miliary calcification in the lung or spleen, and a positive histoplasmin skin test indicate exposure to histoplasmosis. Other important tests include blood studies, biopsy (tissue removed for analysis), and culture of *H. capsulatum* from sputum or other specimens.

How is it treated?

Treatment consists of antifungal therapy, surgery, and supportive care.

Antifungal therapy is most important. Except for primary acute histoplasmosis (which resolves spontaneously and shows no symptoms), histoplasmosis requires high-dose or long-term (10-week) therapy with Fungilin or Diflucan. For a person who also has AIDS, lifelong therapy with Diflucan is indicated.

Supportive care usually includes oxygen for respiratory distress, glucocorticoids for adrenal insufficiency, and parenteral fluids for difficulty swallowing due to oral or laryngeal ulcerations. Histoplasmosis doesn't require the person to be isolated.

What can a person with histoplasmosis do?

- Be aware that Fungilin may cause chills, fever, nausea, and vomiting.
- If you live in an area where the organism is prevalent, watch for early signs of this infection and seek treatment promptly to help prevent histoplasmosis. If you risk occupational exposure to contaminated soil, wear a face mask.

*I*NFECTIOUS MONONUCLEOSIS

What is this condition?

Infectious mononucleosis is an acute infectious disease that mainly affects young adults and children. (In children, it's usually so mild that it's often overlooked.) Typically, it causes fever, sore throat, and swollen glands in the neck. It may also cause liver dysfunction and may increase the levels of certain white blood cells (lymphocytes and

Getting over mononucleosis

If you have mononucleosis, your recovery may take several weeks — usually until your white blood cell count returns to normal. During the acute phase of the illness, stay in bed as much as possible.

If you're a student, you may continue less demanding school assignments and see your friends, but should avoid long, difficult projects until after recovery.

To ease a sore throat, drink milk shakes, fruit juices, and broths and eat cool, bland foods. Gargle with saltwater and take aspirin.

monocytes). The prognosis is excellent, and major complications are rare.

Infectious mononucleosis is fairly common in the United States, Canada, and Europe. It affects both sexes equally. The incidence varies seasonally among college students (most common in the early spring and early fall) but not among the general population.

What causes it?

Infectious mononucleosis is caused by the Epstein-Barr virus, a member of the herpes group. The disease probably spreads by the mouth and throat because about 80% of people carry the Epstein-Barr virus in the throat during the acute phase of the infection and for some time afterward. It can also be transmitted by blood transfusion.

Infectious mononucleosis is probably contagious from before symptoms develop until the fever subsides and the characteristic mouth and throat sores disappear.

What are its symptoms?

The symptoms of mononucleosis mimic those of many other infectious diseases, including hepatitis, German measles, and toxoplasmosis. Typically, warning symptoms occur about 10 days after exposure in children and 30 to 50 days after exposure in adults. These symptoms include headache, malaise, and fatigue.

After 3 to 5 days, people typically develop sore throat, swollen neck glands, and temperature fluctuations, with an evening peak of 101° to 102° F (38.3° to 38.8° C). The spleen and liver may enlarge, and mouth sores and tonsillitis may develop. Early in the illness, the person may get a rash resembling the German measles rash. Jaundice occurs in about 5% of people with mononucleosis.

Symptoms usually subside about 6 to 10 days after onset of the disease but may persist for weeks.

How is it diagnosed?

The doctor diagnoses mononucleosis from the person's signs and symptoms. Lab tests, such as a white blood cell count and Epstein-Barr virus antibodies, may be ordered to confirm it.

How is it treated?

Because infectious mononucleosis resists prevention and antibiotics, treatment is supportive and includes relief of symptoms; bed rest during the acute, feverish period; and aspirin or another salicylate for headache and sore throat. (See *Getting over mononucleosis.*) If severe throat inflammation causes airway blockage, steroids can be used to relieve swelling.

A ruptured spleen marked by sudden abdominal pain requires surgery. About 20% of people with infectious mononucleosis also have streptococcal infection of the throat and tonsils; they should receive antibiotics for at least 10 days.

LEPROSY

What do doctors call this condition?
Besides leprosy, doctors call this condition Hansen's disease.

What is this condition?
Leprosy is a chronic, systemic (generalized) infection characterized by progressive skin lesions. With timely and correct treatment, it has a good prognosis and is rarely fatal. Untreated, however, it can cause severe disability. The lepromatous form of the disease may lead to blindness and deformities.

Leprosy occurs in three distinct forms:
- *Lepromatous leprosy,* the most serious type, causes damage to the upper respiratory tract, eyes, and testicles, as well as the nerves and skin.
- *Tuberculoid leprosy* affects peripheral nerves and sometimes the surrounding skin, especially on the face, arms, legs, and buttocks.
- *Borderline (dimorphous) leprosy* has characteristics of both lepromatous and tuberculoid leprosies. Skin lesions in this type of leprosy are diffuse and poorly defined.

Leprosy is most prevalent in the underdeveloped areas of Asia (especially India and China), Africa, South America, and the islands of the Caribbean and Pacific. About 15 million people worldwide suffer from this disease; approximately 4,000 are in the United States, mostly in California, Texas, Louisiana, Florida, New York, and Hawaii.

Leprosy is most prevalent in the underdeveloped areas of Asia, Africa, South America, and the islands of the Caribbean and Pacific. About 15 million people worldwide suffer from this disease; approximately 4,000 are in the United States.

What causes it?

Leprosy is caused by *Mycobacterium leprae,* a bacterium that attacks skin tissue and peripheral nerves, producing skin lesions, anesthesia, infection, and deformities. Contrary to popular belief, leprosy is not highly contagious. Rather, continuous, close contact is needed to transmit it. In fact, 9 out of 10 persons have a natural immunity to it.

Susceptibility appears highest during childhood and seems to decrease with age. Presumably, transmission occurs through airborne respiratory droplets containing *M. leprae* or by inoculation through skin breaks (with a contaminated hypodermic or tattoo needle, for example). The incubation period is unusually long — 6 months to 8 years.

What are its symptoms?

If the bacteria attack the skin's fine nerves, they cause anesthesia, loss of sweat gland function, and dryness. If they attack a large nerve trunk, they cause motor nerve damage, weakness, and pain, followed by peripheral anesthesia and muscle paralysis or wasting. In later stages, clawhand, footdrop, and eye complications — such as corneal insensitivity and ulceration, conjunctivitis (eye inflammation), light sensitivity, and blindness — can occur. Injury, ulceration, infection, and disuse of the deformed parts cause scarring and contracture.

Lepromatous and tuberculoid leprosies affect the skin in markedly different ways. In lepromatous disease, early lesions are multiple, symmetrical, and reddened, sometimes appearing as macules or papules with smooth surfaces. Later, they enlarge and form plaques or nodules on the earlobes, nose, eyebrows, and forehead, giving the person a leonine appearance. In advanced stages, the entire skin surface is involved. Lepromatous leprosy also causes loss of eyebrows, eyelashes, and oil and sweat gland function.

Upper respiratory lesions cause nosebleed, ulceration of the uvula and tonsils, septal perforation, and nasal collapse. Lepromatous leprosy can lead to an enlarged liver and spleen and inflamed testicles. Fingertips and toes deteriorate as bone resorption follows injury and infection in these insensitive areas.

When tuberculoid leprosy affects the skin, it produces raised, large, reddened plaques or macules with clearly defined borders. As they grow, they become rough, hairless, pale in color, and leave painless scars.

In borderline leprosy, skin lesions are numerous, but smaller, less anesthetic, and less sharply defined than tuberculoid lesions. Untreated, borderline leprosy may deteriorate into lepromatous disease.

How is it diagnosed?

Early clinical indications of skin lesions and muscular and neurologic deficits are usually sufficiently diagnostic in people from areas where the disease is prevalent. Removal and analysis of tissue from skin lesions or peripheral nerves, or smears of the skin or of ulcerated mucous membranes, and blood tests help confirm the diagnosis.

How is it treated?

Treatment consists of antimicrobial therapy using sulfones, primarily oral dapsone. Failure to respond to sulfone or the occurrence of respiratory complications requires use of alternative therapy, such as Rifaden or Rimactane in combination with Lamprine or Trecator-SC. Clawhand, wristdrop, or footdrop may require surgical correction.

Persons suspected of having leprosy may be referred to the Gillis W. Long Hansen's Disease Center in Carville, Louisiana, or to a regional center. At this international research and educational center, people undergo diagnostic studies and treatment and are educated about their disease. People are encouraged to return home as soon as their medical condition permits. The federal government pays the full cost of their medical and nursing care. (See *Coping with leprosy*.)

 SELF-HELP

Coping with leprosy

- Get adequate nutrition and rest. Watch for fatigue, jaundice, and other signs of anemia and hepatitis.
- Take care not to injure an anesthetized leg by putting too much weight on it. Test bath water carefully to prevent scalding. To prevent ulcerations, wear sturdy footwear and soak your feet in warm water after any kind of exercise, even a short walk. Rub feet with Vaseline, oil, or lanolin.
- Although leprosy isn't highly contagious, take precautions against the possible spread of infection. Cover coughs or sneezes with a Kleenex and dispose of it properly.

LOCKJAW

What do doctors call this condition?

Besides lockjaw, doctors call this condition tetanus.

What is this condition?

Lockjaw is an acute exotoxin-mediated infection. Usually, it's generalized; less often, localized. Lockjaw is fatal in up to 60% of unimmunized persons, usually within 10 days of onset. When

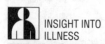

Facts about lockjaw

Occurs worldwide

Lockjaw occurs worldwide, but it's more prevalent in agricultural regions and developing countries that lack mass immunization programs.

Fatal to newborns

Lockjaw is one of the most common causes of newborn deaths in developing countries, where infants of unimmunized mothers are delivered under unsterile conditions.

Danger greater in spring and summer

In America, about 75% of all cases occur between April and September.

symptoms develop within 3 days after exposure, the prognosis is poor. (See *Facts about lockjaw.*)

What causes it?

Lockjaw is caused by the anaerobic bacterium *Clostridium tetani*. Normally, the disease is transmitted through a puncture wound that is contaminated by soil, dust, or animal excretions containing *C. tetani*, or through burns and minor wounds. After *C. tetani* enters the body, it causes local infection and tissue death. It also produces poisons that then enter the bloodstream and lymphatic system and eventually spread to the brain and spinal cord.

What are its symptoms?

The incubation period varies from 3 to 4 weeks in mild lockjaw to under 2 days in severe lockjaw. When symptoms occur within 3 days after injury, death is more likely. If lockjaw remains localized, signs of onset are spasm and increased muscle tone near the wound.

If lockjaw is systemic (generalized), indications include marked increase in muscle tone; hyperactive deep tendon reflexes; rapid heartbeat; profuse sweating; low-grade fever; and painful, involuntary muscle contractions in:

- neck and facial muscles, especially cheek muscles — lockjaw (trismus) and a grotesque, grinning expression called *risus sardonicus*
- somatic muscles — arched-back rigidity and boardlike abdominal rigidity
- intermittent tonic seizures lasting several minutes, causing oxygen deprivation, which may result in cyanosis (bluish skin discoloration) and sudden death by asphyxiation.

Despite such pronounced neuromuscular symptoms, cerebral and sensory functions remain normal. Complications include collapsed lung, pneumonia, pulmonary blood clots, acute stomach ulcers, flexion contractures, and irregular heartbeats.

Lockjaw in newborns is always generalized. The first clinical sign is difficulty in sucking, which usually appears 3 to 10 days after birth. It progresses to total inability to suck with excessive crying, irritability, and stiffening of the muscles in the back of the neck.

How is it diagnosed?

Frequently, the diagnosis must rest on clinical features and a history of injury and no previous tetanus immunization. Blood cultures and tetanus antibody tests are often negative; only one-third of infected people have a positive wound culture. Cerebrospinal fluid pressure may rise above normal. The diagnosis also must rule out meningitis, rabies, phenothiazine or strychnine poisoning, and other conditions that mimic lockjaw.

How is it treated?

Within 72 hours after a puncture wound, a person with no previous history of tetanus immunization first requires tetanus immune globulin or tetanus antitoxin to confer temporary protection and then active immunization with tetanus toxoid. A person who has not received tetanus immunization within 5 years needs a booster injection of tetanus toxoid.

If lockjaw develops despite immediate postinjury treatment, the person will require airway maintenance and a muscle relaxant, such as Valium, to decrease muscle rigidity and spasm. If muscle contractions aren't relieved by muscle relaxants, a neuromuscular blocker may be needed. The person with lockjaw needs high-dose antibiotics (penicillin given intravenously, if he or she isn't allergic to it).

LYME DISEASE

What is this condition?

Lyme disease is a disorder affecting many body systems and organs. It often begins in the summer with a classic skin rash ("bull's-eye" rash) called *erythema chronicum migrans.* Weeks or months later, heart or nervous system abnormalities sometimes develop, possibly followed by arthritis.

Lyme disease was first identified in a group of children in Lyme, Connecticut. Now the disease is known to occur mainly in three parts of the United States:

- in the Northeast, from Massachusetts to Maryland
- in the Midwest, in Wisconsin and Minnesota
- in the West, in California and Oregon.

However, cases have been reported in 43 states and 20 other countries, including Germany, Switzerland, France, and Australia.

What causes it?

Lyme disease is caused by *Borrelia burgdorferi,* a spirochete (spiral-shaped bacterium) carried by a blood-sucking parasite, the minute tick *Ixodes dammini,* or by another tick in the Ixodidae family. The disease occurs when a tick injects spirochete-laden saliva into the bloodstream or deposits fecal matter on the skin. After incubating for 3 to 32 days, the spirochetes fan out through the skin tissue, causing the classic rash. Then they spread to other skin sites or organs by the bloodstream or lymphatic system.

The spirochetes' life cycle isn't completely understood. They may survive for years in the joints or they may trigger an inflammatory response in the host and then die.

What are its symptoms?

Typically, Lyme disease has three stages. The "bull's-eye" rash heralds stage one, often occurring at the site of a tick bite. This rash often feels hot and itchy and may grow to over 19 inches (48 centimeters) in diameter. Within a few days, more skin lesions may erupt, along with a rash on the cheeks, conjunctivitis (eye inflammation), or widespread hives.

In 3 to 4 weeks, lesions are replaced by small red blotches, which remain for several more weeks. Malaise and fatigue are constant, but other findings are intermittent: headache, fever, chills, achiness, and swollen glands. Less common effects are irritation of the meninges (the membranes covering the brain and spinal cord), muscle and bone pain, and hepatitis. A persistent sore throat and dry cough may develop several days before the rash appears.

Weeks to months later, the second stage begins with nervous system abnormalities that usually clear up after days or months. Facial palsy (paralysis) is especially noticeable. Heart abnormalities also may develop.

Stage three begins weeks or years later and is characterized by arthritis. Muscle and bone pain leads to arthritis with marked swelling, especially in the large joints. The person may have recurrent attacks, then experience chronic arthritis with severe cartilage and bone erosion.

How is it diagnosed?

Because it's hard to isolate *B. burgdorferi* in humans and because diagnostic tests aren't conclusive, diagnosis often rests on the "bull's-eye" rash and related findings, especially in areas where the disease is prev-

The tick that causes Lyme disease injects spirochete-laden saliva into the bloodstream or deposits fecal matter on the skin. After incubating for 3 to 32 days, the spirochetes fan out to the skin, causing the classic "bull's-eye" rash, and then spread to other skin sites or organs.

alent. Mild anemia and the results of certain blood tests support the diagnosis.

How is it treated?

For adults, a 10- to 20-day course of Achromycin is the treatment of choice. Penicillin and E-Mycin are alternate drugs. Oral penicillin is usually prescribed for children. Early medication can minimize later complications. When given during the late stages, high-dose intravenous penicillin may be successful.

MALARIA

What is this condition?

Malaria, an acute infectious disease, is caused by protozoa of the genus *Plasmodium: P. falciparum, P. vivax, P. malariae,* and *P. ovale,* all of which are transmitted to humans by mosquitoes. Falciparum malaria is the most severe form of the disease.

When treated, malaria is rarely fatal; untreated, it's fatal in 10% of victims, usually as a result of complications such as disseminated intravascular coagulation.

Untreated primary attacks last from a week to a month, or longer. Relapses are common and can recur sporadically for several years. Susceptibility to the disease is universal.

What causes it?

Malaria literally means "bad air" and for centuries was thought to result from the inhalation of swamp vapors. It is now known that malaria is transmitted by the bite of female *Anopheles* mosquitoes, which abound in humid, swampy areas. When an infected mosquito bites, it injects *Plasmodium* organisms into the wound. These migrate to the liver, where they reproduce, invade red blood cells, and spread throughout the circulatory system. The infected person becomes a carrier of malaria, infecting any mosquito that bites him, thereby continuing the new cycle of transmission.

Plasmodium vivax, P. ovale, and *P. malariae* may persist for years in the liver. These parasites are responsible for the chronic carrier state. Since blood transfusions and street-drug paraphernalia can also

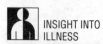
INSIGHT INTO ILLNESS

Malaria in the United States

1970
Malaria affected 4,230 people, mainly American soldiers returning from Vietnam.

1973
Malaria affected only 222 United States residents.

1993
1,150 cases are reported.

spread malaria, drug addicts have a higher incidence of the disease. (See *Malaria in the United States.*)

What are its symptoms?

After an incubation period of 12 to 30 days, malaria produces chills, fever, headache, and muscle pain interspersed with periods of well-being (the hallmark of the benign form of malaria). Paroxysms (acute attacks) occur when red cells rupture and release parasites. Paroxysms have three stages:

- *cold stage,* lasting 1 to 2 hours, ranging from chills to extreme shaking
- *hot stage,* lasting 3 to 4 hours, characterized by a high fever (temperature up to 107° F [41.6° C])
- *wet stage,* lasting 2 to 4 hours, characterized by profuse sweating.

Paroxysms occur every 48 to 72 hours when malaria is caused by *P. malariae* and every 42 to 50 hours when malaria is caused by *P. vivax* or *P. ovale.* All three types have low levels of parasite infestation and are self-limiting as a result of early acquired immunity.

Vivax and ovale malaria also produce an enlarged liver and spleen. Hemolytic anemia is present in all but the mildest infections.

The most severe form of malaria is caused by *P. falciparum,* the only life-threatening strain. This species produces persistent high fever, low blood pressure on standing, and red-blood-cell sludging that leads to capillary obstruction at various sites. Signs and symptoms of obstruction at these sites include the following:

- *brain:* partial paralysis, seizures, delirium, coma
- *lungs:* coughing, coughing up blood
- *viscera:* vomiting, abdominal pain, diarrhea, melena
- *kidneys:* decreased or absent urination, uremia.

How is it diagnosed?

A history showing travel to areas where the disease is prevalent, recent blood transfusion, or drug abuse in a person with high fever of unknown origin strongly suggests malaria. But because symptoms of malaria mimic other diseases, unequivocal diagnosis depends on lab identification of the parasites in red blood cells of peripheral blood smears. The Centers for Disease Control and Prevention can identify blood donors responsible for transmitting malaria by using indirect fluorescent serum antibody tests. However, these tests are unreliable in the acute phase because antibodies can be undetectable for 2 weeks after onset. Specialized lab tests confirm a diagnosis.

How is it treated?

Malaria is best treated with Chlorquin in all forms except Chlorquin-resistant *P. falciparum.* Symptoms and the presence of parasites decrease within 24 hours after such therapy begins, and the person usually recovers within 3 to 4 days. If the person is comatose or vomiting frequently, Chlorquin is given intramuscularly. Rare toxic reactions include gastrointestinal upset, itching, headache, and visual disturbances.

Malaria caused by *P. falciparum* requires treatment with oral Duraquin for 10 days, given concurrently with Daraprim and a sulfonamide such as Microsulfon. Relapses require the same treatment, or Duraquin alone, followed by Achromycin.

The only drug effective against the stage of the disease that affects the liver that's available in the United States is primaquine phosphate, given daily for 14 days. This drug can induce hemolytic anemia, especially in people with a glucose-6-phosphate dehydrogenase deficiency.

Travelers to areas where the disease is prevalent should take special precautions. (See *Avoiding malaria.*)

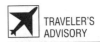

TRAVELER'S ADVISORY

Avoiding malaria

Malaria occurs most often in the tropics of Asia, Africa, and Latin America. Use these guidelines to help you avoid contracting malaria.

Get preventive medications
Obtain medications before traveling to an area where malaria is prevalent.
- If you're spending less than 3 weeks in areas where malaria exists, you'll need to take the drug Chlorquin weekly for 2 weeks before the trip and 6 weeks after it.
- If you're staying longer than 3 weeks, the doctor may prescribe Chlorquin and Fansidar, although this combination can have severe side effects. If you're not sensitive to either component of Fansidar (sufadoxine or pyrimethamine), you may receive a single dose to take if a fever develops.

Take precautions
If you develop a fever during your travels, see a doctor right away, even if you've taken malaria-preventing medications.

Prevent mosquito bites
- Use an insecticide on clothing and skin to keep mosquitoes away.
- Install screens in living and sleeping quarters.

MEASLES

What do doctors call this condition?

Rubeola

What is this condition?

Measles is an acute, highly contagious viral infection that may be one of the most common and most serious of all communicable childhood diseases. Use of the measles vaccine has made measles less common during childhood. As a result, it's becoming more prevalent in adolescents and adults.

In the United States, the prognosis is usually excellent. However, measles is a major cause of death in children in underdeveloped countries.

In temperate zones, the measles incidence is highest in late winter and early spring. Before the availability of measles vaccine, epidemics occurred every 2 to 5 years in large urban areas.

What causes it?

Measles is caused by a virus called a *paramyxovirus*. It's spread by direct contact or through the air. The virus enters the body through the upper respiratory tract.

What are its symptoms?

About 10 to 14 days after exposure to the virus, symptoms begin. Measles is most contagious during a prodromal (warning) phase, about 11 days after exposure to the virus. This phase lasts from 4 to 5 days. Symptoms include fever, light sensitivity, malaise, appetite loss, conjunctivitis (an eye inflammation), nasal congestion, hoarseness, and hacking cough.

At the end of the prodrome, *Koplik's spots*, the hallmark of the disease, appear. These spots look like tiny, bluish gray specks surrounded by a red halo. They appear inside the mouth opposite the molars and occasionally bleed.

About 5 days after Koplik's spots appear, the person's temperature rises sharply, the spots slough off, and a slightly itchy rash appears. This characteristic rash starts as small, flat blemishes behind the ears and on the neck and cheeks. These macules become red, solid, and raised and spread rapidly over the entire face, neck, eyelids, arms, chest, back, abdomen, and thighs. When the rash reaches the feet (2 to 3 days later), it starts to fade in the same sequence it appeared, leaving a brownish discoloration that disappears in 7 to 10 days.

The disease climaxes 2 to 3 days after the rash appears, when the person's temperature climbs to 103° to 105° F (39.4° to 40.5° C) and gets a severe cough, puffy red eyes, and a runny nose. About 5 days after the rash appears, other symptoms disappear and the disease is no longer contagious.

Symptoms are usually mild in people with partial immunity, such as those who've received gamma globulin, and in infants with their mother's antibodies. Young infants, adolescents, adults, and immunocompromised people generally have more severe symptoms and complications than young children.

Atypical measles may appear in people who received the killed measles vaccine. These people get acutely ill with a fever and a rash that's most obvious in the arms and legs, or with respiratory involvement and no rash.

Severe infection may lead to secondary bacterial infection and to autoimmune reaction or organ invasion by the virus, resulting in ear infection, pneumonia, and brain inflammation.

The measles vaccine has reduced the occurrence of measles during childhood. As a result, measles is becoming more prevalent in adolescents and adults.

How is it diagnosed?

The doctor diagnoses measles from the person's signs and symptoms, especially Koplik's spots. Mild measles may resemble other diseases, such as German measles and toxoplasmosis; lab tests are required to rule these out. If necessary, measles virus may be isolated from the blood, nose and throat secretions, and urine during the feverish period. (See *Helping your child cope with measles*.)

MENINGOCOCCAL INFECTIONS

What are these conditions?

Two major meningococcal infections (meningitis and meningo-coccemia) are caused by the gram-negative bacteria *Neisseria meningitidis,* which also causes primary pneumonia, blood-tinged conjunctivitis, endocarditis, sinusitis, and genital infection. Meningococcemia occurs as simple bacteremia, fulminant (sudden and severe) meningococcemia, and rarely, chronic meningococcemia. It often accompanies meningitis.

Meningococcal infections may occur sporadically or in epidemics; virulent infections may be fatal within a matter of hours.

Meningococcal infections occur most often among children (ages 6 months to 1 year) and men, usually military recruits, because of overcrowding.

N. meningitidis has seven serogroups (A, B, C, D, X, Y, Z); group A causes most epidemics. These bacteria are often normally present in the upper respiratory system. Transmission takes place through inhalation of an infected droplet from a carrier. The bacteria then localize in the nasopharynx. Following an incubation period of 3 or 4 days, they spread through the bloodstream to joints, skin, adrenal glands, lungs, and the central nervous system. The tissue damage that results (possibly from effects of bacterial endotoxins) produces symptoms and, in fulminant meningococcemia and meningococcal bacteremia, progresses to hemorrhage, blood clot formation, and localized tissue death.

What are their symptoms?

Clinical features of meningococcal infections vary. Symptoms of *meningococcal bacteremia* include sudden spiking fever, headache, sore

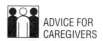

Helping your child cope with measles

- Keep your child in bed and away from other children throughout the contagious period. Provide plenty of fluids.
- Use a vaporizer and keep the child's room warm to reduce respiratory symptoms. However, be aware that cough preparations and antibiotics are generally ineffective.
- If your child is sensitive to light, darken the room or provide sunglasses.
- Reduce fever with aspirin or Tylenol (or another drug containing acetaminophen) and warm sponge baths.
- Be on the lookout for complications, such as ear infection or pneumonia.

throat, cough, chills, muscle pain (in back and legs), joint pain, rapid heart rate, rapid breathing, mild low blood pressure, and a petechial, nodular, or maculopapular rash.

In about 10% to 20% of infected people, this progresses to *fulminant meningococcemia,* with extreme prostration, enlargement of skin lesions, disseminated intravascular coagulation, and shock. Unless it is treated promptly, fulminant meningococcemia results in death from respiratory or heart failure in 6 to 24 hours.

> *Meningococcal infections occur most often among children (ages 6 months to 1 year) and men, usually military recruits, because of overcrowding.*

How are they diagnosed?

Isolation of *N. meningitidis* through a positive blood culture, a cerebrospinal fluid culture, or lesion scraping confirms the diagnosis.

How are they treated?

As soon as meningococcal infection is suspected, treatment begins with large doses of liquid Bicillin, Omnipen, or some cephalosporins, such as Mefoxin or Moxan; or, for the person who is allergic to penicillin, intravenous Chloromycetin.

Therapy may also include Osmitrol for cerebral swelling, intravenous heparin for disseminated intravascular coagulation, Dopastat for shock, and Lanoxin and a diuretic if congestive heart failure develops.

Supportive measures include fluid and electrolyte maintenance, proper breathing (aided by oxygen, if necessary), insertion of an arterial or central venous pressure line to monitor cardiovascular status, and bed rest.

MUMPS

What do doctors call this condition?

Infectious or epidemic parotitis

What is this condition?

Mumps is an acute viral disease that usually strikes children between ages 5 and 9. Its incidence peaks during late winter and early spring. Most children recover completely, although a few experience complications.

What causes it?

Mumps is caused by a virus called a *paramyxovirus*. Found in the saliva of an infected person, the virus spreads through the air or by direct contact. It's present in the saliva from 6 days before to 9 days after the parotid glands (the salivary glands below and in front of the ear) start to swell. (See *Site of parotid inflammation in mumps*.) The infection is probably most contagious during the 48 hours immediately before this swelling begins. A person can get mumps only once; one attack almost always confers lifelong immunity.

What are its symptoms?

Symptoms vary widely, typically arising 14 to 25 days after exposure to the virus. An estimated 30% of susceptible people have no noticeable symptoms.

Mumps usually starts with warning symptoms that last for 24 hours. These include muscle ache, appetite loss, headache, and a slight fever, followed by an earache that's aggravated by chewing, parotid gland tenderness and swelling, a temperature of 101° to 104° F (38.3° to 40° C), and pain when chewing or when drinking sour or acidic liquids such as orange juice.

Complications

One complications of mumps is inflammation of the testicles and epididymis (the duct behind the testicles). This condition occurs in about 25% of males who contract mumps after puberty. It causes sudden testicular swelling and tenderness, redness of the scrotum, lower abdominal pain, nausea, vomiting, fever, and chills. In extremely rare cases, mumps causes sterility in males.

Mumps meningitis (inflammation of the lining of the brain and spinal cord) complicates mumps in 10% of people; it's more common in males. Symptoms include fever, nuchal rigidity (muscle stiffening at the nape of the neck), headache, irritability, vomiting, and drowsiness. Recovery is usually complete.

How is it diagnosed?

The doctor diagnoses mumps from characteristic signs and symptoms — parotid gland enlargement with a history of exposure to mumps. Blood tests for mumps antibodies can verify the diagnosis if the person doesn't have parotid or other salivary gland enlargement.

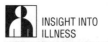

INSIGHT INTO ILLNESS

Site of parotid inflammation in mumps

The familiar painful swelling around the ears indicates diseased salivary (parotid) glands. These can cause ear pain that's aggravated by chewing.

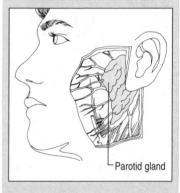

Parotid gland

Helping your child cope with mumps

Promote comfort

- Make sure your child gets plenty of bed rest during the feverish period.
- Apply warm or cool compresses to your child's neck to ease pain.
- To reduce fever and relieve pain, give aspirin or Tylenol (or another drug containing acetaminophen), as directed by your doctor, and provide warm sponge baths.
- Prevent dehydration by encouraging your child to drink plenty of fluids.
- Avoid preparing spicy foods and those that require a lot of chewing.

Don't let it spread

If you have other children, keep in mind that mumps can be prevented. Have your children receive immunization at age 15 months. (Susceptible family members — especially males — who are near or past puberty should also get the vaccine.) Remember, immunization within 24 hours of exposure may prevent or shorten the actual disease. Immunity against mumps lasts 12 years or longer.

How is it treated?

Treatment includes analgesics for pain, aspirin or Tylenol (or another drug containing acetaminophen) for fever, and adequate fluid intake to prevent dehydration from fever and appetite loss. A person who can't swallow may be hospitalized to receive intravenous fluids. (See *Helping your child cope with mumps.*)

PLAGUE

What is this condition?

Plague (sometimes called *black death*) is an acute infection that occurs in several forms. *Bubonic plague,* the most common, causes the characteristic buboes (swollen and sometimes pus-producing lymph glands) that give this infection its name. Other forms include *septicemic plague,* a severe, rapid systemic form, and *pneumonic plague,* which can be primary or secondary to the other two forms. *Primary pneumonic plague* is an acutely fulminant (sudden and severe), highly contagious form that causes acute prostration, respiratory distress, and death — often within 2 to 3 days after onset.

Without treatment, the death rate is about 60% in bubonic plague and approaches 100% in both septicemic and pneumonic plagues. With treatment, the death rate is approximately 18%. One attack confers permanent immunity. (See *Avoiding the plague.*)

What causes it?

Plague is caused by the bacterium *Yersinia pestis* (formerly called *Pasteurella pestis*). It's usually transmitted to a human through the bite of a flea from an infected rodent host, such as a rat, squirrel, prairie dog, or hare. Occasionally, transmission occurs when infected animals or their tissues are handled.

Bubonic plague caused the historic pandemics in Europe and Asia during the Middle Ages, which in some areas killed up to two-thirds of the population. This form is rarely transmitted from person to person. However, if untreated, it may progress to a secondary pneumonic form, which is transmitted by contaminated respiratory droplets (coughing) and is highly contagious.

What are its symptoms?

The incubation period, early symptoms, severity at onset, and clinical course vary in the three forms of plague. In bubonic plague, the incubation period is 2 to 6 days. The milder form begins with malaise, fever, and pain or tenderness in regional lymph nodes, possibly associated with swelling. Lymph node damage (usually under the arms or in the groin) eventually produces painful, inflamed and, possibly, pus-producing buboes. The classic sign of plague is an excruciatingly painful bubo. Bleeding areas may experience tissue death; in the skin, such areas appear dark — hence the name "black death." This infection can progress extremely rapidly: an apparently mildly ill person with symptoms limited to fever and adenitis may be close to death within hours. Plague may also begin dramatically, with a sudden high temperature of 103° F (39.4° C) to 106° F (41.1° C), chills, muscle ache, headache, prostration, restlessness, disorientation, delirium, blood poisoning, and staggering gait. Occasionally, it causes abdominal pain, nausea, vomiting, and constipation, followed by diarrhea (frequently bloody), skin mottling, petechiae, and circulatory collapse.

In *primary pneumonic plague,* the incubation period is 2 to 3 days, followed by a typically acute onset, with high fever, chills, severe headache, rapid heart rate and breathing, shortness of breath, and a productive cough (first mucoid sputum, later frothy pink or red). The disease rapidly causes severe prostration, respiratory distress, and, possibly, death.

Septicemic plague usually develops without overt lymph node enlargement. In this form, the person shows toxicity, high body temperature, seizures, prostration, shock, and disseminated intravascular coagulation. Septicemic plague causes widespread nonspecific tissue damage and is rapidly fatal unless promptly and correctly treated.

How is it diagnosed?

Because plague is rare in the United States, it's often overlooked until after the person dies or multiple cases develop. Characteristic buboes and a history of exposure to rodents strongly suggest bubonic plague.

Stained smears and cultures of *Y. pestis* obtained from a needle aspirate of a small amount of fluid from skin lesions confirm this diagnosis. Diagnosis should rule out tularemia, typhus, and typhoid.

In pneumonic plague, diagnosis requires a chest X-ray to show fulminating pneumonia, and stained smear and culture of sputum to identify *Y. pestis.* Other bacterial pneumonias and psittacosis must be ruled out. Stained smear and blood cultures containing *Y. pestis* are

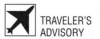
TRAVELER'S
ADVISORY

Avoiding the plague

Danger zones
Wild rodent plague, one form of this deadly disease, is native to the western United States and Canada as well as to South America, the Near East, central and Southeast Asia, north central and southern Africa, and Mexico.

Danger times
Plague tends to occur between May and September; between October and February it usually occurs in hunters who skin wild animals.

Safety measures
To help prevent plague, avoid contact with wild animals — especially sick or dead ones. If you live in or are planning to travel to an area where the disease is prevalent, get immunization with plague vaccine. However, be aware that immunization is only temporarily effective.

diagnostic in septicemic plague. Treatment should begin without waiting for lab confirmation.

How is it treated?

Antimicrobial treatment of suspected plague must begin immediately after blood specimens have been taken for culture and shouldn't be delayed for lab confirmation. Generally, treatment consists of large doses of streptomycin, the drug of choice against *Y. pestis*. Other effective drugs include Achromycin, Chloromycetin or Chloroptic, and, possibly, Kanasig or Kantex; penicillins are ineffective.

In both septicemic and pneumonic plagues, lifesaving antimicrobial treatment must begin within 18 hours of onset. Supportive management aims to control fever, shock, and seizures and to maintain fluid balance.

After antimicrobial therapy has begun, glucocorticoids can combat life-threatening blood poisoning and shock; Valium relieves restlessness; and if the person develops disseminated intravascular coagulation, treatment may include heparin.

What can the family of a person with plague do?

- Be aware that you may need to be quarantined for 6 days of observation if you've had recent contact with the person. Also, you'll be instructed to take Achromycin as a preventive measure.
- Know that people with plague require strict isolation, which may be discontinued 48 hours after antimicrobial therapy begins unless respiratory symptoms develop.

PINWORM

What do doctors call this condition?

Besides pinworm, doctors call this condition enterobiasis, threadworm, or oxyuriasis.

What is this condition?

Pinworm is a benign intestinal disease that is common even in temperate regions with good sanitation. Found worldwide, pinworm is the most prevalent helminthic infection in the United States.

Pinworm infection and reinfection occurs most often in children between ages 5 and 14 and in certain institutionalized groups because of poor hygiene and frequent hand-to-mouth activity. (See *Keeping your child safe from pinworm.*) Crowded living conditions often enhance its spread to several members of a family.

What causes it?

Pinworm is caused by the roundworm *Enterobius vermicularis.* Adult pinworms live in the intestine; female worms migrate to the perianal region to deposit their eggs.

Direct transmission occurs when the person's hands transfer infective eggs from the anus to the mouth. *Indirect transmission* occurs when he or she comes in contact with contaminated articles, such as linens and clothing.

What are its symptoms?

Pinworm that doesn't cause any symptoms is often overlooked. However, intense perianal itching may occur, especially at night, when the female worm crawls out of the anus to deposit her eggs. Itching disturbs sleep and causes irritability, scratching, skin irritation and, sometimes, vaginitis.

How is it diagnosed?

A history of anal itching suggests pinworm; microscopic identification of *Enterobius* eggs recovered from the perianal area with a cellophane tape swab confirms it. A stool sample is generally egg- and worm-free because these worms deposit their eggs outside the intestine and die after migrating to the anus.

How is it treated?

Drug therapy with Combantrin, Entacyl, or Vermox destroys these parasites. Effective eradication requires concurrent treatment of family members and, in institutions, other people.

What can a person with pinworm do?

- If you're taking Combantrin, be aware that this drug colors stools bright red and may cause vomiting. (Your vomit will also be red.) The tablet form of this drug is coated with aspirin and shouldn't be taken by aspirin-sensitive people.

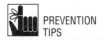 PREVENTION TIPS

Keeping your child safe from pinworm

Because of their hand-to-mouth habits, children ages 5 to 14 are most likely to get pinworm. Here are some tips that may help your child avoid this infection:

- Have your child bathe daily. Showers are preferable to tub baths.
- Make sure your child changes his underwear daily. If possible, also change his bedsheets daily.
- Teach your child proper personal hygiene. Emphasize the importance of washing the hands thoroughly after defecating and before handling food.
- Discourage your child from biting his nails. If he can't stop, have him wear gloves until the infection clears.

■ If you have a history of seizure disorders, tell your doctor. The drug Entacyl may aggravate these disorders and shouldn't be given to someone with such a history.

PNEUMOCYSTIS CARINII *PNEUMONIA*

What is this condition?

Pneumocystis carinii pneumonia is an opportunistic infection that can occur in people with weak immune systems. Because of its association with HIV infection, its incidence has risen dramatically since the 1980s.

Before the advent of preventive treatment, *Pneumocystis carinii* pneumonia was the first clue in about 60% of people that HIV infection was present. It strikes up to 90% of HIV-infected people in the United States at some point during their lifetime. It's the leading cause of death in this group.

This infection is also associated with other conditions that impair the immune system, including organ transplants, leukemia, and lymphoma.

What causes it?

This type of pneumonia is caused by the microorganism *P. carinii.* Although it's usually classified as a protozoan, some researchers think it's more closely related to a fungus. Although it's part of the body's flora (normally occurring fungi and bacteria) in most healthy people, *P. carinii* becomes an aggressive killer in people with weak immune systems.

P. carinii invades the air sacs in both lungs and reproduces outside the cells. Eventually, the lungs fill with these microorganisms and a discharge occurs, impairing breathing. The air sacs then enlarge and thicken progressively, eventually combining into a single mass.

Pneumocystis carinii pneumonia seems to be transmitted mainly through the air, although the microorganism already resides in most people. The time between exposure and the onset of symptoms is probably 4 to 8 weeks.

What are its symptoms?

The person typically has a history of an immunocompromising condition (such as HIV infection, leukemia, or lymphoma) or has undergone a procedure that weakens the immune system (such as organ transplantation).

Pneumocystis carinii pneumonia begins slowly with increasing shortness of breath and a nonproductive cough. Appetite loss, generalized fatigue, and weight loss may follow. A slight, intermittent fever may develop.

Other symptoms include rapid breathing, use of accessory chest muscles to breathe, an abnormal breath sound called *crackles*, and decreased breath sounds (in advanced pneumonia). In an acutely ill person, a bluish discoloration of the skin due to oxygen deprivation may occur.

How is it diagnosed?

Tissue studies confirm *Pneumocystis carinii* pneumonia. In people with HIV infection, initial examination of a sputum specimen (induced by inhaling an ultrasonically dispersed saltwater mist) may be sufficient. But this technique usually isn't effective in people without HIV infection.

Fiberoptic bronchoscopy, in which an instrument is inserted into the airway to allow visualization, is the most commonly used study to confirm this disease. Less often, the doctor will perform invasive procedures to diagnose it.

A chest X-ray may show a characteristic finding called *fluffy infiltrates*, but this may result from other types of pneumonia or adult respiratory distress syndrome.

Before the advent of preventive treatment for Pneumocystis carinii pneumonia, this disease was the first clue in about 60% of people that HIV infection was present. The disease occurs in up to 90% of HIV-infected people in the United States at some point during their lifetime.

How is it treated?

Some people with *Pneumocystis carinii* pneumonia respond to the drugs Pentam or NebuPent. Unfortunately, because of immune system impairment, many people with HIV experience severe side effects to drug therapy. These reactions include bone marrow suppression, thrush (yeast infection of the mouth), fever, toxic liver effects, and anaphylaxis (acute hypersensitivity reaction). Nausea, vomiting, and rashes are common side effects.

Pentam or NebuPent may be taken intravenously or in an aerosol form. However, intravenous Pentam or NebuPent often have severe toxic effects. Although the inhaled form usually is well tolerated, it may not reach crucial areas in the lungs, making it less effective.

Supportive measures, such as oxygen therapy, mechanical ventilation, adequate nutrition, and fluid balance, are important secondary therapies.

POLIO

What do doctors call this condition?

Besides polio, doctors call this condition poliomyelitis or infantile paralysis.

What is this condition?

Polio is an acute communicable disease that ranges in severity from inapparent infection to fatal paralytic illness. With the development of the Salk vaccine, polio has almost been eliminated from developed countries.

Minor polio outbreaks still occur, usually among nonimmunized groups. For example, an outbreak occurred among the Amish of Pennsylvania in 1979. The disease strikes most often during the summer and fall. Once confined mainly to infants and children, polio occurs more often today in people over age 15. Among children, it paralyzes boys most often; adults and girls are at greater risk of infection but not of paralysis.

The prognosis depends largely on the site affected. If the central nervous system is spared, the prognosis is excellent. However, brain and spinal cord infection can cause paralysis and death. The death rate for all types of polio is 5% to 10%.

What causes it?

Polio is caused by the poliovirus, which has three antigenically distinct serotypes — types 1, 2, and 3 — all of which cause polio. These polioviruses are found worldwide and are transmitted from person to person by direct contact with infected oropharyngeal secretions or feces. The incubation period ranges from 5 to 35 days — 7 to 14 days on the average.

What are its symptoms?

Manifestations of polio follow three basic patterns. Inapparent (sub-clinical) infections constitute 95% of all poliovirus infections. Abortive polio (minor illness), which makes up between 4% and 8% of all cases, causes slight fever, malaise, headache, sore throat, pharyngitis, and vomiting. The person usually recovers within 72 hours. Most cases of inapparent and abortive polio go unnoticed.

However, the third type, major polio, involves the brain and spinal cord and takes two forms: nonparalytic and paralytic. In children, the disease often occurs in two phases: recovery from the minor illness stage, followed by onset of major illness. Nonparalytic polio produces moderate fever, headache, vomiting, lack of energy, irritability, and pains in the neck, back, arms, legs, and abdomen. It also causes muscle tenderness and spasms in the extensors of the neck and back, and sometimes in the hamstring and other muscles. Nonparalytic polio usually lasts about a week, with meningeal irritation persisting for about 2 weeks.

Paralytic polio usually develops within 5 to 7 days of the onset of fever. The person displays symptoms similar to those of nonparalytic polio, with asymmetrical weakness of various muscles, loss of superficial and deep reflexes, paresthesia, hypersensitivity to touch, urine retention, constipation, and abdominal expansion. The extent of paralysis depends on the level of the spinal cord lesions, which may be cervical, thoracic, or lumbar.

Bulbar polio, polio that affects the medulla of the brain, is the most perilous type. This form weakens the muscles controlled by the cranial nerves and produces symptoms of brain inflammation. Other symptoms include facial weakness, speech impairment, difficulty chewing, inability to swallow or expel saliva, food regurgitation through the nasal passages, and shortness of breath, as well as abnormal respiratory rate, depth, and rhythm, which may lead to respiratory arrest. Fatal pulmonary edema and shock are possible.

Complications — many of which result from prolonged immobility and respiratory muscle failure — include high blood pressure, urinary tract infection, urolithiasis, atelectasis, pneumonia, myocarditis, cor pulmonale, skeletal and soft-tissue deformities, and paralytic ileus.

Minor polio outbreaks still occur, usually among nonimmunized groups. For example, an outbreak occurred among the Amish of Pennsylvania in 1979.

How is it diagnosed?

Diagnosis requires isolation of the poliovirus from throat washings early in the disease, from stools throughout the disease, and from cerebrospinal fluid cultures in brain and spinal cord infection.

Coxsackievirus and echovirus infections must be ruled out. Routine lab tests are usually within normal limits.

How is it treated?

Treatment is supportive and includes pain relievers to ease headache, back pain, and leg spasms; morphine should not be used because of the danger of additional respiratory suppression. Moist heat applications may also reduce muscle spasm and pain.

Bed rest is necessary only until extreme discomfort subsides; in paralytic polio, this may take a long time. Paralytic polio also requires long-term rehabilitation using physical therapy, braces, corrective shoes and, in some cases, orthopedic surgery.

RABIES

What is this condition?

Rabies is an acute infection of the brain and spinal cord. Getting treatment soon after being bitten by an infected animal may prevent the infection from spreading to the central nervous system. But if symptoms occur, rabies is almost always fatal.

What causes it?

Rabies is caused by a ribonucleic acid virus. Generally, the virus is transmitted to a human through the bite of an infected animal. The virus proliferates in muscle cells at the bite site, then spreads along the affected nerve to the central nervous system and multiplies in the brain. Finally, it moves through the nerves into other tissues, including the salivary glands. Occasionally, the virus is spread through the air or in infected tissue transplants. (See *Facts about rabies.*)

What are its symptoms?

Typically, about 1 to 3 months after the animal bite, the person has local or radiating pain or burning, a cold sensation, itching, and tingling at the bite site. The individual may also have warning signs, such as a slight fever (100° to 102° F [37.7° to 38.8° C]), malaise, headache, appetite loss, nausea, sore throat, and a persistent loose cough.

After this, the person becomes nervous, anxious, irritable, and highly sensitive to touch, light, and loud noise. Other symptoms include dilated pupils; a fast pulse; shallow respirations; and excessive salivation, eye tearing, and sweating.

About 2 to 10 days after the warning signs appear, an *excitation phase* begins. This is marked by agitation, restlessness, anxiety, apprehension, paralysis and deviation of the eyes, pupil dilation or constriction, absence of certain eye reflexes, weak facial muscles, and hoarseness. Other symptoms include a fast or slow heart rate, abnormal breathing, urine retention, and a temperature of about 103° F (39.5° C).

About 50% of affected people exhibit *hydrophobia* (fear of water), which causes them to experience forceful, painful throat muscle spasms, vomiting, and dehydration. Breathing problems and death may follow. Difficulty swallowing causes frothy saliva to drool from the mouth. Eventually, even the sight, mention, or thought of water causes uncontrollable throat muscle spasms and excessive salivation. Between episodes of excitation and hydrophobia, the person usually is cooperative and lucid.

After about 3 days, excitation and hydrophobia subside and the progressively paralyzing, terminal phase of this illness begins. The person has progressive, generalized loss of muscle tone that ultimately leads to collapse of blood vessels, coma, and death.

How is it diagnosed?

Because rabies is fatal unless treated promptly, it should always be suspected in anyone who experiences an animal bite, until proven otherwise.

The most frequently performed diagnostic tests are virus isolation from the person's saliva or throat and examination of blood for fluorescent rabies antibody. To support the diagnosis, the suspected animal is confined for 10 days of observation by a veterinarian. If the animal appears rabid, it should be killed and its brain tissue tested for fluorescent rabies antibody and Negri bodies (oval or round masses that conclusively confirm rabies).

How is it treated?

As soon as possible after exposure to rabies, the wound should be treated and rabies immunization administered. All bite wounds and scratches should be washed thoroughly with soap and water. The person may also need a tetanus-diphtheria shot.

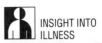

INSIGHT INTO ILLNESS

Facts about rabies

Often caused by wild animals
In North America, dog vaccinations have significantly reduced the risk of rabies. But now, bites by wild animals, such as skunks, foxes, and bats, account for 70% of all cases.

Where you're bitten matters
Your risk of developing rabies depends on the location of the bite. For instance, if you're bitten on the face, your risk is 60%; on the arm, 15% to 40%; and on the leg, about 10%.

The doctor will take steps to control bacterial infection. If the wound must be stitched, special treatment and stitching techniques are used to allow proper wound drainage.

After rabies exposure, a person who hasn't been immunized before must receive rabies immune globulin and human diploid cell vaccine. If the individual *has* received human diploid cell vaccine before and has an adequate rabies antibody titer, he or she doesn't need rabies immune globulin immunization, just a booster for the vaccine.

To help prevent this disease, all household pets that may be exposed to rabid wild animals should be vaccinated. Also, never try to touch wild animals, especially if they appear ill or overly docile — a possible sign of rabies.

RESPIRATORY SYNCYTIAL VIRUS INFECTION

What is this condition?

Respiratory syncytial virus infection is the leading cause of lower respiratory tract infections in infants and young children. It's the major cause of pneumonia, tracheobronchitis, and bronchiolitis in this age-group, and a suspected cause of the fatal respiratory diseases of infancy.

What causes it?

This disease is caused by a subgroup of the myxoviruses resembling paramyxovirus. Blood tests for antibodies seem to indicate that few children under age 4 escape contracting some form of it, even if it's mild. In fact, this is the only viral disease that has its maximum impact during the first few months of life.

This virus creates annual epidemics that occur during the late winter and early spring in temperate climates and during the rainy season in the tropics. The organism is transmitted from person to person by respiratory secretions and has an incubation period of 4 to 5 days.

Reinfection is common, producing milder symptoms than the primary infection. School-age children, adolescents, and young adults with mild reinfections are probably the source of infection for infants and young children.

What are its symptoms?

The symptoms of this infection vary in severity, ranging from mild coldlike symptoms to bronchiolitis or bronchopneumonia, and in a few people, severe, life-threatening lower respiratory tract infections. Generally, symptoms include coughing, wheezing, malaise, sore throat, shortness of breath, and inflamed mucous membranes in the nose and throat.

Middle ear infection is a common complication of respiratory syncytial virus in infants. This disease has also been identified in people with a variety of central nervous system disorders, such as meningitis and myelitis.

How is it diagnosed?

Diagnosis is usually made on the basis of clinical findings and epidemiologic information. Cultures of nasal and pharyngeal secretions may show infection. However, the virus is very changeable, so cultures aren't always reliable. Serum antibody titers may be elevated, but before 6 months of age, maternal antibodies may impair test results. Chest X-rays help detect pneumonia.

Two recently developed serologic techniques are the indirect immunofluorescent and the enzyme-linked immunosorbent assay methods.

How is it treated?

Treatment aims to support respiratory function, maintain fluid balance, and relieve symptoms. Respiratory status is monitored closely. The child may need to undergo percussion, drainage, and suction. A croup tent is used to provide a high-humidity atmosphere.

> *Evidence suggests that few children under age 4 escape contracting some form of respiratory syncytial virus, even if it's mild. In fact, this is the only viral disease that has its maximum impact during the first few months of life.*

*R*OCKY MOUNTAIN SPOTTED FEVER

What is this condition?

Rocky Mountain spotted fever is a rash- and fever-producing illness that's transmitted to humans by a tick bite. Occurring throughout the continental United States, this disease is particularly prevalent in the Southeast and Southwest.

Because Rocky Mountain spotted fever is associated with outdoor activities, such as camping and backpacking, its incidence is usually higher in the spring and summer. The incidence is also higher in children ages 5 to 9, men and boys, and whites.

This disease is fatal in about 5% of cases. The death rate rises when treatment is delayed. It also increases in older people.

What causes it?

Rocky Mountain spotted fever is caused by a virus-like organism, *Rickettsia rickettsii*, which is transmitted by the wood tick (*Dermacentor andersoni*) in the west and by the dog tick (*D. variabilis*) in the east. This disease is transmitted to a human or small animal by a prolonged bite (4 to 6 hours) of an adult tick. Occasionally, it's acquired through inhalation or through breaks in the skin with tick excretions or tissue juices. (This explains why people shouldn't crush ticks between their fingers when removing them from other people and animals.) In most tick-infested areas, 1% to 5% of the ticks harbor *R. rickettsii*.

What are its symptoms?

The incubation period is usually about 7 days, but it can range anywhere from 2 to 14 days. Generally, the shorter the incubation time, the more severe the infection. Symptoms, which usually begin abruptly, include a persistent fever of 102° to 104° F (38.8° to 40° C); a generalized, excruciating headache; and aching in the bones, muscles, joints, and back. In addition, the tongue is covered with a thick white coating that gradually turns brown as the fever persists and rises.

Initially, the skin may simply appear flushed. But between days 2 and 5, eruptions begin around the wrists, ankles, or forehead and, within 2 days, cover the entire body, including the scalp, palms, and soles. The rash consists of red macules 1 to 5 millimeters in diameter that blanch on pressure; if untreated, the rash may become discolored and blistered. By the third week, the skin peels off and may become gangrenous over the elbows, fingers, and toes. The pulse is strong initially, but it gradually becomes rapid (possibly reaching 150 beats per minute) and thready. A rapid pulse and low blood pressure (systolic pressure less than 90) herald imminent death from vascular collapse.

Other signs and symptoms include a bronchial cough, a rapid respiratory rate (as high as 60 breaths per minute), loss of appetite, nausea, vomiting, constipation, abdominal pain, enlarged liver and spleen, insomnia, restlessness and, in extreme cases, delirium. Urine output falls to half of the normal level or less, and the urine is dark and contains albumin.

How is it diagnosed?

The diagnosis generally rests on a history of a tick bite or travel to a tick-infested area and a positive complement fixation test (which shows a fourfold increase in convalescent antibody titer compared with acute titers). Blood cultures should be performed to isolate the organism and confirm the diagnosis.

How is it treated?

Treatment requires careful removal of the tick and administration of antibiotics, such as Chloromycetin or Achromycin, until 3 days after the fever subsides. Treatment also includes measures to relieve symptoms and, in disseminated intravascular coagulation, heparin and platelet transfusion.

What can a person with Rocky Mountain spotted fever do?

■ After recovery, be sure to report any recurrent symptoms to the doctor at once so that treatment can be promptly resumed.

■ Take precautions to prevent a recurrence. (See *Avoiding Rocky Mountain spotted fever.*)

ROSEOLA INFANTUM

What is this condition?

Roseola infantum is an acute, benign infection that usually affects infants and young children (ages 6 months to 3 years). Characteristically, it first causes a high fever and then a rash that accompanies an abrupt drop to normal temperature.

Roseola affects boys and girls alike. It occurs year-round but is most prevalent in the spring and fall. Overt roseola, the most common rash in infants under age 2, affects 30% of all children; inapparent roseola (feverish illness without a rash) may affect the rest.

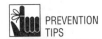

PREVENTION TIPS

Avoiding Rocky Mountain spotted fever

You can prevent this tick-borne illness by following the precautions below.

Avoid infested areas

Stay away from tick-infested areas — woods, meadows, streams, and canyons — if possible. If you must go to a tick-infested area, check your entire body, including scalp, every 3 to 4 hours for attached ticks. Wear protective clothing, such as a long-sleeved shirt, slacks securely tucked into firmly laced boots, and a head covering, such as a cap or a bandana. Apply insect repellant to clothes and exposed skin.

If a tick bites

If you find a tick attached to your body, don't crush it, as this may contaminate the bite wound. To detach the tick, place a drop of oil, alcohol, gasoline, or kerosene on it or hold a lighted cigarette near it.

Take precautions

If you're at high risk (for instance, if you work in a laboratory with rickettsiae, or if you're planning an extended camping trip and will be far from adequate medical facilities), get vaccinated against this illness.

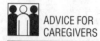

Handling a high fever

If your infant has roseola infantum, his or her temperature may soar as high as 105° F (40.5° C) — and stay there for several days. To ensure your infant's well-being during this temperature peak, follow these guidelines.

Reduce fever

To lower your infant's fever, give warm baths. Dress your infant in lightweight clothes and maintain a normal room temperature.

Prevent dehydration

To avoid this condition, give your infant plenty of fluids.

Watch for seizures

Be aware that some infants have seizures from high fevers. But know that a short seizure accompanying the fever will not cause brain damage. And the seizures will stop once the fever subsides. If the doctor has prescribed Phenobarbital to prevent or relieve seizures, this drug is likely to cause drowsiness. But if it causes stupor, call the doctor immediately.

What causes it?

Roseola infantum presumably is caused by a virus. The mode of transmission isn't known. Only rarely does an infected child transmit roseola to a sibling.

What are its symptoms?

After a 10- to 15-day incubation period, the infant with roseola develops an abruptly rising, unexplainable fever and, sometimes, seizures. Temperature peaks at 103° to 105° F (39.4° to 40.5° C) for 3 to 5 days, then drops suddenly. In the early feverish period, the infant may lose his or her appetite and be irritable and listless but not seem particularly ill.

As the temperature drops abruptly, a maculopapular, nonitching rash develops, which turns white with pressure. The rash is profuse on the infant's trunk, arms, and neck and is mild on the face and legs. It fades within 24 hours. Complications are extremely rare.

How is it diagnosed?

Diagnosis requires observation of the typical rash that appears about 48 hours after fever subsides.

How is it treated?

Because roseola is self-limiting, treatment is supportive and focuses on symptoms: antipyretics to lower fever and, if necessary, anticonvulsants (such as Phenobarbitol) to relieve seizures. (See *Handling a high fever*.)

ROUNDWORM

What do doctors call this condition?

Besides roundworm, doctors call this condition ascariasis.

What is this condition?

Roundworm is an infection that occurs worldwide but is most common in tropical areas with poor sanitation and in Asia, where farmers use human wastes as fertilizer. In the United States, it's more prevalent in the south, particularly among 4- to 12-year-olds.

What causes it?

Roundworm is caused by *Ascaris lumbricoides*, a large roundworm resembling an earthworm. This parasite is transmitted to humans by ingestion of soil contaminated with human feces that harbor *A. lumbricoides* eggs. Such ingestion may occur directly (by eating contaminated soil) or indirectly (by eating poorly washed raw vegetables grown in contaminated soil). Roundworm never passes directly from person to person.

What are its symptoms?

Roundworm produces two phases: early pulmonary and prolonged intestinal. Mild intestinal infection may cause only vague stomach discomfort. The first clue may be vomiting a worm or passing a worm in stools. Severe infection, however, causes stomach pain, vomiting, restlessness, disturbed sleep, and, in extreme cases, intestinal obstruction. Larvas migrating by the lymphatic and the circulatory systems cause various symptoms: For instance, when they invade the lungs, pneumonitis may result.

How is it diagnosed?

The key to diagnosis is identifying the eggs, which are passed in stools, or adult worms, which may be passed rectally or by mouth. When migrating larvas invade lung tissue, X-rays will show characteristic bronchovascular markings.

How is it treated?

Antiascaris drug therapy, the primary treatment, uses Combantrin or Entacyl to temporarily paralyze the worms, permitting the body to expel them. Vermox is also used to prevent the worms from feeding. These drugs are up to 95% effective, even after a single dose. No specific treatment exists for migratory infection because the drugs affect only mature worms.

In intestinal obstruction, nasogastric suctioning is used to control vomiting. Entacyl is administered through the tube and, if vomiting does not occur, a second dose of Entacyl is typically administered orally after 24 hours. If this is ineffective, surgery may be necessary. (See *Protecting yourself against roundworm*.)

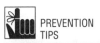 PREVENTION TIPS

Protecting yourself against roundworm

You can avoid another roundworm infection by following directions discussed below.

Cleanliness does it
- Wash your hands thoroughly, especially before eating and after going to the bathroom.
- Bathe daily. Also change your underwear and bed linens every day.

Get the maximum benefit from drug therapy

Take all prescribed medications on time, according to your doctor's directions. Tell your doctor if you experience any side effects. Entacyl, for instance, may cause stomach upset, dizziness, and hives. Combantrin causes red stools and may cause stomach upset, headache, dizziness, and a rash. Vermox may cause stomach pain and diarrhea.

SALMONELLA

What do doctors call this condition?

Salmonellosis

What is this condition?

Salmonella is a common infection in the United States that occurs as enterocolitis, bacteremia (the presence of bacteria in the blood), localized infection, typhoid, or paratyphoid fever. Nontyphoidal forms usually produce mild to moderate illness with low mortality.

Typhoid, the most severe form of salmonella, usually lasts from 1 to 4 weeks. About 3% of persons who are treated and 10% of those who aren't treated die, usually as a result of intestinal perforation or hemorrhage, a cerebral blood clot, blood poisoning, pneumonia, or acute circulatory failure.

An attack of typhoid confers lifelong immunity, although the person may become a carrier. Salmonella occurs 20 times more often in people with AIDS.

What causes it?

Salmonella is caused by gram-negative bacilli of the genus *Salmonella*, a member of the Enterobacteriaceae family. Of an estimated 1,700 serotypes of *Salmonella*, 10 cause the diseases most common in the United States. All 10 can survive for weeks in water, ice, sewage, or food.

Nontyphoidal salmonella generally follows the ingestion of contaminated or inadequately processed foods, especially eggs, chicken, turkey, and duck. Proper cooking reduces the risk of contracting salmonella.

Other causes include contact with infected persons or animals or ingestion of contaminated dry milk, chocolate bars, or drugs of animal origin. Salmonella may occur in children under age 5 from fecal-oral spread. Enterocolitis and bacteremia are common (and more virulent) among infants, elderly people, and people already weakened by other infections. Paratyphoid fever is rare in the United States.

Typhoid results most frequently from drinking water contaminated by excretions of a carrier. Most people with typhoid are under age 30; most carriers are women over age 50. Incidence of typhoid in the

Typhoid, caused by Salmonella, usually results from drinking water contaminated by excretions of a carrier. In the United States, the incidence of typhoid is increasing because of travelers returning from areas where the organism is prevalent.

United States is increasing as a result of travelers returning from areas where the disease is prevalent.

What are its symptoms?

Signs and symptoms of salmonella vary but usually include fever, abdominal pain, and severe diarrhea with enterocolitis. Headache, increasing fever, and constipation are more common with typhoid infection.

How is it diagnosed?

Generally, diagnosis depends on isolation of the organism in a culture, particularly blood (in typhoid, paratyphoid, and bacteremia) or feces (in enterocolitis, paratyphoid, and typhoid). Other appropriate culture specimens include urine, bone marrow, pus, and vomit.

How is it treated?

The choice of an antibiotic for typhoid, paratyphoid, and bacteremia depends on the infecting organism's sensitivity to the specific drug. Treatment may include Amoxil, Chloromycetin and, in severely toxemic people, Bactrim, Cipro, or Rocephin. Localized abscesses may also need surgical drainage. Enterocolitis requires a short course of antibiotics only if it causes septicemia or prolonged fever. Other treatments include bed rest and replacement of fluids and electrolytes. The administration of paregoric, Kaopectate, Motofen, codeine, or small doses of morphine may be necessary to relieve diarrhea and control cramps in people who must remain active.

To *prevent* salmonella, people should always wash their hands thoroughly after defecating and before eating or handling food, and they should refrigerate meat and cooked foods promptly. (Avoid keeping the items at room temperature for any prolonged period.) Lab workers and people who will be traveling to areas where the organism is prevalent should get vaccinated against the disease.

What can a person with salmonella do?

If you have positive stool cultures on discharge from the hospital, use a different bathroom than other family members if possible (while you're on antibiotics). Be sure to wash your hands afterward. Avoid preparing uncooked foods, such as salads, for family members.

SEPTIC SHOCK

What is this condition?

Usually a result of bacterial infection, septic shock leads to inadequate blood flow and circulatory collapse. It occurs most often in hospital patients, especially men over age 40 and women ages 25 to 45. Unless vigorous treatment begins promptly, preferably before symptoms fully develop, septic shock may rapidly progress to death, often within a few hours.

What causes it?

In two-thirds of people, septic shock results from infection with gram-negative bacteria: *Escherichia coli, Klebsiella, Enterobacter, Proteus, Pseudomonas*, and *Bacteroides*; in others, from gram-positive bacteria: *Streptococcus pneumoniae, S. pyogenes*, and *Actinomyces*. Infections with viruses, rickettsiae, chlamydiae, and protozoa may be complicated by shock.

These organisms produce blood poisoning in people whose resistance is already compromised by an existing condition; infection also results from transplantation of bacteria from other areas of the body through surgery, intravenous therapy, and catheters. Septic shock often occurs in people hospitalized for primary infection of the genitourinary, biliary, gastrointestinal, and gynecologic tracts. Other predisposing factors include a weakened immune system, advanced age, injury, burns, diabetes, cirrhosis, and cancer.

What are its symptoms?

The symptoms of septic shock vary according to the stage of the shock, the organism causing it, and the person's age.

- *Early stage:* decreased urine output, sudden fever (over 101° F [38.3° C]), chills, nausea, vomiting, diarrhea, and prostration.
- *Late stage:* restlessness, apprehension, irritability, thirst from decreased blood flow to the cerebral tissue, rapid heart rate, and rapid breathing. Low blood pressure, altered consciousness, and rapid breathing may be the *only* signs among infants and elderly people.

Low body temperature and lack of urination are common late signs. Complications of septic shock include disseminated intravascular coagulation, kidney and heart failure, gastrointestinal ulcers, and liver malfunction.

How is it diagnosed?

Observation of one or more typical symptoms (fever, confusion, nausea, vomiting, rapid breathing) in a person suspected of having an infection suggests septic shock and requires immediate treatment.

In early stages, lab tests indicate respiratory alkalosis; as shock progresses, metabolic acidosis with blood oxygen deficiency develops. Additional lab tests support the diagnosis and determine the type of treatment.

How is it treated?

The doctor's first objective is to monitor and reverse shock by giving intravenous fluids to expand fluid volume and inserting a pulmonary artery catheter to check pulmonary circulation and pulmonary wedge pressure. Administration of whole blood or plasma can raise pulmonary wedge pressure to a satisfactory level. A respirator may be needed to provide proper ventilation to overcome hypoxia. Urinary catheterization allows accurate measurement of hourly urine output.

The doctor will also need to provide immediate intravenous antibiotics to control the infection. Depending on the organism, the antibiotic combination usually includes an aminoglycoside, such as Garamycin or Tobrex for gram-negative bacteria, combined with a penicillin, such as Geocillin or Ticillin. Sometimes treatment includes a cephalosporin such as Zolicef and Unipen for suspected staphylococcal infection instead of Geocillin or Ticillin. Therapy may include Chloromycetin for nonsporulating anaerobes *(Bacteroides)*, although it may cause bone marrow depression, and Cleocin, which may produce pseudomembranous enterocolitis. Appropriate anti-infectives for other causes of septic shock depend on the suspected organism. Other measures to combat infection include surgery to drain and excise abscesses to remove contaminated tissue.

If shock persists after fluid infusion, treatment with vasopressors such as Dopastat maintains adequate blood perfusion in the brain, liver, digestive tract, kidneys, and skin. Other treatment includes intravenous bicarbonate to correct acidosis and intravenous corticosteroids, which may improve blood perfusion and increase cardiac output.

Septic shock is the second leading cause of death from shock. Usually caused by bacterial infection, it results in inadequate blood flow and circulatory collapse.

SHINGLES

What do doctors call this condition?
Besides shingles, doctors call this condition herpes zoster.

What is this condition?
Shingles is an acute inflammation of the dorsal root ganglia on one side of the body, caused by infection with the varicella-zoster herpesvirus, which also causes chickenpox.

Usually occurring in adults, shingles produces localized vesicular skin lesions confined to a dermatome and severe neuralgic (nerve) pain in peripheral areas innervated by the nerves arising in the inflamed root ganglia. (See *Where the shingles rash erupts.*)

The prognosis is good unless the infection spreads to the brain. Eventually, most people recover completely, except for possible scarring and, in corneal damage, visual impairment. Occasionally, neuralgia may persist for months or years.

What causes it?
Shingles results from the reactivation of varicella virus that has lain dormant in the cerebral ganglia or the ganglia of posterior nerve roots following an episode of chickenpox. Exactly how or why this reactivation occurs isn't clear. Some believe that the virus multiplies as it's reactivated and that it's neutralized by antibodies remaining from the initial infection. But if effective antibodies aren't present, the virus continues to multiply in the ganglia, destroys the host neurons, and spreads down the sensory nerves to the skin.

Shingles is found primarily in adults, especially those past age 50. It seldom recurs.

What are its symptoms?
Shingles begins with fever and malaise. Within 2 to 4 days, severe deep pain, itching, and paresthesia or hyperesthesia develop, usually on the trunk and occasionally on the arms and legs in a dermatomal distribution. Pain may be continuous or intermittent and usually lasts from 1 to 4 weeks.

Up to 2 weeks after the first symptoms, small red nodular skin lesions erupt on the painful areas. (These lesions commonly spread unilaterally around the chest or vertically over the arms or legs.)

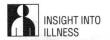

INSIGHT INTO
ILLNESS

Where the shingles rash erupts

The herpes zoster virus infects the nerves that send signals to the skin, eyes, and ears. Each nerve (tagged for its corresponding vertebral source) emanates from the spine, banding and branching about the body to send its signals to a skin area called a *dermatome*.

The shingles rash erupts along the course of the affected nerve, covering the skin in one or several of the dermatomes shown below.

The thoracic (T) and lumbar (L) dermatomes are most commonly affected. But other dermatomes, such as those covering the cervical (C) and the sacral (S) areas can be affected too. In fact, the shingles rash can occur anywhere on the face or body.

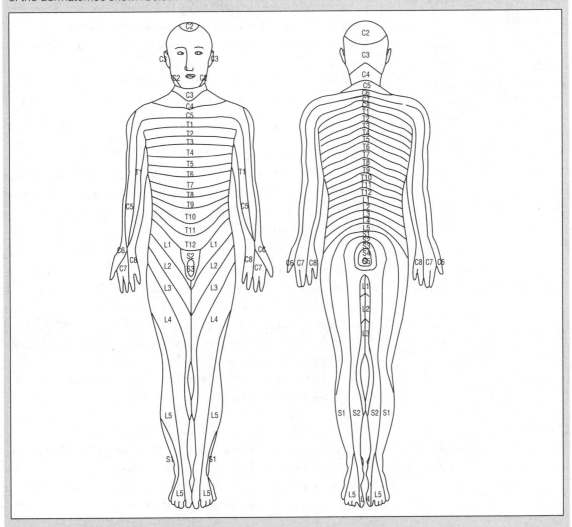

SELF-HELP

Coping with shingles

Don't scratch
Avoid scratching the lesions. If the vesicles rupture, apply a cold compress as directed by the doctor.

Ease the pain
To decrease the pain of oral lesions, use a soft toothbrush, eat a soft diet, and gargle with saltwater.

Be patient
Know that pain caused by the infection will eventually subside.

Sometimes nodules don't appear at all, but when they do, they quickly become vesicles filled with clear fluid or pus. About 10 days after they appear, the vesicles dry and form scabs. When ruptured, such lesions often become infected and, in severe cases, may lead to the enlargement of regional lymph nodes; they may even become gangrenous. Intense pain may occur before the rash appears and after the scabs form.

Occasionally, shingles involves the cranial nerves, especially the trigeminal and geniculate ganglia or the oculomotor nerve, which moves the eye. Geniculate zoster may cause vesicle formation in the external ear canal, ipsilateral facial palsy, hearing loss, dizziness, and loss of taste. Trigeminal ganglion involvement causes eye pain and, possibly, corneal and scleral damage and impaired vision. Rarely, oculomotor nerve involvement causes conjunctivitis (an eye inflammation), extraocular weakness, a drooping eyelid, and paralytic dilation of the pupil.

In postherpetic neuralgia, a complication most common in elderly people, intractable neurologic pain may persist for years. Scars may be permanent.

How is it diagnosed?

Diagnosis of shingles usually isn't possible until the characteristic skin lesions develop. Before then, the pain may mimic appendicitis, pleurisy, or other conditions. Lab tests and a lumbar puncture may help to pinpoint the diagnosis.

How is it treated?

No specific treatment exists. The primary goal of supportive treatment is to relieve itching and neuralgic pain with calamine lotion or another drug to relieve itching; aspirin, possibly with codeine or another pain reliever; and, occasionally, collodion or tincture of benzoin applied to unbroken lesions.

If bacteria have infected ruptured vesicles, the treatment plan usually includes an appropriate systemic antibiotic.

Trigeminal zoster with corneal involvement calls for instillation of Herplex ointment or another antiviral agent. To help a person cope with the intractable pain of postherpetic neuralgia, the doctor may order a systemic corticosteroid — such as cortisone or, possibly, a corticotropin — to reduce inflammation, tranquilizers, sedatives, or tricyclic antidepressants with phenothiazines.

Zovirax seems to stop progression of the rash and prevent visceral complications. In immunocompromised people — both children and adults — Zovirax therapy may be administered intravenously. The drug appears to prevent disseminated, life-threatening disease in some people. (See *Coping with shingles*.)

Toxic Shock Syndrome

What is this condition?

Toxic shock syndrome is an acute bacterial infection. It mainly affects menstruating women under age 30 and is associated with continuous use of tampons during the menstrual period.

Incidence of the infection peaked in the mid-1980s and has since declined, probably because high-absorbency tampons have been taken off the market.

What causes it?

Toxic shock syndrome is caused by toxin-producing, penicillin-resistant strains of *Staphylococcus aureus*.

Although tampons are clearly implicated in this infection, their exact role is uncertain. Theoretically, tampons may contribute to development of toxic shock syndrome by introducing *S. aureus* into the vagina during insertion; absorbing toxin from the vagina; injuring the vaginal mucous membrane during insertion, leading to infection; and providing a favorable environment for the growth of *S. aureus*.

When toxic shock syndrome isn't related to menstruation, it seems to be linked to *S. aureus* infections, such as abscesses, osteomyelitis (a bone infection), and postsurgical infections.

Although tampons are implicated in toxic shock syndrome, their exact role is uncertain.

What are its symptoms?

Typically, the disease produces intense muscle ache, a fever that's above 104° F (40° C), vomiting, diarrhea, headache, decreased level of consciousness, violent shivering attacks, redness of the eyes, and vaginal discharge. Blood pressure drops sharply with hypovolemic shock — a state of physical collapse caused by massive blood loss, impaired circulation, and poor tissue perfusion.

Within a few hours of onset, a deep red rash develops — especially on the palms and soles — and later desquamates (scales and falls off).

Major complications of toxic shock syndrome include persistent neurologic and psychological abnormalities, mild kidney failure, rash, and bluish discoloration of the arms and legs.

How is it diagnosed?

The doctor diagnoses toxic shock syndrome from the person's signs and symptoms and the presence of at least three of the following:

- gastrointestinal effects, including vomiting and profuse diarrhea
- muscular effects, with severe muscle ache or a fivefold or greater increase in creatine kinase, an enzyme in the muscles and brain
- mucous membrane effects such as swelling
- kidney involvement with blood urea nitrogen or creatinine at least twice their normal levels
- liver involvement with elevated levels of bilirubin and other substances
- blood involvement with a platelet count below 100,000 per microliter
- central nervous system effects such as disorientation.

In addition, isolation of S. aureus from vaginal discharge or lesions supports the diagnosis. Negative results on blood tests for Rocky Mountain spotted fever, leptospirosis, and measles help rule out these disorders.

How is it treated?

Treatment consists of intravenous antistaphylococcal antibiotics, such as Bactocill and Unipen. To reverse shock, the person must receive intravenous fluids.

TOXOPLASMOSIS

What is this condition?

Toxoplasmosis, one of the most common infectious diseases, results from the protozoa *Toxoplasma gondii*. Distributed worldwide, it's less common in cold or hot, arid climates and at high elevations. It usually causes localized infection but may produce significant generalized infection, especially in immunodeficient persons or newborns. Congenital toxoplasmosis, characterized by lesions in the central nervous system, may result in stillbirth or serious birth defects.

What causes it?

T. gondii exists in trophozoite forms in the acute stages of infection and in cystic forms (tissue cysts and oocysts) in the latent stages. Ingestion of tissue cysts in raw or uncooked meat (heating, drying, or freezing destroys these cysts) or fecal-oral contamination from infected cats transmits toxoplasmosis. However, toxoplasmosis also occurs in vegetarians who aren't exposed to cats, so other means of transmission may exist. Congenital toxoplasmosis follows transplacental transmission from a chronically infected mother or one who acquired toxoplasmosis shortly before or during pregnancy.

What are its symptoms?

Toxoplasmosis acquired in the first trimester of pregnancy often results in stillbirth. About one-third of infants who survive have congenital toxoplasmosis. The later in pregnancy maternal infection occurs, the greater the risk of congenital infection in the infant. Obvious signs of congenital toxoplasmosis include retinochoroiditis, "water on the brain" or an abnormally small head, cerebral calcification, seizures, lymphadenopathy (lymph node disease), fever, an enlarged liver and spleen, jaundice, and rash. Other defects, which may become apparent months or years later, include eye deviation, blindness, epilepsy, and mental retardation.

Acquired toxoplasmosis may cause localized (mild lymphatic) or generalized (sudden, severe, disseminated) infection. Localized infection produces fever and a mononucleosis-like syndrome (malaise, muscle pain, headache, fatigue, sore throat) and lymphadenopathy. Generalized infection produces encephalitis, fever, headache, vomiting, delirium, seizures, and a diffuse maculopapular rash (except on the palms, soles, and scalp). Generalized infection may lead to myocarditis, pneumonitis, hepatitis, and polymyositis.

How is it diagnosed?

Identification of *T. gondii* from a tissue specimen confirms toxoplasmosis. Blood tests may be useful and, in people with toxoplasmosis encephalitis, a computed tomography scan (commonly called a CAT scan) and magnetic resonance imaging (commonly called an MRI) disclose lesions.

To help prevent toxoplasmosis, people should wash their hands after working with soil, cook meat thoroughly and freeze it promptly if they won't be using it immediately, change cat litter daily, cover children's sandboxes, and keep flies away from food.

How is it treated?

Treatment for acute disease consists of drug therapy with sulfonamides and Daraprim for about 4 weeks and, possibly, Wellcovorin to control side effects. In people who also have AIDS, treatment continues indefinitely. No safe, effective treatment exists for chronic toxoplasmosis or toxoplasmosis occurring in the first trimester of pregnancy.

To help *prevent* toxoplasmosis, people should wash their hands after working with soil (because it may be contaminated with cat oocysts); cook meat thoroughly and freeze it promptly if it's not for immediate use; change cat litter daily (cat oocysts don't become infective until 1 to 4 days after excretion); cover children's sandboxes; and keep flies away from food (flies transport oocysts).

TRICHINOSIS

What do doctors call this condition?

Besides trichinosis, doctors call this condition trichiniasis or trichinellosis.

What is this condition?

Trichinosis is an infection caused by larvae of the intestinal roundworm *Trichinella spiralis*. It occurs worldwide, especially in populations that eat pork or bear meat. Trichinosis may produce multiple symptoms; respiratory, central nervous system, and cardiovascular complications; and, rarely, death.

What causes it?

Transmission occurs through ingestion of uncooked or undercooked meat that contains *T. spiralis* cysts. The cysts are found primarily in pigs and, less often, in dogs, cats, bears, foxes, wolves, and sea animals. Person-to-person transmission does not take place.

Humans get trichinosis by eating uncooked or undercooked meat that contains T. spiralis *cysts found in pigs and other animals. Pigs acquire the cysts by eating table scraps or raw garbage.*

What are its symptoms?

In the United States, trichinosis is usually mild and seldom produces symptoms. When symptoms do occur, they vary with the stage and degree of infection:

- *Stage 1 (invasion):* occurs 1 week after ingestion. Release of larvas and reproduction of adult *T. spiralis* cause loss of appetite, nausea, vomiting, diarrhea, abdominal pain, and cramps.
- *Stage 2 (dissemination):* occurs 7 to 10 days after ingestion. *T. spiralis* penetrates the mucous membranes of the intestine and begins to migrate to striated muscle. Symptoms include swelling, especially of the eyelids or face; muscle pain, particularly in the arms and legs; and, occasionally, itching and burning skin, sweating, skin lesions, a temperature of 102° to 104° F (38.8° to 40° C), and delirium; and, in severe respiratory, cardiovascular, or central nervous system infections, palpitations and sluggishness.
- *Stage 3 (encystment):* occurs during convalescence, generally 1 week later. *T. spiralis* larvas invade muscle fiber and become encysted.

How is it diagnosed?

If trichinosis is suspected, the doctor will ask about the person's recent diet. A history of ingestion of raw or improperly cooked pork or pork products, with typical clinical features, suggests trichinosis. However, infection may be difficult to prove.

Laboratory and diagnostic tests are important in diagnosing trichinosis. Stools may contain mature worms and larvas during the invasion stage. Skeletal muscle biopsies (removal and analysis of tissue) can show encysted larvas 10 days after ingestion and, if available, analyses of contaminated meat also show larvas.

Skin testing may help diagnose trichinosis. Blood tests which measure levels of antibodies confirm this diagnosis.

How is it treated?

The doctor will prescribe a drug called Triasox. This drug effectively combats the parasite during the intestinal stage. If the person has a severe infection (especially central nervous system invasion), the doctor may prescribe glucocorticoids to fight against possible inflammation.

What can a person with trichinosis do?

- Reduce fever with alcohol rubs, tepid baths, cooling blankets, or drugs (such as aspirin or Tylenol).

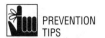

PREVENTION TIPS

Protect yourself against trichinosis

Death to the organism

To help prevent trichinosis, properly cook and store all pork, pork products, and meat from carnivores. To kill the trichinosis organism, internal meat temperatures should reach 150° F (65° C) and its color should change from pink to grey, unless the meat has been cured or frozen for at least 10 days at low temperatures.

A word to travelers

When traveling to foreign countries or very poor areas in the United States, avoid eating pork; pigs in these areas are often fed raw garbage.

- To relieve muscular pain, take pain relievers and stay in bed.
- Continue bed rest into the convalescent stage to avoid a serious relapse and possible death.
- Be aware that possible side effects of Triasox are nausea, vomiting, dizziness, skin inflammation, and fever. (See *Protect yourself against trichinosis,* page 811.)

WHOOPING COUGH

What do doctors call this condition?
Besides whooping cough, doctors call this condition pertussis.

What is this condition?
Whooping cough is a highly contagious respiratory infection. Typically, it causes sudden attacks of an irritating cough, which often ends in a high-pitched whooping sound as the person takes a breath.

Whooping cough occurs throughout the world, usually during early spring and late winter. Half of the victims are unimmunized children under age 2.

Since the 1940s, immunization and aggressive diagnosis and treatment have greatly reduced the death rate from whooping cough in the United States. Children under age 1 who die from the disease usually do so from pneumonia and other complications. Whooping cough is dangerous in elderly people, too, but tends to be less severe in older children and adults.

What causes it?
Whooping cough is usually caused by the coccobacillus *Bordetella pertussis* and occasionally by *B. parapertussis* and *B. bronchiseptica.*

The disease is usually transmitted by directly inhaling contaminated droplets from someone in the acute stage of the disease. It may also spread indirectly through soiled linen and other articles contaminated by respiratory secretions.

What are its symptoms?
About 7 to 10 days after exposure, *B. pertussis* enters the airways, where it causes progressively tenacious mucus. Whooping cough fol-

lows a classic 6-week course that includes three stages, each lasting about 2 weeks.

The catarrhal stage

The first stage typically produces an irritating hacking, nighttime cough; appetite loss; sneezing; listlessness; eye infection; and, occasionally, a slight fever. During this stage, the disease is highly contagious.

The paroxysmal stage

The second stage begins after 7 to 14 days. The paroxysmal stage causes recurrent coughing spells that may expel tenacious mucus. Each cough characteristically ends in a loud, crowing whoop, and choking on mucus may cause vomiting. (Very young infants, however, might not develop the typical whoop.)

The coughing spells may cause complications, such as increased pressure in the veins, nosebleeds, swelling around the eyes, eye hemorrhages, detached retina (and blindness), rectal prolapse, an intestinal or abdominal hernia, seizures, and lung inflammation. In infants, choking spells may cause apnea (periodic absence of breathing), an oxygen deficiency, and metabolic disturbances.

During this stage, people are highly vulnerable to potentially fatal secondary bacterial or viral infections. Such secondary infection (usually a middle ear infection or pneumonia) should be suspected in anyone with a fever during this stage because whooping cough itself seldom causes fever.

The convalescent stage

During this third and final stage, coughing spells and vomiting gradually subside. However, for months afterward, even a mild upper respiratory infection may trigger such coughing.

How is it diagnosed?

The doctor will suspect whooping cough in anyone with classic symptoms — especially during the paroxysmal stage — and will order lab tests to confirm it. Nose and throat swabs and sputum cultures show *B. pertussis* only in the early stages of this disease. The white blood cell count is usually increased, especially in children older than age 6 months and early in the paroxysmal stage.

Since the 1940s, immunization and aggressive diagnosis and treatment have greatly reduced the death rate from whooping cough in the United States.

How is it treated?

A person with whooping cough should be hospitalized (perhaps in the intensive care unit), where he or she will receive fluids and electrolytes. Other treatments include adequate nutrition, codeine and mild sedatives to decrease coughing, oxygen therapy if the person has apnea, and antibiotics to shorten the contagious period and prevent secondary infections.

A person with whooping cough may require respiratory isolation. This means that he or she must stay in a private room with the door closed and that any person entering the room must wear a mask. Respiratory isolation continues for 5 to 7 days after the initiation of antibiotic therapy. Steps may also be taken to ensure a quiet environment to decrease coughing stimulation. The person should be served small, frequent meals.

Vaccination for whooping cough

Because very young infants are particularly vulnerable to whooping cough, immunization — usually with diphtheria and tetanus toxoids (the diphtheria, tetanus, and pertussis vaccine) — is performed at ages 2, 4, and 6 months. Boosters follow at age 18 months and at age 4 to 6.

Although the vaccine causes nervous system damage and other complications, the risk of whooping cough is greater than the risk of these complications. But if the vaccination causes seizures or unusual and persistent crying, this may be a sign of a severe neurologic reaction and the doctor may not order the other doses. The vaccine shouldn't be given to children over age 6 because it can cause a severe fever.

INJURIES

ARM AND LEG FRACTURES

What are these conditions?

A broken arm or leg usually results from an injury. It can damage the muscles, nerves, and other soft tissues.

Most broken bones — especially in children — heal fully, without deformity. But the bones of adults in poor health or with poor circulation may never heal properly. A severe open fracture — one in which the overlying skin is broken — may cause major blood loss and may even lead to life-threatening shock.

What causes them?

Most arm and leg fractures result from major injuries — for example, a fall on an outstretched arm or a skiing accident. In a child who has multiple or repeated episodes of fractures, these injuries may result from abuse.

In someone with a bone-weakening condition, such as osteoporosis, a bone tumor, or a metabolic disease, merely coughing or sneezing can cause a fracture. Prolonged standing, walking, or running can lead to stress fractures of the foot and ankle — a condition seen most often in nurses, postal workers, soldiers, and joggers.

What are their symptoms?

Broken arms and legs may produce any or all of the "5 P's":
- pain and tenderness
- paleness of the overlying skin
- pulse loss
- paresthesia (sensation of numbness and tingling)
- paralysis.

The fracture may impair limb movement, and the injury site may be deformed, swollen, and discolored. Bone fragments rubbing together may cause a crackling noise. Numbness, tingling, and loss of pulses, along with cool, mottled, bluish skin beyond the injury site, may signal poor circulation or nerve damage. In open fractures, there's also an obvious skin wound.

Complications

Broken arms and legs can cause the following complications:
- permanent deformity and limb dysfunction if bones fail to heal (nonunion) or if they heal improperly (malunion)

- localized destruction and infection of bone segments (from poor circulation)
- shock from blood vessel damage (especially with a fractured thigh)
- muscle contractures and kidney stones (from prolonged immobility)
- fat embolism — a serious circulatory problem in which a piece of fat blocks an artery.

How are they diagnosed?

To diagnose a broken arm or leg, the doctor relies on the person's history of a recent injury, gently feels the affected area, and has the person cautiously try to move the extremity below the injury site. To confirm the fracture, the doctor takes X-rays of the injury site and the joints above and below it.

How are they treated?

A broken arm or leg calls for emergency treatment. The limb is splinted above and below the fracture site, an ice pack is applied, and the limb is raised to reduce swelling and pain.

In severe fractures that cause blood loss, direct pressure is applied to control bleeding and fluids are given as soon as possible to prevent or treat shock.

Open fractures call for a tetanus shot, antibiotics, surgery to repair soft-tissue damage, and thorough wound cleansing to help prevent infection and promote healing.

Fracture reduction

Fractures must be reduced—that is, displaced bone segments must be restored to their normal position. After reduction, the broken arm or leg is immobilized by a splint or cast or with traction.

In *closed reduction,* the doctor manually manipulates the bone fragments. The person receives a local anesthetic, a pain reliever, and a muscle relaxant or sedative to promote the muscle stretching needed to realign the bone. (See *How broken bones heal.*)

When closed reduction is impossible, *open reduction* is performed. In this procedure, the surgeon reduces and immobilizes the fracture using rods, plates, or screws. Afterward, a plaster cast is usually applied.

Traction

When a splint or cast won't maintain the reduction, the fracture is immobilized with skin or skeletal traction, using weights and pulleys.

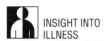

How broken bones heal

A broken bone starts to heal the moment the break occurs. But rigid bone fragments take a long time to reestablish a firm union. That's why you should continue your rehabilitation program, even after your injured bone seems normal again.

Here are the stages your broken bone goes through when it heals.

Blood collects at the site

First, blood collects around the broken bone ends, forming a sticky, jellylike mass called a *clot*. Within 24 hours, a meshlike network forms from the clot. This becomes the framework for growing new bone tissue.

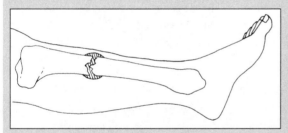

Cells start bone healing

Soon, osteoclasts and osteoblasts — the cells that heal the bone — invade this clot. *Osteoclasts* start smoothing the jagged edges of bone while *osteoblasts* start bridging the gap between the bone ends. Within a few days, these cells form a granular bridge, linking the bone ends.

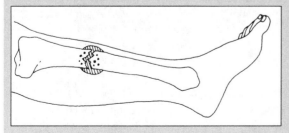

Callus forms

Six to ten days after the injury, the granular bridge of cells becomes a bony mass called a *callus*, which eventually hardens into solid bone.

But for now, the callus is fragile, and abrupt motion can split it. That's why it's so important to keep a broken bone from moving while it's healing.

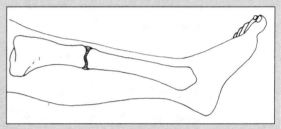

Bone hardens

Three to ten weeks after the injury, new blood vessels start bringing calcium to the area to harden the new bone tissue. This process is called *ossification*, in which the ends of the bones "knit" together.

After ossification, the bone becomes solid and is considered healed. Although the cast may be removed, up to a year may pass before the healed bone is as strong as it was before the break.

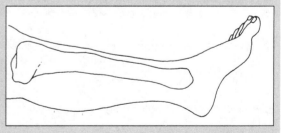

How to care for your cast

Think of your new cast as a temporary body part — one that needs the same attentive care as the rest of you. While you wear your cast, follow these guidelines.

Speeding up drying time
The doctor may apply a cast made of plaster, fiberglass, or a synthetic material. The wet material must dry thoroughly and evenly for the cast to support your broken bone properly. At first, the wet cast will feel heavy and warm. But don't worry — it will get lighter as it dries.

To speed drying, keep the cast exposed to air. Fiberglass and synthetic casts dry soon after application, but plaster casts don't. (A plaster arm or leg cast takes about 24 to 48 hours to dry.) Obviously, drying a plaster cast in less time makes it more comfortable sooner.

When you raise the cast with pillows, make sure the pillows have rubber or plastic covers under the linen case. Place a thin towel between the cast and the pillows to absorb moisture. Never place a wet cast directly onto plastic.

Drying evenly
To make sure the cast dries evenly, change its position on the pillows every 2 hours, using your palms, not your fingertips. (You can have someone else move the cast for you, if necessary.) To avoid creating bumps *inside* the cast — bumps that could cause skin irritation or sores — don't poke at the cast with your fingers while it's wet. Also, be careful not to dent the cast while it's still wet.

Keeping your cast clean
After your cast dries, you can remove dirt and stains with a damp cloth and a gentle abrasive cleanser. Use as little water as possible, and wipe off any moisture that remains when you're done.

Protecting your cast
Avoid knocking your cast against any hard surface. To protect the foot of a leg cast from breakage, scrapes, and dirt, place a piece of used carpet (or a carpet square) over the bottom of the cast. Slash or cut a V-shape at the back, so the carpet fits around the heel when you bring it up toward the ankle. Hold the carpet in place with a large sock or slipper sock. Extending the carpet out beyond the toes a little also will help prevent bumped or stubbed toes.

Preventing snags
To keep an arm cast from snagging clothing and furniture, make a cast cover from an old nylon stocking. Cut the stocking's toe off, and cut a hole in the heel. Then pull the stocking over the cast to cover it. Extend your fingers through the cut-off toe end, and poke your thumb through the hole you cut in the heel. Trim the other end of the stocking to about 1½ inches (4 centimeters) longer than the cast, and tuck the ends of the stocking under the cast's edges.

Caring for your skin
Wash the skin along the cast's edges every day, using a mild soap. Before you begin, protect the cast's edges with plastic wrap. Then wring out a washcloth soaked in soapy water to clean the skin at the cast's edges and as far as you can reach inside the cast. (Avoid getting the cast wet.) Afterward, dry the skin thoroughly with a towel, then massage the skin at and beneath the cast's edges with a towel or pad saturated with rubbing alcohol. (This helps toughen the skin.) To help prevent skin irritation, remove any loose plaster particles you can reach inside the cast.

Relieving itching
No matter how itchy the skin under your cast may feel, *never* try to relieve the itch by inserting a sharp or pointed object into the cast. This could damage

How to care for your cast *(continued)*

your skin and lead to infection. Don't put powder or lotion in your cast, either, or stuff cotton or toilet tissue under the cast's edges. (This may cut down on your circulation.)

Here's a safe technique to relieve itching: Set a handheld blow-dryer on "cool" and aim it at the itchy area.

Staying dry

If you have a plaster cast, you'll need to cover it with a plastic bag before you shower, swim, or go out in wet weather. You can use a garbage bag or a cast shower bag, which you can buy at a drugstore or medical supply store. *Above all, don't get a plaster cast wet.* Moisture will weaken or even destroy it. If the cast gets a little wet, let it dry naturally—for example, by sitting in the sun. Don't cover the cast until it's completely dry.

If you have a fiberglass or synthetic cast, check with your doctor to find out if you may bathe, shower, or swim. If he does allow you to swim, he'll probably tell you to flush the cast with cool tap water after swimming in a chlorinated pool or a lake. (Make sure no foreign material remains trapped inside the cast.)

To dry a fiberglass or synthetic cast, first wrap the cast in a towel. Then prop it on a pad of towels to absorb any remaining water. The cast will air-dry in 3 to 4 hours. To speed drying, use a handheld blow-dryer.

Signing the cast

Family members and friends may want to sign their names or draw pictures on the cast. That's okay, but don't let them paint over large cast areas. Why? Because this could make those areas nonporous and damage the skin beneath them.

In *skin traction,* elastic bandages and sheepskin coverings are used to attach traction devices to the person's skin. In *skeletal traction,* a pin or wire is inserted through the bone beyond the fracture and attached to a weight to allow more prolonged traction.

What can a person with a broken arm or leg do?

- Drink plenty of fluids to help prevent the kidney stones and constipation that may result from immobilization. Call your doctor if you have symptoms of kidney stones: flank pain, nausea, and vomiting.
- Immediately report any symptoms of circulatory problems: skin coldness, numbness, tingling, or discoloration.
- Care for your cast as directed. (See *How to care for your cast.*)
- Start moving around as soon as you can, with the doctor's permission.
- Be aware that after your cast is removed, physical therapy can help restore your mobility.

ASPHYXIA

What is this condition?

In this breathing problem, the blood and the body's tissues don't get enough oxygen and instead accumulate carbon dioxide. Asphyxia results in cardiac arrest and, without prompt treatment, is fatal.

What causes it?

Asphyxia results from any condition or substance that inhibits breathing:

- narcotic abuse, medullary disease or hemorrhage, collapsed lung, or respiratory muscle paralysis
- blocked breathing passages, severe asthma, foreign body aspiration, pneumonia, or near drowning
- compressed windpipe due to a tumor, strangulation, trauma, or suffocation
- inhalation of toxins, as in carbon monoxide poisoning and smoke inhalation.

What are its symptoms?

Depending on the duration and degree of asphyxia, common symptoms include anxiety, agitation and confusion, shortness of breath, cessation of breathing or altered respiratory rate (abnormally slow or fast), seizures, and a fast, slow, or absent pulse.

How is it diagnosed?

Diagnosis rests on the person's history and lab results. Arterial blood gas analysis, the most important test, shows characteristic levels of oxygen and carbon dioxide. Chest X-rays may show a foreign body, pulmonary edema, or atelectasis. Toxicology tests may show drugs, chemicals, or abnormal hemoglobin. Pulmonary function tests may indicate respiratory muscle weakness.

How is it treated?

Asphyxia requires immediate respiratory support — with CPR, an endotracheal tube to allow breathing, and supplemental oxygen as needed — and removal of the underlying cause: bronchoscopy for extraction of a foreign body, a narcotic antagonist like Narcan for narcotic overdose, stomach pumping for poisoning, and withholding of supplemental oxygen for carbon dioxide narcosis caused by excessive oxygen therapy.

BLUNT AND PENETRATING ABDOMINAL INJURIES

What are these conditions?
Blunt and penetrating abdominal injuries may damage major blood vessels and internal organs. Their most immediate life-threatening consequences are hemorrhage and shock; a later threat is infection. The prognosis depends on the extent of injury and the organs damaged but is generally improved by prompt diagnosis and surgical repair.

What causes them?
Blunt injuries usually result from automobile accidents, falls from heights, or athletic injuries; penetrating injuries, from stab and gunshot wounds.

What are their symptoms?
Symptoms vary. Blunt abdominal injuries cause severe pain (which may radiate beyond the abdomen, for instance, to the shoulders), bruises, abrasions, contusions, or distention. They may also result in tenderness, nausea, vomiting, pallor, bluish skin color, rapid heart rate, and shortness of breath. Rib fractures often accompany blunt injuries.

Penetrating abdominal injuries result in obvious wounds (in gunshots, often both entrance and exit wounds) with blood loss, pain, and tenderness.

In both blunt and penetrating injuries, massive blood loss may cause shock. In general, damage to solid abdominal organs (liver, spleen, pancreas, and kidneys) causes hemorrhage; damage to hollow organs (stomach, intestine, gallbladder, and bladder) causes rupture and release of the organs' contents (including bacteria) into the abdomen, which, in turn, produces inflammation. (See *How blunt abdominal injury damages organs,* page 824.)

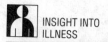

How blunt abdominal injury damages organs

When a blunt object strikes a person's abdomen, it increases pressure within the abdomen. Depending on its force, the blow can tear the liver and spleen, rupture the stomach, bruise the duodenum (the shortest portion of the small intestine), and even damage the kidneys.

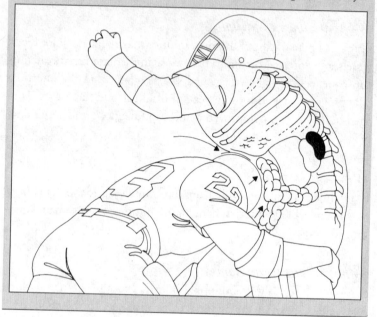

How are they diagnosed?

A history of abdominal injury, signs and symptoms, and lab results confirm the diagnosis and determine which organs have been damaged. Diagnostic tests vary with the person's condition but may include chest and abdominal X-rays, examination of stools and stomach contents for blood, blood and ultrasound studies, and computed tomography scans (commonly called CAT scans).

How are they treated?

Emergency treatment consists of intravenous fluids and blood transfusion to control hemorrhage and prevent shock. Most people with abdominal injuries require surgery after they're stabilized; some people, however, require immediate surgery. Pain relievers and antibiotics increase comfort and prevent infection. If a person has no symptoms, he or she may only require hospital observation for 6 to 24 hours.

*B*LUNT CHEST INJURIES

What are these conditions?

Chest injuries account for one-fourth of all trauma deaths in North America. Many are blunt chest injuries, which include bruising of the heart and fractures of the ribs and sternum (breastbone). These fractures may cause potentially fatal complications, such as hemothorax (blood in the lining around the lungs), pneumothorax (collapsed lung), shock, and ruptured diaphragm.

What causes them?

Most blunt chest injuries result from automobile accidents. Other common causes include sports and blast injuries.

What are their symptoms?

Rib fractures produce tenderness, slight swelling over the fracture site, and pain that worsens with deep breathing and movement; this painful breathing causes the person to breathe shallowly.

Sternal fractures produce persistent chest pain, even at rest. If a fractured rib punctures a lung, it causes pneumothorax, which usually produces severe shortness of breath, bluish skin discoloration, agitation, and extreme pain.

Flail chest

Multiple rib fractures may cause *flail chest,* in which a portion of the chest wall caves in, thus preventing adequate lung inflation. Bruised skin, extreme pain caused by rib fracture and disfigurement, paradoxical chest movements, and rapid, shallow breathing are all signs of flail chest, as are rapid heart rate, low blood pressure, respiratory acidosis, and bluish skin discoloration. (See *How flail chest disrupts the breathing pattern,* page 826.)

Flail chest can also cause tension pneumothorax, a condition in which air enters the chest but can't be ejected during exhalation; this life-threatening buildup of pressure in the chest causes the lung to collapse.

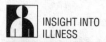
INSIGHT INTO
ILLNESS

How flail chest disrupts the breathing pattern

A blunt injury that makes the chest wall cave in may lead to *flail chest*. In this condition, chest movements —
and the person's breathing pattern — are abnormal during both inhalation and exhalation.

Inhalation
- Injured chest wall collapses in.
- Uninjured chest wall moves out.

Exhalation
- Injured chest wall moves out.
- Uninjured chest wall moves in.

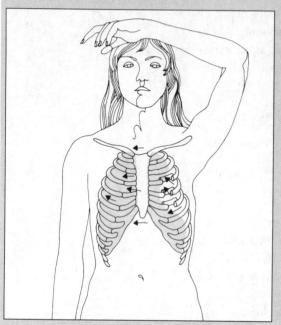

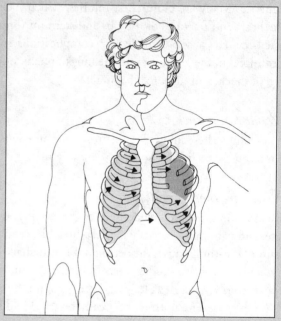

Hemothorax

Hemothorax occurs when blood collects in the lining around the lung, thereby compressing the lung and limiting breathing capacity. It can also result from rupture of large or small pulmonary blood vessels. Massive hemothorax is the most common cause of shock after a chest injury.

Rib fractures may also cause pulmonary contusion (resulting in coughing up blood, reduced oxygen supply to tissue, shortness of breath, and possibly obstruction), large myocardial tears (which can be rapidly fatal), and small myocardial tears.

Laceration (tearing) or rupture of the aorta is nearly always immediately fatal. Rupture of the diaphragm (usually on the left side) causes severe respiratory distress.

Other complications of blunt chest trauma may include cardiac tamponade, pulmonary artery tears, ventricular rupture, and bronchial, tracheal, or esophageal tears or rupture.

How are they diagnosed?

A history of injury with shortness of breath, chest pain, and other typical symptoms suggests a blunt chest injury. To determine its extent, a physical exam and diagnostic tests are needed. For example, chest X-rays may confirm rib and sternal fractures, pneumothorax, flail chest, pulmonary contusions, lacerated or ruptured aorta, tension pneumothorax, ruptured diaphragm, lung compression, or atelectasis with hemothorax. With heart damage, an electrocardiogram may show abnormalities.

Echocardiography, computed tomography scans (commonly called CAT scans), and cardiac and lung scans may show the injury's extent.

How are they treated?

Blunt chest injuries call for an immediate physical exam, control of bleeding, and maintenance of breathing.

For simple rib fractures, the doctor orders mild pain relievers, bed rest, and heat application. For more severe fractures, nerve blocks may be administered to nerves between the ribs. The person with excessive bleeding is intubated.

For pneumothorax, a chest tube is inserted to remove as much air as possible from the pleural cavity and to reexpand the lungs. For tension pneumothorax, the doctor inserts a needle into the chest to release pressure, and then inserts a chest tube to normalize pressure and reexpand the lung.

For flail chest, the lung is reexpanded and the person receives supplemental oxygen and intravenous therapy. For hemothorax, the person is treated for shock with intravenous fluids. If a lot of blood has been lost, the person receives transfusions. Chest tubes are inserted to remove blood.

For pulmonary contusions, the person receives colloids to replace volume and maintain oncotic pressure, along with pain relievers, diuretics and, if necessary, corticosteroids. For suspected heart damage, the person requires intensive care to detect irregular heart rhythms and prevent cardiogenic shock. He or she will also receive oxygen, pain relievers, and drugs to control heart failure or irregular heart rhythms. For myocardial rupture, septal perforation, and other heart lacerations, immediate surgery is mandatory.

Immediate surgery is also required for aortic rupture or laceration. For a ruptured diaphragm, the person receives a nasogastric tube to temporarily decompress the stomach, and then undergoes surgery.

BRAIN CONTUSION

What do doctors call this condition?
Besides brain contusion, doctors call this condition cerebral contusion.

What is this condition?
Brain contusion is a bruising of brain tissue caused by a severe blow to the head. More serious than a concussion, a contusion disrupts normal nerve functions in the bruised area and may cause loss of consciousness, hemorrhage, swelling, and even death.

What causes it?
Brain contusion results from acceleration-deceleration injuries, in which the brain knocks against the skull (acceleration) and then rebounds (deceleration). Such injuries can occur from the force of a blow (a beating with a blunt instrument, for example) or when the head is hurled forward and stopped abruptly (as in an automobile accident when a driver's head strikes the windshield). These injuries can also cause the brain to strike against bones inside the skull, causing bleeding.

What are its symptoms?
The person with a brain contusion may have severe scalp wounds and labored breathing, and may lose consciousness for a few minutes or longer. If conscious, the person may be drowsy, confused, disoriented, agitated, or even violent. Eventually, he or she should return to a relatively alert state, perhaps with temporary speech defects or slight one-sided paralysis or numbness.

More serious than a concussion, a brain contusion disrupts normal nerve functions in the bruised area and may cause loss of consciousness, hemorrhage, edema, and even death.

How is it diagnosed?

An accurate history of the injury and a neurologic exam are the principal diagnostic tools. A computed tomography scan (commonly called a CAT scan) shows damaged tissue, hematomas, and fractures.

How is it treated?

The health care team ensures proper breathing — for example, by tracheotomy or endotracheal intubation — and carefully monitors the person's neurologic and respiratory status. The person may receive intravenous fluids as well as the drug Decadron for several days to control brain swelling. Fluid intake is restricted to reduce volume and brain swelling.

BURNS

What are these conditions?

Major burns are horrifying injuries that require painful treatment and a long rehabilitation period. They're often fatal or permanently disfiguring and incapacitating — both emotionally and physically.

In North America, more than 2 million people suffer burns each year. Of these, 300,000 are burned seriously and over 6,000 die, making burns the continent's third leading cause of accidental death.

What causes them?

Thermal (heat) burns, the most common type, commonly result from fires, car accidents, playing with matches, improperly stored gasoline, space-heater or electrical malfunctions, or arson. Other causes include improper handling of firecrackers, scalding accidents, and kitchen accidents (such as a child climbing on top of a stove or grabbing a hot iron). In children, thermal burns sometimes are traced to abuse by parents.

Chemical burns result from contacting, ingesting, inhaling, or injecting acids, alkalis (such as lye), or vesicants (blistering agents). *Electrical burns* are usually caused by contact with faulty electrical wiring or high-voltage power lines or chewing on electric cords (by young children). *Friction (abrasion) burns* happen when the skin is

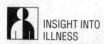

INSIGHT INTO ILLNESS

Classifying burns by degree

Classifying a burn helps the doctor choose appropriate treatment. Burns traditionally have been classified by degree, as follows (although most are a combination of different degrees and thicknesses):

- *First-degree* — Only the epidermis (the outermost skin layer) is damaged. This burn causes redness and pain.
- *Second-degree* — The epidermis and part of the dermis (the underlying skin layer) are damaged, producing blisters and mild to moderate swelling and pain.
- *Third-degree* — Both the epidermis and the dermis are damaged. No blisters appear, but white, brown, or black leathery tissue and clotted blood vessels are visible.
- *Fourth-degree* — Damage extends through deeply charred tissue under the skin to muscle and bone.

rubbed harshly against a coarse surface. *Sunburn,* of course, results from excessive exposure to sunlight.

How are they diagnosed?

A burn is usually obvious from the wound and the person's recent history of contact with a thermal, chemical, electrical, or friction source. To guide treatment, the doctor classifies the burn — usually by depth and size. A more traditional way to classify burns is by degree. (See *Classifying burns by degree.*)

Burn depth

A *partial-thickness burn* damages the epidermis (the skin's outermost layer) and part of the dermis (the underlying layer). A *full-thickness burn* affects the epidermis, dermis, and tissue beneath the skin.

Burn size

The size of a burn is usually expressed as the percentage of body surface area covered by the burn. For example, a burn is considered *major* if the person has third-degree burns on more than 10% of body surface area or second-degree burns on more than 25% of body surface area. A burn is considered *moderate* if the person has third-degree burns on 2% to 10% of body surface area or second-degree burns on 15% to 25% of body surface area.

Other important factors

To help evaluate the burn, the doctor also considers these factors:
- location (burns on the face, hands, feet, and genitalia are most serious because of possible loss of function; burns on the neck can cause a blocked breathing passage; those on the chest can impede lung expansion)
- history of complicating medical problems
- other injuries sustained at the time of the burn
- victim's age (those under age 4 or over age 60 have more complications and, consequently, a higher death rate)
- any lung injury from smoke inhalation.

How are they treated?

Immediate, aggressive treatment increases the person's chances of survival. In many cases, a burn victim is transferred to a specialized burn care unit within 4 hours after the burn.

In *minor burns,* the burned area is immersed in a cool saline solution or covered with cool compresses. The devitalized tissue is surgically cleaned, and the wound is covered with an antibiotic ointment and a dressing. The victim receives pain medication, protection against tetanus, and home care instructions.

In *moderate and major burns,* the victim's airway, breathing, and circulation are stabilized. The health care team assesses for signs of smoke inhalation and respiratory damage, such as singed nasal hairs, burns inside the nostrils, and soot in the mouth or nose. Bleeding is controlled and smoldering clothing is removed. The burns are covered with a clean, dry, sterile bed sheet. Intravenous fluids are given to prevent shock and maintain circulation. A nasogastric tube is inserted to decompress the stomach and prevent the victim from inhaling stomach contents.

Electrical and chemical burns demand special attention. Tissue damage from electrical burns is hard to assess because internal destruction is usually greater than the surface burn would indicate. Electrical burns that ignite the victim's clothes may cause thermal burns as well. If the electric shock caused dangerous heart rhythm disturbances and cardiac and respiratory arrest, CPR must begin at once.

In a chemical burn, the wound is irrigated with large amounts of water or normal saline solution. If the chemical entered the victim's eyes, the eyes are flushed for at least 30 minutes, then covered with a dry, sterile dressing. An emergency eye exam is done. (See *Caring for minor burns.*)

COLD INJURIES

What are these conditions?

Cold injuries result from overexposure to cold air or water. They occur in two major forms: localized injuries such as frostbite and generalized injuries such as hypothermia (a core body temperature below 95° F, or 35° C). Untreated or improperly treated frostbite can lead to gangrene and may require amputation; severe hypothermia can be fatal.

PREVENTION
TIPS

Preventing cold injuries

To prevent frostbite, stay indoors when the temperature drops well below freezing. If you must go outside, follow these guidelines to help avoid frostbite and other cold injuries:

- Wear mittens, not gloves, in cold weather. (Mittens hold the fingers together, keeping them warm.)
- Wear windproof, water-resistant, many-layered clothing.
- Wear two pairs of socks — cotton next to the skin, then wool — and a scarf and a hat that cover your ears to avoid substantial heat loss through the head.
- Before prolonged exposure, don't drink alcohol or smoke, and be sure to get adequate food and rest.
- If caught in a severe snowstorm, find shelter early or increase your physical activity.

What causes them?

Localized cold injuries occur when ice crystals form in the tissues and expand extracellular spaces. With compression of the tissue cell, the cell membrane ruptures.

Frostbite results from prolonged exposure to dry temperatures far below freezing. Hypothermia results from near drowning in cold water and from prolonged exposure to cold temperatures. It causes chemical changes that slow the functioning of most major organs such as the kidneys. (See *Preventing cold injuries.*)

The risk of serious cold injuries, especially hypothermia, is increased by youth, lack of insulating body fat, wet or inadequate clothing, old age, drug abuse, heart disease, smoking, fatigue, hunger and depletion of caloric reserves, and excessive alcohol intake (which draws blood into capillaries and away from body organs).

What are their symptoms?

Frostbite may be superficial or deep. Superficial frostbite affects the skin — especially of the face, ears, arms, legs, and other exposed body areas — and tissue under the skin. Frostbite may go unnoticed at first, but when the person returns to a warm place, he or she will experience burning, tingling, numbness, swelling, and a mottled, blue-gray skin color.

Deep frostbite extends beyond tissue under the skin and usually affects the hands or feet. The skin becomes white until it's thawed; then it turns purplish blue. Deep frostbite also produces pain, skin blisters, tissue deterioration, and gangrene.

Signs and symptoms of hypothermia vary with the disorder's severity:

- *mild hypothermia:* body temperature of 89.6° to 95° F (32° to 35° C), severe shivering, slurred speech, and amnesia
- *moderate hypothermia:* body temperature of 86° to 89.6° F (30° to 32° C), unresponsiveness or confusion, muscle rigidity, peripheral bluish skin discoloration and, with improper rewarming, signs of shock
- *severe hypothermia:* body temperature of 77° to 86° F (25° to 30° C), loss of deep tendon reflexes, and ventricular fibrillation. The person may appear dead, with no palpable pulse or audible heart sounds. The pupils may dilate, and the person may appear to be in a state of rigor mortis. A temperature drop below 77° F (25° C) causes cardiac arrest and death.

How are they diagnosed?

A history of severe and prolonged exposure to cold may make this diagnosis obvious. Nevertheless, hypothermia can be overlooked if outdoor temperatures are above freezing or if the person is comatose.

How are they treated?

Treatment depends on the severity of the injury. In a localized cold injury, treatment consists of rewarming the injured part, supportive measures, and sometimes removal of connective tissue to increase circulation. However, if gangrene occurs, amputation may be necessary. In hypothermia, therapy consists of immediate resuscitative measures, careful monitoring, and gradual rewarming of the body.

CONCUSSION

What is this condition?

By far the most common head injury, a concussion results from a blow to the head. The blow is hard enough to jostle the brain and knock it against the skull, causing temporary nerve dysfunction, but not hard enough to bruise the brain.

Most concussion victims recover completely within 24 to 48 hours. But repeated concussions take a cumulative toll on the brain.

What causes it?

The blow that causes a concussion is usually sudden and forceful — a fall to the ground, a punch to the head, a car accident. (Such a blow sometimes results from child abuse.) Whatever the cause, the resulting injury is mild compared to the damage done by more serious head injuries, such as brain contusions (bruises) and lacerations (tears).

What are its symptoms?

A concussion may cause a brief loss of consciousness, vomiting, and a type of amnesia in which the person not only can't recall what happened just after the injury but also has trouble recalling events that led up to the incident.

What to do after a concussion

You've suffered a concussion that doesn't appear to have caused any serious brain injury. But for safety's sake, follow these instructions.

Watch for symptoms

- Return to the hospital immediately if you experience a persistent or worsening headache, forceful or constant vomiting, blurred vision, any change in personality, abnormal eye movements, staggering gait, twitching, confusion, or excessive sleepiness.
- Don't take anything stronger than Tylenol (or another drug containing acetaminophen) for a headache.
- If vomiting occurs, eat only light meals until it stops. (*Occasional* vomiting is normal after a concussion.)
- Relax for 24 hours. Then, if you feel well, resume normal activities.

Plan for emergencies

Give this note to your parents, guardian, spouse, or roommate: *Wake me every 2 hours during the night, and ask me my name, where I am, and whether or not I can identify you. If you can't awaken me, if I can't answer these questions, or if I have seizures, take me back to the hospital immediately.*

A concussion often causes adults to be irritable or sluggish, to behave out of character, and to complain of dizziness, nausea, or severe headache. Some children have no apparent ill effects, but many grow sluggish and sleepy in a few hours. All of these signs are normal in a concussion. For a few weeks after the injury, the person may have postconcussion syndrome — headache, dizziness, anxiety, and fatigue.

How is it diagnosed?

To rule out more serious head injuries, the doctor obtains a thorough history of the injury and performs a neurologic exam, evaluating the victim's level of consciousness, mental status, nerve and motor functions, reflexes, and orientation to time, place, and person. A computed tomography scan (commonly called a CAT scan) may be done to rule out skull fractures and more serious injuries.

How is it treated?

A thorough history of the injury is crucial to treatment. The health care team obtains the history from the person (if amnesia isn't a factor), the family, eyewitnesses, or ambulance personnel. Of special interest is whether loss of consciousness occurred. If so, the person is monitored closely and checked for other injuries.

If a neurologic exam reveals no abnormalities, the person is observed in the emergency room. If he's stable after 4 or more hours of observation, he's discharged (with a head injury instruction sheet) in the care of a responsible adult. (See *What to do after a concussion*.)

DISLOCATIONS AND SUBLUXATIONS

What are these conditions?

Dislocations displace joint bones so their surfaces totally lose contact; subluxations partially displace the articulating surfaces. Dislocations and subluxations occur at the joints of the shoulders, elbows, wrists, fingers, toes, hips, knees, ankles, and feet; they may accompany fractures of these joints or result in deposition of fracture fragments between joint surfaces. Prompt reduction (restoring the displaced bones to their proper position) can limit the resulting damage to soft tissue, nerves, and blood vessels. (See *Common dislocation*.)

What causes them?

A dislocation or subluxation may be congenital (as in congenital dis-location of the hip), or it may follow trauma or disease of surround-ing joint tissues (for example, Paget's disease).

What are their symptoms?

Dislocations and subluxations produce deformity around the joint, change the length of the involved extremity, impair joint mobility, and cause tenderness. When the injury results from trauma, it is ex-tremely painful and often accompanies joint surface fractures. Even in the absence of accompanying fracture, the displaced bone may damage surrounding muscles, ligaments, nerves, and blood vessels, and may cause bone deterioration.

How are they diagnosed?

The person's history, X-rays, and physical exam rule out or confirm a fracture.

How are they treated?

Immediate reduction (before tissue swelling and muscle spasm make it difficult) can prevent additional damage. Closed reduction consists of manual traction under general anesthesia (or local anesthesia and sedatives). During this procedure, intravenous morphine controls pain, and intravenous Versed controls muscle spasm and facilitates muscle stretching during traction. Some injuries require open reduc-tion under regional block or general anesthesia. Such surgery may in-clude wire fixation of the joint, skeletal traction, and ligament repair.

After reduction, a splint, cast, or traction immobilizes the joint. Generally, immobilizing the fingers or toes for 2 weeks, hips for 6 to 8 weeks, and other dislocated joints for 3 to 6 weeks allows surround-ing ligaments to heal.

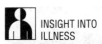
INSIGHT INTO ILLNESS

Common dislocation

These illustrations show the dif-ference between a normal el-bow joint and one that's been dislocated — a common injury.

NORMAL ELBOW JOINT

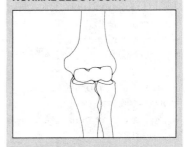

DISLOCATED ELBOW JOINT

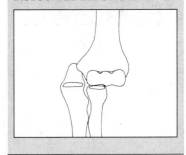

ELECTRIC SHOCK

What is this condition?

Electric shock occurs when an electric current passes through the body. The victim's prognosis depends on the site and extent of dam-

Factors affecting the severity of an electric shock

Electric shock may cause an extremely dangerous heart rhythm disturbance called *ventricular fibrillation,* respiratory paralysis, burns, or death. The severity of the injury depends on the following factors:
- the intensity of the current (amperes, milliamperes, or microamperes)
- the resistance of the tissues it passes through
- the kind of current (AC, DC, or mixed)
- the frequency and duration of current flow.

age, his or her state of health, and the speed and adequacy of treatment. In North America, over 1,000 people die of electric shock each year. (See *Factors affecting the severity of an electric shock.*)

What causes it?

Electric shock usually results from accidental contact with exposed parts of electrical appliances or wiring. (See *Safeguarding your home from electric shock.*) But sometimes it's caused by lightning or the flash of electric arcs from high-voltage power lines or machines.

Electric current can cause injury in three ways:
- true electrical injury as the current passes through the body
- arc or flash burns from current that doesn't pass through the body
- thermal surface burns caused by associated heat and flames.

What are its symptoms?

Severe electric shock usually causes muscle contraction, followed by unconsciousness and loss of reflex control. Sometimes the injury paralyzes the respiratory system. After momentary shock, the muscles contract and the person hyperventilates. Passage of even the smallest electric current — if it passes through the heart — may cause an irregular heart rhythm that eventually progresses to cardiac arrest.

Electric shock from a high-frequency current usually causes burns and localized tissue destruction. Low-frequency currents can also cause serious burns if contact with the current is concentrated in a small area — for example, when a toddler bites into an electric cord.

During the shock, the victim may also suffer bruises, fractures, and other injuries as a result of violent muscle contractions or falls. Later, his kidneys may shut down. A severe electric shock may lead to lasting hearing impairment, cataracts, and vision loss.

How is it diagnosed?

Usually, the cause of electrical injuries is either obvious or suspected. To guide treatment, the doctor tries to find out the voltage of the current source and how long the victim was in contact with it.

How is it treated?

First, the victim must be separated from the current source. If rescuers can't immediately turn off or unplug the source, they pull the victim free with a nonconductive device, such as a loop of dry cloth or rubber, a dry rope, or a leather belt.

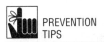

PREVENTION TIPS

Safeguarding your home from electric shock

Electrical hazards in your home can cause a potentially deadly injury. These guidelines can help you identify and correct such hazards:

- If you have small children, put safety guards on all electrical outlets and keep children away from electrical devices.
- Don't use electrical appliances while showering or wet.
- *Never* touch electrical appliances while touching faucets or cold water pipes in the kitchen because these pipes often provide the ground connection for all circuits in the house.
- Check for cuts, cracks, or frayed insulation on electric cords and appliances. Keep these away from hot or wet surfaces and sharp corners.

- Don't set glasses of water, damp towels, or other wet items on electrical equipment. Wipe up accidental spills before they leak into electrical equipment.
- Avoid using extension cords because they may bypass the ground. If they're absolutely necessary, don't place them under carpeting or in areas where they'll be walked on.
- Make sure ground connections on electrical equipment are intact. Line cord plugs should have three prongs; the prongs should be straight and firmly fixed. Check that prongs fit wall outlets properly and that outlets aren't loose or broken. Don't use adapters on plugs.
- If an appliance sparks, smokes, seems unusually hot, or gives you a slight shock, unplug it immediately.

Then emergency treatment begins. Rescuers quickly assess the victim's vital signs. If they don't detect a pulse or breathing, they start CPR at once and continue it until vital signs return or emergency help arrives with life-support equipment. The victim's heart rhythm is monitored continuously and an electrocardiogram is taken.

After the victim arrives at the hospital, intravenous fluids and drugs are typically given to prevent kidney failure and to combat the effects of widespread tissue destruction. Neurologic status is monitored closely because electric shock can damage the central nervous system.

To help prevent infection, the victim may undergo surgical wound cleaning and receive antibiotics. For some wounds, skin grafts or even amputation may be necessary.

*H*EAT *SYNDROME*

What is this condition?

Heat syndrome may result from any environmental or internal condition that increases heat production or impairs heat dissipation.

There are three types of heat syndromes: heat cramps, heat exhaustion, and heatstroke.

What causes it?

Normally, people adjust to high temperatures by complex cardiovascular and neurologic changes. Heat loss offsets heat production to regulate body temperature. The body does this by evaporation (sweating) or by dilation of blood vessels, which cool the body's surface.

However, heat production increases with exercise, infection, and drugs such as amphetamines. Heat loss decreases with high temperatures or humidity, lack of acclimatization, excess clothing, obesity, dehydration, cardiovascular disease, sweat gland dysfunction, and use of certain drugs, such as phenothiazines and anticholinergics. So when heat loss mechanisms fail to offset heat production, the body retains heat and may develop heat syndrome.

Heat syndrome may result from any environmental or internal condition that increases heat production or impairs heat dissipation.

How is it prevented?

Heat illnesses are easily preventable. The following information is especially vital for athletes, laborers, and soldiers in field training:
- Avoid heat syndrome by taking the following precautions in hot weather: wear loose-fitting, lightweight clothing; rest frequently; avoid hot places; and drink plenty of fluids.
- Avoid getting overheated, especially if you're obese, elderly, or taking drugs that impair heat regulation.
- If you've had heat cramps or heat exhaustion, exercise gradually and increase your salt and water intake.
- If you've had heatstroke, be aware that sensitivity to high temperatures may persist for several months.

JAW DISLOCATION OR FRACTURE

What is this condition?

A dislocation of the jaw is a displacement of the temporomandibular joint. A fracture of the jaw is a break in one or both of the two maxillae (upper jawbones) or the mandible (lower jawbone). Treatment can usually restore jaw alignment and function.

What causes it?

Simple fractures or dislocations are usually caused by a manual blow along the jawline. More serious compound fractures often result from car accidents.

What are its symptoms?

Incorrect closure of the jaw is the most obvious sign of dislocation or fracture. Other signs include mandibular pain, swelling, loss of function, and asymmetry. In addition, mandibular fractures can produce numbness and tingling or loss of sensation in the chin and lower lip. Maxillary fractures produce numbness and tingling around the eyes and often accompany fractures of the nose and the eye's orbit.

How is it diagnosed?

Abnormal maxillary or mandibular mobility detected during the physical exam and a history of traumatic injury suggest fracture or dislocation. X-rays confirm it.

How is it treated?

As in all traumatic injuries, steps are taken to preserve the person's airway, breathing, and circulation. Then he or she is evaluated for other injuries and may receive pain relievers.

After the person's condition stabilizes, surgical reduction and fixation by wiring restores mandibular and maxillary alignment. Maxillary fractures may also require reconstruction and repair of soft-tissue injuries.

Teeth and bones are rarely removed during surgery. If the person has lost teeth from the injury, the surgeon will decide whether they can be replanted. If so, they'll be replanted within 6 hours, while they're still capable of living. Viability is increased if the teeth are placed in milk.

NASAL FRACTURE

What is this condition?

The most common facial fracture, a fractured nose usually results from blunt injury and is often associated with other facial fractures.

Caring for a fractured nose

As swelling from the injury increases, you'll find breathing more difficult. The following measures can help you cope:
• Breathe slowly through your mouth.
• In cold weather, cover your mouth with a handkerchief or scarf to help warm the air you inhale.
• Don't blow your nose. This prevents subcutaneous emphysema and intracranial air penetration (and potential meningitis).
• Be aware that bruising should fade after about 2 weeks.

The severity of the fracture depends on the direction, force, and type of the blow. A severe, comminuted fracture (one with several breaks in the bone) may cause extreme swelling or bleeding that may jeopardize the airway and require tracheotomy during early treatment. Inadequate or delayed treatment may cause permanent nasal displacement, septal deviation, and obstruction.

What are its symptoms?
A nosebleed may occur immediately after the injury, and swelling may quickly obscure the break. After several hours, pain, bruises around the eyes, and nasal displacement and deformity are prominent.

How is it diagnosed?
Palpation, X-rays, and clinical findings, such as a deviated septum, confirm a nasal fracture. Diagnosis also requires a full history, including the cause of the injury and the amount of nasal bleeding.

How is it treated?
Treatment restores normal facial appearance and reestablishes the nasal passages after swelling subsides. Reduction of the fracture (restoring the bone fragments to their proper position) corrects alignment; immobilization (intranasal packing and an external splint shaped to fit the nose) maintains it.

Reduction is best accomplished in the operating room under local anesthesia for adults and general anesthesia for children. Severe swelling may delay treatment. (See *Caring for a fractured nose*.)

NEAR DROWNING

What is this condition?
Near drowning refers to surviving — temporarily, at least — the effects of hypoxemia and acidosis that result from a person's submersion in fluid.

Near drowning occurs in three forms: "dry" — the victim doesn't aspirate fluid but suffers respiratory obstruction or lack of oxygen (10% to 15% of cases); "wet" — the victim aspirates fluid and suffers from lack of oxygen or secondary changes due to fluid aspiration (about 85% of cases); and secondary — the victim suffers recurrence of respiratory distress (usually aspiration pneumonia or pulmonary edema) within minutes or 1 to 2 days after the near-drowning incident.

In North America, drowning claims roughly 8,000 lives annually. No statistics are available for near-drowning incidents.

What causes it?

Near drowning results from an inability to swim or, in swimmers, from panic, a boating accident, a heart attack, or a blow to the head while in the water; from drinking heavily before swimming; or from a suicide attempt.

Hypoxemia (insufficient oxygen in the blood) is the most serious consequence of near drowning, followed by metabolic acidosis. Other consequences depend on the kind of water aspirated.

What are its symptoms?

Near-drowning victims can display a host of problems: disrupted breathing, shallow or gasping respirations, chest pain, cardiac standstill, rapid or slow heart rate, restlessness, irritability, lack of energy, fever, confusion, unconsciousness, vomiting, abdominal distention, and a cough that produces a pink, frothy fluid.

How is it diagnosed?

Diagnosis requires a history of near drowning, characteristic signs and symptoms, and detection of abnormal breath sounds with a stethoscope.

How is it treated?

Emergency treatment begins with CPR, administration of oxygen, and stabilization of the neck in case of cervical injury. When the person arrives at the hospital, the airway is assessed and a patent airway is established if necessary. CPR continues and the person may be intubated and receive respiratory assistance, such as mechanical ventilation with positive end-expiratory pressure, if needed.

Much controversy exists about the benefits of drug treatment for near-drowning victims. Such treatment may include baking soda for acidosis, corticosteroids for cerebral swelling, antibiotics to prevent infections, and bronchodilators to ease bronchospasms.

Near drowning results from an inability to swim or, in swimmers, from panic, a boating accident, a heart attack, or a blow to the head while in the water; drinking heavily before swimming; or a suicide attempt.

All near-drowning victims are hospitalized for an observation period of 24 to 48 hours because of the possibility of recurring respiratory distress.

To *prevent* near drowning, swimmers should avoid drinking alcohol before swimming, observe water safety measures, and take a water safety course sponsored by the Red Cross or YMCA.

OPEN WOUNDS

What are these conditions?

Open wounds include abrasions, avulsions, crush wounds, lacerations, missile injuries, and puncture wounds. They often result from home, work, or motor vehicle accidents and from acts of violence.

Abrasions (scrapes) are open surface wounds in which the nerve endings are exposed. In *avulsions,* the injured part is torn away from the body and the wound edges don't close. Avulsions are most common on the nose tip, earlobe, fingertip, and penis. In *crush wounds,* the skin is split and underlying tissues, such as bones, tendons, and nerves, are damaged. In *lacerations,* the skin is torn and the open wound may extend into the deep epithelium (the tissue layer covering the body's surface). *Missile injuries* involve high-velocity tissue penetration. *Puncture wounds* are small-entry wounds that probably damage underlying structures.

What causes them?

Abrasions result from friction. Avulsions occur when the skin is cut, gouged, or completely torn. Crush wounds result when a heavy falling object splits the skin. Lacerations result from penetration with a knife or other sharp object or from a severe blow with a blunt object. Missile injuries typically are caused by gunshot wounds; puncture wounds, by sharp, pointed objects.

How are they diagnosed?

An open wound is usually obvious. The doctor assesses the extent of the injury, looks for obvious bone damage, and evaluates the person's vital signs, level of consciousness, neurologic and musculoskeletal status, and general condition. An accurate history of the injury is obtained from the person or witnesses, including the mechanism and time of the injury and any treatment already provided.

How are they treated?

Most open wounds require emergency treatment. If the person is bleeding, direct pressure is applied to the wound and, if necessary, to arterial pressure points. If the wound is on an arm or a leg, the limb is raised, if possible. (A tourniquet is applied only if there's massive bleeding.) If necessary, surgery is done to repair the wound and related damage.

PENETRATING CHEST WOUNDS

What are these conditions?

Penetrating chest wounds may cause varying degrees of damage to bones, soft tissue, blood vessels, and nerves. They also may result in death, depending on the size and severity of the wound.

Gunshot wounds are usually more serious than stab wounds, because they cause more severe tears and rapid blood loss and because a ricocheting bullet often damages large areas and several organs. With prompt, aggressive treatment, up to 90% of people with penetrating chest wounds recover.

What causes them?

Stab wounds from a knife or an ice pick are the most common penetrating chest wounds; gunshot wounds are a close second. Wartime explosions or firearms fired at close range are the usual source of large, gaping wounds.

What are their symptoms?

In addition to the obvious chest injuries, penetrating chest wounds can also cause:
- a sucking sound as the diaphragm contracts and air enters the chest cavity through the opening in the chest wall
- varying levels of consciousness, depending on the extent of the injury. (A person who is awake and alert may be in severe pain, which will cause splinted respirations, thereby reducing vital capacity.)

Gunshot wounds are usually more serious than stab wounds — because they cause more severe lacerations and result in rapid blood loss and because a ricocheting bullet often damages large areas and several organs.

- rapid heart rate due to anxiety and blood loss
- weak, thready pulse due to massive blood loss and hypovolemic shock.

How are they diagnosed?
An obvious chest wound and a sucking sound during breathing confirm the diagnosis.

How are they treated?
Penetrating chest wounds require immediate support of respiration and circulation, prompt surgical repair, and measures to prevent complications.

PERFORATED EARDRUM

What is this condition?
A perforation of the eardrum is a rupture of the thin membrane that separates the ear canal from the middle ear. Such injury may cause middle ear infection and hearing loss.

What causes it?
The usual cause of a perforated eardrum is an injury: the deliberate or accidental insertion of sharp objects (cotton swabs, bobby pins) in the ear or sudden excessive changes in pressure (explosion, a blow to the head, flying, or diving). The injury may also result from an untreated middle ear infection and, in children, from an acute middle ear infection.

What are its symptoms?
A sudden, severe earache and bleeding from the ear are the first signs of a perforated eardrum. Other symptoms include hearing loss, ringing in the ears, and dizziness. A pus-filled discharge within 24 to 48 hours of injury signals infection.

How is it diagnosed?

Severe earache and bleeding from the ear with a history of traumatic injury strongly suggest a perforated eardrum. The direct visualization of the perforated tympanic membrane with an otoscope confirms it.

How is it treated?

If the ear is bleeding, blood is absorbed with a sterile, cotton-tipped applicator and the person is checked for pus-filled drainage or evidence of cerebrospinal fluid leakage. A culture of the specimen may be ordered.

A sterile dressing is applied over the outer ear, and the person is referred to an ear specialist. A large perforation with uncontrolled bleeding may require immediate surgery to approximate the ruptured edges. Treatment may include a mild pain reliever, a sedative to decrease anxiety, and an oral antibiotic.

What can a person with a perforated eardrum do?

Don't blow your nose or get water in your ear canal until the perforation heals.

POISONING

What is this condition?

In North America, approximately 10 million people are poisoned annually, and more than 4,000 of them die. The prognosis depends on the amount of poison absorbed, its toxicity, and the time interval between poisoning and treatment.

What causes it?

Because of their curiosity and ignorance, children are the main victims of poisoning. Accidental poisoning — usually from ingestion of aspirin or Tylenol (or another drug containing acetaminophen), cleaning agents, insecticides, paints, or cosmetics — is the fourth leading cause of death in children. (See *Protecting your family from accidental poisoning.*)

In adults, poisoning is most common among chemical company employees, particularly those in companies that use chlorine, carbon

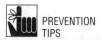 PREVENTION TIPS

Protecting your family from accidental poisoning

Curiosity can be lethal to a child exploring the contents of household containers. Take these basic precautions to reduce poisoning risks in your home.

Medicines

• Store all medicines properly, and keep them out of the reach of children.

• Don't take medicine in front of young children, and don't call medicine "candy" to get them to take it.

• Discard old or expired medications.

• Read the label before taking any medicine.

• Don't take medicines prescribed for someone else, and don't transfer medicines from their original bottles to other containers without labeling them properly.

Household chemicals

• Use toxic sprays only in well-ventilated areas and follow label instructions carefully. Store chemicals properly; don't put unused portions in old food containers.

• Use pesticides carefully and keep the telephone number of the poison control center handy.

Common poisonous plants

Elephant ear philodendron
Symptoms: burning throat, gastro-intestinal distress
Treatment: stomach pumping or induced vomiting, antihistamines and lime juice, treatment of symptoms

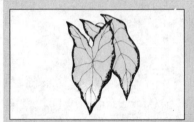

Dieffenbachia
Symptoms: burning throat, swelling, gastrointestinal distress
Treatment: stomach pumping or induced vomiting, antihistamines and lime juice, treatment of symptoms

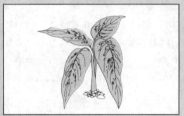

Rhubarb leaves
Symptoms: gastrointestinal and respiratory distress, internal bleeding, coma
Treatment: stomach pumping or induced vomiting with lime water; Kalcinate and forced fluids

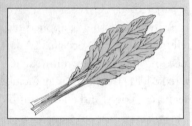

Mistletoe
Symptoms: gastrointestinal distress, slow pulse
Treatment: stomach pumping or induced vomiting, cardiac drugs, potassium, and sodium

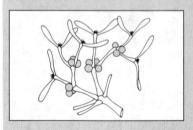

Mushrooms
Symptoms: gastrointestinal, respiratory, and nervous system effects; excessive salivation; sweating; slow pulse; low blood pressure
Treatment: induced vomiting, purging with saline solution, Atropisol

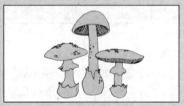

Poinsettia (milky juice)
Symptoms: inflammation, blisters
Treatment: none; condition will disappear after several days

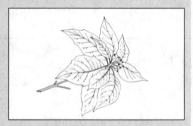

Poison ivy, poison sumac, poison oak (sap)
Symptoms: allergic skin reactions; if ingested, gastrointestinal distress, liver and kidney damage
Treatment: if ingested, balms, morphine, fluids, high-protein, low-fat diet; for skin reactions, antihistamines, topical drugs to reduce fever

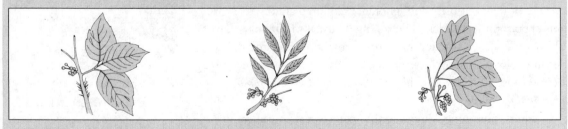

Poisonous parts of the plant are shaded. If the poisonous part can't be shown, it appears in parentheses after the name.

dioxide, hydrogen sulfide, nitrogen dioxide, and ammonia, and in companies that ignore safety standards. Other causes of poisoning in adults include improper cooking, canning, and storage of food; ingestion of, or skin contamination from, plants; and drug overdose (usually barbiturates). (See *Common poisonous plants.*)

What are its symptoms?
Symptoms vary according to the poison.

How is it diagnosed?
A history of internal or external contamination by a poisonous substance and typical clinical features suggest the diagnosis. Poisoning is suspected in any unconscious person with no history of diabetes, seizure disorders, or traumatic injury.

Lab studies (including drug screens) of poison levels in the mouth, vomit, urine, feces, or blood or on the victim's hands or clothing confirm the diagnosis. If possible, the poisoned person or his family should bring the container holding the poison to the emergency room for comparison study. In inhalation poisoning, chest X-rays may show pulmonary infiltrates or swelling; in petroleum distillate inhalation, X-rays may show aspiration pneumonia.

How is it treated?
Treatment includes emergency resuscitation, prevention of further absorption of poison, continuing supportive or symptomatic care and, when possible, a specific antidote. If barbiturate, glutethimide, or tranquilizer poisoning causes hypothermia, a hyperthermia blanket is used to control the person's temperature.

*P*OISONOUS SNAKEBITES

What are these conditions?
Each year, poisonous snakes bite about 7,000 people in North America. Such bites are most common during summer afternoons, in grassy or rocky habitats.

Poisonous snakebites are medical emergencies. However, with prompt, correct treatment, they need not be fatal.

What causes them?

The most common poisonous snakes in North America are pit vipers and coral snakes. Both of these snakes are nocturnal, but pit vipers are more active, so their bites are more common.

Pit vipers include rattlesnakes, water moccasins (cottonmouths), and copperheads. They have a pitted depression between their eyes and nostrils, and two fangs ¾ of an inch to 1¼ inches (1.9 to 3.2 centimeters) long. Because fangs may break off or grow behind old ones, some snakes may have one, three, or four fangs.

The fangs of coral snakes are short but have teeth behind them. Coral snakes have distinctive red, black, and yellow bands (yellow bands always border red ones), tend to bite with a chewing motion, and may leave multiple fang marks, small lacerations, and much tissue destruction.

What are their symptoms?

Most snakebites occur on the arms and legs, below the elbow or knee. Bites to the head or trunk are most dangerous, but any bite into a blood vessel is dangerous, regardless of location.

Pit viper bites

Most poisonous pit viper bites cause immediate and progressively severe pain and swelling (the entire limb may swell within a few hours), local elevation in skin temperature, fever, skin discoloration, red or purple skin spots, bruises, blebs, blisters, bloody wound discharge, and localized tissue death.

Pit viper bites may cause local and facial numbness and tingling, bundling and twitching of skeletal muscles, seizures (especially in children), extreme anxiety, difficulty speaking, fainting, weakness, dizziness, excessive sweating, occasional paralysis, mild to severe respiratory distress, headache, blurred vision, marked thirst and, in severe envenomation, coma and death. Pit viper venom may also impair blood clotting and cause vomiting of blood, blood in the urine and stools, bleeding gums, and internal bleeding. Other symptoms of pit viper bites include nausea, vomiting, diarrhea, rapid heart rate, lymphadenopathy, low blood pressure, and shock. (See *First aid for poisonous snakebites*.)

Coral snakebites

The reaction to coral snakebites is usually delayed — perhaps up to several hours. These bites cause little or no local pain, swelling, or deterioration. However, because their venom is toxic to the nervous

Each year, poisonous snakes bite about 7,000 people in North America... Poisonous snakebites are medical emergencies.

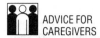

ADVICE FOR
CAREGIVERS

First aid for poisonous snakebites

After a poisonous snakebite, prompt, appropriate first aid can reduce venom absorption and prevent severe symptoms. To help ensure proper care of a snakebite victim, follow these guidelines:

- If possible, identify the snake, but don't waste time trying to find it.
- Immediately immobilize the victim's affected limb below heart level. Have him lie on his back to slow venom metabolism and absorption, and instruct him to remain as quiet as possible.
- If you have a snakebite kit, administer Antivenin.
- If the victim is more than 1 hour away from a hospital, wash the skin over the fang marks.

Applying a tourniquet

Experts disagree about whether a constrictive tourniquet (band) should be placed on the affected limb. But if the victim is far from a medical facility, this may be appropriate.

Important: The use of a tourniquet should never delay Antivenin administration.

If a tourniquet is indicated, apply it so that it's slightly constrictive but loose enough to allow a finger between the band and the skin. Place it about 4 inches (10 centimeters) above the fang marks or just above the first joint between the bite and the victim's trunk. Once the tourniquet is in place, don't remove it until the victim is examined by a doctor.

Caution: Don't apply a tourniquet if more than 30 minutes have elapsed since the bite. And never keep a tourniquet on for more than 2 hours. The victim may lose his limb if the tourniquet is too tight or if it's in place too long.

After applying the tourniquet, check the victim's pulses beyond the tourniquet regularly. If needed, loosen the tourniquet slightly to maintain circulation.

Caring for a pit viper bite

Within 15 minutes of a pit viper bite, make an incision through the fang marks approximately ½ inch (1.3 centimeters) long and ⅛ inch (0.3 centimeter) deep. Be especially careful if the bite is on the hand, where blood vessels and tendons are close to the skin surface.

If you don't have Antivenin, apply suction (preferably with a bulb syringe or, if necessary, with your mouth) to the wound for up to 2 hours.

Important: An incision and suction are effective only in pit viper bites and only within 15 minutes of the bite. Also, *don't* apply mouth suction if you have oral ulcers, if the victim is close to a medical facility, or if Antivenin can be given promptly.

Some important *don'ts*

- *Don't* give the victim any food, beverage, or medication by mouth. Alcoholic drinks and stimulants are especially dangerous because they speed venom absorption.
- *Don't* apply ice to a snakebite because it will increase tissue damage.

system, a reaction can progress swiftly, producing such effects as local numbness and tingling, drowsiness, nausea, vomiting, difficulty swallowing and speaking, marked salivation, drooping eyelid, blurred vision, pupil contraction, respiratory distress and possible respiratory failure, loss of muscle coordination and, perhaps, shock and cardiovascular collapse, leading to death.

How are they diagnosed?

The person's history and account of the injury, observation of fang marks, snake identification (when possible), and progressive symptoms of envenomation all point to poisonous snakebite.

Lab tests, which usually include blood and urine studies, help identify the extent of poisoning and provide guidelines for supportive treatment. The person may also have a chest X-ray. In severe cases, an electrocardiogram may evaluate heart function and an electroencephalogram may be used to detect brain wave changes.

How are they treated?

Prompt treatment of a snakebite can prevent severe consequences. Most snakebite victims are hospitalized for only 24 to 48 hours. Treatment usually consists of Antivenin administration, but minor snakebites may not require Antivenin. Other treatments include tetanus toxoid or human tetanus immune globulin; various broad-spectrum antibiotics; and, depending on the person's respiratory status, the severity of pain, and the type of snakebite, Tylenol, codeine, morphine, or Demerol. (Narcotics are prohibited in coral snakebites.)

Usually, snakebites that cause tissue death need surgical wound cleaning after 3 or 4 days. Intense, rapidly progressive swelling requires removal of damaged tissue within 2 or 3 hours of the bite; extreme envenomation may require limb amputation and subsequent reconstructive surgery, rehabilitation, and physical therapy.

SKULL FRACTURES

What are these conditions?

Skull fractures are fractures of one or more bones of the head. They're considered serious neurosurgical conditions not so much because of damage to the skull itself but because they may lead to brain damage.

Classifying fractures

Skull fractures may be *simple* (closed) or *compound* (open). They are also usually described as linear, comminuted, or depressed. Some fractures, such as cranial vault fractures or basilar fractures, are described in terms of their location.

A *linear fracture* is a common hairline break that doesn't displace bone fragments and seldom requires emergency treatment. It's the least likely fracture type to be fatal. A *comminuted fracture* splinters or crushes the bone into several fragments. A *depressed fracture* pushes the bone toward the brain. It's considered serious only if it compresses underlying structures. A child's thin, elastic skull allows a depression without a fracture.

A *cranial vault fracture* involves the domelike part of the skull, whereas a *basilar fracture* occurs at the base of the skull. Because of the danger of grave complications and meningitis (inflammation of the brain lining), basilar fractures are usually far more serious than cranial vault fractures.

What causes them?

Skull fractures are caused by a blow to the head. Car accidents, bad falls, and severe beatings (especially in children) top the list of causes.

What are their symptoms?

Linear fractures associated only with concussion don't cause loss of consciousness. But a fracture that bruises or lacerates the brain may cause the classic signs of brain injury: agitation, irritability, loss of consciousness, labored breathing or other respiratory changes, abnormal reflexes, altered pupil responses, and motor abnormalities.

If a person with a skull fracture remains conscious, he's apt to complain of a persistent, localized headache. A skull fracture may also cause brain swelling, which may impede the normal flow of impulses to the brain and eventually result in respiratory distress. Also, the person may have an altered level of consciousness, progressing to unconsciousness or even death.

If jagged bone fragments pierce far enough into the brain, bleeding or hematomas (collections of trapped blood) may occur within the brain. When this happens, the victim experiences muscle weakness or paralysis on one side of the body, unequal pupils, dizziness, seizures, projectile vomiting, decreased pulse and breathing rates, and progressive unresponsiveness.

Fractures of the sphenoid bone (at the front of the skull base) may damage the optic nerve, causing blindness. Fractures of the temporal bone (along the lower sides of the skull) may cause one-sided deafness or facial paralysis.

A basilar fracture often produces bleeding from the nose, throat, or ears; bruising under the conjunctiva (outer eye lining) and under

If a person with a skull fracture remains conscious, he's apt to complain of a persistent, localized headache. A skull fracture also may cause brain swelling, which may impede the normal flow of impulses to the brain and eventually result in respiratory distress.

the skin around the eyes ("raccoon eyes"); and bruising behind the ear, sometimes with bleeding behind the eardrum. In this fracture, spinal fluid or even brain tissue may leak from the nose or ears.

Depending on the extent of brain damage, a skull fracture may have lasting effects, such as epilepsy, hydrocephalus ("water on the brain"), and organic brain syndrome (which may result in such abnormalities as delirium, withdrawal, and dementia). Children may tire easily and develop headaches, giddiness, neuroses, and behavior disorders.

The victim of a skull fracture may also have scalp wounds, such as scrapes, bruises, and tears. If the scalp has been scraped or torn away, bleeding may be heavy because the scalp contains many blood vessels. Occasionally, bleeding is so heavy that the victim goes into shock.

How are they diagnosed?

A skull fracture is suspected in anyone with a brain injury until clinical evaluation proves otherwise. The doctor obtains a thorough history of the traumatic injury and orders a computed tomography scan (commonly called a CAT scan) and magnetic resonance imaging (known as an MRI) to try to locate the fracture and assess brain damage. A neurologic exam is crucial to evaluate brain function, level of consciousness, pupil response, motor function, and deep tendon reflexes.

To detect spinal fluid leakage, the health care team checks for drainage from the victim's nose and ears and checks the bedsheets for a blood-tinged spot surrounded by a lighter ring.

How are they treated?

Most linear skull fractures require only supportive treatment, including mild pain relievers (such as Tylenol) and cleaning of any wounds. If the person hasn't lost consciousness, he or she is observed in the emergency room for at least 4 hours. After this, if vital signs are stable and if the neurosurgeon concurs, the person is discharged with an instruction sheet to follow for 24 to 48 hours of observation at home.

More severe vault fractures, especially depressed fractures, usually require a craniotomy. In this operation, the surgeon makes an opening into the skull to elevate or remove fragments that have been driven into the brain and to remove foreign bodies and dead tissue. Doing this reduces the risk of infection and further brain damage. Other treatments for severe vault fractures include antibiotics to prevent infection and, in severe hemorrhage, blood transfusions.

Basilar fractures call for immediate use of antibiotics to prevent meningitis from spinal fluid leakage. Also, the person is observed closely for hematomas and hemorrhages. Surgery may be necessary.

Both basilar and vault fractures often call for Decadron, a steroid that helps to reduce brain swelling and minimize brain damage. Tylenol or another mild pain reliever is also given. (See *When a person with a skull fracture returns home.*)

Spinal injuries

What are these conditions?
Spinal injuries include fractures, contusions, and compressions of the vertebral column, usually the result of traumatic injury to the head or neck. The real danger lies in possible spinal cord damage.

What causes them?
Most serious spinal injuries result from motor vehicle accidents, falls, diving into shallow water, and gunshot wounds; less serious injuries, from lifting heavy objects and minor falls. Spinal dysfunction may also result from hyperparathyroidism and abnormal growths.

What are their symptoms?
The most obvious symptom of spinal injury is muscle spasm and back pain that worsens with movement. In cervical fractures, pain may produce point tenderness; in dorsal and lumbar fractures, it may radiate to other body areas such as the legs.

If the injury damages the spinal cord, signs and symptoms range from mild numbness and tingling to decreased sensation, quadriplegia (paralysis of the limbs), and shock.

The degree of functional disability depends on the level at which the cord was damaged. For example, an injury at the uppermost level of the spinal cord (known as C1) may cause a person to lose most or all sensory and motor function. This person will depend on others for daily functions, such as dressing, eating, and drinking, and will require mechanical ventilation to breathe and a wheelchair. However, if damage is in a different area of the spinal cord, the person may retain partial sensory or motor function. At best, he or she will be able to function independently or with minimal assistance.

How are they diagnosed?

Typically, the diagnosis is based on the person's history, a physical exam, X-rays and, possibly, a lumbar puncture (spinal tap), a computed tomography scan (commonly called a CAT scan), and magnetic resonance imaging (commonly called an MRI).

The history may reveal a traumatic injury, a cancerous lesion, an infection that could produce a spinal abscess, or an endocrine disorder.

The physical exam, which includes a neurologic evaluation, determines if there is cord damage and locates the level of injury. Spinal X-rays, the most important diagnostic measure, may locate a spinal fracture.

In spinal compression, a lumbar puncture may show increased cerebrospinal fluid pressure from a lesion or trauma; a CAT scan or MRI can locate the spinal mass.

How are they treated?

The primary treatment after spinal injury is immediate immobilization to stabilize the spine and prevent spinal cord damage; other measures are supportive. Cervical injuries require immobilization, using sandbags on both sides of the person's head, a hard cervical collar, or skeletal traction with skull tongs or a halo device.

Treatment of stable lumbar and dorsal fractures consists of bed rest on firm support (such as a bed board), pain relievers, and muscle relaxants until the fracture stabilizes (usually in 10 to 12 weeks). Later treatment includes exercises to strengthen the back muscles and a back brace or corset to provide support while walking. An unstable lumbar or dorsal fracture requires a plaster cast, a turning frame, and, in severe fracture, a laminectomy and spinal fusion.

When the damage results in compression of the spinal column, neurosurgery may relieve the pressure. If the cause of compression is a cancerous lesion, chemotherapy and radiation may relieve it. Surface wounds accompanying the spinal injury require a tetanus shot unless the person has recently been immunized.

If the injury causes permanent sensory and motor impairment, the person will require long-term measures. These may include bowel and bladder management (see *Understanding and preventing dysreflexia*); assistance with mobility, including an electric or manual wheelchair; assistance with dressing and eating; a mechanical ventilator; job retraining; and extensive psychological counseling.

SELF-HELP

Understanding and preventing dysreflexia

Because of your spinal cord injury, you're at risk for dysreflexia. Take a few minutes to learn about this response and how to prevent it.

What is dysreflexia?

It's a response caused by excessive sympathetic nervous system activity. The sympathetic nervous system controls how your body responds to a crisis: It raises blood pressure, speeds the heart rate, and prepares the body to fight or flee.

But in dysreflexia, pain sensations and other sensory messages from below the level of your injury can't reach your brain. This triggers an exaggerated sympathetic response that may cause an emergency. For example, your blood pressure could rise to a dangerous level and you could have seizures or a stroke.

What triggers dysreflexia?

An overfilled bladder or rectum is the most common cause. Other causes include:

- pain
- an infection or stones in the urinary tract
- sexual activity
- pressure on the testicles or the head of the penis
- skin irritation (such as a sore or cut)
- tight clothing or shoes
- an upset stomach
- a sudden change of position
- heat from the sun or a hot bath
- certain medications
- strong uterine contractions.

Recognizing and responding to an attack

Before an attack, you may have early warning signals, including blurred vision, spots before your eyes, chest pain, or a metallic taste in your mouth.

If you notice any of these, stay alert for signs of a full-blown attack: a sudden pounding headache, a stuffy nose, anxiety, and goosebumps on your skin above the spinal cord injury level. Also watch for a drooping eyelid on one side of your face, with a lack of sweating on the same side.

If you have any of these signs or symptoms, act quickly — your life may be in danger. Here's what to do (with the help of a caregiver if necessary):

- Call your doctor at once and follow his instructions exactly.
- Take the medications in your dysreflexia kit (if you have one) to lower your blood pressure.
- Sit down, or lie in bed with your head elevated.
- Empty your bladder. If you're using an indwelling catheter, look for — and remove — any kinks or clogs in the tubing. (If you routinely perform Credé's maneuver, *don't* do it at this time.)
- Check your skin for irritation, such as a rash, a burn, or an embedded foreign object. If you see a foreign object, remove it.

Preventing dysreflexia

To prevent attacks, you must avoid known triggers. Dysreflexia can occur many years after your spinal cord injury, so you'll need to follow these precautions for the rest of your life:

- Empty your bladder frequently. Routinely check the area over your bladder for fullness. (Your nurse will show you how.) If you use an indwelling catheter, inspect the tubing often for kinks and clogs.
- Establish good bowel habits. Use a stool softener if recommended.
- Try to prevent skin irritation and infections. Regularly check your skin for redness or embedded foreign objects.
- Don't smoke in bed. A cigarette burn can trigger an attack.
- If you're having pain, ask your nurse about pain-relief measures.
- Before getting into the tub or shower, make sure the water is lukewarm, not hot. (Have your caregiver do this if you can't sense temperature.)

SPRAINS AND STRAINS

What are these conditions?

A *sprain* is a complete or incomplete tear in the supporting ligaments surrounding a joint. A *strain* is an injury to a muscle or tendon. Both injuries usually heal without surgery.

What causes them?

A sprain typically results from a sharp twist. An *acute strain* is the immediate result of vigorous muscle overuse or overstress; a *chronic strain* results from repeated overuse.

What are their symptoms?

A sprain causes local pain (especially during joint movement), swelling, loss of mobility (which may not occur until several hours after the injury), and bruising from blood entering surrounding tissues. A sprained ankle is the most common joint injury.

An acute strain causes a sharp, brief pain (the person may have heard a snapping noise) and rapid swelling. When the sharp pain subsides, the muscle is tender. After several days, bruising appears. A chronic strain causes stiffness, soreness, and generalized tenderness, although these symptoms don't occur until several hours after the injury.

How are they diagnosed?

Typically, sprains and strains are diagnosed from a history of recent injury or chronic overuse, the person's symptoms, physical exam results, and an X-ray to rule out fractures.

How are they treated?

Sprains are treated by controlling pain and swelling and immobilizing the injured joint to promote healing. Immediately after the injury, swelling is controlled by raising the joint above heart level and applying ice intermittently for 12 to 48 hours. To prevent cold injury, a towel is placed between the ice pack and the skin.

To immobilize the joint, the doctor applies an elastic bandage or cast or, if the sprain is severe, a soft cast or splint. For a severe injury, the doctor may prescribe codeine or another pain medication. A sprained ankle may require training in how to walk with crutches. People with sprains seldom require hospitalization.

SELF-CARE

How to apply an elastic bandage

An elastic bandage compresses the tissues around a sprain or a strain to help prevent swelling and provide support. The directions below explain how to wrap an elastic bandage around an ankle. You can modify them for wrapping your knee, wrist, elbow, or hand.

Step 1
With one hand, hold the loose end of the elastic bandage on top of your foot between your instep and toes. With the other hand, wrap the bandage twice around your foot, gradually moving toward your ankle. Make sure to overlap the bandage in a spiral fashion.

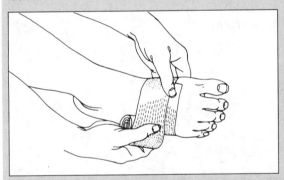

Step 2
After wrapping your foot twice, move your hand to support your heel. Use your other hand to wrap the bandage in a figure-eight fashion, leaving your heel uncovered.

To do this, angle the bandage up, cross it over the foot, and pass it behind the ankle. Next, angle the bandage down, cross it over the top of your foot, and pass it under your foot to complete the figure-eight turn. Do this step twice. (See the illustration at the top of the next column.)

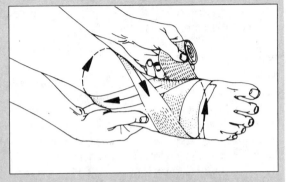

Step 3
Now circle the bandage around your calf, moving toward your knee. Overlap the elastic as you wrap. Stop just below the knee. Don't wrap downward. Secure the end of the bandage with a metal clip or adhesive tape.

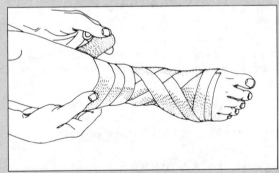

Comfort and safety tips
Aim for a snug, not a tight, fit. Never wrap the bandage so tightly that it restricts or cuts off your circulation. If you're stretching the bandage material, chances are you're wrapping it too tightly.

Promote circulation by removing and rewrapping your bandage at least twice daily.

Remove the bandage immediately if you have any numbness or tingling. When these symptoms disappear, you can reapply the bandage. If numbness or tingling doesn't stop, call your doctor.

SELF-HELP

Taking care of your knees

Now that you've hurt your knee, you're more likely to hurt it again. Here are some tips for preventing a new injury and for recognizing and caring for a knee injury should you hurt yourself again.

Preventing knee injuries

- Build up your leg muscles. Remember, the stronger your leg muscles — especially your quadriceps (front thigh muscles) and hamstrings (back thigh muscles) — the less vulnerable your knees. Try isometric exercise, weight training (using Nautilus or similar equipment), or sports, such as swimming or biking. Consult your doctor about which exercise or equipment is best for you.
- Maintain a normal weight for your height and frame. Being overweight increases your risk of injuring your knee again.
- Don't engage in sports until your strength returns and you can fully bend and stretch your knee without pain or swelling. If you start too soon, you're likely to injure your knee again.
- Until your knee fully heals, wrap it with tape or an elastic bandage when you exercise or play sports. Although this won't add strength, it may remind you to be cautious.
- Wear smooth-soled athletic shoes if you play sports on artificial turf. Don't wear cleats—they boost your injury risk by anchoring your foot to the playing surface with each step. This means your leg has less "give" when your knee comes in contact with a person, an object, or the ground.
- If you take up a new sport, choose one that fits your skills and experience, and work into it slowly. Warm up carefully with conditioning exercises, and don't try to do too much too soon. Remember — tired muscles are weak muscles. Without muscle support, your risk of another injury increases.

Recognizing a knee injury

You know your knee is injured and you should see a doctor when you:
- have pain and swelling
- feel something moving abnormally inside your knee
- wobble or sense that your knee is unstable
- hear (or someone else hears) a "pop" in your knee
- sense numbness or tingling in your toes or feet.
Important: Call your doctor without delay if this happens, even if you're not in pain.

Caring for a knee injury

If you do injure your knee again, remember the acronym "RICE," which stands for **r**est, ice, **c**ompression, **e**levation. Follow these steps to reduce pain and swelling:
- Rest your knee by getting off your feet and staying off them for at least 24 hours.
- Apply an ice pack to your knee for about 20 minutes every half hour for a day or more.
- Use a compression device, such as an elastic bandage, to support injured tissues and reduce swelling. Take care not to restrict your circulation by wrapping the bandage too tightly.
- Elevate your knee — ideally above heart level. This also helps control swelling.
- Call your doctor. Depending on your injury's severity, he may suggest removing fluid from your knee (for severe swelling and inflammation). Or he may recommend rest and isometric exercises, starting 1 to 2 days after the injury, and more active exercise, starting once pain and swelling decrease.

Acute strains are treated with pain medication and application of ice for up to 48 hours, then heat. If the muscle is completely ruptured, surgery may be required. Chronic strains usually don't need treatment, but heat application, nonsteroidal anti-inflammatory drugs (such as Advil), or a pain reliever containing a muscle relaxant can reduce discomfort.

What can a person with a sprain or strain injury do?
- Elevate the affected joint for 48 to 72 hours after the injury. (While sleeping, elevate the joint with pillows.) Apply ice intermittently for 12 to 48 hours.
- If an elastic bandage has been applied, reapply it by wrapping from below to above the injury, forming a figure eight. For a sprained ankle, apply the bandage from your toes to midcalf. Remove the bandage before going to sleep. Loosen it if it makes your leg pale, numb, or painful. (See *How to apply an elastic bandage,* page 857.)
- Call the doctor if pain worsens or persists. (See *Taking care of your knees.*) An additional X-ray may detect a fracture originally missed.
- Know that an immobilized sprain usually heals in 2 to 3 weeks; then you can gradually resume normal activities. However, if torn ligaments don't heal properly and cause recurrent dislocation, you may need surgery.

TRAUMATIC AMPUTATION

What is this condition?
Traumatic amputation is the accidental loss of a body part, usually a finger, toe, arm, or leg. In complete amputation, the part is totally severed; in partial amputation, some soft-tissue connection remains. The prognosis has improved as a result of early and improved emergency and critical care management, new surgical techniques, early rehabilitation, improved prosthesis (artificial limb) fitting, and new prosthesis design. New limb reimplantation techniques have been moderately successful, but incomplete nerve regeneration remains a major limiting factor.

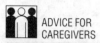

ADVICE FOR
CAREGIVERS

Saving a severed part

Suppose a family member or coworker has just lost a finger. Do you know the correct way to save the severed finger for reimplantation? What will you do if the finger is only partially amputated?

Preserving a completely amputated body part

Wrap the severed finger in saline-soaked gauze (or a clean towel), pack it in a clean plastic bag, and seal the plastic bag.

Then fill a second plastic bag with ice, place the first bag inside the ice-filled bag, seal the package, label it with the victim's name, and take it to the hospital with him. This is the first step in preserving a body part for possible reimplantation.

Once in the hospital, the body part will be cleaned and kept ice-cold until the doctor is ready to reconnect it. (Cooling delays tissue deterioration.) If reimplantation isn't planned, the part will be sent to the pathology department and disposed of according to the victim's wishes.

Caring for a partially amputated body part

If the finger is partially severed, wrap it in a clean towel and apply pressure to help control the bleeding, while keeping the finger as close as possible to its normal anatomic position.

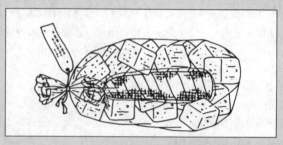

Place the victim's towel-wrapped hand in a clean plastic bag and seal it. Then fill a second plastic bag with ice. Place the bag-wrapped hand inside the ice-filled bag and seal it before having someone bring the victim to the hospital.

In the hospital, the wound will be irrigated, with the finger kept in its normal position, if possible. (The severed part should remain attached to the body, if only by a thread of skin.) Then the finger and hand will be rewrapped in a watertight bag. The injured hand will be slipped into a second bag containing ice. If necessary, the victim will be taken to a reimplantation center.

What causes it?

Traumatic amputations usually result directly from factory, farm, or power tools or from motor vehicle accidents.

How is it diagnosed?

Every traumatic amputee requires careful monitoring of vital signs. If amputation involves more than just a finger or toe, assessment of airway, breathing, and circulation is also required.

How is it treated?

Because the greatest immediate threat after traumatic amputation is blood loss and hypovolemic shock, emergency treatment consists of measures to control bleeding, fluid replacement with normal saline solution and colloids, and blood replacement as needed. (See *Saving a severed part.*)

Reimplantation remains controversial, but it's becoming more common and successful because of advances in microsurgery. If reconstruction or reimplantation is possible, surgical intervention attempts to preserve usable joints. When arm or leg amputations are done, the surgeon creates a stump to be fitted with a prosthesis. A rigid dressing permits early prosthesis fitting and rehabilitation.

WHIPLASH

What do doctors call this condition?
Acceleration-deceleration cervical injuries

What is this condition?
Whiplash results from sharp hyperextension and flexion of the neck that damages muscles, ligaments, disks, and nerve tissue. The prognosis is excellent; symptoms usually subside with appropriate treatment.

What causes it?
Commonly, whiplash results from rear-end automobile accidents. Fortunately, the padded headrests, air bags, and seat belts with shoulder harnesses required in new cars have reduced the risk of this type of injury.

What are its symptoms?
Although symptoms may develop immediately, they're often delayed 12 to 24 hours if the injury is mild. Whiplash produces moderate to severe pain in the front and back of the neck. Within several days, the pain in the front diminishes, but the pain in the back of the neck persists or even intensifies, causing people to seek medical attention if they didn't do so before. Whiplash may also cause dizziness, walking disturbances, vomiting, headache, rigidity and muscle asymmetry in the neck, and rigidity or numbness in the arms.

What can a person with whiplash do?

- Watch for possible drug side effects. Avoid alcohol if you're receiving Valium or narcotics.
- Rest for a few days and avoid lifting heavy objects.
- Return to the hospital immediately if you experience persistent pain or develop numbness, tingling, or weakness on one side.

How is it diagnosed?

Full cervical spine X-rays are required to rule out cervical fractures. If the X-rays are negative, the physical exam focuses on motor ability and sensation below the cervical spine to detect signs of nerve root compression.

How is it treated?

In all suspected spinal injuries, the spine is assumed to be injured until proven otherwise. A person with suspected whiplash or other injuries requires careful transportation from the accident scene. To ensure this, the person is placed in a supine position on a spine board with his or her neck immobilized with tape and a hard cervical collar or sandbags. Until an X-ray rules out cervical fracture, the person is moved as little as possible.

Treatment of symptoms includes:

- a mild pain reliever (such as aspirin with codeine or Advil) and possibly a muscle relaxant (such as Valium, Flexeril, or Paraflex) taken with Tylenol
- hot showers or warm compresses on the neck to relieve pain
- immobilization with a soft, padded cervical collar for several days or weeks
- in severe muscle spasms, short-term cervical traction.

GENETIC DISORDERS

ALBINISM

What is this condition?

In this rare condition, a shortage of a brown or black pigment called *melanin* affects the skin and eyes. At times, just the eyes are affected. When the condition affects only the eyes, it impairs vision. When it affects both the eyes and skin, it also makes the person extremely sensitive to sunlight and more likely to get skin cancer.

What causes it?

Albinism is genetic, transmitted by recessive inheritance. This means that parents with the genetic trait for albinism can pass the disorder on to their children, but don't have the disorder themselves.

Normally, cells called *melanocytes* produce melanin. Within melanocytes are melanin-containing granules called *melanosomes*, which absorb the sun's ultraviolet light, protecting the skin and eyes from its dangerous effects. In *tyrosinase-negative albinism,* the most common form, the melanosomes don't contain melanin because they lack the enzyme that triggers its production. In *tyrosinase-positive albinism,* a less common form, melanosomes contain tyrosine, but a defect in the tyrosine transport system impairs melanin production. In *tyrosinase-variable albinism* (extremely rare), an unidentified enzyme defect probably impairs synthesis of melanin.

Tyrosinase-negative albinism affects 1 in every 34,000 persons in the United States and is equally common among whites and blacks. Tyrosinase-positive albinism affects more blacks than whites. Native Americans have a high incidence of both forms.

What are its symptoms?

Light-skinned whites with tyrosinase-negative albinism have pale skin and hair color ranging from white to yellow; their pupils look red because the iris is translucent. Blacks with the same disorder have hair that may be white, faintly tinged with yellow, or yellow-brown. Both whites and blacks with tyrosinase-positive albinism grow darker as they age. For instance, their hair may become straw-colored or light brown and their skin cream-colored or pink. People with tyrosinase-positive albinism may also have freckles and moles that may need to be removed.

At birth a child with tyrosinase-variable albinism has white hair, pink skin, and gray eyes. As the child grows, the hair becomes yellow, the irises may darken, and the skin may even tan slightly.

The skin of a person with albinism is easily damaged by the sun. It may look weather-beaten and is more likely to have precancerous and cancerous growths. The person also may have eye problems, such as light sensitivity, near-sightedness, and strabismus (a deviation of the eye).

How is it diagnosed?

The doctor diagnoses albinism by examining the person and taking a family history. The skin and hair follicles are examined under a microscope to determine how much pigment is present. Other tests may be done to tell which form of albinism the person has.

How is it treated?

After making a diagnosis of albinism, the doctor will teach the child and his or her parents about ways to be protected from exposure to sunlight and how to identify signs of sun-induced skin damage (excessive drying of skin, crusty lesions on exposed skin, changes in skin color). The person should wear full-spectrum sunblocks, dark glasses, and appropriate protective clothing. (See *Helping a child cope with albinism.*)

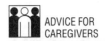

ADVICE FOR CAREGIVERS

Helping a child cope with albinism

- If the child's appearance causes social and emotional problems, psychiatric counseling may be needed. Such counseling may also be appropriate for the family if they have problems accepting the disorder. Early infant-parent bonding can help parents work through any feelings of guilt and depression.
- The parents should learn about cosmetic measures (glasses with tinted lenses, makeup foundation) that can lessen disfigurement as their child ages.
- The parents should be aware that their child will need frequent eye exams to determine how to correct visual defects. Genetic counseling can provide information about the chances of albinism occurring in other family members.

CLEFT LIP AND PALATE

What are these conditions?

Cleft lip and cleft palate are deformities in which the palatine shelves (the front and sides of the face and roof of the mouth) don't unite completely. In cleft palate, for instance, the mouth is only partially separated from the nasal cavity. These conditions arise during the second month of the mother's pregnancy.

Cleft deformities fall into four categories: clefts of the lip (which may involve one or both sides of the face); clefts of the palate (which occur along the center, or midline); clefts of the lip, alveolus (saclike structure), and palate involving one side of the face; and clefts of the lip, alveolus, and palate involving both sides. (See *Cleft lip and palate*, page 866.)

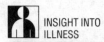

Cleft lip and palate

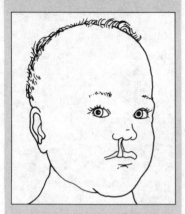

This illustration shows complete, unilateral cleft of the lip and palate, a condition more common in males than females.

Cleft lip with or without cleft palate is more common in males; cleft palate alone is more common in females. Cleft lip and cleft palate occur in 1 in every 800 newborns.

What causes them?

Some cases of cleft lip and palate result from genetic problems such as chromosomal flaws; others are isolated birth defects. The incidence of cleft deformities is higher in children who have family members with the disorder. If normal parents have a baby with a cleft, the risk for subsequent offspring is 5%; if they have two children with it, the risk is 12%.

What are their symptoms?

Congenital clefts of the face occur most commonly in the upper lip. They range from a simple notch to a complete cleft (fissure) from the lip edge through the floor of the nostril, on either side of the midline, but rarely along the midline itself.

A cleft palate may be partial or complete. A complete cleft includes the soft palate, the bones of the maxilla (upper jaw), and the alveolus on one or both sides of the premaxilla (a part of the nose that fuses with the maxilla during embryonic development). A double cleft runs from the soft palate forward to either side of the nose, separating the maxilla and premaxilla into free-moving segments. The tongue and other muscles can displace these segments, enlarging the cleft.

How are they diagnosed?

These abnormalities are obvious when the baby is examined. Cleft lip, with or without cleft palate, is obvious at birth. More severe defects are sometimes seen with diagnostic prenatal ultrasound. Cleft palate without cleft lip may not be detected until a mouth exam is done or until feeding difficulties arise.

How are they treated?

The infant will have surgery to correct the abnormality, but the timing of surgery varies. Some plastic surgeons repair cleft lips within the first few days after birth. This makes it easier to feed the baby and makes the baby more acceptable to the parents. (See *How to feed an infant with a cleft lip or palate.*) However, many surgeons delay lip repairs for 8 to 10 weeks and sometimes as long as 6 to 8 months to allow time for maternal bonding and, most importantly, to rule out

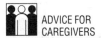

ADVICE FOR
CAREGIVERS

How to feed an infant with a cleft lip or palate

Your infant's condition may cause feeding problems. To make sure he or she gets enough nutrition for normal growth and development, choose the correct feeding method and position, and experiment with different feeding devices.

Breast-feeding
Breast-feeding is the best feeding method for an infant with a cleft lip — if the cleft doesn't prevent effective sucking. Breast-feeding an infant with a cleft palate or one who has just had corrective surgery is impossible. After surgery, the infant can't suck for up to 6 weeks. However, if you wish, you may use a breast pump to express breast milk and then feed it to the baby from a bottle.

Using special devices
An infant with a cleft palate has an excellent appetite but may have trouble feeding because of air leaks around the cleft and regurgitation through the nose. He or she may feed better from a nipple with a flange

that blocks the cleft, a lamb's nipple (a big, soft nipple with large holes), or just a regular nipple with enlarged holes.

When feeding, hold your infant in a near-sitting position, with the flow directed to the side or back of his tongue. Burp the infant frequently because he or she tends to swallow a lot of air. Check the lower part of the nose regularly; sometimes, sores develop on the nasal septum (area between the nostrils), a painful condition that could make the infant refuse to suck. If this happens, direct the nipple to the side of the mouth to give the delicate skin time to heal. After each feeding, gently clean the cleft area with a cotton-tipped applicator dipped in half-strength hydrogen peroxide or water.

associated congenital abnormalities. Cleft palate repair is usually completed by age 12 to 18 months. Still other surgeons repair cleft palates in two steps, repairing the soft palate between ages 6 and 18 months and the hard palate as late as age 5. In any case, surgery is performed only after the infant has gained weight and is infection free.

Surgery may be impossible if the child has a wide "horseshoe defect." Instead, a contoured speech bulb is attached to the back portion of a denture to block the nasopharynx (the portion of the throat just behind the nose) and help the child develop intelligible speech.

The child also will need speech therapy. Because the palate is essential to speech formation, structural changes, even in a repaired cleft, can permanently affect speech patterns. In addtion, many children with cleft palates have hearing problems because of middle ear damage or infections.

CYSTIC FIBROSIS

What is this condition?

Cystic fibrosis is a disorder of the exocrine glands (glands that open through ducts onto the surface of the skin) that affects many of the body's organs. A chronic disease, it has no known cure, at least not yet.

The incidence of cystic fibrosis is highest in people of northern European ancestry and lowest in Blacks, Native Americans, and people of Asian ancestry. The disease affects both sexes equally.

What causes it?

Cystic fibrosis is inherited. (See *How the cystic fibrosis gene is transmitted,* page 870.) Researchers recently identified the gene responsible for the disease.

Symptoms of the disease result from abnormally thick secretions of mucus, which block ducts in the glands. The sweat glands and the glands in the lungs and pancreas are most affected.

What are its symptoms?

Symptoms of cystic fibrosis may appear soon after birth or may take years to develop. The most striking involve the sweat glands, the lungs, and the digestive system. The sweat of a person with cystic fibrosis contains greater-than-normal amounts of sodium and chloride. This chemical imbalance may deplete the body of sodium and chloride, eventually causing heart rhythm problems and shock, especially in hot weather.

Lung and related problems

Lung blockages cause symptoms such as wheezy respirations, a dry cough, difficulty breathing or shortness of breath, and abnormally fast breathing. Eventually, these problems may lead to a collapsed lung and emphysema, a condition in which the lungs overinflate and lose their normal elasticity.

Children with cystic fibrosis have a barrel chest, a bluish tinge to the skin, and clubbed fingers and toes. They suffer recurring bouts of bronchitis and pneumonia and may have polyps in their nasal passages and sinusitis (sinus inflammation).

Reproductive problems
Males may lack sperm in the semen and become sterile. Females may have problems with menstruation but can reproduce. Many infants and children with cystic fibrosis have a sunken rectum because of malnutrition and wasting away of the tissues supporting the rectum.

Pancreas problems
In the pancreas, cystic fibrosis causes a condition called *pancreatic insufficiency.* Symptoms of this condition include too little insulin production, sugar intolerance, and glycosuria (sugar in the urine). Some people with cystic fibrosis have enough pancreatic function for normal digestion; they tend to fare better than others.

In some people, cirrhosis and high pressure in certain veins may cause the veins at the lower end of the esophagus to swell. The person then may vomit blood and have an enlarged liver.

About 75% of the people with cystic fibrosis have a defect in one gene. Researchers are still investigating the cause for the other 25%.

Problems in infants
A newborn with cystic fibrosis may have an abnormal condition called *meconium ileus,* in which the child doesn't excrete meconium, a dark green material found in the intestine at birth. The infant then has symptoms of a blocked intestine, such as a swollen abdomen, vomiting, constipation, and dehydration. Eventually, blocked ducts in the pancreas deplete certain enzymes, which in turn prevents fat and protein absorption in the intestinal tract. The undigested food then passes from the body in frequent, bulky, foul-smelling, and pale stools that are high in fat.

This malabsorption leads to poor weight gain, poor growth, a huge appetite, a swollen abdomen, thin arms and legs, and sallow, lax skin. Unable to absorb fats, the child lacks the fat-soluble vitamins — A, D, E, and K. This in turn impairs blood clotting, slows bone growth, and delays sexual development.

How is it diagnosed?
The doctor will diagnose cystic fibrosis if a person has:
- two clearly positive sweat tests along with one of the following: an obstructive lung disease, confirmed pancreatic insufficiency or failure to thrive, and a family history of cystic fibrosis
- chest X-rays showing early signs of obstructive lung disease
- stool specimen lacking the enzyme trypsin, which suggests pancreatic insufficiency.

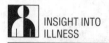

INSIGHT INTO
ILLNESS

How the cystic fibrosis gene is transmitted

If your child has cystic fibrosis, you'll probably be concerned about how the causative gene is transmitted, and you may be concerned that you'll have another child with the disease. Here's what you should know.

Understanding gene types

Cystic fibrosis results from an autosomal recessive gene. Genes are either dominant or recessive. The weaker recessive genes express themselves only when paired with another recessive gene. At conception, an embryo normally gets two genes — one from each parent. If both parents carry the recessive gene for cystic fibrosis, each child has a one-in-four (25%) chance of having the disease.

As shown in the illustration, *C* refers to the dominant gene, and *c* represents the recessive gene. The unaffected noncarrier — *C/C* — inherits the dominant gene from each parent and won't have cystic fibrosis. *C/c* and *c/C* are unaffected carriers; each child inherits one dominant gene and one recessive gene for cystic fibrosis. Because both genes must be recessive for cystic fibrosis to develop, these children won't have the disease, but they can pass the recessive gene to their children.

The affected person — *c/c* — inherits the recessive gene from both parents, has cystic fibrosis, and will pass the recessive cystic fibrosis gene on, if he or she has children.

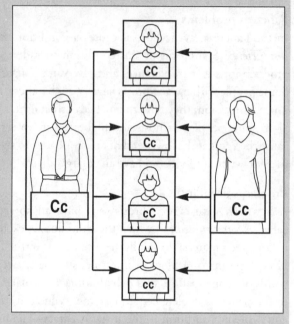

Testing for the cystic fibrosis gene

Special labs can perform prenatal testing for parents of children with cystic fibrosis. About 75% of people with cystic fibrosis have the cystic fibrosis gene. Researchers are still discovering the other 25% of mutations of the gene. For up-to-date information, consult a genetic counselor.

To support the diagnosis, the doctor may also order these other tests:

- DNA testing can now locate the genetic defect responsible for cystic fibrosis (the ΔF_{508} deletion), found in about 75% of persons with cystic fibrosis. (However, the disease can cause more than 100 other genetic mutations.) This test can also be used to identify people who carry the gene for cystic fibrosis and to diagnose the disease prenatally in families with a previously affected child.

- If the person's lungs are especially affected, lung function tests help to identify respiratory problems.
- A liver enzyme test may show liver insufficiency.
- A sputum culture reveals bacteria typically found in people with cystic fibrosis.
- Measurement of the amount of albumin (a protein) in the blood helps assess nutritional status.
- Measurement of the amounts of various electrolytes can show if the person is dehydrated.
- Measurement of serum glucose level indicates high or low blood sugar.

How is it treated?

The goal of treatment is to help the child lead as normal a life as possible. The Cystic Fibrosis Foundation can help provide emotional support and other aid to the child and family. Medical treatment depends on which body organs are involved.

Treating lung problems

- To manage lung problems, the doctor will instruct the parents or other caregivers to perform physical therapy for the chest, postural drainage (special body positioning), and breathing exercises several times daily to help remove lung secretions. The child shouldn't take antihistamines because they may dry the mucous membranes, making it difficult or impossible to expel mucus. Before postural drainage, the doctor may recommend aerosol therapy (intermittent nebulizer treatments) to help loosen secretions.
- Dornase alfa, a genetically engineered lung enzyme given by aerosol nebulizer, helps thin mucus in the lungs, improving lung function and reducing the risk of lung infection.

   If the child has a lung infection, he or she will require:
- loosening and removal of secretions containing mucus and pus, using an intermittent nebulizer and postural drainage to relieve blockages; some doctors recommend use of a mist tent, although this is controversial because mist particles may get trapped in the esophagus and stomach and never even reach the lungs
- antibiotics
- oxygen therapy, as needed, and use of air conditioners and humidifiers.

Clinical trials of aerosol gene therapy show promise in reducing the lung problems associated with cystic fibrosis.

Getting the right nutrients

▪ To combat the child's electrolyte loss in sweat, the parents should salt the child's food generously and, during hot weather, have the child take salt tablets.

▪ To offset the lack of pancreatic enzymes, the child should take oral pancreatic enzymes with meals and snacks, eat a diet low in fat but high in protein and calories, and take supplements of vitamins A, D, E, and K.

Undergoing other procedures

Recently, some people with cystic fibrosis have received lung transplants to reduce the effects of the disease.

DOWN SYNDROME

What do doctors call this condition?

Trisomy 21

What is this condition?

Down syndrome — the first disorder known to be caused by a chromosome problem — typically results in mental retardation, abnormal facial features, and other distinctive physical abnormalities. It's often associated with heart defects and other disorders that are present at birth.

Life expectancy for a person with Down syndrome has risen significantly because of better treatment for complications (heart defects, tendency toward respiratory and other infections, acute leukemia). But many of those born with heart disease die before age 1.

What causes it?

Down syndrome usually results from trisomy 21, a genetic abnormality in which chromosome 21 has 3 copies instead of the normal 2 because of nondisjunction of the ovum or, sometimes, the sperm. This results in what doctors call a *karyotype* (chromosome pattern) of 47 chromosomes, instead of the normal 46.

Overall, Down syndrome occurs in 1 in 800 to 1,000 live births, but its incidence rises with advanced parental age, especially when the mother is age 34 or older at delivery or the father is older than age

42. At age 20, a mother has about 1 chance in 2,000 of having a child with Down syndrome; by age 49, she has 1 chance in 12. Although women over age 35 account for fewer than 5% of all births, they bear 20% of the children with Down syndrome.

What are its symptoms?

The physical signs of Down syndrome (especially poor muscle tone) are usually apparent at birth. Mental retardation is obvious as the infant grows older. Typically, the child has abnormalities of the skull and face, such as slanting, almond-shaped eyes with epicanthic folds (vertical skin fold over the inner angle of the eye); a protruding tongue; a small mouth and chin; a single horizontal crease in the palm; small white spots called *Brushfield spots* on the iris; strabismus (deviation of the eyes); a small skull; a flat bridge across the nose; slow tooth development with abnormal or absent teeth; a flattened face; small ears; a short neck; and cataracts.

Other signs of Down syndrome include dry, sensitive, inelastic skin; umbilical hernia; short stature; and short arms and legs, with broad, flat, squarish hands and feet. These people may have clinodactyly (a small little finger that curves inward), a wide space between the first and second toe, and abnormal fingerprints and footprints. Poor muscle tone in the arms and legs impairs reflex development, posture, coordination, and balance.

The person's IQ may range from 30 to 70. However, his or her social performance usually is beyond that expected for mental age. Intellectual development slows with age.

Commonly, people with Down syndrome have congenital heart disease, duodenal atresia (absence or blockage of a portion of the small intestine), megacolon (massive enlargement of the colon, a part of the large intestine), and pelvic bone abnormalities. Their genitalia are poorly developed and puberty is delayed. Females may menstruate and be fertile. Males are infertile with low testosterone levels; in many, the testicles don't descend. These people are prone to thyroid disorders, leukemia, and infections.

How is it diagnosed?

At birth, the newborn's physical features (especially poor muscle tone) suggest Down syndrome, but no one physical feature is diagnostic in itself.

A chromosome analysis showing the specific abnormality can confirm Down syndrome. Amniocentesis (analysis of fluid in the

Meeting the physical and emotional needs of a child with Down syndrome

If your child has Down syndrome, you can improve his or her physical and emotional development by following these guidelines.

Providing stimulation and care

▪ As a newborn, your child may have trouble sucking and may be less demanding and seem less eager to eat than other babies. Be patient when feeding the baby, and make sure to provide a balanced diet.

▪ Hold and nurture your child as much as possible.

▪ Make sure your child gets plenty of exercise and environmental stimulation. Ask your doctor about infant stimulation classes, which may begin in the early months of life.

▪ Set realistic goals for your child. Although his or her mental development may seem normal at first, this is not a sign of future progress. By the time the child is 1 year old, development clearly will lag behind that of normal children. To help chart the child's progress, the doctor may use the Denver Developmental Screening Test. View your child's successful achievements positively, even though he or she is slow.

▪ Remember the emotional needs of your other children.

Seeking advice and support

▪ Seek genetic and psychological counseling, if appropriate, to help evaluate your risk of having another child with Down syndrome. If you're considering having another child, your doctor may recommend prenatal testing.

▪ For more support, ask your doctor or nurse for the names of national or local Down syndrome organizations and support groups.

uterus) allows prenatal diagnosis and is recommended for pregnant women past age 34, even if the family history is negative. Amniocentesis is indicated for a pregnant woman of any age when either she or the father carries a translocated chromosome.

How is it treated?

Down syndrome has no known cure. Surgery to correct heart defects and other related congenital abnormalities and antibiotic therapy for recurrent infections have improved life expectancy considerably. Plastic surgery may be done to correct the characteristic facial traits, especially the protruding tongue. Beyond improved appearance, benefits of such surgery may include improved speech, a reduced chance of dental cavities, and fewer orthodontic problems. Most people with Down syndrome are now cared for at home and attend special education classes; if they're profoundly retarded, they may be put in an institution if supervised housing is unavailable. As adults, some may work in a sheltered workshop. (For information on caring for a child with Down syndrome at home, see *Meeting the physical and emotional needs of a child with Down syndrome.*)

HEMOPHILIA

What is this condition?

Hemophilia is an inherited bleeding disorder in which certain blood clotting factors are deficient or nonfunctioning. In a hemophiliac, even a minor injury can lead to severe bleeding.

The most common form, hemophilia A (classic hemophilia), affects over 80% of all hemophiliacs. It results from a deficiency of clotting factor VIII. Hemophilia B, which is also called *Christmas disease*, affects about 15% of hemophiliacs and results from a deficiency of clotting factor IX.

Thanks to treatment advances, many hemophiliacs now live normal life spans. Overall, people with mild hemophilia, which doesn't cause spontaneous bleeding and joint deformities, tend to fare better than those with more severe disease. Some hemophiliacs can even safely undergo surgery at special treatment centers.

In hemophilia, even a minor injury can lead to severe bleeding.

What causes it?

Hemophilia A and B are inherited as X-linked recessive traits. This type of disorder occurs only in males and is transmitted only by a female carrier.

Female carriers have a 50% chance of passing on the gene to each daughter, who would then be a carrier, and a 50% chance of passing on the gene to each son, who would be born with hemophilia. (See *Answers to parents' questions about hemophilia inheritance*, page 876.)

What are its symptoms?

Hemophilia causes abnormal bleeding, which may be mild, moderate, or severe, depending on the degree of clotting factor deficiency. Often, mild hemophilia isn't diagnosed until adulthood, because this person has prolonged bleeding only after a major injury or surgery. After surgery, bleeding continues as a slow ooze or stops and starts again for up to 8 days.

Severe hemophilia, in contrast, causes spontaneous bleeding. Often, the first sign occurs when a newborn bleeds excessively after cir-

STRAIGHT
TALK

Answers to parents' questions about hemophilia inheritance

No one in either of our families ever had hemophilia. How did our son get hemophilia?

In 20% to 25% of families with a hemophiliac, there's no family history of the disorder. Evidently, there's a high mutation (change) rate in the genes that produce clotting factors VIII and IX. The mutation may occur in the child, in either parent, or elsewhere in the family tree.

What are our chances of having another child with hemophilia?

Each son of a carrier has a 50% chance of being a hemophiliac, and each daughter has a 50% chance of being a carrier. Your hemophilia treatment center can tell you more about testing and probability.

Our son has hemophilia. Does this mean his children will have it, too?

If your son marries a carrier, your grandsons may have hemophilia. If your son marries someone who isn't a carrier, your grandsons won't have hemophilia and they won't pass on the gene. All of their sisters will be carriers, though, and your great-grandsons may have hemophilia. The diagram below shows how a sex-linked recessive disorder is passed on. The diagram's second row (the second generation) shows that each son of a carrier has a 50% chance of having hemophilia, and each daughter has a 50% chance of being a carrier. The last two rows represent the third generation if the second-generation offspring mate with normal partners.

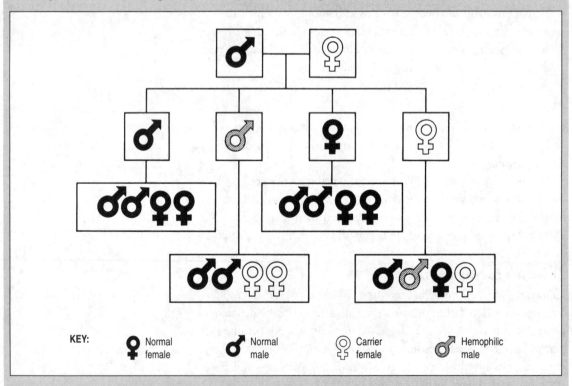

cumcision. Later, spontaneous bleeding or severe bleeding after a minor injury may cause large hematomas — collections of trapped blood — in the skin and muscles. With severe hemophilia, the person also bleeds into joints and muscles, suffering pain, swelling, extreme tenderness, and, possibly, permanent deformity.

Moderate hemophilia causes symptoms similar to severe hemophilia. Fortunately, though, the person has only occasional episodes of spontaneous bleeding.

Bleeding near peripheral nerves (those not located in the brain or spinal cord) may cause nerve inflammation and degeneration, pain, abnormal sensations, and muscle wasting. If bleeding impairs blood flow through a major vessel, it can decrease blood supply to the affected part, with possible gangrene (local death of soft tissues). Bleeding in the throat, tongue, heart, brain, and skull may all lead to shock and even death.

How is it diagnosed?

Typically, hemophilia is diagnosed in a person who experiences prolonged bleeding after injury or surgery (including tooth extractions), or who has episodes of spontaneous bleeding into the muscles or joints.

Tests of specific blood clotting factors can diagnose the type and severity of hemophilia. A family history of hemophilia also helps the doctor diagnose hemophilia (although about 20% of hemophiliacs have no family history of the disease).

A person with hemophilia A usually has the following findings:

- factor VIII assay 0% to 30% of normal
- prolonged activated partial thromboplastin time
- normal platelet count and function, bleeding time, and prothrombin time.

A person with hemophilia B typically has these findings:

- deficient factor IX assay
- baseline coagulation (blood clotting) results similar to those seen with hemophilia A, with normal clotting factor VIII.

In hemophilia A or B, the degree of clotting factor deficiency indicates the severity of the disease:

- mild hemophilia — factor levels 5% to 40% of normal
- moderate hemophilia — factor levels 1% to 5% of normal
- severe hemophilia — factor levels less than 1% of normal.

How is it treated?

Although hemophilia isn't curable at this time, treatment can prolong life and prevent crippling deformities. Correct treatment quickly stops bleeding by increasing the levels of deficient blood clotting factors. This, in turn, helps prevent disabling deformities that result from repeated bleeding into muscles and joints.

A person with hemophilia A may receive substances known as *antihemophilic factors* to raise clotting factor levels above normal. Often, this permits normal blood clotting. A person with hemophilia B may receive clotting factor IX concentrate during bleeding episodes to increase clotting factor IX levels.

A person with hemophilia who undergoes surgery must be managed carefully by a hematologist (a specialist in the study of blood) who's an expert in hemophilia care. Before and after surgery, the person must receive replacements of the deficient clotting factor. Such replacement may be necessary even for minor surgery such as a tooth extraction. This person also may receive epsilon-aminocaproic acid, a drug that inhibits oral bleeding.

To manage the disease, a hemophiliac must learn how to avoid injury, manage minor bleeding, and recognize bleeding that requires immediate medical help. (For advice for parents of a hemophiliac, see *What to do if your child has hemophilia.*)

What can a person with hemophilia do?

After you're diagnosed, the doctor may refer you to a hemophilia treatment center for evaluation. The center will devise a treatment plan for your primary physician and will serve as a resource for other medical and school personnel, dentists, or others involved in your care. Always follow your doctor's instructions.

How to manage bleeding episodes

- Seek medical help. Chances are, the doctor will give you the deficient clotting factor or plasma — possibly in repeated infusions until the bleeding stops.
- Apply cold compresses or ice bags to the injured part, and raise it.
- To prevent bleeding from recurring, minimize physical activity for 48 hours after the bleeding is under control.
- If you're in pain, take an analgesic, such as Tylenol or another drug containing acetaminophen, or a drug prescribed by your doctor. *Don't take aspirin or aspirin-containing medication* because these may make the bleeding worse.

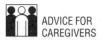

ADVICE FOR
CAREGIVERS

What to do if your child has hemophilia

By following these guidelines, you can help prevent complications of hemophilia and safeguard your child's health.

Monitor for health and safety
- Notify the doctor immediately — even after a minor injury — especially if your child has injured his head, neck, or abdomen. Such injuries may require special blood factor replacement. Also, check with the doctor before your child has surgery or a tooth extraction.
- Stay alert for signs of severe internal bleeding, such as severe pain or swelling in a joint or muscle; stiffness; decreased joint movement; severe stomach pain; blood in the urine; black, tarry stools; and severe headache.

Be aware of risks
- Be aware that your child is at risk for hepatitis because he receives blood components. Early signs of this infection may appear 3 weeks to 6 months after the child gets the blood components. They include headache, fever, decreased appetite, nausea, vomiting, stomach tenderness, and pain over the liver area (the area under the rib cage and in the center of the stomach).
- *Never give your child aspirin.* It can make bleeding worse. Give Tylenol or another drug containing acetaminophen instead.
- If your child received blood products before such products were routinely screened for HIV, he may be HIV-positive. Ask the doctor about periodic HIV testing.
- If you have daughters, arrange for them to have genetic screening and testing to determine if they're hemophilia carriers. Affected males should have counseling, too.

Follow home health guidelines
- Make sure your child wears a medical identification bracelet at all times.
- Make sure your child practices regular, careful toothbrushing to prevent the need for dental surgery. Provide a soft toothbrush.
- Protect your child from injury, but avoid unnecessary restrictions that could hinder his development. For example, instead of forbidding a toddler from playing, sew padded patches into the knees and elbows of his clothing to protect these joints during falls. Forbid an older child to play contact sports, such as football, but encourage him to swim or play golf.
- Apply cold compresses or ice bags to an injured area and elevate it, or apply light pressure to a bleeding site. To prevent bleeding from recurring, restrict your child's activity for 48 hours after bleeding is under control.
- If you've been trained to administer blood factor components at home to avoid frequent hospitalization, make sure you know proper venipuncture and infusion techniques. Don't delay treatment during bleeding episodes. Keep blood factor concentrate and infusion equipment on hand at all times, even on vacation.
- Make sure your child keeps routine medical appointments at the local hemophilia center.
- For more information, contact the National Hemophilia Foundation.

What to do if you're bleeding into a joint
- Suspect bleeding into a joint if you have pain, swelling, tingling, and warmth in a joint (such as the knee, elbow, ankle, shoulder, hip, or wrist).
- Immediately raise the joint.

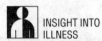

INSIGHT INTO
ILLNESS

Spermatogenic mistake

In Klinefelter's syndrome, fertilization by a sperm with X and Y chromosomes produces an XXY zygote (developing ovum), instead of a pair of X chromosomes, as in normal females, or an X and a Y, as in normal males.

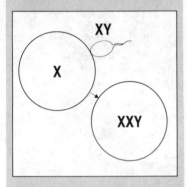

- To restore joint mobility, the doctor may tell you to perform range-of-motion exercises at least 48 hours after the bleeding is controlled. Avoid weight-bearing exercise (such as walking) until the bleeding stops and the swelling subsides.

KLINEFELTER'S SYNDROME

Klinefelter's syndrome is a relatively common genetic abnormality that affects only males. It often causes abnormal breast enlargement and learning disabilities, and usually becomes apparent at puberty, when the secondary sex characteristics develop. The testicles fail to mature, and degenerative testicular changes begin, eventually leading to a permanent inability to father children.

What causes it?
Klinefelter's syndrome usually results from one extra X chromosome. (See *Spermatogenic mistake.*) The syndrome appears in about 1 in every 600 males. Also, it accounts for roughly 1 in every 100 institutionalized mentally retarded males. Its incidence increases with maternal age.

What are its symptoms?
Klinefelter's syndrome may not be apparent until puberty, or later in mild cases. If the person is not mentally retarded, infertility may be the only abnormality. The syndrome's characteristic features include a small penis and prostate; small, firm testicles; sparse facial and abdominal hair; feminine distribution of pubic hair; sexual dysfunction (impotence, lack of libido); and, in fewer than 50% of affected males, breast enlargement.

Absence of sperm and infertility result from abnormalities in the testicles. Klinefelter's syndrome is also associated with osteoporosis (loss of bone mass), abnormal body build (long legs with a short, obese trunk), tall stature, learning disabilities characterized by poor verbal skills and, in some people, personality impairment. It's also associated with an increased incidence of pulmonary disease, varicose veins, and breast cancer.

How is it diagnosed?

The doctor diagnoses Klinefelter's syndrome from typical clinical features, but only a chromosome analysis can definitively confirm it.

How is it treated?

Depending on the severity of the syndrome, treatment may include mastectomy for persistent breast enlargement and supplemental testosterone to induce the secondary sexual characteristics of puberty. The testicular changes that lead to infertility can't be prevented.

Psychotherapy with sexual counseling is needed if sexual dysfunction causes emotional maladjustment. If a person with the rare, mosaic form of the syndrome is fertile, genetic counseling is essential because he may transmit this chromosomal abnormality as well as others.

NEUROFIBROMATOSIS

What do doctors call this condition?

Von Recklinghausen's disease

What is this condition?

Sometimes called *Elephant Man's disease,* neurofibromatosis is an inherited developmental disorder of the nervous system, muscles, bones, and skin. It causes formation of many neurofibromas (soft tumors) and café-au-lait spots (flat, darkened skin areas).

About 80,000 Americans have neurofibromatosis; in many others, this disorder is overlooked because symptoms are mild. The disease occurs in about 1 in 3,000 births. The prognosis varies, although spinal or brain tumors can shorten the life span.

What causes it?

Neurofibromatosis is present at birth, but symptoms generally appear during childhood or adolescence. Sometimes progression stops as the person matures, but it may accelerate at puberty, during pregnancy, or after menopause. It's often associated with meningiomas, suprarenal medullary secreting tumors, kyphoscoliosis, vascular and lymphatic moles, and eye and kidney abnormalities.

In some people, the disease is transmitted genetically as an autosomal dominant trait; in others, it occurs as a new genetic mutation. People with neurofibromatosis have a 50% risk that their children will have this disease.

What are its symptoms?

Symptoms result from an overgrowth of certain elements in the skin, central nervous system, and other organs. Such overgrowth produces neurofibromas — multiple pedunculated (stemlike) nodules of varying sizes on the nerve trunks of the arms and legs and on the nerves of the head, neck, and body. Symptoms generally get worse during puberty and pregnancy. Effects vary with the location and size of the tumors. They include:

- neurologic impairment that results from tumors of the intracranial area, spine, eighth cranial nerve, and eye region — and in 10% of these people, seizures, blindness, deafness, developmental delays, mental deficiency, and obstructive hydrocephalus ("water on the brain")
- skin lesions — typically, six or more café-au-lait spots, especially if the lesions are present in the underarm areas, neck, and perineum; hard and soft fibromas and lipomas on the skin and in tissue under the skin; pigmented hairy moles; extra hair growth on the small of the back; and deep furrows of the skin over the scalp
- skeletal involvement — scoliosis, severe kyphoscoliosis, macrocephaly, short stature, and spinal fusion defects
- endocrine abnormalities — acromegaly, cretinism, hyperparathyroidism, myxedema, precocious puberty, and growth retardation
- kidney damage — high blood pressure and pheochromocytoma
- peripheral nerve involvement — pain, disfigurement, paresis, and spinal cord compression.

Complications of neurofibromatosis include congenital tibial pseudoarthrosis; neurofibrosarcoma (cancer of the nerve sheath), which occurs in up to 8% of people with the disease; and cancerous changes in the tumors themselves.

How is it diagnosed?

The doctor diagnoses the condition from typical clinical findings, especially neurofibromas and café-au-lait spots. He or she will probably order X-rays and a computed tomography scan (commonly called a CAT scan) to determine the presence of a widening internal auditory meatus and intervertebral foramen. Myelography is used to identify spinal cord tumors, and a lumbar puncture (spinal tap) with analysis of cerebrospinal fluid will show characteristic changes in a person with spinal neurofibromas and acoustic tumors.

How is it treated?

Treatment involves surgery to remove intracerebral or intraspinal tumors, when possible, and correction of kyphoscoliosis. Cosmetic surgery for disfiguring or disabling growths may be done, although regrowth is likely. (See *How to cope with neurofibromatosis.*)

PHENYLKETONURIA

What do doctors call this condition?

Phenylalaninemia, phenylpyruvic oligophrenia

What is this condition?

Commonly called by its abbreviation *PKU*, phenylketonuria is an inborn error in the metabolism of phenylalanine, one of the essential amino acids. This error causes high levels of phenylalanine in the blood, resulting in brain damage and mental retardation.

What causes it?

PKU is a genetic disorder transmitted by an autosomal recessive gene. (See *Understanding PKU gene transmission,* page 884.) People with PKU don't have enough phenylalanine hydroxylase, an enzyme that helps to convert phenylalanine to tyrosine in their livers. As a result, phenylalanine accumulates in the blood, causing mental retardation. The exact mechanism causing retardation is unclear.

In the United States, PKU occurs once in about 14,000 births. (About one person in 60 is a carrier with no symptoms.) It has a low incidence in Finland, in Japan, among Jews of Eastern European ancestry, and among Blacks.

What are its symptoms?

An infant with PKU appears normal at birth, but by age 4 months starts to show signs of arrested brain development, including mental retardation and, later, personality disturbances (schizoid and antiso-

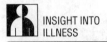

INSIGHT INTO
ILLNESS

Understanding PKU gene transmission

If your infant has PKU, you'll probably want to know how he or she got the disorder and whether you could have other children with it.

Genes fall into two classifications: dominant and recessive. PKU results from transmission of an auto-somal recessive gene. Traits from a recessive gene express themselves only when paired with another recessive gene. The recessive gene that causes PKU ensures that the body cannot convert the enzyme phenylalanine for normal growth and development.

At conception, an embryo normally receives two genes for phenylalanine conversion — one from each parent. If both parents carry one dominant and one recessive gene for phenylalanine conversion, each offspring has a 25% chance of having PKU, a 25% chance of being an unaffected non-carrier, or a 50% chance of being an unaffected PKU carrier.

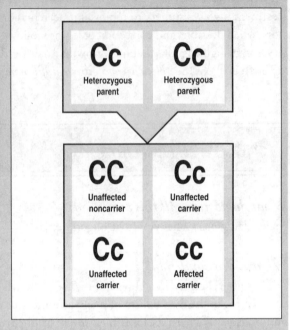

KEY
C: dominant gene for normal phenylalanine conversion
c: recessive gene for PKU

cial personality patterns and uncontrollable temper). Such a child may have a lighter complexion than unaffected siblings and often has blue eyes. The child may also have an abnormally small head; eczema or dry, rough skin; and a musty odor from skin and urine. About 80% of these children have abnormal brain-wave (electroencephalo-gram) patterns, and about one-third have seizures, which usually start when they're age 6 to 12 months.

Children with this disorder show a sharp decrease in IQ in their first year. They're usually hyperactive and irritable and make purpose-less, repetitive motions. They have increased muscle tone and an awkward gait.

Although levels of phenylalanine in the blood are near-normal at birth, they start to rise within a few days. By the time they reach significant levels, brain damage has begun. The damage, which is irreversible, probably is complete by age 2 or 3. However, early detection and treatment can minimize the damage.

How is it diagnosed?

Most states require PKU screening at birth; the Guthrie screening test on a capillary blood sample reliably detects PKU. However, since phenylalanine levels may be normal at birth, the infant should be reevaluated after he or she has received the first feedings, after about 24 to 48 hours.

How is it treated?

The child with PKU must restrict dietary intake of the amino acid phenylalanine to keep phenylalanine blood levels between 3 and 9 milligrams per deciliter of blood. Because most natural proteins contain 5% phenylalanine, they must be limited in the child's diet. An enzymatic hydrolysate of casein (the principal protein in milk), such as Lofenalac powder, is substituted for milk in the diets of affected infants. This milk substitute contains a minimal amount of phenylalanine, normal amounts of other amino acids, and added amounts of carbohydrate and fat. Dietary restrictions should probably continue throughout life.

Such a diet requires careful monitoring. Because the body doesn't make phenylalanine, overzealous dietary restriction can cause phenylalanine deficiency, leading to lack of energy, loss of appetite, anemia, skin rashes, and diarrhea. (See *What you should know about your child's PKU diet,* page 886.) The person with PKU needs frequent tests for urine phenylpyruvic acid and blood phenylalanine levels to evaluate the diet's effectiveness.

Preventing this condition

- Infants should be routinely screened for PKU because detection and control of this condition soon after birth can prevent severe mental retardation.
- Females with PKU who reach reproductive age should have genetic counseling because recent research indicates that their children may have a higher-than-normal incidence of brain damage, mental retardation, microcephaly, and major congenital malformations, especially of the heart and central nervous system. Such damage may be minimized with a low-phenylalanine diet before conception and during pregnancy.

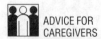

ADVICE FOR
CAREGIVERS

What you should know about your child's PKU diet

Until about age 6, your child will need a special diet to develop normally. Above all, he or she will need to avoid most foods and fluids containing phenylalanine — mainly protein sources, such as dairy products, eggs, and meats. *Don't stop this diet until the doctor tells you it's no longer needed.* Stopping it early could cause permanent brain damage in your child.

Tell your child's teachers, friends' parents, babysitters, and other caregivers about the condition. Make sure they know which foods can and can't be eaten. Also, keep appointments to check your child's phenylalanine levels. Test results will show how well your child's diet is working.

Here are some tips to help your child comply with this diet.

Using milk substitutes
- Give your child a milk substitute made especially for infants and children with PKU. Some brand names are Lofenalac and Phenyl-free.
- If the doctor advises you to add cow's milk or regular infant formula to make sure your child gets certain essential nutrients, follow the doctor's directions precisely. Measure the exact amount — never more — of recommended milk or formula.

Avoiding NutraSweet
- Read all food and drug labels. Make sure the products don't contain the artificial sweetener NutraSweet, a phenylalanine derivative.
- Watch out for "sugar-free" products. NutraSweet may be used to sweeten them.

Adding solid foods
- Choose solid foods carefully. The doctor will tell you how and when to add solid foods to your child's diet.

- Include low-phenylalanine foods, such as cereal, low-protein bread, and pasta; fats and oils (for example, in potato chips); and vegetables. Avoid high-phenylalanine foods, such as cheese, eggs, milk, regular bread, fish, meat, poultry, peas, beans, and nuts.
- Never assume a new food is safe for your child to eat. Always talk to the doctor or dietitian if you have questions about a new food.

Dealing with discouragement
- The difficult dietary restrictions may cause your child to experience psychological and emotional problems. To keep your child from feeling deprived or different from friends — and help him or her stay on the diet — offer special treats. For instance, you can make special ice-cream, milk-shake, and pudding treats using a synthetic milk substitute. Ask a dietitian for ideas and recipes.
- As your child grows older and is supervised less closely, you'll have less control over what he or she eats. The child will be more likely to deviate from the restricted diet, increasing the risk of further brain damage. Allow some choices in the kinds of low-protein foods the child wants to eat; this will help make him or her feel trusted and more responsible.

Practicing moderation
- Don't restrict your child's diet more than the doctor advises. Your child needs some phenylalanine to grow normally and to avoid phenylalanine deficiency (which can also cause serious health problems).
- Be careful not to give your child large amounts of low-phenylalanine foods. This can cause phenylalanine to build up in the blood.

SICKLE CELL ANEMIA

What is this condition?

Sickle cell anemia is an inherited blood disorder in which the red blood cells roughen and become sickle-shaped, clogging blood vessels and impairing circulation. It results from a defective hemoglobin molecule (called *hemoglobin S*).

The person with sickle cell anemia suffers chronic ill health, with easy fatigue, swollen joints, and shortness of breath on exertion. He or she may have periodic painful attacks called *sickle cell crisis* and long-term complications.

No cure exists at this time, and few people with the disease live to middle age. However, by taking penicillin as a preventive measure, they can decrease their risk of getting serious bacterial infections that weaken their health.

What causes it?

Sickle cell anemia results when a person inherits the gene that produces hemoglobin S from two healthy parents who each carry the defective gene (called *sickle cell trait*). The trait alone rarely causes symptoms.

Sickle cell anemia is most common in tropical Africans and in people of African descent. About 1 in 10 Americans of African descent carries the abnormal gene. If two such carriers have children, each child has a 25% chance of developing sickle cell disease. (See *How sickle cell anemia is inherited,* page 888.)

Overall, 1 in every 400 to 600 black children has sickle cell anemia. This disease also occurs in Puerto Rico, Turkey, India, the Middle East, and the Mediterranean region. Some researchers think the defective gene has persisted because in areas where malaria is endemic, the sickle cell trait is beneficial, providing resistance to malaria.

How hemoglobin S causes sickling

The abnormal hemoglobin in the red blood cells of people with sickle cell disease becomes insoluble whenever the blood has too little oxygen. This makes the red cells become rigid, rough, and elongated, forming a crescent or sickle shape. Such sickling can produce hemolysis (cell destruction). These abnormal red blood cells tend to pile up in capillaries and smaller blood vessels, thickening the blood. This, in turn, blocks circulation, causing pain, localized tissue death, and

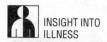

INSIGHT INTO
ILLNESS

How sickle cell anemia is inherited

As this chart shows, when both parents have sickle cell anemia, all of their offspring will have sickle cell anemia. Also, childbearing — if possible at all — is dangerous for the mother.

When one parent has sickle cell anemia and the other is normal, all of their offspring will have the sickle cell trait, which means they'll be carriers of sickle cell anemia.

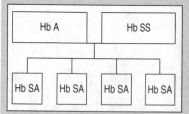

If one parent has normal hemoglobin and the other parent has sickle cell anemia, all offspring will have the sickle cell trait.

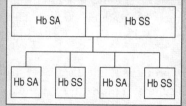

If one parent has sickle cell trait and the other parent has sickle cell anemia, the offspring will have a 50% chance of having sickle cell anemia and an equal chance of having sickle cell trait.

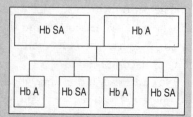

If one parent has sickle cell trait and the other has normal hemoglobin, the offspring will have a 50% chance of having normal hemoglobin and the same chance of having the sickle cell trait.

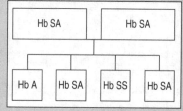

If both parents have the sickle cell trait, the offspring will have a 25% chance of having normal hemoglobin; a 25% chance of having sickle cell anemia; and a 50% chance of having the sickle cell trait.

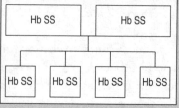

If both parents have sickle cell anemia, all of the offspring will have sickle cell anemia.

KEY: Hb A = normal hemoglobin; Hb SS = sickle cell anemia; Hb SA = sickle cell trait

swelling. Such blockage causes changes that worsen the sickling and result in more blockages.

What are its symptoms?

Typically, the person has a rapid heart rate, an enlarged heart and liver, heart murmurs, localized death of lung tissue, chronic fatigue, shortness of breath on exertion or even at rest, jaundice, pallor, joint swelling, aching bones, chest pain, and leg ulcers (especially around the ankles). Also, the person is especially prone to infection.

Symptoms usually don't arise until after 6 months of age, because large amounts of fetal hemoglobin protect infants for the first few months after birth. Low socioeconomic status and related problems, such as poor nutrition and education, may delay diagnosis and treatment.

Vaso-occlusive crisis

Infection, stress, dehydration, and conditions that reduce oxygen in the blood — strenuous exercise, high altitude, unpressurized aircraft, cold, and drugs that constrict the blood vessels — may all provoke periodic crises.

Vaso-occlusive crisis (also called *infarctive crisis*) is the hallmark of sickle cell disease. These painful crises usually arise periodically after age 5 and occur when the sickle cells block blood vessels, robbing tissues of oxygen and sometimes causing localized tissue death.

During this crisis, the person has severe pain in the stomach, chest, muscles, or bones and may have worsening jaundice, dark urine, or a slight fever.

In people who've had the disease for a long time, the spleen may become so damaged and scarred that it shrinks. This can make the person highly vulnerable to *Streptococcus pneumoniae* sepsis, a serious infection that can be fatal without prompt treatment.

After the crisis subsides (in 4 days to a few weeks), infection may occur. Signs of infection include lack of energy, sleepiness, fever, and apathy.

Aplastic crisis

An aplastic crisis (also called *megaloblastic crisis*) results from bone marrow depression and is associated with infection, usually viral. It's marked by pallor, lack of energy, sleepiness, shortness of breath, possible coma, markedly decreased bone marrow activity, and breakdown of red blood cells.

Acute sequestration crisis

Infants between ages 8 months and 2 years may have an acute sequestration crisis, in which massive amounts of red blood cells suddenly become trapped in the spleen and liver. This rare crisis causes lack of energy and pallor and, if untreated, commonly progresses to shock and death.

Hemolytic crisis

A hemolytic crisis is quite rare and usually occurs in people who also have a disorder called *glucose 6-phosphate dehydrogenase deficiency.* It probably results from complications of sickle cell anemia such as infection — not from the disease itself. In hemolytic crisis, the liver degenerates, becoming congested and enlarged. This crisis worsens chronic jaundice, although increased jaundice doesn't always point to a hemolytic crisis.

Symptoms of a crisis

Any of these crises may cause the following symptoms:
- pale lips, tongue, palms, or nail beds
- lack of energy
- listlessness
- sleepiness, with difficulty awakening
- irritability
- severe pain
- temperature over 104° F (13° C), or a fever of 100° F (12.5° C) that lasts for 2 days.

Long-term complications

Typically, a child with sickle cell anemia is small for his age and experiences delayed puberty. (However, fertility isn't impaired.) If he reaches adulthood, his body build tends to be spiderlike — narrow shoulders and hips, long arms and legs, curved spine, barrel chest, and elongated skull. An adult usually has complications from localized areas of tissue death, such as retinopathy (a disorder of the retina) and nephropathy (a kidney disorder). The person may not be able to survive infection or repeated blockages of small blood vessels that lead to tissue death in major organs.

How is it diagnosed?

The doctor will diagnose sickle cell anemia if the person has a family history of the disease along with typical signs and symptoms. He or she may order a test called *hemoglobin electrophoresis,* which can confirm sickle cell anemia by showing hemoglobin S or other hemoglobin abnormalities. (To provide sickle cell disease screening, umbilical cord blood samples typically are taken at birth from at-risk newborns.)

Other lab studies usually show a low red blood cell count, elevated white blood cell and platelet counts, a decreased erythrocyte sedimentation rate, increased serum iron level, and decreased red blood cell survival. The hemoglobin level may be low or normal.

In a young child, the doctor will also look for an enlarged spleen. However, as the child grows older, the spleen shrinks.

How is it treated?

Treatment starts before age 4 months with preventive penicillin. If the person's hemoglobin count drops suddenly or if his condition worsens rapidly, he'll need to be hospitalized to get a transfusion of packed red blood cells.

Recently, a drug called *hydroxyurea* has been shown to ease pain associated with sickle cell anemia. At this writing, the use of this drug for sickle cell anemia has yet to be approved by the Food and Drug Administration.

During a sequestration crisis, the doctor may order sedatives, pain relievers, blood transfusions, and supplemental oxygen, as well as large amounts of oral or intravenous fluids.

What can a person with sickle cell anemia do?

During a crisis, you'll need supportive measures and may even need to be hospitalized. (For guidelines on recognizing, managing, and preventing a crisis, see *What to do during a vaso-occlusive crisis*, page 892.)

Guidelines during pregnancy and surgery

If you're pregnant or must undergo surgery, you'll need to take special precautions:

- If you're a woman with sickle cell anemia, be sure to seek birth control counseling from a gynecologist because you're at risk for problems during pregnancy. However, using oral contraceptives is also risky. If you do become pregnant, be sure to eat a balanced diet, and talk to the doctor about the possible benefits of a folic acid supplement.
- During general anesthesia, special steps may be necessary to ensure optimal breathing and to prevent hypoxic crisis. Make sure the surgeon and anesthesiologist know you have sickle cell anemia. The doctor may order a transfusion of packed red blood cells before surgery.
- Teenage boys and men with sickle cell anemia may develop sudden, painful episodes of priapism (prolonged or constant erection of the penis). Such episodes are common and can have serious reproductive consequences. Consult your doctor when these episodes occur.

SELF-HELP

What to do during a vaso-occlusive crisis

A person with sickle cell anemia is at risk for a serious complication called *vaso-occlusive crisis*. If this crisis occurs, the tips below can help you treat it and maybe prevent it from recurring.

What causes it?
Some things that cause a crisis are:
- infection, such as a cold or the flu
- dehydration — from not drinking enough fluid or from sweating, vomiting, or diarrhea
- low oxygen level — for example, from a visit to the mountains
- temperature extremes.

Recognizing a crisis
Suspect a crisis if you have:
- pain, especially in the stomach area, chest, muscles, or bones
- paleness, usually around the lips, tongue, and fingernails
- unusual sleepiness or irritability
- a low-grade fever that lasts for 2 days
- dark urine.

Responding to a crisis
First, call the doctor and describe your symptoms. For a mild crisis, the doctor may suggest home care. Here's what you can do to manage the crisis at home:
- Apply warm, moist compresses to painful areas. Cover yourself with a blanket to prevent a chill. *Never* use ice packs or cold compresses. These could be harmful.
- Ease pain with Tylenol, Panadol, or another drug containing acetaminophen.

- Stay in bed. Sit up if that's more comfortable.
- Make sure to drink lots of fluids so you won't get dehydrated.
- Call the doctor if your symptoms persist or worsen. If dehydration or severe pain occurs, you may need to be hospitalized.

Preventing a crisis
Although these precautions aren't foolproof, they may help prevent another crisis. Follow these do's and don'ts.

Do's
- Stay up-to-date with immunizations.
- Prevent infections by taking meticulous care of wounds, eating well-balanced meals, getting regular dental checkups, and maintaining proper tooth and gum care.
- Seek treatment for any infection.
- Drink fluids at the first sign of a cold or other infection.

Don'ts
- Avoid tight clothing that could block circulation.
- Never exercise strenuously or excessively. This could trigger a crisis.
- Avoid drinking lots of ice water or exposing yourself to sizzling hot or freezing cold temperatures.
- Steer clear of mountain climbing, unpressurized aircraft, and high altitudes.

TAY-SACHS DISEASE

What do doctors call this condition?
Amaurotic familial idiocy

What is this condition?
The most common of the lipid (fat) storage diseases, Tay-Sachs disease results from a congenital enzyme deficiency. It's characterized by progressive mental and motor deterioration and is usually fatal before age 5, although some juveniles and adults with hexosaminidase A deficiency have been noted.

Tay-Sachs disease is quite rare and appears in fewer than 100 infants born each year in the United States. However, it strikes persons of Eastern European Jewish ancestry about 100 times more often than the general population; it occurs in about 1 in 3,600 live births in this ethnic group. About 1 in 30 Eastern European Jews and French Canadians are heterozygous carriers. If 2 such carriers have children, each of their offspring has a 25% chance of having Tay-Sachs disease.

What causes it?
Tay-Sachs disease is an autosomal recessive disorder in which the enzyme hexosaminidase A is deficient. This enzyme is necessary for breaking down gangliosides, which are water-soluble fats containing carbohydrates such as sugar. Gangliosides are found primarily in central nervous system tissues. Without hexosaminidase A, accumulating lipid pigments enlarge and progressively destroy central nervous system cells.

What are its symptoms?
A newborn with Tay-Sachs disease appears normal at birth, although he or she may have an exaggerated Moro embrace reflex (this type of reflex is produced by a sudden stimulus such as striking a table and is seen normally up to age 3 to 4 months).

By age 3 to 6 months, the infant becomes apathetic and responds to loud sounds only. Neck, trunk, arm, and leg muscles grow weaker, and soon the child can't sit up or lift his or her head. The infant has difficulty turning over, can't grasp objects, and has progressive vision loss.

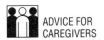

ADVICE FOR
CAREGIVERS

How to cope when your child has Tay-Sachs

If your child has this disease, follow these guidelines to help you cope.

Giving home care
If you're caring for your child at home, make sure you understand how to perform suctioning, postural drainage (special body positioning to drain fluids), and tube feeding, as well as how to give good skin care to prevent bedsores.

Meeting emotional needs
If you're feeling stress and guilt because of your child's illness and the emotional and financial burden it places on the family, don't hesitate to seek psychological counseling.

Seeking information
- Go for genetic counseling. Amniocentesis should be done early in any future pregnancies.
- If you have other children, have them undergo screening to determine if they're carriers. If you have grown children who are are carriers, they should have genetic counseling. However, be aware that there's no danger of transmitting the disease to their children unless they marry another Tay-Sachs carrier.
- For more information, contact the National Tay-Sachs and Allied Diseases Association.

By age 18 months, the infant is usually deaf and blind and has seizures, generalized paralysis, and spastic movement. Pupils are dilated and don't react to light. Decerebrate rigidity, resulting from brain damage, and a vegetative state follow. The child suffers recurrent bronchopneumonia after age 2 and usually dies before age 5. A child who survives may develop ataxia (lack of muscle coordination) and progressive motor retardation between ages 2 and 8.

How is it diagnosed?

Typical clinical features point to Tay-Sachs disease, but blood analysis showing deficient hexosaminidase A is the key to diagnosis. An eye exam showing optic nerve atrophy and a distinctive cherry-red spot on the retina supports the diagnosis.

Diagnostic screening is essential for all couples when at least one member is of Eastern European Jewish or French Canadian ancestry and for others with a family history of the disease. A blood test evaluating hexosaminidase A levels can identify carriers. Amniocentesis or chorionic villus sampling can detect hexosaminidase A deficiency in the fetus.

How is it treated?

Tay-Sachs disease has no known cure. Supportive treatment includes tube feedings using nutritional supplements, suctioning and postural drainage (special body positioning) to remove pharyngeal secretions, skin care to prevent bedsores in bedridden children, and mild laxatives to relieve constipation caused by central nervous system disorders. Anticonvulsants usually fail to prevent seizures. Because these children need constant physical attention, their parents often have full-time, skilled home health care or place them in long-term, special care facilities. (See *How to cope when your child has Tay-Sachs*, page 893.)

APPENDIX

Appendix: Mental and Emotional Disorders

WHAT IS THIS CONDITION?	WHAT ARE ITS SYMPTOMS?	HOW IS IT TREATED?
Alcoholism Chronic, uncontrolled alcohol use that disrupts health, relationships, and responsibilities	• Daily or episodic need to drink to function normally • Inability to stop drinking or to drink less • Amnesia (blackouts) after drinking • Violent behavior while intoxicated • Denial of the problem and hostility when confronted • Frequent mood swings or depression • Masking of odor with mouthwash, mints, or aftershave • Social, family, and work problems • Upset stomach • Frequent infections • Poor personal hygiene • Unexplained injuries, such as bruises, cigarette burns, or fractures	• Abstinence • Detoxification • Psychotherapy (group therapy, family therapy, behavior modification) • Involvement in a self-help group such as Alcoholics Anonymous • Hospitalization in acute alcohol intoxication • Possible drug therapies include medications to ease withdrawal symptoms, Antabuse to discourage drinking, tranquilizers to relieve anxiety, and antipsychotics to control hyperactivity and psychosis.
Attention-deficit hyperactivity disorder Inability to focus attention on key tasks or to engage in passive activities (or both), which disrupts routine family, social, school, and employment performance; thought to be a physiologic brain disorder involving neurotransmitter levels in the brain. This disorder is present at birth but rarely diagnosed before age 4 or 5 unless symptoms are severe. It's more common in males and is usually first noticed in school, where disruptive classroom behavior or learning and organizational difficulties prompt evaluation.	• Moodiness, inattentiveness, boredom, laziness, forgetfulness, impulsiveness, poor organizational ability • Tendency to daydream and be easily distracted by extraneous thoughts, sights, or sounds • Failure to pay attention to details or follow instructions • Tendency to make careless mistakes • Avoidance of tasks that require sustained mental effort • Uneven performance at school or job (even if highly intelligent) • Tendency to move from one incomplete project, thought, or task to another	No cure exists. Treatment seeks to lessen symptoms and help the individual cope with the condition. Depending on the severity of symptoms, treatment may include: • education about the disorder and its effects • behavior modification, including use of coaching, external structure, planning and organizing systems, and supportive psychotherapy • drug therapy to lessen symptoms.
Autism A severe, pervasive developmental disorder marked by unresponsiveness to social contact, deficits in intelligence and language development, ritualistic and compulsive behaviors, limited capacity for appropriate activities and interests, and bizarre responses to the environment. The cause of autism is unknown. It is a rare disorder, affecting 4 or 5 out of every 10,000 children. It's much more common in males, often occurring in firstborn males.	Symptoms usually appear before age 30 months but may go unnoticed until the child enters school. *In infants:* • Unresponsiveness (reacts to attention with rigid, screaming resistance or indifference) • Delayed development (may not smile or lift arms to be picked up, forms no attachments, does not learn typical games) *In children:* • Under- or overreaction to stimuli	Treatment begins early and is prolonged, probably requiring a structured environment throughout life. Treatment may be provided at home or in a special school, day care, or psychiatric facility. Therapy includes: • behavior modification to encourage social adjustment and speech development • reducing self-destructive behavior • family counseling • possibly drug therapy.

Mental and Emotional Disorders *(continued)*

WHAT IS THIS CONDITION?	WHAT ARE ITS SYMPTOMS?	HOW IS IT TREATED?
Autism *(continued)*	▪ Severe language impairment (mute or meaningless speech) ▪ Lack of fantasy or adult role-playing ▪ Repetitive activities (for example, always lining up toys in the same manner) ▪ Bizarre behavior (rituals, fits)	

Anorexia nervosa
Self-starvation induced by distorted body image and an intense and irrational fear of gaining weight.
  This disorder affects women almost exclusively, typically in adolescence or early adulthood. Social attitudes equating slimness with beauty are probably a contributing factor.
	▪ Preoccupation with appearance and body size, with frequent expressions of dissatisfaction
	▪ Fear of gaining weight that persists even when the person is emaciated
	▪ Morbid dread of being fat
	▪ Anger and ritualistic behavior
	▪ Paradoxical obsession with food; for example, preparing elaborate meals for others
	▪ Tendency to exercise compulsively, induce vomiting, or abuse laxatives or diuretics
	▪ Depression
		With early diagnosis and the person's cooperation, the outlook is good.
		  Treatment involves the following:
		▪ medical care to help the person gain weight
		▪ nutritional counseling to correct malnutrition
		▪ individual, group, or family therapy to deal with psychological dysfunction and control compulsive binge eating and purging
		▪ hospitalization if condition is serious.

Bipolar disorder
A group of disorders marked by severe pathologic mood swings from euphoric hyperactivity (mania) to sadness and depression. In Type I disorder, the person has alternating episodes of mania and depression. Type II disorder involves recurrent episodes of depression with occasional manic episodes.
  The problems typically start between ages 20 and 35 but may occur anytime after adolescence. With age, episodes recur more frequently and last longer. Men and women are affected equally.
	Manic episodes:
	▪ Euphoria, expansiveness, or irritability with little control over actions and responses
	▪ Hyperactivity, elaborate plans, buying sprees, sexual promiscuity
	▪ Tendency to dress in unusual clothing
	▪ Poor personal hygiene
	▪ Reduced sleeping and eating
	▪ Rapid and poorly organized talking, easy distractibility
	Depressive episodes:
	▪ Overall negative attitude
	▪ Sluggishness
	▪ Weight loss
	▪ Worsening physical health
	▪ Extreme concern about health
	▪ Social withdrawal
	▪ Slow responses or speech
		Drug therapy with lithium is widely used. Therapy may also include anticonvulsants and antidepressants.
		  The person should be watched for severe depression because 20% of people with bipolar disorder commit suicide.

Bulimia nervosa A pattern of binge eating followed by feelings of guilt and self-deprecation. These feelings lead the person to compensate by taking extreme measures, such as inducing vomiting, abusing laxatives or diuretics, or fasting. This disorder affects women almost exclusively, typically in adolescence	▪ Distorted body image ▪ Episodes of binge eating (tendency to eat until interrupted by abdominal pain, sleep, or another person) ▪ Peculiar eating habits or rituals ▪ Frequent use of diuretics or laxatives ▪ Vomiting that causes hoarseness	Physical and psychological symptoms must be treated simultaneously. Psychotherapy seeks to stop the binge-purge cycle and promote control over eating. Treatment includes: ▪ behavior modification therapy ▪ individual and family therapy *(continued)*

Mental and Emotional Disorders *(continued)*

WHAT IS THIS CONDITION?	WHAT ARE ITS SYMPTOMS?	HOW IS IT TREATED?
Bulimia nervosa *(continued)* or early adulthood. It may occur simultaneously with anorexia nervosa. Contributing factors may include family conflict, sexual abuse, cultural emphasis on physical appearance, and parental obesity.	• Hyperactivity • Frequent weight fluctuations • Thin, emaciated appearance • Excessive exercise • Exaggerated sense of guilt • Depression	• antidepressants • participation in a self-help group.
Conversion disorder Loss of a physical function (such as ability to move, see, or swallow), without physiologic cause, to resolve a psychological conflict. This disorder may affect either sex at any age. It is not life-threatening and is usually of short duration.	• Recent stressful event • Sudden onset of a single debilitating symptom that neutralizes the affected body part • Physical exam results that fail to reveal a physical cause for the symptom • Lack of concern for loss of function	• Psychotherapy • Family therapy • Relaxation therapy • Behavioral therapy • Hypnotherapy
Delusional disorders Fixed, false beliefs (for example, feelings of persecution) that have a plausible basis in reality. These disorders typically begin between ages 40 and 55, though they may start earlier. Men and women are affected equally. Chronic delusions interfere with social and marital relationships but seldom impair intellectual or occupational function. If diagnosed in early stages, delusional disorders can be treated successfully.	• Problems with social and marital relationships • Depression • Social isolation • Relentless criticism of, or placing unreasonable demands on, others • Denial or rationalization • Chronic jealousy or suspicion • Evasiveness or talkativeness • Contradictory, jumbled, or irrational responses • Excessive vigilance when entering a room	• Psychotherapy for mood and behavior disturbances • Antipsychotic drugs to reduce psychotic symptoms (hallucinations, delusions) • Antidepressants and antianxiety drugs • Developing a support system (especially for older, isolated individuals)
Depersonalization disorders Persistent or repeated episodes of detachment, during which self-awareness is altered or lost. The person sees this change as a barrier between self and the outside world. The sensation may be restricted to a single limb or may involve the whole self. Though the person rarely loses touch with reality completely, episodes cause severe distress.	• Anxiety • Depression, fear of going insane • Feelings of detachment • Expressed concerns about mind and body • Feeling that life is not real • Obsessive contemplation • Difficulty speaking • Lost sense of time • Dizziness • Prolonged recall time	Psychotherapy helps the person recognize the traumatic cause of the disorder and the resulting anxiety, and teaches him or her to use reality-based coping strategies rather than detachment.
Dissociative amnesia A sudden inability to recall important personal information (typically events) following severe psychosocial stress, often a threat of physical injury or death. The disorder may strike after the person thinks about or engages in unacceptable behavior, such as an extramarital affair.	• Perplexed and disoriented appearance • Inability to remember key events or even to recognize that his or her memory is impaired • Aimless wandering	Psychotherapy helps the person recognize the traumatic cause of the disorder and the resulting anxiety, and teaches appropriate coping techniques.

Mental and Emotional Disorders *(continued)*

WHAT IS THIS CONDITION?	WHAT ARE ITS SYMPTOMS?	HOW IS IT TREATED?
Dissociative fugue Disorder marked by wandering or traveling, and often adopting a new personality while mentally blocking out an extremely stressful event, such as a combat experience, disaster, or violent confrontation. Afterward, he or she fails to recall what happened. The fugue state is usually brief (lasting hours to days), but it can last for months and carry the person far from home. The outlook for recovery is good and recurrences are rare.	• Sudden, unexpected travel away from home • Sudden appearance of a new, less inhibited personality • Person may move and establish new relationships elsewhere • History may include episodes of violent behavior	Psychotherapy helps the person recognize the traumatic event that triggered the fugue state and develop appropriate coping strategies.
Dissociative identity disorder Complex disturbance of identity and memory marked by the existence of two or more distinct, fully integrated personalities in the same person. The personalities alternate in dominance and each has unique memories, behavior patterns, and social relationships. One personality rarely knows of the others. The cause is unknown; however, some form of emotional trauma is often involved.	• Peculiar behavior • Inability to recall events • Sudden change in facial expression, voice, or behavior following stressful events	Psychotherapy seeks to unite the personalities and prevent future splitting. Treatment is usually intensive and prolonged.
Generalized anxiety disorder Uncontrollable, unreasonable worry, without a specific cause, that persists for 6 or more months and interferes with normal daily life. Unlike fear (a reaction to a specific external danger), anxiety is an apprehensive reaction to an internal threat (such as an unacceptable impulse or a repressed thought). Occasional anxiety is normal; overwhelming anxiety can be debilitating.	• Tendency to become easily fatigued • Feelings of anger or fear • Loss of appetite • Restlessness • Inability to concentrate • Poor anxiety control • Headaches • Muscular tension, aches • Rapid pulse, shortness of breath • Rigid movements • Sleep disturbances • Trembling, spasms	Treatment usually consists of a combination of drug therapy and psychotherapy. The psychotherapy has two goals: • to help the person identify and deal with the cause of the anxiety • to eliminate the environmental factors that trigger it.
Hypochondriasis Unrealistic interpretation of the severity and significance of aches and pains. The person becomes preoccupied with fear of having a serious disease. The fear persists despite the doctor's reassurance to the contrary and severely interferes with work and relationships.	• Misinterpretation of one's own physical sensations as signs of serious illness • Multiple complaints about a single organ system • Vague complaints and preoccupation with normal body functions • Extensive knowledge about illness, diagnosis, and treatment because of past contact with doctors	To help the person lead a productive life despite this condition, the doctor will state clearly that the person doesn't have a serious disease but that continued medical follow-up will help monitor his or her symptoms. Follow-up is important to detect real illness. (Up to 30% of these people do develop an organic disease eventually.)

(continued)

Mental and Emotional Disorders *(continued)*

WHAT IS THIS CONDITION?	WHAT ARE ITS SYMPTOMS?	HOW IS IT TREATED?
Major depression Persistently sad, discontented mood. Causes disturbances in sleep and appetite, sluggishness, and an inability to experience pleasure. Major depression strikes people in all racial, ethnic, and socioeconomic groups. It affects both sexes but is more common in women. A chronic physical disorder can lead to depression. Major depression can profoundly interfere with relationships and work and in some cases may lead to suicide.	■ Sad mood and a loss of interest or pleasure in daily activities ■ Lack of self-esteem or ability to cope ■ Anger, anxiety ■ Inability to concentrate or think clearly ■ Appetite or sleep disturbances ■ Suicidal thinking, preoccupation with death ■ History of life problems or losses	Depression is difficult to treat, especially in children, adolescents, elderly people, and the chronically ill. The favored methods are drug therapy, electroconvulsive (shock) therapy, and psychotherapy. When a depressed person is incapacitated, suicidal, or psychotic or when antidepressant drugs don't work, electroconvulsive therapy may be recommended.
Obsessive-compulsive disorder Obsessive thoughts and compulsive behaviors that result from the person's repeated efforts to control overwhelming anxiety, guilt, or unacceptable impulses. An *obsession* is a repetitive idea, thought, or image that is intrusive and causes major anxiety. A *compulsion* is a ritualistic and involuntary defensive behavior that reduces the person's anxiety.	■ Persistent and involuntary thoughts or words ■ Repetitive worry about a tragic event ■ Repeating or counting images, words, or objects in the environment ■ Symptoms may interfere with social and work activity or the person may appear normal and restrict compulsive acts to private time.	Treatment with a combination of medication and talk therapy brings improvement in 60% to 70% of cases. ■ Effective medications include clomipramine, clonazepam, fluoxetine, paroxetine, sertraline, and fluvoxamine. ■ Effective behavioral therapies include aversion therapy, thought stopping, switching, flooding; implosion therapy; and response prevention. ■ Self-help measures include avoidance of unwanted thoughts with active diversional activities, relieving stress by channeling emotional energy into sports and creative endeavors, and relaxation and breathing techniques to help reduce anxiety.
Pain disorder Persistent complaints of pain with no evident physical cause. Symptoms are either inconsistent with the normal reaction of the nervous system, or they mimic a disease, such as angina, that isn't present. Although the pain has no physical cause, it is real to the person. Pain disorder is more common in women than in men and often strikes in their 30s and 40s. The pain usually is chronic, often interfering with relationships or work. The cause of pain disorder is unknown, but it may be related to severe stress or conflict.	■ Chronic, persistent complaints of pain without a physical basis ■ A long history of visits to medical facilities, without much pain relief ■ Familiarity with pain medications because of frequent hospitalizations ■ Faking symptoms ■ Pain that does not follow anatomic pathways ■ Failure to display typical nonverbal signs of pain, such as grimacing or guarding	Treatment aims to ease the pain and help the person live with it, avoiding invasive tests and surgery. ■ Supportive (non-drug) pain-relief measures include hot or cold packs, physical therapy, distraction techniques, massage, or electrical nerve stimulation. ■ Measures to reduce anxiety include antidepressants and regular follow-up appointments with a doctor.

Mental and Emotional Disorders *(continued)*

WHAT IS THIS CONDITION?	WHAT ARE ITS SYMPTOMS?	HOW IS IT TREATED?
Panic disorder Repeated episodes of intense apprehension, terror, and impending doom; anxiety in its most severe form. Unpredictable at first, these panic attacks may come to be linked with specific situations or tasks. The disorder often goes with agoraphobia (fear of public places). Men and women get it equally, but combined panic disorder and agoraphobia strikes about twice as many women. Untreated panic disorder can persist for years, with good and bad periods. The person is at high risk for drug or alcohol abuse to relieve his or her fear.	■ Repeated episodes of unexpected apprehension, fear or, rarely, intense discomfort ■ Attacks that may last for minutes or hours and leave the person shaken, fearful, and exhausted ■ Episodes that occur several times a week, sometimes even daily ■ Periods of anxiety between attacks ■ During a panic attack, signs of intense anxiety, such as fast breathing, fast heartbeat, trembling, and profuse sweating	A person with panic disorder may respond to behavioral therapy, supportive psychotherapy, or drug therapy, singly or in combination. Psychotherapy teaches the person to view anxiety-provoking situations more realistically and to recognize panic symptoms as a misinterpretation of harmless physical sensations. Drug therapy includes antianxiety drugs, beta blockers (for relief of symptoms), and antidepressants.
Personality disorders Chronic, inflexible, and maladaptive behavior that causes social discomfort and interferes with relationships and jobs. Most people with these disorders aren't treated. When they do get help, it's usually as outpatients or when the disorder is linked to an episode of another mental disorder. Personality disorders typically start around adolescence or early adulthood and persist throughout life.	■ Each specific disorder produces its own symptoms. For example, borderline personality disorder is marked by instability in personal relationships. Antisocial personality disorder is marked by disregard for the rights of others. ■ In general, long-standing difficulties arise in relationships (ranging from dependency to withdrawal) and at work (from compulsive perfectionism to intentional sabotage). ■ Convinced that his or her behavior is normal, the person avoids responsibility for its consequences, often blaming others.	Personality disorders are difficult to treat. Successful therapy requires a trusting relationship in which the therapist can use a direct approach. The type of therapy depends on the person's symptoms. ■ Drug therapy is ineffective but may be used to relieve acute anxiety and depression. ■ Family and group therapy usually are effective. ■ Hospital inpatient group therapies can be effective in crisis situations and possibly for long-term treatment of borderline personality disorders.
Phobias Persistent and irrational fear of a specific object, activity, or situation that causes the person to have a compelling desire to avoid the perceived hazard. The person recognizes that the fear is out of proportion to any actual danger but can't control it or explain it away. Three types of phobias are: ■ agoraphobia, the fear of being alone or in an open space ■ social phobia, the fear of embarrassing oneself in public ■ specific phobia, the fear of a single, specific object, such as animals or heights.	■ Signs of severe anxiety when confronted with the feared object or situation — for example, in agoraphobia, dizziness, a sensation of falling, a feeling of unreality (depersonalization), loss of bladder or bowel control, vomiting, or cardiac distress when the person leaves home or crosses a bridge ■ Possible loss of self-esteem and feelings of weakness, cowardice, or ineffectiveness if the person routinely avoids the feared object or activity; also possibly signs of mild depression	Because phobic behavior may never be completely cured, the goal of treatment is to help the person function effectively, using the following: ■ antianxiety and antidepressant drugs to help relieve symptoms in people with agoraphobia ■ systematic desensitization, a behavioral therapy; may be more effective than drugs, especially with instruction and suggestion. ■ self-help practices, including relaxation techniques, such as listening to music and meditating ■ exercise and creative activities to channel excess energy and relieve stress

(continued)

Mental and Emotional Disorders *(continued)*

WHAT IS THIS CONDITION?	WHAT ARE ITS SYMPTOMS?	HOW IS IT TREATED?
Posttraumatic stress disorder The presence of psychological consequences that persist for at least 1 month after an unusually traumatic event. This disorder can follow almost any distressing event. Psychological trauma accompanies the physical trauma and involves intense fear and feelings of helplessness and loss of control. Posttraumatic stress disorder can be acute, chronic, or delayed. When the precipitating event is caused by other people, the disorder is more severe and more persistent. It can happen at any age, even during childhood.	• Pangs of painful emotion and unwelcome thoughts • Intrusive memories (flashbacks) • Difficulty falling or staying asleep • Frequent nightmares of the traumatic event and aggressive outbursts on awakening • Emotional numbing • Chronic anxiety or panic attacks (with physical signs and symptoms) • Rage and survivor guilt, use of violence to solve problems, depression and suicidal thoughts, phobic avoidance of situations that arouse memories of the traumatic event	Treatment goals include reducing symptoms, preventing chronic disability, and promoting occupational and social rehabilitation. Specific treatments may include behavioral techniques (such as relaxation therapy to decrease anxiety and induce sleep or progressive desensitization), antianxiety and antidepressant drugs, and psychotherapy (supportive, insight, or cathartic) to minimize the risks of dependency and a chronic disorder. Support groups are highly effective.

Psychoactive drug abuse and dependence
Use of legal or illegal drugs that cause physical, mental, emotional, or social harm. Examples include narcotics (such as heroin and codeine), stimulants (such as cocaine and amphetamines), depressants (such as barbiturates), antianxiety agents (such as Valium), and hallucinogens (such as LSD and PCP).
   Drug abuse can occur at any age and often leads to addiction. It is caused by a combination of low self-esteem, peer pressure, inadequate coping skills, and curiosity.
	Chronic drug abuse, especially intravenous use, can lead to life-threatening complications, such as AIDS, tetanus, and a range of heart, respiratory, nervous system, digestive system, and muscle and skeletal conditions.	Treatment aims to relieve symptoms and varies with the drug taken. The person may receive fluid replacement, nutritional and vitamin supplements, detoxification with the same or a similar drug, sedatives to induce sleep, drugs to relieve stomach distress, and antianxiety drugs for severe agitation, especially in cocaine abusers.
		   Treatment of drug dependence is three-pronged and includes detoxification, short- and long-term rehabilitation, and aftercare to foster a lifetime of abstinence, usually with the help of Narcotics Anonymous or a similar self-help group.

Schizophrenia
Characterized by disturbances (for at least 6 months) in thought content and form, perception, behavior, sense of self, relationships, and physical behavior. Psychiatrists recognize five types: paranoid, disorganized, catatonic, undifferentiated, and residual schizophrenia.
   Schizophrenia affects 1% to 2% of the U.S. population to varying degrees and strikes both sexes equally, usually in adolescence or early adulthood.
	Symptoms vary widely, depending on the type and phase (prodromal, active, or residual) of the illness, and include:
	• delusions
	• hallucinations
	• disorganized speech
	• grossly disorganized behavior or a catatonic state
	• ambivalence — strong positive and negative feelings, leading to emotional conflict.
		Treatment may combine drug therapy, long-term psychotherapy for the person and his or her family, psychosocial rehabilitation, vocational counseling, and the use of community resources.
		   The primary treatment for more than 30 years, antipsychotic drugs appear to work by blocking some brain chemicals. These drugs reduce the number of psychotic symptoms, such as hallucinations and delusions, and relieve anxiety and agitation.
		   Other psychiatric drugs, such as antidepressants and antianxiety drugs, may control associated signs and symptoms.

Mental and Emotional Disorders *(continued)*

WHAT IS THIS CONDITION?	WHAT ARE ITS SYMPTOMS?	HOW IS IT TREATED?
Somatization disorder Presence of numerous symptoms over several years that suggest physical disorders but that doctors can't account for. Somatization disorder usually is chronic, gets worse in times of stress, and is involuntary (the person consciously wants to feel better). It usually begins in adolescence and is seldom diagnosed in males. Both genetic and environmental factors contribute to the development of somatization disorder.	▪ Physical complaints presented in a dramatic, vague, or exaggerated way ▪ A history of multiple medical evaluations by different doctors at different institutions — sometimes simultaneously — without significant findings ▪ Anxiety and depression ▪ Common physical complaints, including paralysis or blindness, stomach pain, reproductive difficulties (such as painful menstruation or erectile dysfunction), chronic back pain, chest pain, dizziness, or palpitations	The goal of treatment is to help the person learn to live with the symptoms. After diagnostic evaluation has ruled out organic causes, the person should be told that she has no serious illness currently but will receive care for her genuine distress and ongoing medical attention for her symptoms. The most important aspect of treatment is a continuing supportive relationship with a health care provider who will help the person live with her symptoms. The person should have regular appointments to review her complaints and the effectiveness of her coping strategies.
Tic disorders Characterized by involuntary, spasmodic, repetitive, and purposeless physical movements or vocalizations. All tics are similar physiologically but differ in severity and prognosis. They include Tourette syndrome, chronic motor or vocal tic disorder, and transient tic disorder. They are classified as motor or vocal and as simple or complex. Tic disorders begin before age 18 and are three times more common in boys than in girls. Transient tics usually go away on their own, but Tourette syndrome is chronic, with better and worse periods. Although their exact cause is unknown, tic disorders affect some families, suggesting a genetic cause.	*Tourette syndrome:* ▪ Multiple motor tics and one or more vocal tics ▪ Violent twitching or movement of the face, arms, other body parts ▪ Bizarre speech, explosive sounds, or compulsive shouting of obscene words *Chronic motor or vocal tic disorder:* ▪ Single or multiple motor or vocal tics, but not both, that happen regularly ▪ Tic interferes with relationships, work, or other functions *Transient tic disorder:* ▪ Single or multiple motor or vocal tics, or both ▪ Tics occur regularly, every day, but don't last more than a year	Behavior modification may help treat some tic disorders. Psychotherapy can help the person uncover underlying conflicts and issues as well as deal with the problems caused by the tics. Tourette syndrome is best treated with medications (haloperidol) and psychotherapy. No medications are helpful in treating transient tics. Self-help measures include: ▪ trying to identify and eliminate any avoidable stress and learning positive new ways to deal with anxiety ▪ talking about the illness, understanding that the movements are involuntary, and avoiding guilt or self-blame.

INDEX